A Clinician's Guide to Asthma

A Clinician's Guide to Asthma

Edited by Jordan Long

AMERICAN
MEDICAL PUBLISHERS
www.americanmedicalpublishers.com

American Medical Publishers,
41 Flatbush Avenue,
1st Floor, New York,
NY 11217, USA

Visit us on the World Wide Web at:
www.americanmedicalpublishers.com

ISBN: 978-1-63927-455-0

Cataloging-in-Publication Data

A clinician's guide to asthma / edited by Jordan Long.
p. cm.
Includes bibliographical references and index.
ISBN 978-1-63927-455-0
1. Asthma. 2. Asthma--Treatment--Guidebooks. 3. Bronchi--Diseases.
4. Lungs--Diseases, Obstructive. 5. Respiratory allergy. I. Long, Jordan.
RC591 .C55 2022
616.238--dc23

Table of Contents

Preface

Asthma is a chronic inflammatory condition that affects the airways of the lungs. In asthma, airway hyper-responsiveness leads to recurring episodes of breathlessness, chest tightness, wheezing and coughing. There is no precise way to diagnose asthma. It is usually suspected on review of symptoms, whether these occur or worsen with exercise, or on exposure to allergens, viral infections or air pollution. Spirometry can be used to support a diagnosis. By avoiding exposure to air pollution, tobacco smoke, perfume and other chemical irritants, and respiratory infections, asthmatic episodes can be managed. Medications for asthma include fast-acting or long-acting. They are generally prescribed depending on the frequency of the symptoms and the severity of the illness. Bronchodilators, mast cell stabilizer, inhalatory corticosteroids and leukotriene antagonists are recommended for the management of asthma. Different approaches, evaluations, methodologies and advanced studies on asthma have been included in this book. It brings forth some of the unexplored aspects of this condition. Students, researchers, experts and all associated with pulmonology will benefit alike from this book.

After months of intensive research and writing, this book is the end result of all who devoted their time and efforts in the initiation and progress of this book. It will surely be a source of reference in enhancing the required knowledge of the new developments in the area. During the course of developing this book, certain measures such as accuracy, authenticity and research focused analytical studies were given preference in order to produce a comprehensive book in the area of study.

This book would not have been possible without the efforts of the authors and the publisher. I extend my sincere thanks to them. Secondly, I express my gratitude to my family and well-wishers. And most importantly, I thank my students for constantly expressing their willingness and curiosity in enhancing their knowledge in the field, which encourages me to take up further research projects for the advancement of the area.

Editor

1

p-STAT6, PU.1, and NF-κB are involved in allergen-induced late-phase airway inflammation in asthma patients

Deimante Hoppenot[1*], Kestutis Malakauskas[1,2], Simona Lavinskiene[1,2] and Raimundas Sakalauskas[1]

Abstract

Background: Previous *in vitro* and animal studies demonstrated that transcription factors p-STAT6 and PU.1 are required to induce interleukin (IL)-9 secretion by T helper (Th) 9 cells. It is believed that n factor-kappaB (NF-κB) plays a role in eosinophil survival. The importance of these transcription factors in the pathogenesis of allergic asthma (AA) in humans is poorly understood. We evaluated p-STAT6 and PU.1 expression in peripheral blood Th9 cells and NF-κB expression in eosinophils during late-phase airway inflammation in AA patients.

Methods: Nineteen adults with AA and 14 adult healthy individuals (HI) were examined. Peripheral blood collected 24 h before (baseline) and 24 h after bronchial allergen challenge. $CD4^+$ cells and eosinophils were isolated by high-density gradient centrifugation and magnetic separation. The percentage of Th9 cells and apoptotic eosinophils was estimated by flow cytometry. p-STAT6 and PU.1 expression was expressed as mean fluorescence intensity (MFI) in Th9 cells. NF-κB levels were expressed as MFI in peripheral blood eosinophils. Serum IL-9 and IL-5 levels were determined by enzyme-linked immunosorbent assay.

Results: At baseline, MFI of p-STAT6 and PU.1 in peripheral blood Th9 cells and MFI of NF-κB in eosinophils and, serum IL-5 and IL-9 levels were greater in AA patients ($P < 0.05$). Decreased eosinophil apoptosis was seen in the AA group compared with HI ($P < 0.05$). MFI of p-STAT6, PU.1, and NF-κB and serum levels of IL-5 and IL-9 were increased in the AA group 24 h after challenge compared with baseline ($P < 0.05$). In the AA group, a correlation between serum IL-9 and Th9 cells ($r = 0.7$, $P = 0.001$) and MFI of PU.1 ($r = 0.6$, $P = 0.01$) 24 h after bronchial allergen challenge was observed. A correlation between Th9 cells and MFI of p-STAT6 ($r = 0.45$, $P = 0.03$) as well as MFI of PU.1 ($r = 0.5$, $P = 0.02$) 24 h after challenge was only observed in AA patients. A correlation between the MFI of NF-κB and eosinophil apoptosis was observed in AA patients 24 h before ($r = -0.46$, $P = 0.02$) and after ($r = -0.5$, $P = 0.02$) challenge.

Discussions: p-STAT6 and PU.1 may be associated with Th9 cells and IL-9 production, whereas NF-κB and IL-5 may be associated with reduced eosinophil apoptosis in allergen-induced late-phase airway inflammation.

Keywords: Allergic asthma, Th9 cells, Interleukin-9, Eosinophil apoptosis, Transcription factors

* Correspondence: deimante@gmail.com
[1]Department of Pulmonology and Immunology, Medical Academy, Lithuanian University of Health Sciences, Kaunas, Lithuania
Full list of author information is available at the end of the article

Background

The mechanisms of allergic asthma (AA) pathogenesis remain poorly understood despite modern investigational methods [1]. AA is a heterogeneous disease because the environmental stimuli, exposure to allergens, and involvement of different cells types and cytokines that participate in asthma pathogenesis are different between individuals. $CD4^+$ T helper cells (Th) [2, 3] and eosinophils [4, 5] are involved in the pathogenesis of AA. The differentiation of $CD4^+$ Th cells to different subsets depends on the type of cytokines present in the local environment and other stimuli. Interleukin-4 (IL-4) induces CD4+ T-cell proliferation and differentiation into Th2 cells that play an important role in asthma pathogenesis [6]. IL-12 induces the development of Th1 cells, which are important in cell-mediated immunity and phagocyte-dependent protective responses [7]. Transforming growth factor-β (TGF-β1), IL-6, IL-1β, and IL-23 are required for the differentiation of Th17 cells [8], which are associated with an increased number of airway neutrophils and a more severe asthma course. More recently, a newly identified T helper cell subset, Th9 cells, were identified and shown to develop under the influence of TGF-β and IL-4 stimuli [9, 10]. Th9 cells are thought to be an unstable subset that produce mainly IL-9 and are involved in allergic inflammation, some autoimmune diseases [11], and antitumor immune responses *in vivo* [12]. It was recently shown that Th9 cells differentiated from atopic children secrete greater amounts of IL-9 in bronchial lavage than those from non-atopic children [13]. Moreover, IL-9 is an important growth factor for repetitively stimulated T-cell lines and induces lung eosinophilia after allergen stimuli. Transcription factors often regulate the expression of different cytokines and are essential for the regulation of gene expression. Usually one or several specific transcription factors are key for subset-specific differentiation, and other transcription factors are shared between several subsets. Th9 cell development has been less studied than other CD4+ T helper subsets, but studies have shown that Th9 cells develop under stimulation of IL-4-activated signal transducer and activator of transcription protein-6 (STAT6). IL-4 and STAT6 are required to repress the expression of *Foxp3*, which induces a *Treg* phenotype and can repress IL-9 production [9, 10, 14]. STAT6 induces interferon regulatory factor 4 (IRF4) that is important for Th9 development [15]. Basic leucine zipper transcription factor is required for IL-9 production in both human and mouse Th9 cells and cooperates with IRF4 in binding to and activating the *Il9* locus [16]. IL-4 and STAT-6 activate the GATA3 gene, which is a main Th2 cell type regulator. E26 transformation-specific (ETS) family transcription factor PU.1 is a transcription factor that promotes switching between Th2 and Th9 phenotypes. PU.1 plays an important role in the development of Th9 memory cells and Th9 immunity [17].

Eosinophils develop from CD34+ pluripotent progenitor cells under certain stimuli and in many cases participate in the pathogenesis of AA. Progenitor CD34+ cells express high numbers of IL-5 receptors (IL-5R) and IL-5 generated by Th2 cells during asthma act on the bone marrow to enhance the production of eosinophils [18, 19]. Degranulated eosinophils release cytotoxic substances that damage airway epithelial cells [20]. IL-3, IL-5, and granulocyte-macrophage colony-stimulating factor prolong eosinophil survival *in vitro* by delaying apoptosis [21], while more recent studies have shown that IL-9 possesses eosinophil viability-enhancing effects [22]. Nuclear factor-kappaB (NF-κB) is believed to be an important transcription factor that mediates eosinophil survival because the inhibition of NF-κB in humans and animals induces eosinophil apoptosis [23].

This study investigated the role of the transcription factors PU.1, STAT-6, and NF-κB in allergen-induced inflammation in adult AA patients to try and mimic real-life conditions because the importance of these transcription factors in AA pathogenesis in humans has not been completely elucidated. The aim of this study was to evaluate STAT6 and PU.1 expression in peripheral blood Th9 cells and NF-κB expression in eosinophils during late-phase airway inflammation in AA patients after inhaled allergen bronchial challenge.

Methods

The research protocol described below was approved by the Regional Biomedical Research Ethics Committee of the Lithuanian University of Health Sciences (BE-2-23). The study was registered in the U.S. National Institutes of Health trial registry ClinicalTrials.gov with identifier NCT02214303.

Study population

We examined 33 nonsmoking adults (16 men and 17 women; median age, 26 years; interquartile range (IQR), 8) of which 19 patients had mild or moderate persistent AA and 14 were healthy individuals (HI). Asthma was diagnosed according to the revised 2012 GINA criteria [24]. All the study participants were recruited from the Department of Pulmonology and Immunology, Hospital of the Lithuanian University of Health Sciences, Kaunas. In all cases, informed consent was obtained using a written consent form and was signed by the study individuals. All participants were screened for inclusion and exclusion criteria. Inclusion criteria were patients with AA who had a clinical history of disease for ≥1 year, with current symptoms, and positive results of the skin prick test (≥3 mm) with *Dermatophagoides pteronyssinus*

(*D. pteronyssinus*), birch pollen allergens, or five grass mixture allergens. All study subjects had refrained from using inhaled, nasal, or oral steroids for at least 1 month, long-acting $\beta 2$ agonists for at least 48 h, and short-acting $\beta 2$ agonists for at least 12 h before the lung function test. Use of antihistamines and antileukotrienes were stopped 7 days before the skin prick test and the lung function test. Baseline forced expiratory volume in 1 s (FEV_1) was greater than 70 % of the predicted value in all patients. All healthy controls had normal spirometric values without airway hyperresponsiveness, no history of lung or other systemic immune diseases, and were nonatopic. None of the study participants had a history of smoking (Table 1).

Study design

Study individuals were seen at the screening visit where their eligibility for the study was checked based on inclusion and exclusion criteria. This visit included physical examination, spirometry, measurement of airway responsiveness to methacholine, and skin prick testing. At 24 h before bronchial allergen challenge, spirometry was performed and peripheral blood was collected from all eligible study subjects. An allergen (*D. pteronyssinus*, birch, or five grass mixture) for the bronchial challenge test in patients with AA was chosen according to the results of skin prick testing and clinical data in patients' medical records. In the case of multiple positive results of the skin prick test, an allergen that most probably caused bronchoconstriction previously was chosen for specific bronchial challenge. All healthy volunteers were challenged with a *D. pteronyssinus* allergen. Bronchial allergen challenge was performed at 8:00 in the morning, and spirometry was reassessed every 10 min within the first hour and then every hour for the subsequent 6 h. Physical examination, spirometry, and peripheral blood collection were performed again 24 h after bronchial allergen challenge. A flow chart of the study is presented in Fig. 1.

Table 1 Demographic and clinical characteristics of study population

Characteristics	Allergic asthma patients $n = 19$	Healthy subjects $n = 14$
Age, median (range), years	25 (18–36)	27 (20–35)
Sex (male/female), n	10/9	7/6
Wheal diameter induced by allergen, median (range), mm	6.8 (5–11)	–
Sensitization to *D. pteronyssinus*/birch/5 grass mixture allergen, n	12/4/3	–
PD_{20}, geometric mean (range), mg	0.13 (0.03–0.42)	–
FEV_1, mean ± SD (range), % of predicted	97 ± 10 (82–118)	102 ± 8 (95–122)
Maximum fall in FEV_1 after bronchial allergen challenge during the first hour, median (range), %	27 (22–34)*	2 (3–8)

FEV_1, forced expiratory volume in the first second
PD_{20}, provocative dose of methacholine causing a 20 % fall in FEV_1
*$P < 0.05$ versus healthy individuals

Measurement of airway responsiveness to methacholine

Methacholine was nebulized into a 10-L reservoir with a pressure nebulizer (Pari Provocation I; Pari, Stanberg, Germany). Aerolized methacholine was inhaled through a one-way valve at 5-min intervals starting with 15-μg methacholine dose and doubling it until a 20 % decrease in FEV_1 from the baseline or the total cumulative dose of 3.87 mg was achieved. The bronchoconstricting effect of each dose of methacholine was expressed as a percentage of decrease in FEV_1 from the baseline value. The provocative dose of methacholine causing a ≥ 20 % fall in FEV_1 (PD_{20}) was calculated from the log dose–response curve by linear interpolation of two adjacent data points [25, 26].

Skin prick testing

Standardized *D. pteronyssinus*, *D. farinae*, cat and dog dander, 5 mixed grass pollen, birch pollen, mugwort, *Alternaria*, *Aspergillus*, and *Cladosporium* allergen extracts for skin prick testing were used (Stallergenes S.A., France) for all study individuals. Histamine hydrochloride (10 mg/mL) was used as a positive control, and physiological saline, as a negative control. After 15–20 min, the diameters of wheals were measured. The result was expressed as the mean of the longest diameter of the wheal and the longest diameter perpendicular to it. Reactions larger than 3 mm and at least half the size of that produced by histamine were considered as positive [27].

Bronchial allergen challenge

Bronchial allergen challenge was performed with *D. pteronyssinus*, birch, or five grass mixture allergens (Stallergenes SA, Antony Cedex, France) at different concentrations (0.1, 1.0, 10.0, and 33.3 IR/mL) using a KoKo DigiDoser nebulizer (Sunrise Medical, Somerset, PA, USA) [28]. A freeze-dried lyophilized allergen was diluted with nonphenol saline. The results of the test were considered positive if there was a fall in FEV_1 of 20 % or more from the baseline value. Spirometry was reassessed every 10 min within the first hour and then every hour for the subsequent 6 h (in case of a late asthmatic reaction occurrence). Spirometry was also performed 24 h after bronchial allergen challenge. For patients with pollinosis, bronchial allergen challenge was not performed during the birch pollen and grass pollen season.

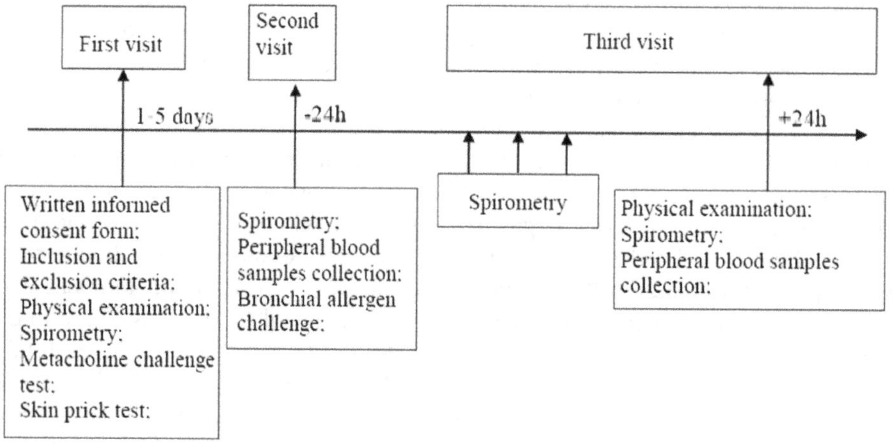

Fig. 1 The flowchart of the study

CD4+ T cells isolation from peripheral blood and intracellular pStat6 and PU.1 staining in Th9 cells

Peripheral blood lymphocytes were isolated from peripheral blood samples on Ficoll-Paque gradient and resuspended in RPMI 1640 (Sigma- Aldrich, USA) containing L-glutamine autologous plasma. CD4 T cells were separated from all mononuclear cells (PBMCs) using a magnetic separation kit (Miltenyi, USA). PBMCs were resuspended in cold MACS buffer (containing: PBS pH 7.2, 0.5 % bovine serum albumin [BSA] and 2 mM EDTA by diluting MACS BSA Stock Solution 1:20 in autoMACSR Rinsing Solution) (40 μL per 10^7 total cells) and incubated with Biotin-Antibody Cocktail (CD8, CD14, CD15, CD16, CD19, CD36, CD56, CD123, TCRγ/δ, and CD235a (Glycophorin A) (10 μL per 10^7 total cells) for 5 min. After incubation, 20 μL of Anti-Biotin MicroBeads (conjugated to monoclonal anti-biotin antibodies [isotype: mouse IgG1]) per 10^7 total cells was added, mixed, and incubated for additional 10 min at 4 °C. A LS column (Miltenyi Biotec, USA) was prepared during this time by placing it in the magnetic field of MACS Separator and washing it with 2 mL of MACS buffer. A preseparation filter (30 μm Miltenyi Biotec, USA) was rinsed with MACS buffer and placed on the top of the column. The cells were then applied to the preseparation filter/LS column, and the magnetically labeled non-CD4 T cells depleted by retaining them on a column in the magnetic field of a Separator, while the unlabeled CD4 T cells passed through the column. The cell fraction was eluted with 5 mL of MACS buffer.

Cell fractions were centrifuged (400 *g*, 10 min, 4 °C), and the pellet resuspended in 1 mL of RPMI 1640. Two million cells per mL were activated for 5 h at 37 °C with phorbol-12-myristate-13-acetate (Sigma-Aldrich) and ionomycin (Invitrogen, USA) in the presence of a protein transport inhibitor (BD GolgiStopTM, BD Biosciences, USA) to avoid cytokine secretion. After the activation, the cells were fixed with BD CytofixTM fixation buffer (BD Biosciences). Permeabilization of the fixed cells was performed by adding BD Perm/WashTM buffer (BD Biosciences) and stained by adding human IFN-GMA Alexa 488, TGF-β Alexa 488, IL-17A Alexa 488, IL-4 Alexa 488, IL-9 PERCP-CY5.5, pStat6 PE, PU.1 primary antibody, and secondary IgG2a + b PE. Flow cytometry was performed on a FACSCalibur flow cytometer (BD Biosciences). Results are reported as the mean fluorescence intensity (MFI) of intracellular p-STAT6 and PU.1 in Th9 cells ($CD4^+$ $IL\text{-}9^+$ $IFN\gamma^-$ $TGF\beta_1^-$ $IL\text{-}4^-$ $IL\text{-}17^-$ cells).

Eosinophil isolation from peripheral blood and intracellular NF-κB staining

Peripheral blood samples (20 mL) were diluted by adding the same volume of PBS. The suspension was carefully layered over Ficoll-Paque (ρ = 1.077 g/mL) in conical tubes and centrifuged at 1000 *g* for 30 min at 20 °C in a swinging bucket rotor without brake. A layer with mononuclear cells (PBMCs) was removed and used for Th cell isolation. Granulocytes were separated by hypotonic lysis of erythrocytes. Later, the granulocyte pellet was resuspended in cold MACS buffer (containing: PBS pH 7.2, 0.5 % BSA, and 2 mM EDTA by diluting MACS BSA Stock Solution 1:20 in autoMACSR Rinsing Solution) (40 μL per 10^7 total cells) and incubated with Biotin-Antibody Cocktail (biotin-conjugated monoclonal antibodies against CD2, CD14, CD16, CD19, CD56, CD123, and CD235a (Glycophorin A) (10 μL per 10^7 total cells) for 10 min. After incubation, 20 μL of Anti-Biotin MicroBeads (conjugated to monoclonal anti-biotin antibodies [isotype: mouse IgG1]) per 10^7 total cells was added, mixed, and incubated for additional 15 min at 4 °C. A LS column (Miltenyi Biotec, USA) was prepared during this time by placing it in the magnetic field of MACS Separator and washing it with 2 mL of MACS buffer. A preseparation filter (30 μm Miltenyi Biotec, USA) was rinsed with MACS buffer and placed on the top of the column. The cells were then applied to the preseparation filter/LS column, and the magnetically labeled non-eosinophils depleted by retaining them on a column in the magnetic field of a Separator, while the nonlabeled eosinophils passed through the column. The cell fraction was eluted with 5 mL of MACS buffer.

Cell fractions were centrifuged (400 *g*, 10 min, 4 °C), and the pellet resuspended in 1 mL of RPMI 1640. Two million cells per mL were activated for 5 h at 37 °C with phorbol-12-myristate-13-acetate (Sigma-Aldrich) and ionomycin (Invitrogen, USA) in the presence of a protein transport inhibitor (BD GolgiStopTM, BD Biosciences, USA) to avoid cytokine secretion. After the activation, the cells were fixed with BD CytofixTM fixation buffer (BD Biosciences). Permeabilization of the fixed cells was performed by adding BD Perm/WashTM buffer (BD Biosciences) and stained by adding 20 μL of Alexa Fluor® 647 Mouse anti-NF-κB p65 (pS529) from BD, cat.no 558422 which recognizes the phosphorylated serine 529 (pS529) in the transactivation domain of the human NF-κB p65 subunit. NF-κB in general is an ubiquitously expressed transcription factor. Optimal activation of NF-κB requires phosphorylation (e.g. serine phosphorylation) in the transactivation domain of p65.

Flow cytometry was performed on a FACSCalibur flow cytometer (BD Biosciences). Results are reported as the MFI of intracellular NF-κB expression in peripheral blood eosinophils.

The peripheral blood cell analysis was performed on an automated hematology analyzer (Sysmex XE-5000, Japan) at the Department of Laboratory Medicine, Hospital of Lithuanian University of Health Sciences Kaunas Clinics.

Detection of cytokines in serum

Serum cytokine levels were measured by the enzyme-linked immunosorbent assay (ELISA) according to the manufacturer's instructions: the minimal detectable doses of IL-9 and IL-5 were 0.1 ng/mL (Abcam, USA) and 5 pg/mL (Abcam, USA), respectively.

Apoptosis assay

Isolated eosinophils were resuspended in the annexin-binding buffer (pH 7.4) containing 50 mM HEPES, 700 mM NaCl, and 12.5 mM $CaCl_2$ (Invitrogen, USA) and incubated with fluorescein isothiocyanate-labeled (FITC)-annexin V (Invitrogen, USA) and propidium iodide (PI) for 15 min at room temperature in the dark. After the incubation, apoptosis was analyzed by flow cytometry using the CellQuest software (BD Biosciences, USA). Apoptotic cells were quantified as the percentage of the total population that was positive for FITC, but negative for PI. Necrotic cells were positive for PI.

Statistical analysis

Statistical analysis was performed by using the Statistical Package for the Social Sciences, version 20.0 for Windows (IBM SPSS Statistics 20.0, USA). The normality assumption of data was verified with the Shapiro–Wilks test. All the data were distributed not normally and were presented as median and ranges or interquartile range. Because of a skewed distribution of the variables, non-parametric tests were used. We analyzed two dependent groups: one group comprised the same allergic asthma patients 24 h before and 24 h after bronchial allergen challenge; the second dependent group consisted of the same healthy control individuals 24 h before and 24 h after bronchial allergen challenge. The changes in data before and after bronchial challenge in dependent groups were evaluated for statistical significance by the Wilcoxon test for paired analyses. Differences between two independent groups were evaluated using the Mann–Whitney U test. The Spearman rank test was used to assess relationships between variables. Statistical significance was assumed when $P < 0.05$.

Results

Characteristics of study population

No significant age and sex differences were documented when both groups were compared. Only AA patients showed positive skin prick test results. In the AA group, 12 patients were sensitized to *D. pteronyssinus,* four patients to birch pollen allergens, and three patients to five grass mixture allergens. Five patients had positive skin prick test results for several inhalant allergens: birch pollen, five grass mixture allergens, mugwort, and *Alternaria.* Three patients had positive skin prick test results for *D. pteronyssinus* and five grass mixture allergens. Demographic and clinical data of the study population are presented in Table 1. Baseline FEV_1 (% of predicted) did not differ when comparing both groups. A significant reduction in FEV_1 after bronchial allergen challenge during the first hour was only observed in AA patients.

At the baseline, AA patients had a significantly higher peripheral blood eosinophil count compared with the HI group ($P < 0.01$). The absolute peripheral blood eosinophil number significantly increased in the AA group 24 h after bronchial challenge compared with the baseline values ($P < 0.05$). There were no significant differences in peripheral blood leukocyte, lymphocyte, and neutrophil counts before and after bronchial challenge when comparing the AA and HI groups (Additional file 1: Table S1).

Peripheral blood Th9 cells and serum IL-9

At 24 h after bronchial allergen challenge, the percentage of Th9 cells (Additional file 2: Figure S1) was higher in the AA group compared with the control group and baseline values (1.32 % [0.78–2.12 %] vs. 0.11 % [0.05–0.22 %] and 0.64 % [0.22–1.21 %], respectively, $P < 0.05$) (Fig. 2a). At the baseline, the percentage of Th9 cells was greater in the AA group compared with the HI group ($P < 0.05$). There was no significant difference in the percentage of Th9 cells in the HI group before or after bronchial allergen challenge.

At the baseline, the serum IL-9 level was significantly higher in the AA than the HI group (66.5 ng/mL [31.3–82.4] vs. 36.3 ng/mL [28.2–42.9], respectively, $P < 0.05$). At 24 h after bronchial allergen challenge, the serum IL-9 level was significantly increased in the AA group compared with the baseline value and the HI group (87.4 ng/mL [51.41–114.2] vs. 66.5 ng/mL [31.25–82.4] and 38.9 ng/mL [32.6–46.3], respectively, $P < 0.01$) (Fig. 2b). In the AA group, the percentage of Th9 cells and serum IL-9 levels correlated with those at 24 h before ($r = 0.52$, $P = 0.02$) and 24 h after ($r = 0.69$, $P = 0.001$) bronchial allergen challenge.

STAT6 and PU.1 transcription factors in Th9 cells

At 24 h after bronchial allergen challenge, there was a significantly higher mean MFI of p-STAT6 in Th9 cells in the AA group compared with the baseline value and the HI group (84.6 MFI [67.2–105.5] vs. 51.7 MFI [34.9–84.9] and 30.2 MFI [21.1–38.12], respectively; $P < 0.01$). The mean MFI of p-STAT6 was also higher in the AA group compared with the HI group at the baseline (51.7 MFI [34.9–84.9] vs. 27.4 MFI [20.3–34.2], $P < 0.01$) (Fig. 3a–c). At 24 h after bronchial allergen inhalation, the MFI of PU.1 in Th9 cells was higher compared with the baseline data and the HI group (98.6 MFI [68.45–115.68] vs. 65.2 MFI [51.3–80.1] and 42.4 MFI [36.51–52.4], respectively; $P < 0.01$). The mean MFI of PU.1 remained unchanged after bronchial allergen challenge in the HI group (38.7 MFI [28.4–55.6] vs. 42.4 MFI [36.5–52.4], respectively; $P > 0.05$) (Fig. 4a–c). The percentage of Th9 cells correlated with p-STAT6 ($r = 0.45$, $P = 0.03$), and the serum IL-9 level correlated with PU.1 ($r = 0.6$, $P = 0.01$) and the percentage of Th9 cells ($r = 0.7$, $P = 0.001$) after bronchial allergen challenge in the AA group only. Moreover, there was a significant correlation between PU.1 and Th9 cells in the AA group 24 h after allergen challenge ($r = 0.5$, $P = 0.02$). There was no significant correlation between the percentage of Th9 cells and serum IL-9 level or p-STAT6 and PU.1 in the HI group.

Peripheral blood eosinophil apoptosis, serum IL-5, and NF-κB expression

Serum IL-5 levels were significantly greater in the AA group than the HI group 24 h before bronchial allergen challenge (42.3 pg/mL [28.7–55.6] vs. 16.2 pg/mL [14.2–18.5], $P < 0.01$) (Additional file 3: Figure S2). At 24 h after bronchial allergen challenge, serum IL-5 levels were significantly increased in the AA group compared with the baseline value and the HI group (78.9 pg/mL [54.9–90.2] vs. 42.3 pg/mL [28.7–55.6] and 16.2 pg/mL [14.6–19.3], respectively; $P < 0.01$). There was no significant difference in the serum IL-5 level before and after bronchial allergen challenge in the HI group.

At the baseline, a significantly lower percentage of peripheral blood apoptotic eosinophils was observed in the AA group compared with the HI group (3.45 % [2.1–5.4 %] vs. 7.9 % [5.0–10.2 %] $P < 0.001$). At 24 h after bronchial allergen provocation, the percentage of apoptotic eosinophils decreased in the AA group compared with the baseline value and the HI group (2.2 % [0.9–3.12 %] vs. 3.5 % [2.1–5.4 %] and 8.0 % [6.6–9.1 %], respectively; $P < 0.001$). Eosinophil survival in the HI group remained the same even 24 h after bronchial allergen challenge (Fig. 5a). Correlation between the percentage of apoptotic peripheral blood eosinophils and serum IL-5 levels was only observed in AA patients 24 h after bronchial allergen challenge ($R = -0.78$, $P = 0.03$), but there was no significant correlation in this group 24 h before allergen bronchial challenge. In addition, we did not observe a correlation between the percentage of apoptotic peripheral blood eosinophils and serum IL-5 levels in the HI group at any time point.

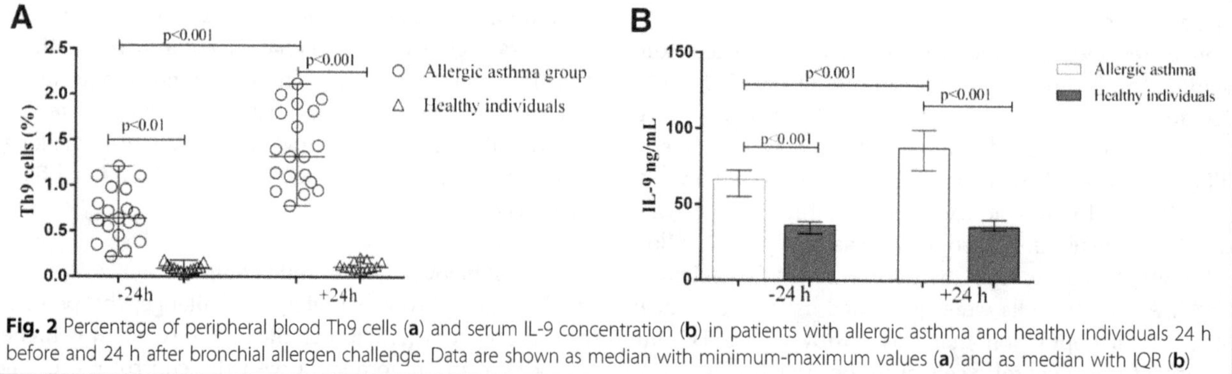

Fig. 2 Percentage of peripheral blood Th9 cells (**a**) and serum IL-9 concentration (**b**) in patients with allergic asthma and healthy individuals 24 h before and 24 h after bronchial allergen challenge. Data are shown as median with minimum-maximum values (**a**) and as median with IQR (**b**)

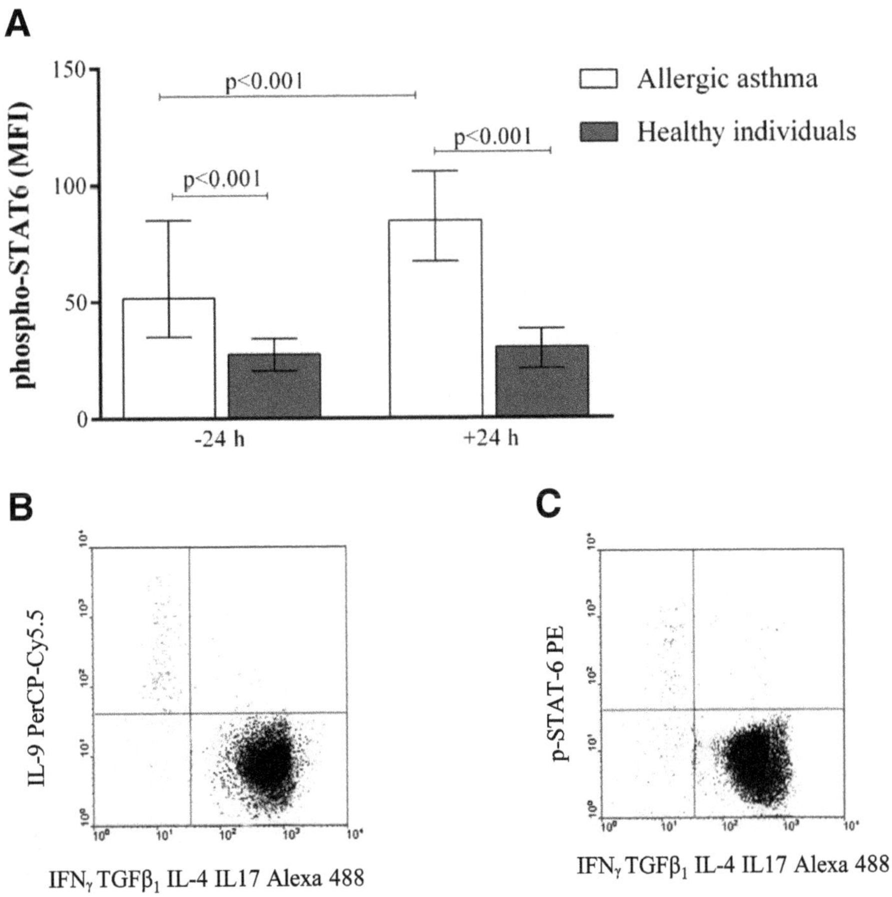

Fig. 3 Diagram (**a**) represents the mean fluorescence intensity of p-STAT6 in Th9 cells in peripheral blood CD4$^+$ cells in allergic asthma and healthy individuals 24 h before and 24 h after bronchial allergen challenge. Data are shown as median (minimum-maximum values). Dot plot (**b**) represents Th9 expression and dot plot (**c**) represents p-STAT6 expression in Th9 cells in one allergic asthma patient after bronchial allergen challenge

Our data showed a greater MFI of NF-κB in eosinophils in the AA group 24 h after bronchial allergen challenge compared with the baseline value and the HI group (99.3 MFI [79.5–153.5] vs. 51.4 MFI [39.2–70.26] and 27.8 MFI [17.2–34.15], respectively; $P < 0.001$) (Fig. 5b). There was no change in NF-κB in the HI group. Furthermore, we observed significant negative correlations between the MFI of NF-κB and eosinophil apoptosis 24 h before ($r = -0.52$, $P = 0.02$) and after ($r = -0.46$, $P = 0.02$) allergen provocation.

Discussion

Our study has shown that p-STAT6 and PU.1 may be important for Th9 cells and IL-9 production, whereas NF-κB and IL-5 were associated with reduced eosinophil apoptosis in allergen-induced late-phase airway inflammation in AA patients.

A decade ago it was assumed that IL-4 and TGF-β could induce IL-9 production from CD4+ T cells [29], and this theory was proved by two independent groups [9, 10]. Only a few CD4+ T-cell subsets are stable; often, CD4+ T-cell subsets acquire new characteristic features typical of different phenotypes dependent upon the type of stimulating cytokine, and one polarized phenotype can switch to another polarized phenotype [30]. Th9 cells are a CD4+ cell subset with great plasticity and flexibility. Th9 cells require both IL-4 and TGF-β stimulation because IL-4 alone stimulates the development of CD4$^+$ T cells into Th2 cells, and TGF-β alone induces *Treg* cells. Th9 cells have lower *Foxp3* expression than *Treg* cells, lack Th2 cytokine production, and produce high levels of IL-9. The plasticity of CD4+ T cells might be explained by the presence of specific transcription factors [31]: Th2 and Th9 cell phenotypes share common factors such as STAT6, PU.1, GATA3, c-maf, and IRF4. Environmental factors activate the expression of only one or several transcription factors, which induce another CD4+ T-cell phenotype. Although the number of Th9 cells is low and Th9 cells are closely related to Th2 cells, these cells can be considered a unique and separate CD4$^+$ T-cell subset. There is a lack of studies and consensus regarding Th9 cells; therefore, further

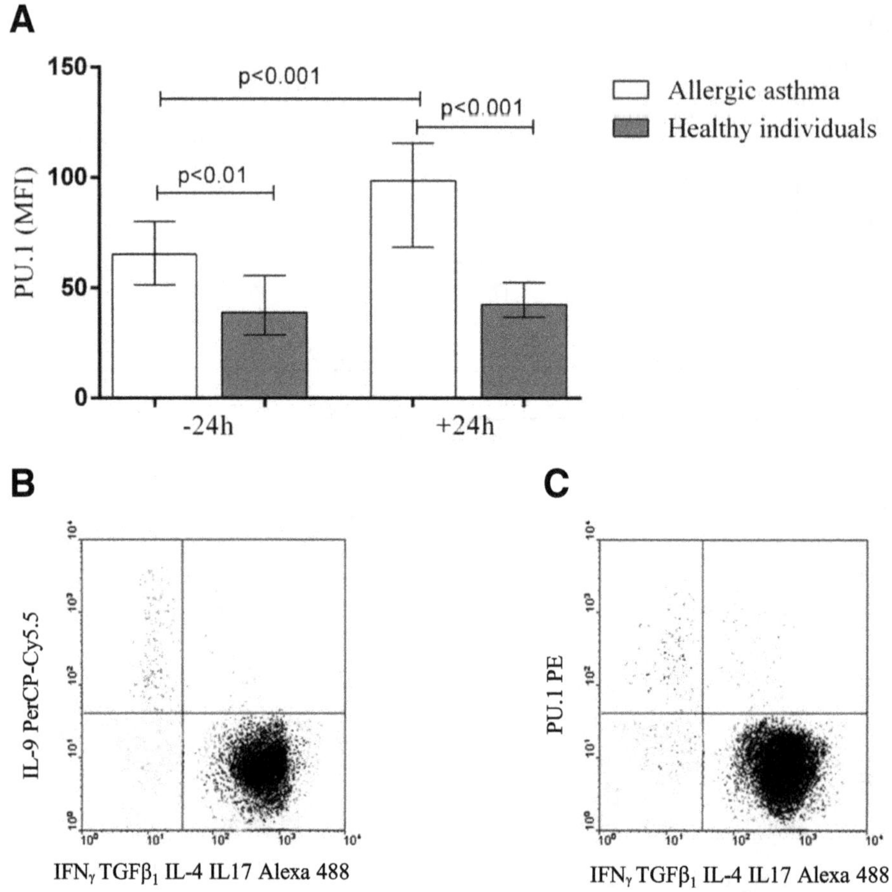

Fig. 4 Diagram (**a**) represents the mean fluorescence intensity of transcription factor PU.1 in Th9 cells among peripheral blood CD4$^+$ cells in allergic asthma and healthy individuals before and after bronchial allergen challenge. Data are shown as median (minimum-maximum values). Dot plot (**b**) represents Th9 expression and dot plot (**c**) represents PU.1 expression in Th9 cells in one allergic asthma patient after bronchial allergen challenge

studies on this new cell subset, especially in humans, are needed. Many studies have used mouse models, which are useful for the investigation of responses to inhaled allergens. Murine models allow the application of a broad range of immunological tools as well as gene deletion *in vivo*. Studies of Th9 cells showed that both human and murine Th9 cells do not express cytokines characteristic of other CD4+ T-cell subsets except for IL-9; however, some authors believe Th9 cells also produce IL-10. However, in contrast to murine Th9 cells, IL-10 is not expressed by human Th9 cells [10, 32, 33]. Other studies have suggested the importance of Th9 cells in airway allergic inflammation [14, 34–36], although some issues remain to be resolved. To study Th9 cells and their transcription factors as well as the role of eosinophils in AA, we decided to challenge study individuals with an inhaled specific allergen as this provocation model imitates natural allergen exposure in humans.

There is some evidence that PU.1, a TS-family transcription factor, is required for the generation of Th9 cells. In the study by Chang et al., naive T cells from wild-type and PU.1 knockout mice were differentiated under conditions favorable for the development of Th9 cells [36]. It was found that IL-9 protein secretion, IL-9 mRNA expression, and IL-9 intracellular staining were decreased in Th9 cultures that lacked PU.1 expression. This abovementioned study showed that PU.1 bound to sites in the *Il9* promoter specifically in Th9 cells and promoted the switch between Th2 and Th9 phenotypes. PU.1 protein is encoded by the *SPI1* gene in humans, and in the same study, the inhibition of *SPI1* expression in human Th9 cell cultures resulted in a significantly lower production of IL-9 [36]. To identify associations between human Th9 cells and PU.1, we applied the bronchial challenge test to AA patients using an inhaled specific allergen as this provocation model imitates natural allergen exposure quite well. We investigated PU.1 expression using flow cytometry analysis of Th9 cells

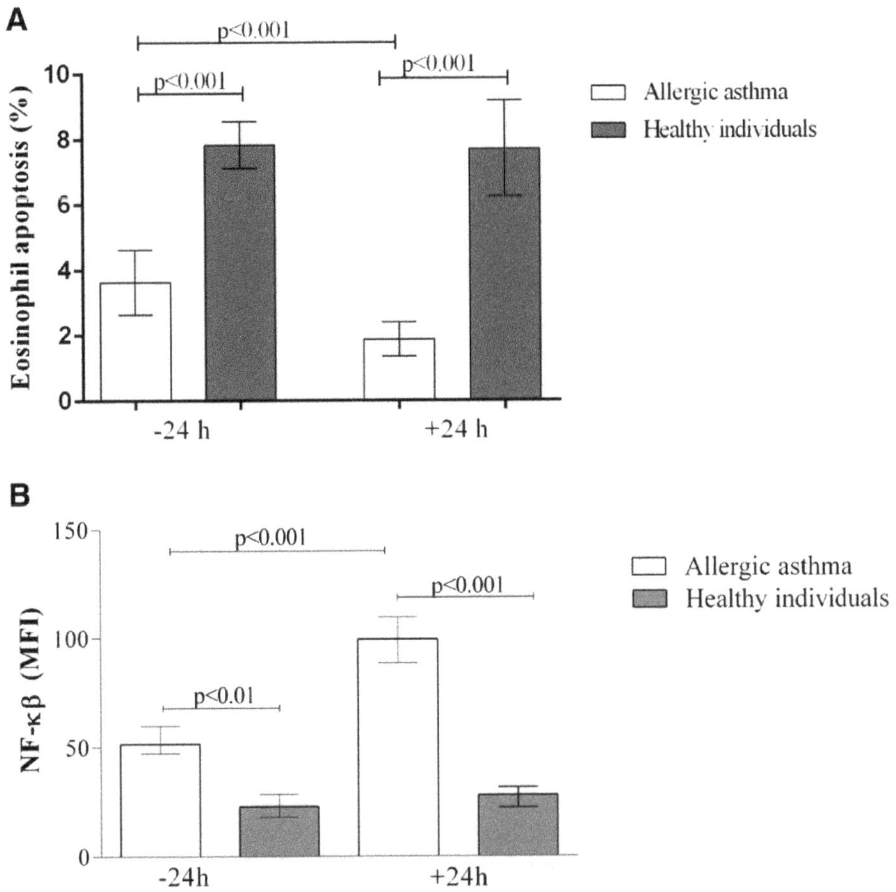

Fig. 5 Peripheral blood eosinophil apoptosis (**a**) and mean fluorescence intensity of NF-κB in peripheral blood eosinophils (**b**) in patients with allergic asthma and healthy individuals before and after bronchial allergen challenge. Data are shown as median with minimum-maximum values (**a**) and median with IQR (**b**)

from human peripheral blood and found a higher expression of this transcription factor in AA patients compared with the control group, and the expression was more prominent 24 h after allergen exposure. Moreover, the MFI of PU.1 only correlated well with the percentage of Th9 cells and serum IL-9 levels in the AA group 24 h after bronchial allergen challenge. These data support the findings from other studies that PU.1 is important in Th9 cell differentiation.

STAT6 belongs to the family of transcription factors that activate gene transcription in response to a particular cytokine. It is a cytoplasmic protein that is activated by tyrosine phosphorylation by cytokine receptor-associated JAK (Janus) kinases after cytokine exposure. IL-4 activates STAT6 and the expression of a very specific gene program that regulates viability, proliferation, and differentiation of the responding cell. STAT6 only recognizes phosphorylated tyrosines on the cytoplasmic tail of the IL-4 receptor α chain and does not interact with phospho-tyrosines on the IFN-γ receptor [37]. JAK kinases, Jak1 and Jak3, bind to the α and γ IL-4R chains, respectively, and are responsible for the subsequent phosphorylation of the IL-4 receptor itself as well as STAT6. The phosphorylated STAT6 monomers then dimerize, translocate to the nucleus, and bind DNA to activate transcription [38]. STAT6 is required for the modification of TGF-β-induced *Treg* development because Th9 cells develop when TGF-β and IL-4 act together. Mice expressing constitutively active STAT6 are predisposed to allergic disease [39]. We found greater pSTAT6 expression in IL-9-producing cells from AA patients compared with the HI group. A correlation between serum IL-9 levels and pSTAT6 as well as between the percentage of Th9 cells and pSTAT6 indicated the importance of this transcription factor in the development and function of Th9 cells.

IL-9 is a signature cytokine of Th9 cells. Th2 cells, mast cells, natural killer cells, Th17 cells, and Treg cells under some conditions produce less clinically important amounts of IL-9. It was shown that IL-9 increased the expression of IL-5R on eosinophils and inhibited eosinophil apoptosis, enhancing eosinophil development and promoting eosinophil maturation in synergy with IL-5 [22, 39]. Expression of IL-9 in transgenic mice under the control of a lung-specific promoter resulted in severe airway inflammation with eosinophils and lymphocytes as well as mast cell hyperplasia [40]. We investigated serum IL-9 levels in patients with AA and HI before and after allergen challenge and found higher serum IL-9 levels in patients with AA, which increased further after allergen provocation. The IL-9 level correlated with the percentage of peripheral blood Th9 cells 24 h after allergen challenge in AA patients. These findings indicate the important role of IL-9 and Th9 cells in allergen-induced late-phase airway inflammation.

TGF-β-, IL-4-, and T-cell receptor-induced transcription factors (including NF-κB non-canonical pathway) co-stimulate acute *Il9* expression. The *Il9* promoter region has multiple NF-κB binding sites [31, 41]. Moreover, TGF-β activates NF-κβ, which reduces eosinophil apoptosis and in this way prolongs eosinophil survival [42, 43]. In a recent study by Kankaanranta et al., cultures of peripheral blood eosinophils from healthy, atopic, or asthmatic donors (patients were allowed to continue usual treatment with inhaled steroids or antihistaminic drugs) were investigated, and the data demonstrated a major role for NF-κB in the TNF-β-induced inhibition of eosinophil apoptosis [44]. Inhibition of NF-κB leads to decreased airway eosinophilia in mice [45]. As delayed eosinophil apoptosis in asthma is a major cause of prolonged eosinophil inflammation [46, 47], we investigated peripheral blood eosinophil apoptosis 24 h before and after bronchial allergen challenge. We found a significantly higher percentage of apoptotic eosinophils and higher serum IL-5 levels in the AA group compared with the HI group at the baseline. However, the percentage of apoptotic eosinophils correlated with NF-κB expression in the AA group 24 h after bronchial allergen challenge but did not correlate with the IL-5 levels. Serum IL-5 levels were also increased in AA patients after challenge. The HI group did not show any significant changes in serum IL-5 levels or peripheral blood eosinophil apoptosis. Our data support evidence from previous studies that NF-κB and IL-5 are important in prolonging eosinophil survival.

Conclusions

In summary, our data show associations between p-STAT6, PU.1, and Th9 cells in adult AA patients. In addition, associations between eosinophil NF-κB, serum IL-5, and peripheral blood eosinophil apoptosis in late-phase airway inflammation in AA patients were observed.

Additional files

Additional file 1: Table S1. Changes in peripheral blood cells before and after bronchial allergen challenge in allergic asthma patients and healthy individuals.

Additional file 2: Figure S1. Dot plot representing lymphocytes by size and granularity (A); T lymphocytes gated by expressing $CD4^+$ (B); Th9 expression (C).

Additional file 3: Figure S2. The serum IL-5 concentration in patients with allergic asthma and healthy individuals before and after bronchial allergen challenge.

Abbreviations

AA: Allergic asthma; STAT-6: Signal transducer and activator of transcription protein-6; NF-κB: Nuclear factor kappa-light-chain-enhancer of activated B cells; IL: Interleukin; Th: T helper lymphocyte; IFN-γ: Interferon gamma; TGF-β: Transforming growth factor beta; FEV_1: Forced expiratory volume in one second; IL-5Rα: IL-5 receptor α-chain; FVC: Forced vital capacity; HI: Healthy individuals; PBMCs: Peripheral blood mononuclear cells; GM-CSF: Granulocyte-macrophage colony-stimulating factor; EDTA: Ethylenediaminetetraacetic acid.

Competing interests

The authors declare that they do not have any competing interests.

Authors' contributions

All authors were involved in the design of the study, analysis, and interpretation of results. DH and SL carried out experiments in the laboratory. DH contributed to the recruitment and clinical characterization of patients. RS contributed to the design and coordination of the study. KM initiated the study and participated in its design and coordination as well as helped to draft the manuscript. All authors read and approved the final manuscript.

Acknowledgments

A large part of this study was supported by the Research Council of Lithuania (project number LIG-08/2012). Funding was also received from the Scientific Foundation of the Lithuanian University of Health Sciences. We thank laboratory assistants Ieva Janulaityte and Auguste Vadisiute from the Laboratory of Pulmonology, Department of Pulmonology and Immunology, Medical Academy, Lithuanian University of Health Sciences for their great contribution to the study. We also thank Jurgita Grigiene for help with the English language editing of this manuscript.

Author details

Department of Pulmonology and Immunology, Medical Academy, Lithuanian University of Health Sciences, Kaunas, Lithuania. [2]Laboratory of Pulmonology, Department of Pulmonology and Immunology, Medical Academ, Lithuanian University of Health Sciences, Kaunas, Lithuania.

References

1. Eder W, Ege MJ, von Mutius E. The asthma epidemic. N Engl J Med. 2006;355(21):2226–35.
2. Durrant DM, Metzger DW. Emerging roles of T helper subsets in the pathogenesis of asthma. Immunol Invest. 2010;39(4–5):526–49.
3. Wan YY. Multi-tasking of helper T cells. Immunology. 2010;130(2):166–71.
4. Trivedi SG, Lloyd CM. Eosinophils in the pathogenesis of allergic airways disease. Cell Mol Life Sci. 2007;64(10):1269–89.
5. Kroegel C. The role of eosinophils in asthma. Lung. 1990;168(Suppl):5–17.
6. Paul WE. Interleukin 4: signalling mechanisms and control of T cell differentiation. Ciba Found Symp. 1997;204:208–16. discussion 216–209.
7. Jacobson NG, Szabo SJ, Weber-Nordt RM, Zhong Z, Schreiber RD, Darnell Jr JE, et al. Interleukin 12 signaling in T helper type 1 (Th1) cells involves tyrosine phosphorylation of signal transducer and activator of transcription (Stat)3 and Stat4. J Exp Med. 1995;181(5):1755–62.
8. Korn T, Bettelli E, Oukka M, Kuchroo VK. IL-17 and Th17 Cells. Annu Rev Immunol. 2009;27:485–517.
9. Veldhoen M, Uyttenhove C, van Snick J, Helmby H, Westendorf A, Buer J, et al. Transforming growth factor-beta 'reprograms' the differentiation of T helper 2 cells and promotes an interleukin 9-producing subset. Nat Immunol. 2008;9(12):1341–6.
10. Dardalhon V, Awasthi A, Kwon H, Galileos G, Gao W, Sobel RA, et al. IL-4 inhibits TGF-beta-induced Foxp3+ T cells, and together with TGF-beta, generates IL-9+ IL-10+ Foxp3(−) effector T cells. Nat Immunol. 2008;9(12):1347–55.

11. Jabeen R, Kaplan MH. The symphony of the ninth: the development and function of Th9 cells. Curr Opin Immunol. 2012;24(3):303–7.
12. Lu Y, Hong S, Li H, Park J, Hong B, Wang L, et al. Th9 cells promote antitumor immune responses in vivo. J Clin Invest. 2012;122(11):4160–71.
13. Yao W, Tepper RS, Kaplan MH. Predisposition to the development of IL-9-secreting T cells in atopic infants. J Allergy Clin Immunol. 2011;128:1357–60.
14. Goswami R, Jabeen R, Yagi R, Pham D, Zhu J, Goenka S, et al. STAT6-dependent regulation of Th9 development. J Immunol. 2012;188(3):968–75.
15. Staudt V, Bothur E, Klein M, Lingnau K, Reuter S, Grebe N, et al. Interferon-regulatory factor 4 is essential for the developmental program of T helper 9 cells. Immunity. 2010;33(2):192–202.
16. Jabeen R, Goswami R, Awe O, Kulkarni A, Nguyen ET, Attenasio A, et al. Th9 cell development requires a BATF-regulated transcriptional network. J Clin Invest. 2013;123(11):4641–53.
17. Ramming A, Druzd D, Leipe J, Schulze-Koops H, Skapenko A. Maturation-related histone modifications in the PU.1 promoter regulate Th9-cell development. Blood. 2012;119(20):4665–74.
18. Hamid QA, Minshall EM. Molecular pathology of allergic disease: I: lower airway disease. J Allergy Clin Immunol. 2000;105(1 Pt 1):20–36.
19. Wardlaw AJ. Molecular basis for selective eosinophil trafficking in asthma: a multistep paradigm. J Allergy Clin Immunol. 1999;104(5):917–26.
20. Ricci M, Matucci A, Rossi O. Bronchial asthma: pathogenetic mechanisms and genetic aspects. Recenti Prog Med. 1997;88(11):530–40.
21. Tai PC, Sun L, Spry CJ. Effects of IL-5, granulocyte/macrophage colony-stimulating factor (GM-CSF) and IL-3 on the survival of human blood eosinophils in vitro. Clin Exp Immunol. 1991;85(2):312–6.
22. Gounni AS, Gregory B, Nutku E, Aris F, Latifa K, Minshall E, et al. Interleukin-9 enhances interleukin-5 receptor expression, differentiation, and survival of human eosinophils. Blood. 2000;96(6):2163–71.
23. Fujihara S, Jaffray E, Farrow SN, Rossi AG, Haslett C, Hay RT. Inhibition of NF-kappa B by a cell permeable form of I kappa B alpha induces apoptosis in eosinophils. Biochem Biophys Res Commun. 2005;326(3):632–7.
24. Bateman ED, Hurd SS, Barnes PJ, Bousquet J, Drazen JM, FitzGerald M, et al. Global strategy for asthma management and prevention: GINA executive summary. Eur Respir J. 2008;31(1):143–78.
25. Pellegrino R, Viegi G, Brusasco V, Crapo RO, Burgos F, Casaburi R, et al. Interpretative strategies for lung function tests. Eur Respir J. 2005;26(5):948–68.
26. Baur X, Huber H, Degens PO, Allmers H, Ammon J. Relation between occupational asthma case history, bronchial methacholine challenge, and specific challenge test in patients with suspected occupational asthma. Am J Ind Med. 1998;33(2):114–22.
27. Dreborg S. The skin prick test in the diagnosis of atopic allergy. J Am Acad Dermatol. 1989;21(4 Pt 2):820–1.
28. Liu L, Jarjour NN, Busse WW, Kelly EA. Enhanced generation of helper T type 1 and 2 chemokines in allergen-induced asthma. Am J Respir Crit Care Med. 2004;169(10):1118–24.
29. Schmitt E, Germann T, Goedert S, Hoehn P, Huels C, Koelsch S, et al. IL-9 production of naive CD4+ T cells depends on IL-2, is synergistically enhanced by a combination of TGF-beta and IL-4, and is inhibited by IFN-gamma. J Immunol. 1994;153(9):3989–96.
30. Hegazy AN, Peine M, Helmstetter C, Panse I, Frohlich A, Bergthaler A, et al. Interferons direct Th2 cell reprogramming to generate a stable GATA-3(+)T-bet(+) cell subset with combined Th2 and Th1 cell functions. Immunity. 2010;32(1):116–28.
31. Perumal NB, Kaplan MH. Regulating Il9 transcription in T helper cells. Trends Immunol. 2011;32(4):146–50.
32. Wong MT, Ye JJ, Alonso MN, Landrigan A, Cheung RK, Engleman E, et al. Regulation of human Th9 differentiation by type I interferons and IL-21. Immunol Cell Biol. 2010;88(6):624–31.
33. Putheti P, Awasthi A, Popoola J, Gao W, Strom TB. Human CD4 memory T cells can become CD4 + IL-9+ T cells. PLoS One. 2010;5(1), e8706.
34. Zhao P, Xiao X, Ghobrial RM, Li XC. IL-9 and Th9 cells: progress and challenges. Int Immunol. 2013;25(10):547–51.
35. Jones CP, Gregory LG, Causton B, Campbell GA, Lloyd CM. Activin A and TGF-beta promote T(H)9 cell-mediated pulmonary allergic pathology. J Allergy Clin Immunol. 2012;129(4):1000–10. e1003.
36. Chang HC, Sehra S, Goswami R, Yao W, Yu Q, Stritesky GL, et al. The transcription factor PU.1 is required for the development of IL-9-producing T cells and allergic inflammation. Nat Immunol. 2010;11(6):527–34.
37. Wurster AL, Tanaka T, Grusby MJ. The biology of Stat4 and Stat6. Oncogene. 2000;19(21):2577–84.
38. Sehra S, Bruns HA, Ahyi AN, Nguyen ET, Schmidt NW, Michels EG, et al. IL-4 is a critical determinant in the generation of allergic inflammation initiated by a constitutively active Stat6. J Immunol. 2008;180(5):3551–9.
39. Louahed J, Zhou Y, Maloy WL, Rani PU, Weiss C, Tomer Y, et al. Interleukin 9 promotes influx and local maturation of eosinophils. Blood. 2001;97(4):1035–42.
40. Temann UA, Geba GP, Rankin JA, Flavell RA. Expression of interleukin 9 in the lungs of transgenic mice causes airway inflammation, mast cell hyperplasia, and bronchial hyperresponsiveness. J Exp Med. 1998;188(7):1307–20.
41. Xiao X, Balasubramanian S, Liu W, Chu X, Wang H, Taparowsky EJ, et al. OX40 signaling favors the induction of T(H)9 cells and airway inflammation. Nat Immunol. 2012;13(10):981–90.
42. Ward C, Chilvers ER, Lawson MF, Pryde JG, Fujihara S, Farrow SN, et al. NF-kappaB activation is a critical regulator of human granulocyte apoptosis in vitro. J Biol Chem. 1999;274(7):4309–18.
43. Temkin V, Levi-Schaffer F. Mechanism of tumour necrosis factor alpha mediated eosinophil survival. Cytokine. 2001;15(1):20–6.
44. Kankaanranta H, Ilmarinen P, Zhang X, Adcock IM, Lahti A, Barnes PJ, et al. Tumour necrosis factor-alpha regulates human eosinophil apoptosis via ligation of TNF-receptor 1 and balance between NF-kappaB and AP-1. PLoS One. 2014;9(2), e90298.
45. Edwards MR, Bartlett NW, Clarke D, Birrell M, Belvisi M, Johnston SL. Targeting the NF-kappaB pathway in asthma and chronic obstructive pulmonary disease. Pharmacol Ther. 2009;121(1):1–13.
46. Kankaanranta H, Lindsay MA, Giembycz MA, Zhang X, Moilanen E, Barnes PJ. Delayed eosinophil apoptosis in asthma. J Allergy Clin Immunol. 2000;106(1 Pt 1):77–83.
47. Wedi B, Raap U, Lewrick H, Kapp A. Delayed eosinophil programmed cell death in vitro: a common feature of inhalant allergy and extrinsic and intrinsic atopic dermatitis. J Allergy Clin Immunol. 1997;100(4):536–43.

2

Effect of inhaled corticosteroid particle size on asthma efficacy and safety outcomes

Céline El Baou[1,11*], Rachael L. Di Santostefano[2,9], Rafael Alfonso-Cristancho[3,4], Elizabeth A Suarez[5,10], David Stempel[2], Mark L Everard[6] and Neil Barnes[7,8]

Abstract

Background: Inhaled corticosteroids (ICS) are the primary treatment for persistent asthma. Currently available ICS have differing particle size due to both formulation and propellant, and it has been postulated that this may impact patient outcomes. This structured literature review and meta-analysis compared the effect of small and standard particle size ICS on lung function, symptoms, rescue use (when available) and safety in patients with asthma as assessed in head-to-head randomized controlled trials (RCTs).

Methods: A systematic literature search of MEDLINE was performed to identify RCTs (1998–2014) evaluating standard size (fluticasone propionate-containing medications) versus small particle size ICS medication in adults and children with asthma. Efficacy outcomes included forced expiratory volume in 1 s (FEV_1), morning peak expiratory flow (PEF), symptom scores, % predicted forced expiratory flow between 25 and 75% of forced vital capacity ($FEF_{25-75\%}$), and rescue medication use. Safety outcomes were also evaluated when available.

Results: Twenty-three independent trials that met the eligibility criteria were identified. Benefit-risk plots did not demonstrate any clinically meaningful differences across the five efficacy endpoints considered and no appreciable differences were noted for most safety endpoints. Meta-analysis results, using a random-effects model, demonstrated no significant difference between standard and small size particle ICS medications in terms of effects on mean change from baseline FEV_1 (L) (−0.011, 95% confidence interval [CI]: −0.037, 0.014 [$N = 3524$]), morning PEF (L/min) (medium/low doses: −3.874, 95% CI: −10.915, 3.166 [$N = 1911$]; high/high-medium doses: 5.551, 95% CI: −1.948, 13.049 [$N = 749$]) and $FEF_{25-75\%\ predicted}$ (−2.418, 95% CI: −6.400; 1.564 [$N = 115$]).

Conclusions: Based on the available literature, no clinically significant differences in efficacy or safety were observed comparing small and standard particle size ICS medications for the treatment of asthma.

Keywords: Inhaled corticosteroids, Particle size, Asthma, Systematic review, Meta-analysis

* Correspondence: celine.elbaou@phastar.com
[1]GSK, Middlesex, Stockley Park, Uxbridge, UK
[11]PHASTAR, Chiswick, London, UK
Full list of author information is available at the end of the article

Background

Asthma is a common chronic lung condition characterized by inflammation of the airways, and defined by episodes of wheezing, chest tightness, shortness of breath, and coughing [1]. Treatment with regular daily inhaled corticosteroids (ICS) is highly effective at reducing symptoms and the risk of asthma exacerbation and is the primary therapy for control of chronic asthma in both adults and children [1]. The clinical effects of daily ICS are recognized in national and international guidelines as they eliminate or reduce chronic symptoms of asthma, prevent exacerbations, maximize lung function, reduce the need for rescue β_2-agonist treatment, and enable normal activity with few side effects at low and medium dose [1, 2].

Delivery of drug to the lungs is influenced by a number of factors including inspiratory flow and particle size. Current aerosol delivery systems generally deliver polydispersed aerosols with the majority of particles in the range 1–5 μm in diameter [3]. Particles <1 μm are generally exhaled while most particles >5 μm are usually deposited in the upper airways. However, altering the characteristics of the aerosol even within this narrow window of 1–5 μm can alter the pattern of deposition within the lungs. As control of asthma by ICS requires delivery to both small and large airways, the differing particle size of ICS medications could potentially impact both efficacy and safety outcomes [4, 5]. Traditional chlorofluorocarbon (CFC) pressurized metered dose inhalers (pMDIs) were all suspension-based formulations but following the CFC transition and the advent of hydrofluoroalkane (HFA) propellants, a variety of new suspension-based and solution-based formulations have been developed. Solution-based pMDIs differ from traditional suspension-based pMDIs in that the respirable particles are only generated after actuation as the propellant evaporates from the liquid plume [6, 7]. The characteristics of the particles generated with solution-based pMDIs vary from formulation to formulation, with some generating extra-fine particles with mass median aerodynamic diameter (MMADs) of <2 μm while others generate particles with MMADs more comparable with traditional HFA-suspension pMDIs (MMADs of 2–5 μm).

Two of the most widely prescribed ICS treatments are fluticasone propionate (FP) and beclometasone dipropionate (BDP), which are chemically and structurally similar but differ in their pharmacodynamic properties [5]. For patients not controlled on ICS alone, both the United States and European guidelines recommend the additional use of a long-acting β_2-agonist (e.g. salmeterol, formoterol, etc.) in a fixed-dose combination device. FP and FP/salmeterol (FP/SAL) are formulated as HFA-suspensions, while BDP, BDP-formoterol (BDP-F), and a more recent ICS, ciclesonide (CIC) are formulated as HFA-solutions which generate extra-fine aerosols [5]. Thus, FP and FP/SAL are considered standard particle size ICS (2–5 μm), while BDP, BDP-F and CIC are considered small particle ICS (<2 μm).

It has been postulated that the use of ICS medications with a smaller particle size may confer additional clinical benefits to patients with asthma compared with medications with particles of a standard size as they are able to access the smaller airways resulting in increased efficacy [8].

The objective of this systematic literature review and meta-analysis was to evaluate the impact of particle size on clinical outcomes of patients with asthma by comparing the effect of small and standard size particle ICS on lung function, symptoms, rescue use (when available) and safety as assessed in head-to-head randomized controlled trials (RCTs).

Methods

Details on the methods of the analysis and inclusion criteria were specified in advance and documented in a protocol (GSK Clinical Study Register ID: 202012, data on file), and are summarized below.

Inclusion criteria, information source, search and study selection

Studies eligible for inclusion in the systematic review were published RCTs comparing FP-containing therapy (standard particle size) with ICS preparations of small particle size in adults and children with asthma. Specifically, treatments evaluated included FP and FP/SAL versus ICS small particle size comparators (BDP, BDP-F or CIC). Abstracts for potential inclusion in the systematic review were identified from the MEDLINE database using the following search terms in PubMed: disease: asthma; exposure: fluticasone, Flovent®, Flixotide®, Advair®, Seretide®. Abstracts in English published between January 1, 1998 and January 13, 2014 were considered.

All identified citations were downloaded and duplicate citations were removed to yield a number of unique hits. Citations were assessed in a multi-stage screening process as outlined in Fig. 1. During Screening Stage One, studies/abstracts were excluded if they included only patients with allergic rhinitis, compared ICS medications other than FP or FP/SAL versus BDP, BDP-F, or CIC, were placebo-controlled, were not a primary epidemiologic/clinical study or were considered 'gray literature' (meeting abstracts, letters, websites). Other exclusion criteria included: restricted population (e.g. pregnant women); comparisons of the same ICS at different dosages; no efficacy or safety data. Citations were designated as 'Exclude', 'Include' or 'Doubt' and a record of these decisions was maintained. Abstracts marked as 'Doubt' were cross-reviewed by a second epidemiologist.

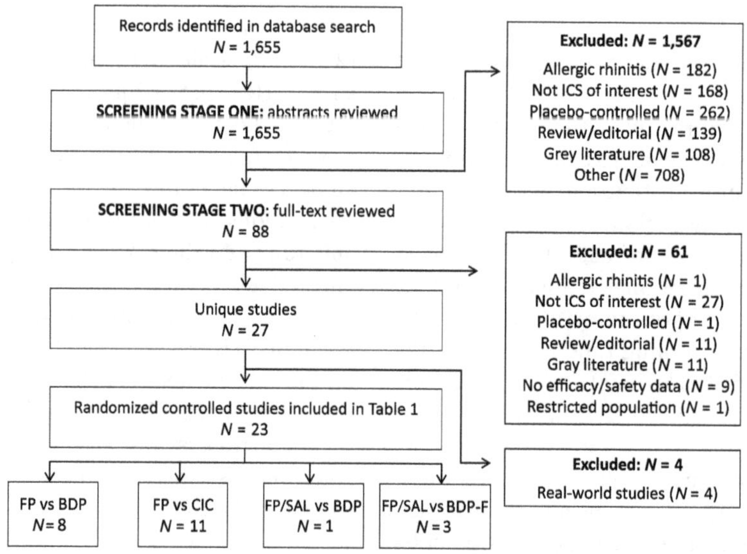

Fig. 1 Flow diagram showing implementation of search and screening strategies. BDP, beclometasone dipropionate, BDP-F, beclometasone dipropionate/formoterol fumarate; CIC, ciclesonide; FP, fluticasone propionate; FP/SAL, fluticasone propionate/salmeterol; ICS, inhaled corticosteroid

In Screening Stage Two, full text articles of the titles identified as 'Include' in Screening Stage One were reviewed and screened against the exclusion criteria listed above. The remaining studies were utilized for extraction.

Data extraction and data items

Study/patient characteristics and interventions were abstracted from the selected studies. Information on the following efficacy outcome measures were also extracted: forced expiratory volume in 1 s (FEV_1), morning peak expiratory flow (PEF), asthma symptom scores (on 4–9-point scale where a lower score corresponded to fewer symptoms), % predicted forced expiratory flow between 25 and 75% of forced vital capacity (FVC; $FEF_{25-75\%}$), and rescue medication use per day. In addition to the common lung function measure in asthma studies (FEV_1 and PEF), $FEF_{25-75\%}$ was chosen as an efficacy measure as it is a more sensitive indicator for small airway obstruction than FEV_1 [9], and thus more likely to demonstrate variations in efficacy if the smaller particles were meeting the small airways. To characterize available safety data, the following endpoints were considered: any adverse events (AEs; at least one), local steroid effects (oral candidiasis, hoarseness), upper respiratory tract infections, growth and bone metabolism, and serum cortisol levels to assess adrenal suppression.

Assessment of risk of bias

Funnel plots were used to detect biases in the identification and selection of studies. The funnel plot is a technique used to investigate the possibility of biases in the identification and selection phases. In a funnel plot, the estimated effect size of the intervention from individual studies (mean difference) is plotted on the horizontal axis against the standard error of the intervention effect estimate or sample size on the vertical axis. If there are no biases, the graph will tend to have a symmetrical funnel shape centered on the average effect of the studies. All studies were included and additional sources of bias were not formally assessed.

Planned analysis and statistical methods

Aggregated clinical data from the completed systematic review were summarized in standardized electronic extraction forms, with comparative data also entered into spreadsheets. Clinical statisticians transferred relevant extracted data into SAS (Statistical Analysis Software, Cary, NC) or R (R Foundation for Statistical Computing, Vienna, Austria) for calculation of appropriate statistics and data displays.

The objective of this analysis was to determine if there were any clinically significant differences in the comparative efficacy or safety of FP-containing medications with smaller particle ICS-containing comparators; this was evaluated in the form of a benefit-risk interval plot and/or meta-analysis, when appropriate. The data were extracted on the intent-to-treat (ITT) population as defined in each individual trial. The original publications gave treatment doses as either emitted or delivered; these same doses were reported within this manuscript for consistency.

Treatment comparisons were made using absolute treatment differences between FP-containing formulations and small particle ICS, including 95% confidence intervals (CI). For continuous measures, adjusted mean differences were used, when available. When standard errors (SE) and/or CIs were not directly available, they were estimated using available data [10]. For binary measures, the absolute risk difference and its 95% CI were calculated using the normal approximation to the binomial distribution.

Formal meta-analysis was conducted for efficacy endpoints when there was sufficient sample size and homogeneity across trials. Due to this approach, there was no adjustment for multiple testing. If there was no significant evidence of heterogeneity across the studies, both fixed and random effects models were performed. The statistical heterogeneity of the meta-analysis was assessed by means of the Cochran Q, chi-square test and the I2 statistic with 95% CI. When the assessments such as Cochran Q or chi-square test showed that heterogeneity existed, the results of the random effects model were selected. Results in children (12 years and younger) and adolescents/adults were analyzed separately. Meta regression was used to adjust for differences across studies as appropriate. Additional sensitivity analyses were performed when appropriate.

Where meta-analysis was not feasible, benefit-risk interval plots were produced to visually display the estimated differences between treatments and their 95% CIs for different endpoints on the same graph across studies; irrespective of differences in study designs, endpoints and units.

Results

The search of the PubMed database identified 1655 potentially relevant articles: 1567 were excluded, mainly because they were placebo-controlled, evaluated allergic rhinitis or did not evaluate an ICS of interest; 88 full-text articles were reviewed and 23 RCTs were included in the final analysis (Fig. 1) [4, 11–32].

Eight studies evaluated FP versus BDP, 11 evaluated FP versus CIC, one evaluated FP/SAL versus BDP and three evaluated FP/SAL versus BDP-F (Table 1). No studies evaluating FP versus BDP-F and FP/SAL versus BDP or CIC were identified. Information for children (6 to 15 years in age) was only available in four studies [15, 18, 26, 27]; one of which utilized a spacer in each arm [18]. No other studies (adults or children) were found to use a spacer.

The main efficacy endpoints evaluated in the studies were FEV_1 and PEF (Table 1). The predominant safety endpoints were overall incidence of AEs and urinary cortisol levels.

Fluticasone propionate versus beclometasone dipropionate

In the eight identified trials comparing conventional suspension-based FP pMDIs with the 'ultra fine' solution-based BDP formulations similar doses have been used in each arm (Table 1). This is in accordance with GINA guidelines reporting the clinically comparable doses of HFA-FP and HFA-BDP [1]. Hence these comparisons will address the issue of whether differences in particle size results in a change in the efficacy or safety profile.

The majority of the RCTs reported no significant difference in efficacy outcome measures between FP and BDP. Two of the eight RCTs reported significant differences in $FEF_{25-75\%}$ between FP and BDP; one demonstrating improvement with FP [18] and the other with BDP [16] (Table 1).

The majority of RCTs reported no significant difference in AEs or other safety markers between the two treatments. Overnight urinary cortisol/creatinine production was suppressed more in patients using BDP compared with patients on FP (1000 µg/day FP versus BDP: geometric mean fold difference 1.97 [95% CI: 1.28, 3.02]; $p < 0.05$) [12]. No significant difference was found in cortisol levels in three studies, either in levels at the end of the treatment period or in change from baseline [11, 13, 14].

Fluticasone propionate versus ciclesonide

With few exceptions in 10 identified RCTs, CIC was found to be non-inferior or not statistically different from FP for numerous efficacy endpoints (Table 1). Notably, in a trial by Pedersen et al. in children aged 6–11 years, non-inferiority of CIC to FP (88 µg twice daily) was observed with regard to change in FEV_1 from baseline over 12 weeks of treatment with 160 µg but not 80 µg once daily [27]. A similar trial in children aged 6–15 years comparing the same doses found that CIC did not show non-inferiority in the change from baseline in morning or afternoon PEF following 12 weeks of treatment [26]. One trial of adult patients, by Cohen et al., found greater improvement in lung function among patients receiving FP compared with patients receiving CIC, specifically in mean ± SD % predicted FEV_1 (0.5 ± 4.3 versus −3.0 ± 4.6, respectively; $p = 0.021$) and $FEF_{25-75\%}$ (0.6 ± 5.6 versus −3.6 ± 6.0, respectively; $p = 0.034$) [4].

Results for differences in urinary cortisol levels (adjusted for creatinine) were variable, with greater adrenal suppression among patients receiving FP (compared with CIC) reported in an ITT analysis restricted to patients with normal creatinine levels ($p = 0.006$) [26]. In a small crossover study, patients on FP 2000 µg/day had significantly lower mean overnight 10-h urinary cortisol than patients on CIC (CIC versus FP: geometric mean fold difference 1.5 [95% CI: 1.1, 2.0]; $p < 0.05$) [24]. One

Table 1 Characteristics of RCTs included in the analysis

Reference	Study design and treatment duration	Study population	Treatment group	Comparison group	Efficacy outcome measures (as change from baseline at end of treatment unless otherwise indicated)	Significant results between groups (treatment versus comparison)
Fluticasone propionate (FP) versus beclometasone dipropionate (BDP)						
Aubier, 2001[11]	Open-label, parallel-group 8 weeks	Adults (18–75 years) with ≥4-week clinical history of moderate to severe asthma from 31 medical centers	BDP 800 µg/day via HFA-pMDI (n = 101 ITT) High dose	FP 1000 µg via HFA-pMDI (n = 97 ITT) High dose	AM PEF (L/min), PM PEF (L/min), FEV_1 (L), patients free from daily asthma symptoms (%), patients using SABA rescue medication (%)	Equivalence demonstrated for AM PEF: CI within ±25 L/min
Currie, 2002[12]	Single-blind, crossover 3 weeks per Tx period	Patients (mean [SE] age = 38 [4] years) with mild to moderate asthma	FP 500 µg/d via HFA-pMDI (n = 20 ITT) Medium dose	BDP 500 µg/d via HFA-pMDI (n = 20 ITT) Medium dose	Methacholine PD_{20} (µg), exhaled tidal NO (ppb), FEV_1 (% predicted), AM PEF (L/min)	None
			FP 1000 µg/d via HFA-pMDI (n = 20 ITT) High dose	BDP 1000 µg/d via HFA-pMDI (n = 20 ITT) High dose	Methacholine PD_{20} (µg), exhaled tidal NO (ppb), FEV_1 (% predicted), AM PEF (L/min)	None
Fairfax, 2001[13]	Double-blind, double-dummy, parallel-group 6 weeks	Patients 18–65 years with at least a 4-week past history of clinically diagnosed asthma from 30 general practice sites	BDP 400 µg/d via HFA-pMDI (n = 88 ITT) Medium dose	FP 400 µg/d via CFC-pMDI (84 ITT) Medium dose	PEFR (L/min), FEV_1 (L)	Equivalence demonstrated for AM PEFR: CI within ±25 L/min
Ohbayashi, 2008[14]	Double-crossover (results presented from parallel-group analysis of first stage of study) 3 months per Tx	Patients (FP group mean age (years): 61.0 ± 17.4; BDP group mean age: 67.9 ± 13.1) with mild to moderate persistent asthma controlled with FP Diskus for ≤6 months	FP dose dependent on patient, via Diskus (n = 25)	BDP Same dose as FP, via HFA-pMDI (n = 24)	VC, FVC, FEV_1, MEFR, PEF (all % predicted), $FEF_{50\%}$ (L/s), $FEF_{75\%}$ (L/s)	None
Robroeks, 2008[15]	Crossover 3 months per Tx	Children (6–12 years) with moderate persistent asthma from outpatient clinic	BDP 200 µg/d via HFA-pMDI (n = 30) Low dose	FP 200 µg/d via DPI (n = 30) Low dose	Absolute measures at end of treatment: FEV_1, FVC, MEF_{50} (all % predicted), FEV_1/VC (%)	None
Thongngarm, 2005[16]	Open-label 3 months	Patients (≥18 years) with 6-month history of asthma	BDP 320 µg/d via HFA-pMDI (n = 20 ITT) Medium dose	FP 330 µg/d via CFC-pMDI (n = 10 ITT) Medium dose	FEV_1, FVC, $FEF_{25–75\%}$ (all % predicted), CV (L), CV-VC, post-bronchodilator TLC, TGV, RV, FEV_1, FVC, $FEF_{25–75\%}$ (all % predicted), AM PEF, night-time awakening, shortness of breath, chest tightness, wheezing, cough, phlegm (all symptoms/day), albuterol use (puffs/day)	BDP users had larger improvement in $FEF_{25–75\%}$ (% predicted), CV, CV-VC, phlegm and albuterol use
Tunon-de-Lara, 2007[17]	Open, parallel-group 84 days	Patients with mild or moderate asthma	BDP 400 µg/d via HFA-pMDI (n = 11 PP) Medium dose	FP 500 µg/d via Diskus (n = 14 PP) Medium dose	FEV_1, FVC, SVC, SVC-FVC, FEV_1/FVC, FEV_1/LCV, $FEF_{50\%}$ and $FEF_{25–75\%}$ (all % predicted)	None
Van Aalderen, 2007[18]	Double-blind, double-dummy, parallel-group 6 weeks	Patients (5–12 years) with asthma dx ≥ 3 months from 6 sites	BDP 200 µg/d via HFA-pMDI (n = 139 ITT) Low dose	FP 200 µg/d via CFC-pMDI (n = 140 ITT)	AM PEF, PM PEF, FEV_1, FVC, $FEF_{25–75\%}$ (all % predicted), symptom-free days (%), nights without sleep disturbance	Noninferior: lower CL > −5 (% predicted) for AM PEF;

Table 1 Characteristics of RCTs included in the analysis *(Continued)*

				Low dose	(%), β_2-agonist therapy, mean (puffs/day)	FP users had greater improvement in $FEF_{25-75\%}$ (% predicted)
Fluticasone propionate versus extra-fine ciclesonide (CIC)						
Bateman, 2008[19]	Open-label, parallel-group 24 weeks	Outpatient adults and adolescents (12–75 years) with asthma in Europe	CIC 640 μg/d via HFA-pMDI (*n* = 255 ITT) High dose	FP 660 μg/d via HFA-pMDI (*n* = 273 ITT) High dose	FEV_1 (mL), FVC (L), PEF (L/min), AM PEF (L/min), asthma symptom score, rescue medication use (puffs/day) Absolute measures at end of treatment: Asthma symptom-free days, rescue medication-free days, asthma symptom and rescue medication-free days	Noninferior: lower CL above −200 mL for FEV_1; Noninferior: lower CL above −0.2 L for FVC; Noninferior: lower CL above -25 L/min for PEF and AM PEF
Boulet, 2007[20]	Open-label, parallel-group 12 weeks	Adult and adolescent (12–75 years) patients with asthma from 59 Tx centers	CIC 320 μg/d via MDI (*n* = 233 ITT) Medium dose	FP 400 μg/d via DPI (*n* = 239 ITT) Medium dose	FEV_1 (mL), FEV_1 (% predicted), FVC (L), SVC (L), AM PEF (L/min), PM PEF (L/min), daytime asthma symptom score, total asthma symptom score, rescue medication use (puffs/day)	Noninferior: lower CL above −200 mL for FEV_1; Noninferior: lower CL above −0.2 L for FVC; Noninferior: lower CL above −25 L/min for AM PEF and PM PEF
Buhl, 2006[21]	Multicenter, double-blind, double-dummy, parallel-group 12 weeks	Adult and adolescent (12–75 years) patients with asthma from 57 Tx centers	CIC 160 μg/d (*n* = 266 ITT) Low dose	FP 176 μg/d via HFA-pMDI (*n* = 263 ITT) Low dose	FEV_1 (L), FVC (L), AM PEF (L/min), daytime symptom score, night-time symptom score, total asthma symptom score (day + night score), rescue medication use (puffs/day)	Noninferior: lower CL above -0.2 L for FEV_1 and FVC; Noninferior: lower CL above -25 L/min for AM PEF
Cohen, 2011[4]	Double-blind, double-dummy, parallel-group 65 days	Adult patients with asthma (18–60 years) recruited from outpatient clinics of pulmonology departments in the Netherlands	CIC 160 μg/d via HFA-pMDI (*n* = 19) Low dose	FP 200 μg/d via HFA-pMDI (*n* = 18) Low dose	FEV_1 (% predicted), FVC (L), SVC (L), FVC/SVC (L), $FEF_{50\%}$ (L/s), $FEF_{25-75\%}$ (% predicted)	FP users had greater improvement in FEV_1 and $FEF_{25-75\%}$ (% predicted)
Dahl, 2010[22]	Double-blind, double-dummy, 2-arm, parallel-group 24 weeks	Adult and adolescent patients (12–75 years) with mild to moderate asthma from 48 centers internationally	CIC 80 μg/d via HFA-pMDI (*n* = 240 ITT) Low dose	FP 200 μg/d via HFA-pMDI (*n* = 240 ITT) Low dose	FEV_1 (L), FVC (L), AM PEF (L/min) Absolute measures at end of treatment: Days with asthma control (%), asthma exacerbations requiring Tx (%)	Noninferior: lower CL above -0.2 L for FEV_1 and FVC; Noninferior: lower CL above -25 L/min for AM PEF
Lee, 2004[23]	Double-blind, double-dummy, crossover 4 weeks per Tx	Non-smoking patients with mild-to-moderate persistent asthma	CIC 400 μg/d via HFA-pMDI (*n* = 19) High dose	FP 500 μg/d via HFA-pMDI (*n* = 19) Medium dose	NO (ppb), FEV_1 (L), FEV_1 (% predicted), $FEF_{25-75\%}$ (L/s), $FEF_{25-75\%}$ (% predicted), methacholine PD_{20} (mg/ml), AM PEF (L/min), PM PEF (L/min), NO (ppb), AM and PM asthma symptom score, AM and PM rescue medication use (puffs/day)	None
Lee, 2005[24]	Double-blind, double-dummy, crossover 4 weeks per Tx	Adult patients (mean age 47 years) with moderate, persistent asthma stable for 3 months	CIC 1600 μg/d via HFA-pMDI (*n* = 14) High dose	FP 2000 μg/d via HFA-pMDI (*n* = 14) High dose	Absolute measures at end of treatment: FEV_1 (L), FEV_1 (% predicted), $FEF_{25-75\%}$ (L/s), $FEF_{25-75\%}$ (% predicted), AM PEF (L/min), PM PEF (L/min), AM and PM asthma symptom score, AM and PM rescue meds (puffs/	None

Table 1 Characteristics of RCTs included in the analysis *(Continued)*

					d), exhaled nitric oxide (ppb), methacholine PC_{20} (mg/mL)	
Magnussen, 2007[25]	Double-blind, double-dummy, 3-arm, parallel-group 12 weeks	Patients at least 12 years of age with asthma from 91 sites	CIC 80 µg/d via HFA-pMDI (*n* = 278 ITT) Low dose	FP 178 µg/d via HFA-pMDI (*n* = 259 ITT) Low dose	FEV_1 (mL), FVC (L), PEF (L/min), asthma symptom score, daytime and night-time symptom score, rescue medication use (puffs/day)	Noninferior: lower CL above -200 mL for FEV_1; Noninferior: limit NR for FVC and PEF
			CIC 160 µg/d via HFA-pMDI (*n* = 270 ITT) Low dose	FP 178 µg/d via HFA-pMDI (*n* = 259 ITT) Low dose	FEV_1 (mL), FVC (L), PEF (L/min), asthma symptom score, daytime and night-time symptom score, rescue medication use (puffs/day)	Noninferior: lower CL above -200 mL for FEV_1; Noninferior: limit NR for FVC and PEF
Pedersen, 2006[26]	Multicenter, double-blind, double-dummy, 2-arm, parallel-group 12 weeks	Children (6–15 years) with asthma from 51 sites	CIC 160 µg/d via HFA-pMDI (*n* = 254 ITT) Low dose	FP 178 µg/d via HFA-pMDI (*n* = 257 ITT) Low dose	FEV_1 (L), PEF (L/min), AM PEF (L/min), PM PEF (L/min), asthma symptom score sum, asthma symptom free days, rescue medication-free days	Noninferior: lower CL greater than −0.1 L for FEV_1; Not noninferior: lower CL less than −12.5 L/min for PEF, AM PEF and PM PEF
Pedersen, 2009[27]	Double-blind, double-dummy, 3-arm, parallel-group 12 weeks	Children (6–11 years) with asthma from 50 internationa centers	CIC 80 µg/d via HFA-pMDI (*n* = 234 ITT) Low dose	FP 178 µg/d via HFA-pMDI (*n* = 245 ITT) Low dose	FEV_1 (L), AM PEF (L/min), asthma symptom score sum, rescue medication use Absolute measures at end of treatment: Asthma exacerbations (%)	Noninferior: lower CL greater than −0.1 L for FEV_1; Not noninferior: lower CL less than −12.5 L/min for AM PEF; Noninferior: upper CL less than 0.30 for asthma symptom score sum
			CIC 160 µg/d via HFA-pMDI (*n* = 232 ITT) Low dose	FP 178 µg/d via HFA-pMDI (*n* = 245 ITT) Low dose		Noninferior: lower CL greater than −0.1 L for FEV_1; Noninferior: lower CL greater than −12.5 L/min for AM PEF; Noninferior: upper CL less than 0.30 for asthma symptom score sum
Van der Molen, 2010[28]	Multicenter, parallel-group (series of 3 studies) 12–24 weeks	Health patients with asthma? aged 12–75 years	CIC 320 µg/d via pMDI (*n* = 224 ITT) Medium dose	FP 400 µg/d via DPI (*n* = 228 ITT) Medium dose	No efficacy outcomes; only safety outcomes available	
			CIC 640 µg/d via pMDI (*n* = 244 ITT) High dose	FP 750 µg/d via pMDI (*n* = 254 ITT) High dose		
			CIC 640 µg/d via pMDI (*n* = 250 ITT) High dose	FP 1000 µg/d via pMDI (*n* = 237 ITT) High dose		
Fluticasone propionate/salmeterol versus extra-fine beclometasone dipropionate						
Fowler, 2002[29]	Double-blind, double-dummy, parallel-group 8 weeks	Patients with asthma aged 16–70 years	BDP 400 µg/d via HFA-pMDI (*n* = 20) Medium dose	FP/SAL 200/100 µg/d via DPI (*n* = 19) Low dose	Absolute measures at end of treatment: Methacholine PD_{20} (µg), FEV_1 (L), FEV_1 (% predicted), $FEF_{25-75\%}$ (L/s), $FEF_{25-75\%}$ (% predicted), AM PEF (L/min), PM PEF (L/min),	FP/SAL users had higher post-study methacholine PD_{20}, FEV_1 (L), FEV_1 (% predicted), post-study AM/PM PEF

Table 1 Characteristics of RCTs included in the analysis *(Continued)*

					tidal exhaled NO (ppb), symptom score, reliever use (puffs/d)	
Fluticasone propionate/salmeterol versus extra-fine beclometasone dipropionate/formoterol fumarate						
Papi, 2007[30]	Double-blind, 2-arm parallel-group 12 weeks	Patients with asthma aged 18–65 years from 12 outpatient respiratory clinics in Europe	BDP-F 400/24 μg/d via pMDI (*n* = 115 ITT) Medium dose	FP/SAL 500/100 μg/d via pMDI (*n* = 113 ITT) Medium dose	AM pre-dose PEF, AM PEF and PM PEF (all L/min), FEV_1 (L), FVC (L), Absolute measures at end of treatment: Daytime and night-time symptom score, symptom-free days (%), day time use of rescue medication (puffs)	Noninferior: lower CL above -20 L/min for AM pre-dose PEF; BDP-F users had greater improvement in FVC
Papi, 2012[31]	Prospective, controlled, 2-arm parallel-group 24 weeks	Patients with asthma aged 18–65 years from 67 respiratory clinics in Europe	BDP-F 400/24 μg/d via pMDI (*n* = 206 ITT) Medium dose	FP/SAL 500/100 μg/d via Diskus DPI (*n* = 216 ITT) Medium dose	Absolute measures at end of treatment: AM PEF (L/min), FEV_1 (L), FEV_1 (% predicted), PEF (L/min), PEF (% predicted), daytime and night-time symptom score, symptom-free days (%), patients with controlled asthma, asthma exacerbations and severe asthma exacerbations (all %)	Equivalent: CI falls within –20 to +20 L/min for AM PEF
Scichilone, 2010[32]	Double-blind, double-dummy, parallel-group 12 weeks	Adult patients with asthma (18–50 years) in Italy	BDP-F 400/24 μg/d via HFA-pMDI (*n* = 15) Medium dose	FCS 500/100 μg/d via pMDI (*n* = 15) Medium dose	Absolute measures at end of treatment: Pre-dose FEV_1 (L), $FEF_{25-75\%}$ (L/s), PD_{20} FEV_1 methacholine (μg)	None

AM, morning; *CFC*, chlorofluorocarbon; *CI*, confidence interval; *CL*, clearance; *CV-VC*, closing volume/vital capacity; *DPI*, dry powder inhaler; *dx*, diagnosis; *ER*, emergency room; *FEF*, forced expiratory flow; FEV_1, forced expiratory volume in 1 sec; *FVC*, forced vital capacity; *HFA-pMDI*, hydrofluoroalkane-pressurized metered dose inhaler; *ITT*, intent-to-treat; *NO*, nitric oxide; *NR*, not reached; *PEFR*, peak expiratory flow rate; *PM*, evening; *PP*, per protocol; ppb, part per billion; *RV*, residual volume; *SABA*, short-acting beta agonists; *SVC*, slow vital capacity; *TGV*, thoracic gas volume; *TLC*, total lung capacity; *Tx*, treatment trial assessed side effect perception using a 100-point scale, and observed that patients on CIC had either a smaller increase in perceived side effects or a decrease over the treatment period from baseline compared with patients receiving FP (between-treatment least squares mean (±SE) in total Inhaled Corticosteroid Questionnaire Scores: CIC 320 μg once-daily versus FP 200 μg twice-daily (12 weeks): −2.52 ± 0.82, $p = 0.0011$; CIC 320 μg twice-daily versus FP 500 μg twice-daily (24 weeks): −2.05 ± 0.79, $p = 0.0047$ [28].

Fluticasone propionate/salmeterol versus beclometasone dipropionate

One trial was identified that compared the efficacy of BDP (400 μg/day) and FP/SAL (200 μg/100 μg/day) as a step-down therapy after high-dose ICS (dry powder inhaler [DPI]-BDP 2000 μg/day) (Table 1) [29]. Lung function measures were compared between treatment groups at the end of the 8-week treatment period instead of comparing the change from baseline in each group. Methacholine PD_{20}, post-study FEV_1 (measured and % of predicted), morning and afternoon PEF were all significantly greater in patients on FP/SAL than in patients on BDP (methacholine PD_{20} (μg): 149.9 [95% CI: 114.3, 196.5] versus 71.2 (95% CI: 54.7, 92.8]; FEV_1 (L): 2.46 [95% CI: 2.39, 2.53] versus 2.26 [95% CI: 2.20, 2.33], $p < 0.05$; FEV_1 (% predicted): 77 [95% CI: 75, 79] versus 70 (95% CI: 68, 72], $p < 0.05$; morning PEF (L/min): 434 [95% CI: 424, 445] versus 402 [95% CI: 391, 411], $p < 0.05$; evening PEF (L/min): 436 [95% CI: 425, 446] versus 408 [95% CI: 398, 418]; $p < 0.05$). No differences were found in $FEF_{25-75\%}$, symptom scores, or reliever medication use [29]. No significant differences were found between treatment groups for serum cortisol levels, urinary cortisol/creatinine ratio, or serum osteocalcin [29].

Fluticasone propionate/salmeterol versus beclometasone dipropionate-formoterol

Three RCTs compared the efficacy of FP/SAL with BDP-F (Table 1) [30–32]. One trial in adults with asthma found significantly greater improvement in FVC in patients receiving BDP-F than in those receiving FP/SAL (0.46 ± 0.51 L versus 0.34 ± 0.44 L, respectively; $p = 0.040$); however, no differences were found for any other efficacy parameters [30].

Two RCTs were identified that compared the safety of BDP-F with FP/SAL; no differences in AEs or urinary cortisol/creatinine ratio were observed between the two treatments [30, 31].

Meta-analysis

Meta-analysis methods could only be applied for the efficacy endpoints of FEV_1, PEF, and $FEF_{25-75\%}$ (Fig. 2). Other efficacy and safety endpoints were not considered for the meta-analysis due to heterogeneity, potential publication bias, and disparity of endpoint definitions and/or timing of collection. In adults, the random effects models showed no significant differences between small and standard size particle ICS for change in FEV_1 (−0.011 L, 95% CI: −0.037, 0.014; $p = 0.394$), or $FEF_{25-75\%}$ (−2.418, 95% CI: −6.400, 1.564; $p = 0.234$) (Figs. 2a and c).

Meta-regression analysis showed that the only treatment effect modifier present for morning PEF was dose level (high versus low); however, high dose versus medium dose or high hose versus high-medium dose did not show a statistically significant difference. This suggested that it may not be appropriate to use either meta-regression or meta-analysis with all of the data in the final model. Instead, the morning PEF endpoint was analyzed as two separate subgroups (high/high-medium doses and medium/low doses). The random effects models showed no significant differences between small and standard size particle ICS for change in morning PEF (medium/low doses: −3.874 L/min, 95% CI: −10.915, 3.166; high/high-medium doses: 5.551 L/min, 95% CI: −1.948, 13.049) (Figs. 2bi and ii).

For each endpoint, the heterogeneity test showed that there was no between-study variation, suggesting that fixed effects models were also appropriate. The random effects models, which provide a more conservative approach, were retained as primary models. Similar to the random effects model, no significant differences were observed for change in FEV_1 and morning PEF using a fixed effects model ($p = 0.394$ and $p = 0.097$, respectively). Even though the analysis of both data subgroups for the morning PEF data led to the same conclusion, the results for the mean differences between medium/low (−4.223 L/min) and high/high-medium (5.551 L/min) dose levels appeared to be in opposite directions (Figs. 2bi and ii). Treatment differences in $FEF_{25-75\%}$ were found to be significantly in favor of FP using a fixed effects model (−2.853 L/min; 95% CI −5.579, −0.127; $p = 0.040$), though not in the random effects model (−2.418, 95% CI: −6.400, 1.564; $p = 0.234$) (Fig. 2c). The heterogeneity test and I^2 (p-value = 0.174 and $I^2 = 39.6\%$) showed no significant between-study-variation. However, definitive conclusions could not be drawn from these treatment differences due to the small number of studies ($N = 4$) evaluated, which also explains the wider CIs for the results of the random effects model. In children, the small number of studies with disparate endpoints and results did not allow for meta-analysis.

Sensitivity analyses were performed for FEV_1, the high/high-medium dose subgroup data for morning PEF, and $FEF_{25-75\%}$, by excluding trials with crossover design [23] or with multiple arms (only in the case of FEV_1) [25]. The results of the sensitivity analyses for FEV_1 and

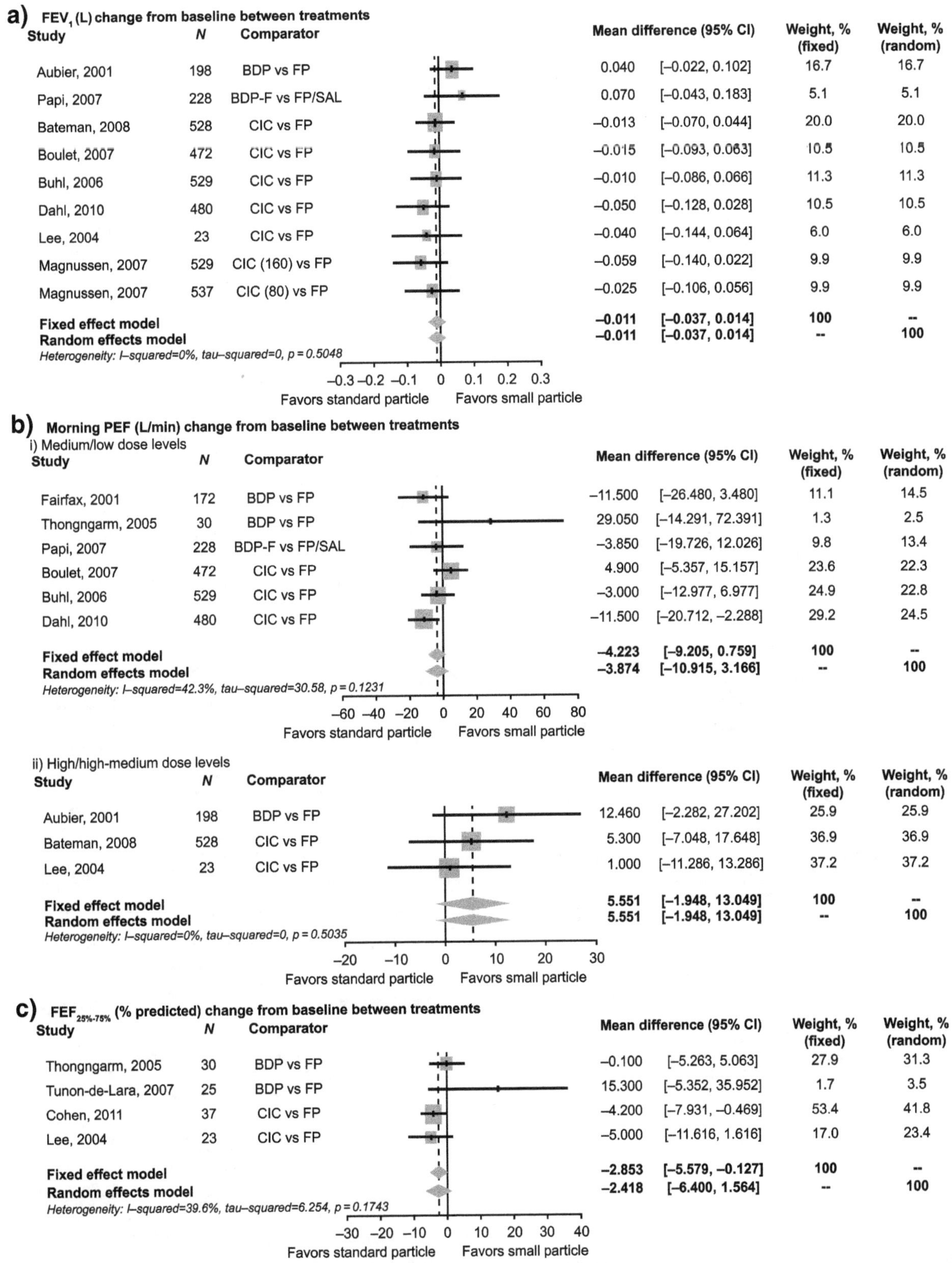

Fig. 2 (See legend on next page.)

(See figure on previous page.)
Fig. 2 Pooled effects for efficacy endpoints with 95% CI of eligible studies comparing small versus standard size particle ICS medications. Mean difference in change from baseline between treatments for (**a**) FEV_1, (**b**) morning PEF and (**c**) $FEF_{25\%-75\%}$. BDP, beclometasone dipropionate, BDP-F, beclometasone dipropionate/formoterol fumarate; CI, confidence interval; CIC, ciclesonide; $FEF_{25-75\%}$, % predicted forced expiratory flow between 25% and 75% of forced vital capacity; FEV_1, forced expiratory volume in 1 s; FP, fluticasone propionate; FP/SAL, fluticasone propionate/salmeterol; PEF, peak expiratory flow

the morning PEF were similar to the results of the final model. However, the results of the sensitivity analysis for $FEF_{25-75\%}$ (excluding Lee et al. [22]), were found to differ from the final model. There was a statistically significant treatment difference between standard size and small size particles on $FEF_{25-75\%}$ in the final fixed effect model (−2.853 L/min; 95% CI −5.579, −0.127; $p = 0.040$) but not in the sensitivity analysis (−2.414 L/min; 95% CI −5.406, 0.578; $p = 0.114$). These conflicting conclusions may be due to small patient sample sizes.

Benefit-risk plots

The benefit-risk plots included effect estimates from all individual studies included in the analysis of each efficacy and safety endpoint. For adult/adolescent patients (aged ≥12 years), the effect on total asthma symptom score and rescue medication use was only assessed for FP versus CIC. No clinically meaningful differences were noted across the five efficacy endpoints considered (FEV_1, morning PEF, and $FEF_{25-75\%}$, asthma symptoms and rescue medication use) in both adults (Fig. 3) and children (Fig. 4).

No appreciable differences were noted for most safety endpoints (AEs, local steroid effects, upper respiratory tract infections, growth and bone metabolism, and adrenal suppression) in both adults and children (Figs. 3 and 4); most studies though were not designed to test treatment differences for safety endpoints. Patients receiving FP experienced more local steroid effects at the upper airways than those receiving CIC; this was likely due to the fact that CIC is administered as a pro-drug which is only activated in the lower airways. The cortisol levels data were variable, with no clear differentiation between treatments.

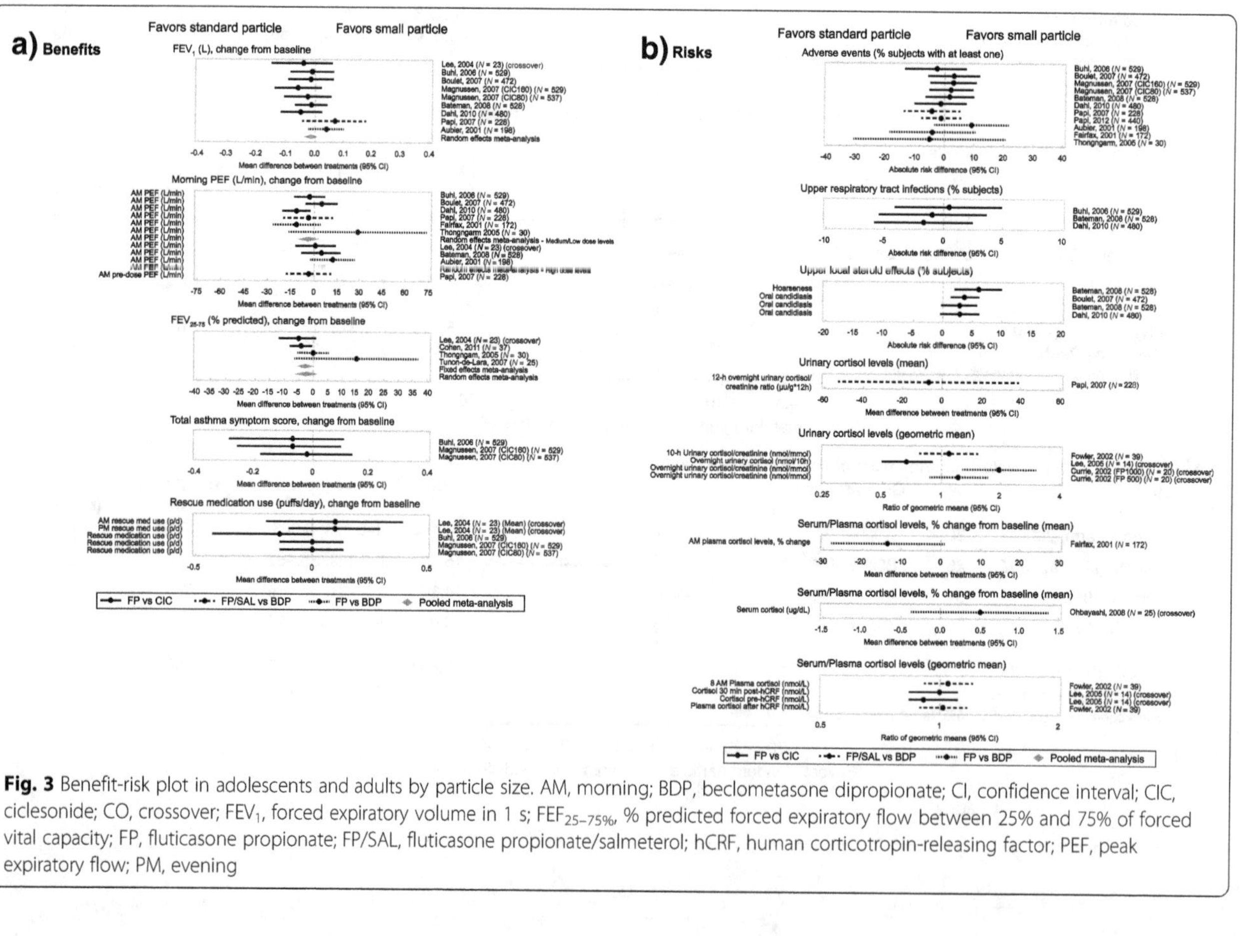

Fig. 3 Benefit-risk plot in adolescents and adults by particle size. AM, morning; BDP, beclometasone dipropionate; CI, confidence interval; CIC, ciclesonide; CO, crossover; FEV_1, forced expiratory volume in 1 s; $FEF_{25-75\%}$, % predicted forced expiratory flow between 25% and 75% of forced vital capacity; FP, fluticasone propionate; FP/SAL, fluticasone propionate/salmeterol; hCRF, human corticotropin-releasing factor; PEF, peak expiratory flow; PM, evening

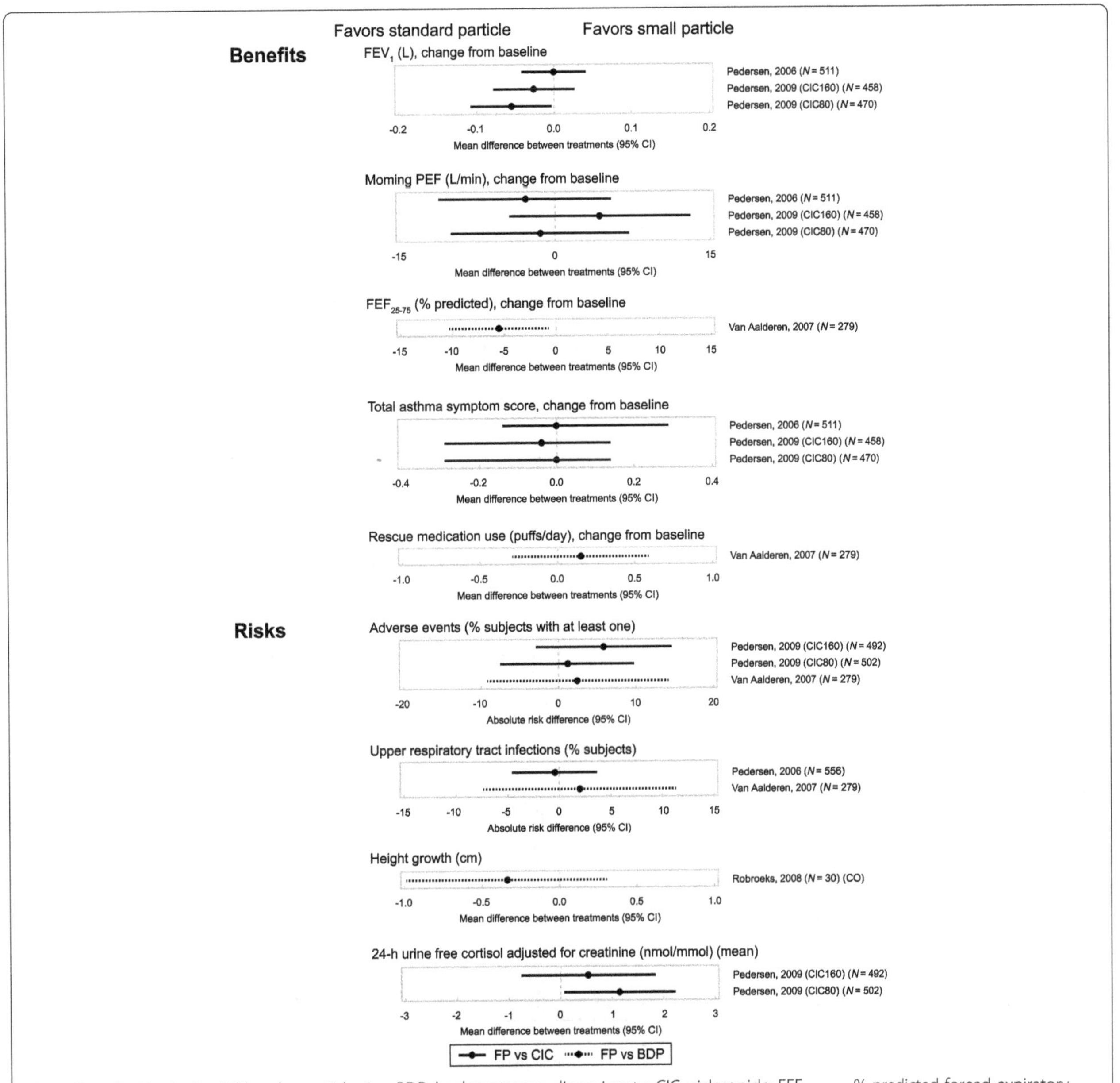

Fig. 4 Benefit-risk plot in children by particle size. BDP, beclometasone dipropionate; CIC, ciclesonide; $FEF_{25-75\%}$, % predicted forced expiratory flow between 25% and 75% of forced vital capacity; FEV_1, forced expiratory volume in 1 s; FP, fluticasone propionate; PEF, peak expiratory flow

Publication bias Based on the funnel plots and the test of asymmetry (p-values ranging from 0.225–0.822) (Fig. 5), the FEV_1, morning PEF and $PEF_{25-75\%}$ data did not exhibit asymmetry, which suggests that there is neither publication bias nor a systematic difference between smaller and larger studies ('small study effects').

Discussion

Summary

In this meta-analysis of studies in adults and adolescents, no significant differences were observed between standard size (FP and FP/SAL) and small size (BDP, CIC and BDP-F) particles ICS for change in FEV_1, morning PEF or $FEF_{25-75\%}$ using the random effects model. Similarly, no significant differences were observed between standard size and small size particles ICS in the subgroup analysis according to dose for morning PEF. However, it was observed that the result of the medium/low dose analysis for morning PEF was slightly in favor of standard particles (i.e. standard size particles ICS demonstrated better efficacy) versus small particles while the converse was true for high/high-medium dose analysis. This observed difference in the subgroup analyses suggests that dose level may be the effect modifier for morning PEF.

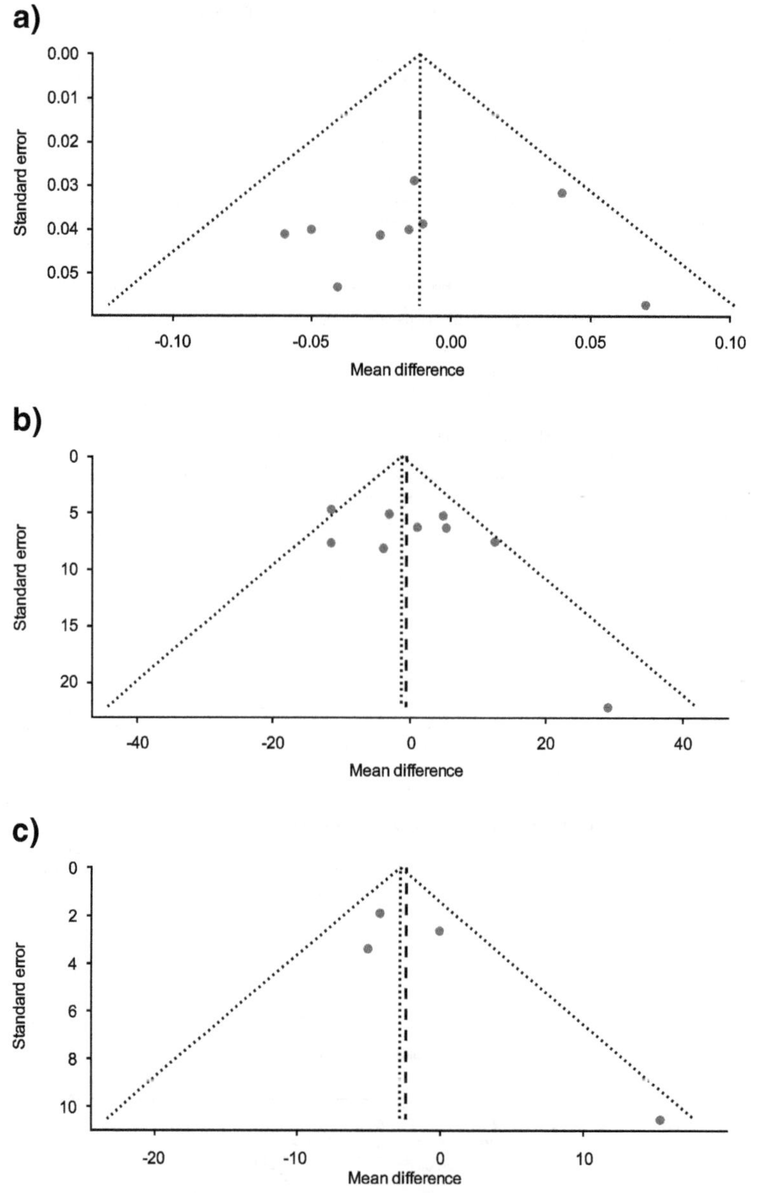

Fig. 5 Funnel plots for studies included in the (**a**) FEV_1, (**b**) morning PEF and (**c**) $FEF_{25-75\%}$ endpoints meta-analyses. **a**. Linear regression test of funnel plot asymmetry: $t = -0.2342$, $df = 7$, p-value $= 0.822$. **b**. Linear regression test of funnel plot asymmetry: $t = 1.332$, $df = 7$, p-value $= 0.225$. **c**. Linear regression test of funnel plot asymmetry $t = 1.547$, $df = 6$, p-value $= 0.262$. $FEF_{25-75\%}$, % predicted forced expiratory flow between 25% and 75% of forced vital capacity; FEV_1, forced expiratory volume in 1 s; PEF, peak expiratory flow

$FEF_{25-75\%}$ was chosen as an efficacy endpoint as it is a more sensitive indicator for disease in the small airways than FEV_1 [9], and thus more likely to demonstrate variations in efficacy if the smaller particles were meeting the small airways. However, there is ongoing debate as to the role of $FEV_{25-75\%}$ values in assessing asthma control and phenotype-driven treatment [33, 34]. Although there were no significant differences in $FEF_{25-75\%}$ for different particle sizes using the random effect model (mostly due to the small number of studies), a statistically significant difference in favor of standard particles was seen when the fixed effects model was used because the heterogeneity tests were not significant. However, this statistical difference was not clinically significant.

In terms of specific treatment comparisons, little or no differences in (FEV_1 and PEF) were reported for FP versus CIC, FP/SAL versus BDP-F, and FP versus BDP. There were no significant differences in $FEF_{25-75\%}$ for FP versus CIC; however, evidence of increased efficacy in $FEF_{25-75\%}$ was demonstrated in one trial with FP versus BDP [18] while the opposite was shown in another [16]. The results of this study also showed no significant differences in asthma symptoms and use of rescue medications between small and standard size ICS. However, these results should be treated with caution as these parameters were only evaluated between FP and CIC and not for FP versus BDP.

For the safety endpoints considered, no appreciable differences were observed for most endpoints though it should be noted that the majority of studies were not designed to test treatment differences for safety endpoints. Adult/adolescent patients experienced more local steroid effects with standard particles than small particles. The observation that the local steroid effects at the upper airways favored small particles was likely due to the fact that CIC is administered as a pro-drug which is only activated in the lower airways. Overall, the cortisol data were variable with no clear differentiations between particle sizes.

Particle size, lung deposition, and clinical outcomes

Although there is a relationship between smaller particle size and increased delivery to the distal lung [35, 36], the current study demonstrated that increased deposition in the distal lung does not appear to translate into improved clinical outcomes for patients with asthma. These results are unsurprising for a number of reasons, not least because an increased proportion of the inhaled dose is likely to deposit in the distal respiratory compartment beyond the conducting airways. Based on current understanding, the effect of using an aerosol with smaller particle size or a 'finer' aerosol is both to increase the dose reaching the lungs by reducing the oropharyngeal deposition and to increase the proportion of that dose depositing distally. While simplistically this increased distal deposition might be considered to result in increased deposition in the 'small airways', it is important to recognize the increased deposition in fact occurs in the respiratory compartment beyond the conducting airways.

In considering the impact of ICS with different particle sizes it is important to understand the factors influencing the pattern of deposition of an aerosol in the complex 3D structure formed by the conducting airways (large and small) and pulmonary/alveolar compartments of the lung. Current mathematical modeling methods combined with 3D imaging suggest that the vast majority of inhaled aerosol (>90%) inhaled during tidal breathing is delivered to the pulmonary/alveolar compartment beyond the conducting airways, and this will increase with the modified inspiratory breath when using a pMDI (with or without a holding chamber) [37, 38]. Hence for a given dose administered to the conducting airways (large, medium, and small), the dose delivered more distally will be relatively greater with the 'finer' aerosol. With such a small proportion of the aerosol depositing in the conducting airways it is unlikely that there will be a major change in the concentration of aerosol at the epithelial surface of the conducting airways. This is particularly true of the small conducting airways which have a much greater relative surface area than the more central airways.

Another point of consideration is the conjecture that 'finer' aerosols will penetrate more effectively in the face of airways narrowing. However, any perceived advantage of finer aerosols in accessing the blocked/narrowed airways would be transient in nature as it has been shown that the blockage is resolved very rapidly in the vast majority of patients with asthma when they commence ICS treatment [39].

Based on the results of this study and discussions above, it is evident that the key issue should be the evaluation of the 'therapeutic index' of different drug-device combinations rather than a comparison of aerosol particle sizes for controlling asthma. Unfortunately, there is no robust method for assessing this. As previously mentioned, apart from particle size, drug deposition within the lung is dependent on other factors such as inhaler device and inhalation technique, which varies between patients [36, 40, 41]. Thus, these factors make it impossible to know what lung doses will be achieved when an individual patient uses a particular drug-device combination, even under controlled conditions [42]. Consequently current guidelines advocate titration of ICS dosages against symptoms and spirometric data [2]. Using the lowest effective dose ensures maximum efficacy and minimizes the risk of side effects. The guidelines do not distinguish between corticosteroids formulations and this approach is supported by this systematic review.

A number of observational studies and historical matched cohort analyses have recently been published comparing the outcomes and cost of treatment with small versus standard size particle ICS in patients with asthma [43–46]. In general, the studies found that asthma treatment outcomes were similar or better with small size particle ICS (BDP) compared with standard size particle ICS (FP). However, such studies are usually confounded by variables that are not present in RCTs. For example, observational studies often rely on prescription data (which does not necessarily translate to actual dosage taken) or are not able to quantify past exposure of some drugs. Furthermore, control for asthma severity in these studies was often indirect via rescue medication and hospitalizations. Another factor that might confound the results of these studies is the lack of patient randomization.

Most of the individual clinical studies included in this review may not have been powered to detect clinically meaningful differences but statistically significant differences. This meta-analysis offered the opportunity to increase the sample size and power to calculate pooled estimates for treatment differences. Despite this increased power to detect statistical differences, the relevance and clinical meaningfulness of these results must be determined beyond the results showing statistical significance.

A potential limitation of literature reviews/meta-analyses pertains to publication bias. Searches of databases such as PubMed or EMBASE yield long lists of studies that have been published. Such searches are unlikely to yield a representative sample because studies that show a 'positive' result are more likely to be published than those that do not. However, based on the funnel plots and the test of asymmetry, the FEV_1, morning PEF and $FEF_{25-75\%}$ data did not exhibit asymmetry, which suggests that publication bias is not likely to be a limiting factor in this study.

Another potential limitation is that the present study did not explore whether other parameters of inflammation such as fractional exhaled nitric oxide [47] were differentially affected by particle size. Similarly, endpoints such as asthma exacerbations, which together with lung function and asthma symptoms indicate sub-optimal asthma control [1], was also not assessed in the present study.

Conclusion

In summary, the results of this systematic review do not support the suggestion that smaller size particle ICS are intrinsically more 'effective' than larger standard size particle ICS on the endpoints of lung function, asthma symptoms and rescue medication use. Markers of inflammation and asthma exacerbation were not assessed in this meta-analysis and so the ability of small particle treatments to differentially affect these outcomes were not possible to ascertain. No study to date has clearly addressed the key issue of the relative therapeutic index of the different drug-delivery combinations though there are robust data that regular (>80% of doses) use of these treatments at licenced doses is effective and well tolerated.

Abbreviations

AE: Adverse event; AM: Morning; BDP: Beclometasone dipropionate; BDP-F: Beclometasone dipropionate-formoterol; CFC: Chlorofluorocarbon; CI: Confidence interval; CIC: Ciclesonide; CL: Clearance; CO: crossover; CV-VC: Closing volume/vital capacity; DPI: Dry powder inhaler; dx: Diagnosis; ER: Emergency room; FEF: Forced expiratory flow; FEV_1: Forced expiratory volume in 1 s; FP: Fluticasone propionate; FP/SAL: Fluticasone propionate-salmeterol combination; FVC: Forced vital capacity; hCRF: human corticotropin-releasing factor; HFA: Hydrofluoroalkane; HFA-pMDI: Hydrofluoroalkane-pressurized metered dose inhaler; ICS: Inhaled corticosteroids; ITT: Intent-to-treat; MMAD: Mass median aerodynamic diameter; NO: Nitric oxide; NR: Not reached; PEF: Peak expiratory flow; PEFR: Peak expiratory flow rate; PM: Evening; PMDI: Pressurized metered dose inhalers; PP: Per protocol; ppb: Part per billion; RCT: Randomized controlled trial; RV: Residual volume; SABA: Short-acting beta agonists; SE: Standard error; SVC: Slow vital capacity; TGV: Thoracic gas volume; TLC: Total lung capacity; Tx: Treatment

Acknowledgments

All authors meet the criteria for authorship set forth by the International Committee for Medical Journal Editors. The authors wish to acknowledge the following individuals for their critical review during the development of the outlines and first draft of this manuscript: David Hinds, Daniel Parks, and Michael Gibbs (all employees of GSK). The authors also acknowledge Maggie Davis (GSK employee) for editorial input, data review, and coordination of author review cycles. Initial drafting of the outline was conducted by Tracy Taylor Sandell of TaylorWrit Communications Ltd, UK, funded by GSK. Editorial support in the form of editorial suggestions to draft versions of this paper, assembling tables and figures, collating author comments, copyediting, and referencing, was provided by Karen Yee PhD, of Fishawack Indicia Ltd, UK, and was funded by GSK.

Funding

Financial support for the conduct of this study and preparation of the article was provided by GSK. Staff from GSK were involved in the study design, analysis and interpretation of data, in the preparation of the article, and in the decision to submit the article for publication.

Authors' contributions

RDS participated in study conception and design, data acquisition and interpretation. CEB participated in study conception and design, data acquisition (involved in meta-analyses), analysis and interpretation. RA-C contributed to the study concept and design, and data acquisition (conducted meta-analyses). EAS participated in data acquisition (planned and conducted literature review, wrote literature review report, performed preliminary data extraction, critically reviewed material). DS participated in study conception and design; data acquisition, analysis and interpretation. MLE contributed to data analysis and interpretation. NB participated in study conception and design; data acquisition, analysis and interpretation. All authors read and approved the final manuscript.

Competing interests

CEB was contracted by GSK during the conduct of this analysis. RDS was a full-time employee of GSK during the conduct of this analysis and is currently a shareholder. RA-C, DS, and NB are full-time employees and shareholders of GSK. MLE previously received honoraria for presentations/attending advisory boards as well as support for attending conferences from a number of companies producing inhaled corticosteroid products including GSK, AstraZeneca, 3 M, Orion, and Chiesi. EAS does not have any conflict of interest to declare.

Consent for publication

Not applicable.

Author details

[1]GSK, Middlesex, Stockley Park, Uxbridge, UK. [2]GSK, Research Triangle Park, NC, USA. [3]GSK, Upper Providence, PA, USA. [4]University of Washington, School of Medicine, Seattle, WA, USA. [5]New England Research Institutes, Watertown, MA, USA. [6]The University of Western Australia, Crawley, WA 6009, Australia. [7]GSK, Brentford, UK. [8]William Harvey Research Institute, Barts and The London School of Medicine and Dentistry, London, UK. [9]Current affiliation: Janssen Pharmaceuticals, Titusville, NJ, USA. [10]Current affiliation: University of North Carolina at Chapel Hill, Chapel Hill, NC, USA. [11]PHASTAR, Chiswick, London, UK.

References

1. Global Strategy for Asthma Management and Prevention. Available from: http://ginasthma.org/gina-reports/. Accessed May 2016.
2. British guideline on the management of asthma. Available from: https://www.brit-thoracic.org.uk/standards-of-care/guidelines/btssign-british-guideline-on-the-management-of-asthma/. Accessed May 2016.
3. Usmani OS. Small-airway disease in asthma: pharmacological considerations. Curr Opin Pulm Med. 2015;21(1):55–67.

4. Cohen J, Postma DS, Douma WR, et al. Particle size matters: diagnostics and treatment of small airways involvement in asthma. Eur Respir J. 2011;37(3):532–40.
5. Dyer MJ, Halpin DM, Stein K. Inhaled ciclesonide versus inhaled budesonide or inhaled beclomethasone or inhaled fluticasone for chronic asthma in adults: a systematic review. BMC Fam Pract. 2006;7:34.
6. Grainger CI, Saunders M, Buttini F, et al. Critical characteristics for corticosteroid solution metered dose inhaler bioequivalence. Mol Pharm. 2012;9(3):563–9.
7. Buttini F, Miozzi M, Balducci AG, et al. Differences in physical chemistry and dissolution rate of solid particle aerosols from solution pressurised inhalers. Int J Pharm. 2014;465(1–2):42–51.
8. Gentile DA, Skoner DP. New asthma drugs: small molecule inhaled corticosteroids. Curr Opin Pharmacol. 2010;10(3):260–5.
9. Lipworth B. Targeting the small airways asthma phenotype: if we can reach it, should we treat it? Ann Allergy Asthma Immunol. 2013;110(4):233–9.
10. Cochrane Handbook for Systematic Reviews of Interventions Version 5.1.0 [updated March 2011]. The Cochrane Collaboration, 2011. Available from: http://community.cochrane.org/handbook. Accessed May 2016.
11. Aubier M, Wettenger R, Gans SJ. Efficacy of HFA-beclomethasone dipropionate extra-fine aerosol (800 microg day(−1)) versus HFA-fluticasone propionate (1000 microg day(−1)) in patients with asthma. Respir Med. 2001;95(3):212–20.
12. Currie GP, Fowler SJ, Wilson AM, et al. Airway and systemic effects of hydrofluoroalkane fluticasone and beclomethasone in patients with asthma. Thorax. 2002;57(10):865–8.
13. Fairfax A, Hall I, Spelman R. A randomized, double-blind comparison of beclomethasone dipropionate extrafine aerosol and fluticasone propionate. Ann Allergy Asthma Immunol. 2001;86(5):575–82.
14. Ohbayashi H, Adachi M. Hydrofluoroalkane-beclomethasone dipropionate effectively improves airway eosinophilic inflammation including the distal airways of patients with mild to moderate persistent asthma as compared with fluticasone propionate in a randomized open double-cross study. Allergol Int. 2008;57(3):231–9.
15. Robroeks CM, van de Kant KD, van Vliet D, et al. Comparison of the anti-inflammatory effects of extra-fine hydrofluoroalkane-beclomethasone vs fluticasone dry powder inhaler on exhaled inflammatory markers in childhood asthma. Ann Allergy Asthma Immunol. 2008;100(6):601–7.
16. Thongngarm T, Silkoff PE, Kossack WS, et al. Hydrofluoroalkane-134A beclomethasone or chlorofluorocarbon fluticasone: effect on small airways in poorly controlled asthma. J Asthma. 2005;42(4):257–63.
17. Tunon-de-Lara JM, Laurent F, Giraud V, et al. Air trapping in mild and moderate asthma: effect of inhaled corticosteroids. J Allergy Clin Immunol. 2007;119(3):583–90.
18. van Aalderen WM, Price D, De Baets FM, et al. Beclometasone dipropionate extrafine aerosol versus fluticasone propionate in children with asthma. Respir Med. 2007;101(7):1585–93.
19. Bateman ED, Linnhof AE, Homik L, et al. Comparison of twice-daily inhaled ciclesonide and fluticasone propionate in patients with moderate-to-severe persistent asthma. Pulm Pharmacol Ther. 2008;21(2):264–75.
20. Boulet LP, Bateman ED, Voves R, et al. A randomized study comparing ciclesonide and fluticasone propionate in patients with moderate persistent asthma. Respir Med. 2007;101(8):1677–86.
21. Buhl R, Vinkler I, Magyar P, et al. Comparable efficacy of ciclesonide once daily versus fluticasone propionate twice daily in asthma. Pulm Pharmacol Ther. 2006;19(6):404–12.
22. Dahl R, Engelstatter R, Trebas-Pietras E, et al. A 24-week comparison of low-dose ciclesonide and fluticasone propionate in mild to moderate asthma. Respir Med. 2010;104(8):1121–30.
23. Lee DK, Haggart K, Currie GP, et al. Effects of hydrofluoroalkane formulations of ciclesonide 400 microg once daily vs fluticasone 250 microg twice daily on methacholine hyper-responsiveness in mild-to-moderate persistent asthma. Br J Clin Pharmacol. 2004;58(1):26–33.
24. Lee DK, Fardon TC, Bates CE, et al. Airway and systemic effects of hydrofluoroalkane formulations of high-dose ciclesonide and fluticasone in moderate persistent asthma. Chest. 2005;127(3):851–60.
25. Magnussen H, Hofman J, Staneta P, et al. Similar efficacy of ciclesonide once daily versus fluticasone propionate twice daily in patients with persistent asthma. J Asthma. 2007;44(7):555–63.
26. Pedersen S, Garcia Garcia ML, Manjra A, et al. A comparative study of inhaled ciclesonide 160 microg/day and fluticasone propionate 176 microg/day in children with asthma. Pediatr Pulmonol. 2006;41(10):954–61.
27. Pedersen S, Engelstatter R, Weber HJ, et al. Efficacy and safety of ciclesonide once daily and fluticasone propionate twice daily in children with asthma. Pulm Pharmacol Ther. 2009;22(3):214–20.
28. van der Molen T, Foster JM, Caeser M, et al. Difference between patient-reported side effects of ciclesonide versus fluticasone propionate. Respir Med. 2010;104(12):1825–33.
29. Fowler SJ, Currie GP, Lipworth BJ. Step-down therapy with low-dose fluticasone-salmeterol combination or medium-dose hydrofluoroalkane 134a-beclomethasone alone. J Allergy Clin Immunol. 2002;109(6):929–35.
30. Papi A, Paggiaro P, Nicolini G, et al. Beclomethasone/formoterol vs fluticasone/salmeterol inhaled combination in moderate to severe asthma. Allergy. 2007;62(10):1182–8.
31. Papi A, Nicolini G, Crimi N, et al. Step-down from high dose fixed combination therapy in asthma patients: a randomized controlled trial. Respir Res. 2012;13:54.
32. Scichilone N, Battaglia S, Sorino C, et al. Effects of extra-fine inhaled beclomethasone/formoterol on both large and small airways in asthma. Allergy. 2010;65(7):897–902.
33. Ciprandi G, Cirillo I, Pasotti F, Luigi F, Ricciardolo M. FEF_{25-75}: A marker for small airways and asthma control. Ann Allerg Asthma Im. 2013;111(3):233.
34. Lipworth B. Author response. Ann Allerg Asthma Im. 2013;111(3):234.
35. van den Berge M, ten Hacken NH, Cohen J, et al. Small airway disease in asthma and COPD: clinical implications. Chest. 2011;139(2):412–23.
36. Usmani OS, Barnes PJ. Assessing and treating small airways disease in asthma and chronic obstructive pulmonary disease. Ann Med. 2012;44(2):146–56.
37. Tossici-Bolt L, Fleming JS, Conway JH, et al. An analytical technique to recover the third dimension in planar imaging of inhaled aerosols–2 estimation of the deposition per airway generation. J Aerosol Med. 2007; 20(2):127–40.
38. Majoral C, Fleming J, Conway J, et al. Controlled, parametric, individualized, 2D and 3D imaging measurements of aerosol deposition in the respiratory tract of healthy human volunteers: in vivo data analysis. J Aerosol Med Pulm Drug Deliv. 2014;27(5):349–62.
39. Brown HM, Storey G, George WH. Beclomethasone dipropionate: a new steroid aerosol for the treatment of allergic asthma. Br Med J. 1972;1(5800):585–90.
40. Haughney J, Price D, Barnes NC, et al. Choosing inhaler devices for people with asthma: current knowledge and outstanding research needs. Respir Med. 2010;104(9):1237–45.
41. Scheuch G, Kohlhaeufl MJ, Brand P, et al. Clinical perspectives on pulmonary systemic and macromolecular delivery. Adv Drug Deliv Rev. 2006;58(9–10):996–1008.
42. Everard ML. CFC transition: the emperor's new clothes. Each class of drug deserves a delivery system that meets its own requirements. Thorax. 2000; 55(10):811–4.
43. Colice G, Martin RJ, Israel E, et al. Asthma outcomes and costs of therapy with extrafine beclomethasone and fluticasone. J Allergy Clin Immunol. 2013;132(1):45–54.
44. van Aalderen WMC, Grigg J, Guilbert TW, et al. Small-particle inhaled corticosteroid as first-line or step-up controller therapy in childhood asthma. J Allergy Clin Immunol Pract. 2015;3(5):721–31.
45. Price D, Martin RJ, Barnes N, et al. Prescribing practices and asthma control with hydrofluoroalkane-beclomethasone and fluticasone: a real-world observational study. J Allergy Clin Immunol. 2010;126(3):511–8.
46. Lage MJ, Gross GN, Brewster C, et al. Outcomes and costs of patients with persistent asthma treated with beclomethasone dipropionate hydrofluoroalkane or fluticasone propionate. Adv Ther. 2009;26(8):762–75.
47. Dweik RA, Boggs PB, Erzurum SC, et al. An official ATS clinical practice guideline: interpretation of exhaled nitric oxide levels (FENO) for clinical applications. Am J Respir Crit Care Med. 2011;184(5):602–15.

3

Efficacy of budesonide/formoterol maintenance and reliever therapy compared with higher-dose budesonide as step-up from low-dose inhaled corticosteroid treatment

Christine R. Jenkins[1*], Göran Eriksson[2], Eric D. Bateman[3], Helen K. Reddel[4], Malcolm R. Sears[5], Magnus Lindberg[6] and Paul M. O'Byrne[5]

Abstract

Background: Asthma management may involve a step up in treatment when symptoms are not well controlled. We examined whether budesonide/formoterol maintenance and reliever therapy (MRT) is as effective as higher, fixed-dose budesonide plus as-needed terbutaline in patients requiring step-up from Step 2 treatment (low-dose inhaled corticosteroids), stratified by baseline reliever use.

Methods: A *post-hoc* analysis utilized data from three clinical trials of 6–12 months' duration. Patients aged ≥12 years with symptomatic asthma uncontrolled despite Step 2 treatment were included. Severe exacerbation rate, lung function and reliever use were analysed, stratified by baseline reliever use (<1, 1–2 and >2 occasions/day).

Results: Overall, 1239 patients were included. Reductions in severe exacerbation rate with budesonide/formoterol MRT versus fixed-dose budesonide were similar across baseline reliever use levels, and were statistically significant in patients using 1–2 (42%, $p = 0.01$) and >2 (39%, $p = 0.02$) reliever occasions/day, but not <1 reliever occasion/day (35%, $p = 0.11$). Both treatments significantly increased mean FEV_1 from baseline; improvements were significantly greater for budesonide/formoterol MRT in all reliever use groups. Reductions in reliever use from baseline were significantly greater with budesonide/formoterol MRT versus fixed-dose budesonide in patients using 1–2 and >2 reliever occasions/day (−0.33 and −0.74 occasions/day, respectively).

Conclusions: Treatment benefit with budesonide/formoterol MRT versus higher, fixed-dose budesonide plus short-acting β_2-agonist was found in Step 2 patients with relatively low reliever use, supporting the proposal that budesonide/formoterol MRT may be useful when asthma is uncontrolled with low-dose inhaled corticosteroid.

Keywords: Asthma, Bronchodilators, Corticosteroids, Respiratory therapy, Therapy

* Correspondence: christine.jenkins@sydney.edu.au
[1]Department of Thoracic Medicine, Concord Hospital and The George Institute for Global Health, PO Box M201Missenden Rd, Sydney, NSW 2050, Australia
Full list of author information is available at the end of the article

Background

Mild asthma comprises approximately 70% of asthma in the community [1], and accounts for a significant economic burden [2]. Despite this, the principal focus of most research has been in patients with more severe asthma. The long-term goals of asthma management are to achieve good control of symptoms and to minimise future risk to the patient, including exacerbations [3]. Whilst poor symptom control is a well-known predictor of risk of exacerbations [4], even patients with well controlled asthma symptoms may continue to experience exacerbations, and require interventions to reduce this risk.

The Global Initiative for Asthma (GINA) report recommends control-based asthma management, with pharmacological and non-pharmacological treatments adjusted in a continuous cycle based on assessment of symptom control and risk factors; a step up in treatment is recommended if asthma symptoms are not well controlled or if exacerbations continue despite good adherence and correct technique with the patient's existing inhaled treatment [3]. The recommended treatment at Step 2 is low-dose inhaled corticosteroid (ICS) as maintenance treatment plus as-needed short-acting β_2-agonist (SABA) as reliever medication [3]. It was established in the 1990s that, for those needing a step up in treatment, maintenance therapy with a low-dose ICS/long-acting β_2-agonist (ICS/LABA) plus as-needed SABA as reliever was more effective than a two- or four-fold higher dose of ICS [5, 6]; hence, the preferred Step 3 options are either low-dose ICS/formoterol, such as budesonide/formoterol (BUD/FORM), as both maintenance and reliever therapy (MRT), or conventional maintenance treatment with low-dose ICS/LABA plus as-needed SABA as reliever. An alternative Step 3 option is a two- or even four-fold higher dose of ICS plus as-needed SABA as reliever [3]. The latter is equally recommended with maintenance low-dose ICS/LABA in the US guidelines (Expert Panel Report 3) [7], and is the recommended Step 3 treatment in the International Union Against Tuberculosis and Lung Disease guidelines [8].

We have previously shown in a *post-hoc* analysis of five studies that, in patients with sub-optimal asthma control despite GINA Step 2, 3 or 4 treatment, BUD/FORM MRT is more effective in improving symptom control and reducing exacerbations than higher-dose ICS [9]. However, most patients in these studies had poor symptom control at entry, with mean reliever use of 1.7 to 2.4 occasions/day, which is well above the criterion of SABA use of ≥3 occasions/week at which a step-up would normally be considered.

Thus, it is relevant to question whether BUD/FORM MRT is effective in patients with milder, less poorly controlled disease at study entry, i.e. those with less frequent reliever use while taking low-dose ICS (≤400 µg/day BUD equivalent). This *post-hoc* analysis evaluated the efficacy of BUD/FORM MRT in improving exacerbation rate, lung function and reliever use compared with reference treatment of a higher, fixed dose of BUD plus as-needed SABA in such patients, stratified by baseline reliever use.

Methods

Study design

This retrospective, *post-hoc* analysis included data from double-blind, randomized, parallel-group studies of 6 [10] and 12 [11, 12] months' duration. The detailed methodologies have been published elsewhere [10–12]. Briefly, the clinical studies investigated the efficacy of BUD/FORM 160–320/9 µg/day MRT (Symbicort SMART™; AstraZeneca, Lund, Sweden) compared with fixed-dose BUD 320–640 µg/day as maintenance therapy and the SABA, terbutaline 0.4 mg, as needed. A fixed dose of BUD/FORM 160/9 µg maintenance therapy plus terbutaline 0.4 mg as-needed treatment arm was investigated as a comparator only in one [12] of three studies and was not included in the present analysis for this reason. All study drugs were administered using Turbuhaler® (AstraZeneca, Lund, Sweden) dry powder inhaler as delivered doses. Patients were permitted to take a maximum of 10 as-needed occasions/day of BUD/FORM or terbutaline before contacting the investigator for reassessment. The studies were performed in accordance with the Declaration of Helsinki and Good Clinical Practice guidelines. Approval from regulatory agencies and ethics committees was obtained at all centres. All patients gave written informed consent.

Patients

Patients aged 12–80 [10, 11] and 4–80 [12] years and with a diagnosis of asthma were enrolled in the clinical studies. Inclusion criteria comprised: a forced expiratory volume in 1 s (FEV_1) of 60–100% predicted in two studies [10, 12], and FEV_1 50–90% predicted in the third study [11]; baseline bronchodilator reversibility of ≥12%; and, in two studies [11, 12], at least one exacerbation in the 12 months prior to enrolment. Patients were required to have a minimum of 7 [10] and 12 [11, 12] as-needed occasions of terbutaline during the last 10 days of run-in for enrolment, but no more than 10 occasions on any day. All patients received ICS (200–1600 µg/day) for ≥3 months and at a constant dose for 30 days prior to study entry.

In the present *post-hoc* analysis, patients with asthma aged ≥12 years who were receiving Step 2 treatment (low-dose ICS, ≤400 µg/day BUD equivalent, and no long-acting β_2 agonist therapy) were included. Outcomes were analysed across a range of baseline reliever use levels: <1, 1–2 and >2 occasions/day. These cut-points were chosen for clinical simplicity rather than based on statistical distribution.

Efficacy evaluations

A severe exacerbation was defined as hospitalization/ emergency department treatment due to asthma worsening or the need for oral steroid treatment of asthma (as judged by the investigator). FEV_1 measurements were assessed by spirometry at enrolment and all clinic visits, and in accordance with the European Respiratory Society recommendations [13]. Use of reliever medication (terbutaline or BUD/FORM according to randomised allocation) was recorded by patients using diary cards.

Statistical analysis

Efficacy analysis was carried out for each study variable to determine whether BUD/FORM MRT was more efficacious than fixed-dose BUD by baseline reliever use (<1, 1–2 and >2 occasions/day). Severe exacerbation rates were analysed using Poisson regression with treatment and study as factors, and presented as p values and 95% confidence intervals (CI). On-treatment FEV_1 [14] and reliever use were analysed as treatment average change from baseline using analysis of covariance (ANCOVA) with treatment, study and baseline as fixed factors; least-square mean [LSM] treatment differences and 95% CI were calculated. In addition, the proportion of patients on both treatments with baseline reliever use ≥1 and >2 occasions/day who achieved a reduction in mean reliever use to thresholds of <0.5 and <1 occasion/ day was analysed using Fisher's exact test; patients with baseline reliever use ≥1 occasions/day comprise those from both the 1–2 and >2 occasions/day baseline reliever use subgroups. P values <0.05 were considered statistically significant. Statistical analysis was performed using standard statistical software (SAS v9.2, SAS Institute Inc., NC, USA).

Results

Patients

In total, 1239 patients (BUD/FORM MRT = 626; fixed-dose BUD = 613) were included in this *post-hoc* analysis. Baseline data for these patients are presented in Table 1. Baseline characteristics between randomization groups were comparable, including lung function, reliever use and ICS dose, but as expected baseline lung function was lower in the groups with highest baseline reliever use (Table 1).

Severe exacerbations

The percentage of patients with a severe exacerbation generally increased with increasing baseline reliever use for both treatments (Table 2). In all baseline reliever use groups, the percentage of patients with a severe exacerbation was lower with BUD/FORM MRT than fixed-dose BUD (Table 2).

Severe exacerbation rates for patients treated with BUD/FORM MRT and fixed-dose BUD stratified by baseline reliever use levels are shown in Table 2. In the group using reliever on <1 occasion/day at baseline, there was a 35% reduction in severe exacerbations for BUD/FORM MRT versus fixed-dose BUD (mean 0.09 vs 0.14 severe exacerbations per year, respectively; Table 2), but this effect did not reach statistical significance (rate ratio = 0.65 [95% CI: 0.38, 1.11]; $p = 0.11$; Fig. 1). In the baseline reliever use 1–2 occasions/day group, exacerbation rates for patients treated with BUD/FORM MRT and fixed-dose BUD were mean 0.09 and 0.16 exacerbations per year, respectively (Table 2), corresponding with a 42% reduction in severe exacerbations (rate ratio = 0.58 [95% CI: 0.38, 0.88]; $p = 0.01$; Fig. 1) for BUD/ FORM MRT compared with fixed-dose BUD. Among patients with reliever use >2 occasions/day at baseline, patients treated with BUD/FORM MRT had fewer severe exacerbations than those treated with fixed-dose BUD (mean 0.22 vs 0.37 exacerbations per year, Table 2), corresponding with a 39% lower reduction in severe exacerbations (rate ratio = 0.61 [95% CI: 0.40, 0.93]; $p = 0.02$; Fig. 1).

FEV_1

Both BUD/FORM MRT and fixed-dose BUD significantly improved mean FEV_1 from baseline in all three reliever use groups; for both treatments, improvements from baseline were greatest in patients with baseline reliever use >2 occasions/day (Table 2). For all reliever use groups, improvements from baseline in mean FEV_1 were significantly greater for BUD/ FORM MRT compared with fixed-dose BUD (treatment differences: <1 occasion/day = +0.11 L [95% CI: 0.04, 0.17], $p = 0.001$; 1–2 occasions/day = +0.11 L [95% CI: 0.06, 0.16], $p < 0.0001$; >2 occasions/day = +0.10 L [95% CI: 0.02, 0.17], $p = 0.01$; Fig. 2).

Reliever use

Both BUD/FORM MRT and fixed-dose BUD reduced reliever use from baseline in all three baseline reliever use groups (Table 2); reductions were greater with increasing baseline reliever use and were most prominent in patients using >2 occasions/day. In patients using <1 reliever occasion/day at baseline, reductions in reliever use for BUD/FORM MRT compared with fixed-dose BUD were not statistically significant; treatment difference = -0.03 occasions/day, $p = 0.68$ (Table 2, Fig. 3). Among patients using 1–2 and >2 reliever occasions/day at baseline, reductions in mean reliever use were significantly greater for BUD/FORM MRT than fixed-dose

Table 1 Patients' baseline and demographic data, stratified by baseline reliever use (<1, 1–2 and >2 occasions/day)

	BUD/FORM MRT (All patients) (*n* = 626)	Fixed-dose BUD (All patients) (*n* = 613)	Baseline reliever use subgroup					
			<1 occasion/day		1–2 occasions/day		>2 occasions/day	
			BUD/FORM MRT (*n* = 168)	Fixed-dose BUD (*n* = 155)	BUD/FORM MRT (*n* = 257)	Fixed-dose BUD (*n* = 253)	BUD/FORM MRT (*n* = 201)	Fixed-dose BUD (*n* = 205)
Male, n (%)	254 (40.6)	227 (37.0)	71 (42.3)	58 (37.4)	104 (40.5)	100 (39.5)	79 (39.3)	69 (33.7)
Age, year	37.0 (15.9)	38.3 (16.5)	35.6 (15.7)	37.5 (16.0)	36.0 (16.2)	37.7 (17.0)	39.4 (15.5)	39.6 (16.1)
Duration of asthma, years[a]	10	9	7	8	10	10	11	10
Dose of inhaled corticosteroid, μg/day BUD eqv	357.8 (70.2)	356.1 (70.8)	339.9 (84.6)	325.4 (88.1)	359.9 (71.0)	367.2 (63.2)	370.1 (51.0)	365.6 (57.4)
Pre-BD FEV_1 % predicted	73.6 (10.9)	73.0 (10.7)	74.0 (11.2)	74.0 (11.1)	74.8 (10.6)	73.4 (10.6)	71.7 (10.6)	71.7 (10.5)
Post-BD FEV_1 % predicted	88.5 (12.6)	88.0 (12.9)	89.4 (12.9)	89.0 (13.6)	89.5 (11.7)	88.5 (12.4)	86.5 (13.2)	86.8 (12.8)
Baseline pre-BD FEV_1, L	2.41 (0.7)	2.35 (0.7)	2.51 (0.7)	2.47 (0.7)	2.46 (0.7)	2.41 (0.8)	2.26 (0.7)	2.19 (0.7)
Baseline FEV_1 reversibility, %	14.9 (7.5)	15.0 (7.8)	15.4 (7.0)	15.0 (8.0)	14.7 (7.6)	15.0 (7.9)	14.9 (7.9)	15.1 (7.6)
Current smoker/ ex-smoker, n (%)	117 (18.7)	114 (18.6)	26 (15.5)	24 (15.5)	52 (20.2)	47 (18.6)	39 (19.4)	43 (21.0)

Data are given as mean (SD), unless otherwise stated

Patients treated with BUD/FORM MRT comprised 254 patients from the STEAM study, [10] 171 patients from the STEP study, [11] and 201 patients from the STAY study [12]

Patients treated with fixed-dose BUD comprised 255 patients from the STEAM study, [10] 161 patients from the STEP study, [11] and 197 patients from the STAY study [12]

[a]Median

BD bronchodilator, *BUD* budesonide, *eqv* equivalent, *FEV_1* forced expiratory volume in 1 s, *FORM* formoterol, *MRT* maintenance and reliever therapy, *SD* standard deviation

Table 2 Clinical outcomes for patients treated with BUD/FORM MRT or fixed-dose BUD, stratified by baseline reliever use (<1, 1–2 and >2 occasions/day)

	BUD/FORM MRT (All patients) (*n* = 626)	Fixed-dose BUD (All patients) (*n* = 613)	Baseline reliever use subgroup					
			<1 occasion/day		1–2 occasions/day		>2 occasions/day	
			BUD/FORM MRT (*n* = 168)	Fixed-dose BUD (*n* = 155)	BUD/FORM MRT (*n* = 257)	Fixed-dose BUD (*n* = 253)	BUD/FORM MRT (*n* = 201)	Fixed-dose BUD (*n* = 205)
Severe exacerbations								
Patients with severe exacerbation, n (%)	38 (6.1)	72 (11.7)	8 (4.8)	11 (7.1)	11 (4.3)	24 (9.5)	19 (9.5)	37 (18.0)
Rate, exacerbations per year	0.14	0.23	0.09	0.14	0.09	0.16	0.22	0.37
FEV_1								
FEV_1, L	2.62 (0.8)	2.46 (0.7)	2.69 (0.7)	2.55 (0.7)	2.66 (0.8)	2.50 (0.8)	2.51 (0.8)	2.34 (0.7)
Change from baseline in FEV_1, L	0.21 (0.3)	0.11 (0.3)	0.18 (0.3)	0.08 (0.3)	0.20 (0.3)	0.10 (0.3)	0.25 (0.4)	0.16 (0.4)
Reliever use								
Treatment period reliever use, occasions/day	0.84 (1.2)	1.27 (1.5)	0.43 (0.7)	0.50 (0.8)	0.60 (0.7)	0.93 (1.0)	1.50 (1.7)	2.28 (1.7)
Change from baseline in reliever use, occasions/day	−1.00 (1.3)	−0.65 (1.3)	−0.15 (0.7)	−0.15 (0.8)	−0.89 (0.8)	−0.56 (1.0)	−1.84 (1.6)	−1.14 (1.7)

Data are given as mean (SD), unless otherwise stated

BUD budesonide, *FORM* formoterol, *MRT* maintenance and reliever therapy

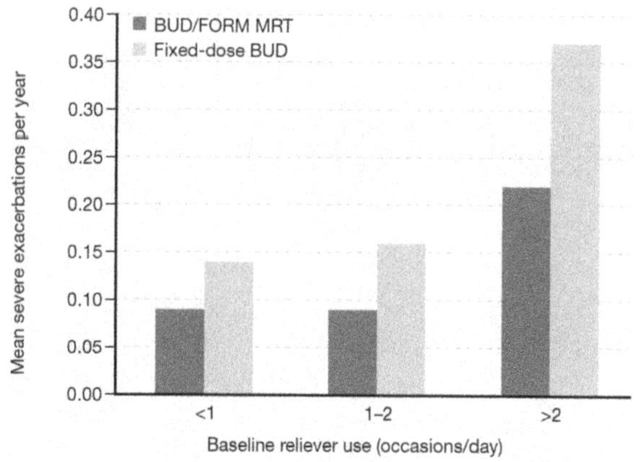

	<1	1–2	>2
RR	0.65	0.58	0.61
95% CI	0.38, 1.11	0.38, 0.88	0.40, 0.93
P value	0.11	0.01	0.02

Fig. 1 Severe exacerbation rates by treatment in patients with baseline reliever use (<1, 1–2 and >2 occasions/day). Rate ratios (95% CI) and statistical comparisons are for BUD/FORM MRT compared with fixed-dose BUD. *BUD* budesonide, *CI* confidence intervals, *FORM* formoterol, *MRT* maintenance and reliever therapy, *RR* rate ratio

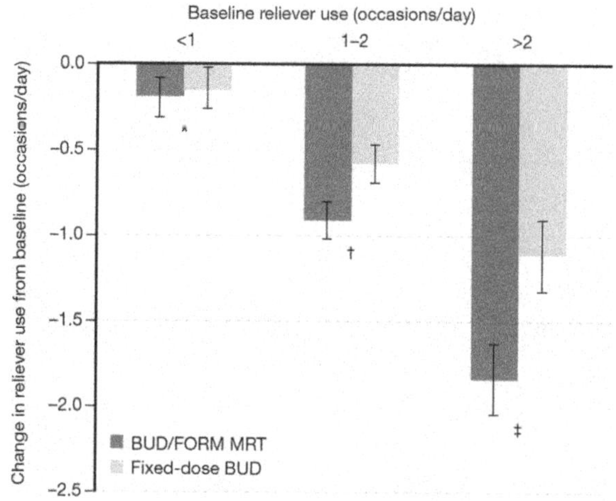

Fig. 3 Least square mean improvements in on-treatment reliever use from baseline in patients treated with BUD/FORM MRT or fixed-dose BUD, stratified by baseline reliever use (<1, 1–2 and >2 occasions/day). The error bars represent 95% CI. Statistical comparisons are for BUD/FORM MRT compared with fixed-dose BUD. *BUD* budesonide, *CI* confidence intervals, *FORM* formoterol, *MRT* maintenance and reliever therapy. * −0.03 occasions/day (95% CI: −0.20, 0.13), $p = 0.68$; † −0.33 occasions/day (95% CI: −0.48, −0.18), $p < 0.0001$; ‡ −0.74 occasions/day (95% CI: −1.03, −0.45), $p < 0.0001$

BUD; 1–2 occasions/day: treatment difference = -0.33 occasions/day, $p < 0.0001$; >2 occasions/day: treatment difference = -0.74 occasions/day, $p < 0.0001$ (Table 2, Fig. 3).

For patients with baseline reliever use ≥1 and >2 occasions/day, the proportion of patients who achieved a reduction in mean reliever use to thresholds of <0.5 and <1 occasion/day was significantly greater with BUD/FORM MRT than fixed-dose BUD (all $p <$ 0.0001, Additional file 1: Table S1).

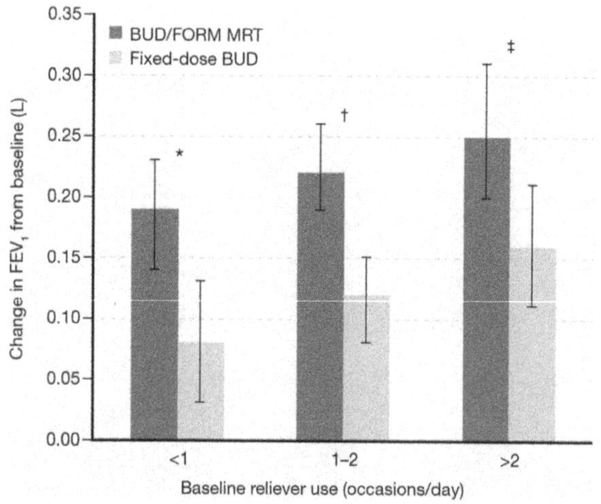

Fig. 2 Least square mean improvements in mean FEV_1 from baseline in patients treated with BUD/FORM MRT or fixed-dose BUD, stratified by baseline reliever use (<1, 1–2 and >2 occasions/day). The error bars represent 95% CI. Statistical comparisons are for BUD/FORM MRT compared with fixed-dose BUD. *BUD* budesonide, *CI* confidence intervals, *FORM* formoterol, *FEV_1* forced expiratory volume in 1 s, *MRT* maintenance and reliever therapy. * +0.11 L (95% CI: 0.04, 0.17), $p = 0.001$; † +0.11 L (95% CI: 0.06, 0.16), $p < 0.0001$; ‡ +0.10 L (95% CI: 0.02, 0.17), $p = 0.01$

Discussion

The efficacy of BUD/FORM MRT for reducing exacerbations in at-risk patients with uncontrolled asthma across a range of baseline treatment steps is well established [9]. The present *post-hoc* analysis, based on patients using Step 2 treatment (low-dose ICS, ≤400 μg/day BUD equivalent) at entry into three double-blind, randomized, parallel-group studies [10–12], and stratifying by baseline reliever use (<1, 1–2 and >2 occasions/day), suggests that the benefit from MRT is seen even in patients with milder asthma and impaired asthma control, most of whom had a history of at least one exacerbation in the previous year. The magnitude of difference in severe exacerbations for MRT compared with higher-dose ICS was similar regardless of baseline reliever use, reducing the proportion of patients having a severe exacerbation by 35–42%; however, statistical significance was not reached in the lowest stratum. Furthermore, this reduction in exacerbation risk with BUD/FORM MRT was achieved with a maintenance dose of ICS approximately two-[10, 11] to four-[12] fold lower than with fixed-dose BUD. This finding supports the value of MRT treatment in this milder category of asthma in terms of reducing exacerbation risk. Importantly, exacerbation reduction may still be important in this group of patients with low exacerbation rates since a significant proportion of asthma deaths occur in patients with so-called mild asthma [15–17].

This study also considers a problem common in clinical practice, that is, the situation in which patients use higher than recommended levels of reliever use before they or their physicians step up treatment [18]. The recommended approach in patients with mild asthma who remain uncontrolled and require reliever medication ≥3 occasions/week [3] despite maintenance treatment with low-dose ICS (<400 µg/day BUD equivalent) and as-needed SABA as reliever, is to check adherence and inhaler technique, and then to step up treatment to low-dose ICS/formoterol (budesonide or beclomethasone) MRT *or* low-dose maintenance ICS/LABA plus as-needed SABA [3]. A third option is medium-dose ICS plus as-needed SABA as reliever. Frequent reliever use is a marker for sub-optimal asthma control and is associated with an increased risk of an exacerbation [4]. The latter has been confirmed in many studies, and a recent comparison of BUD/FORM MRT with conventional maintenance BUD/FORM and as-needed SABA showed that baseline reliever use was a significant predictor of severe exacerbations within the following 12 months [19].

Improvements in measures of daily asthma control (lung function, reliever use) were also seen for BUD/FORM MRT compared with fixed-dose BUD. Given that the comparator was ICS alone, it is not surprising that improvements in on-treatment FEV_1 [14] from baseline were significantly greater for BUD/FORM MRT than fixed-dose BUD (treatment differences 0.10–0.11 L). However, although statistically significant, improvements in FEV_1 of 0.10–0.11 L are relatively small despite these patients having mean 15% FEV_1 reversibility and low prebronchodilator FEV_1 at baseline. That the magnitude of reduction in reliever use with BUD/FORM MRT was smallest in patients with lower baseline reliever use suggests that these patients may have milder underlying asthma or may disregard some symptoms, or that reliever use at such low levels may be a relatively insensitive marker of treatment effect. Despite this, our exacerbation data suggest that there is still potential for clinical benefit by reducing their risk of adverse outcomes. Further to the mean changes in reliever use, BUD/FORM MRT significantly increased the proportion of patients with baseline usage ≥1 and >2 occasions/day whose reliever use fell below 0.5 occasions/day (3.5 occasions/week), usage above which a step-up in treatment would normally be considered.

One mechanism by which BUD/FORM MRT may reduce exacerbations even in patients with infrequent reliever use is by improving adherence with ICS-containing medication. Poor adherence is associated with significant asthma-related morbidity but, despite this, patients with milder asthma may not take daily maintenance treatment on symptom-free days [20, 21], which supports the rationale for the use of MRT in patients with reliever use of <1 occasion/day. The use of a single combination inhaler for ICS/LABA MRT simplifies asthma management and ensures that reliever treatment provides both immediate symptom relief and a rapid anti-inflammatory effect, preventing symptoms from developing into an exacerbation. There is also an established scientific rationale for giving an ICS and a LABA together as they have complementary actions on the pathophysiology of asthma and may act synergistically at a molecular level [22, 23].

We acknowledge that the *post-hoc* design of this analysis is a limitation and future prospective, well-designed trials are required to confirm these findings in patients with milder asthma and lower baseline reliever use. The use of ICS/LABA as-needed in mild asthma is currently being evaluated in the ongoing SYGMA studies [24]. In the present analysis, the selection only of patients on Step 2 treatment at entry, and sub-division by baseline as-needed reliever use, reduced the power of the analyses, with only around 150–250 patients qualifying in each sub-group. Additionally, all patients satisfied the regulatory requirement for significant bronchodilator reversibility at entry, and the studies had minimum reliever use requirements of 7 [10] and 12 [11, 12] occasions in the last 10 days of run-in, so the results cannot and should not be extrapolated to patients with well controlled asthma (e.g., with reliever use <3 occasions/week). Finally, patients in two of the studies were required to have had at least one exacerbation in the previous 12 months and may thus represent a group of patients at higher risk than others at this step of treatment.

Conclusions

In conclusion, BUD/FORM MRT and a higher, fixed dose of BUD plus SABA improved lung function, and reduced reliever use and exacerbation rate, in patients whose asthma was uncontrolled on Step 2 treatment at study entry. Treatment benefit for exacerbations with BUD/FORM MRT compared with a higher, fixed-dose BUD plus SABA was found in these patients across all levels of baseline reliever use, and was statistically significant in those with a baseline reliever use of 1–2 and >2 occasions/day. These results support the beneficial effects of BUD/FORM MRT in patients whose asthma is not well-controlled with low-dose ICS, even when their background use of reliever is relatively low.

Abbreviations
BD: Bronchodilator; BUD/FORM: Budesonide/formoterol; CI: Confidence interval; FEV_1: Forced expiratory volume in 1 second; GINA: Global Initiative for Asthma; ICS: Inhaled corticosteroids; LABA: Long-acting β_2-agonist; MRT: Maintenance reliever therapy; RR: Rate ratio; SABA: Short-acting β_2-agonist; SD: Standard deviation

Acknowledgements
Shaun Foley, inScience Communications, Springer Healthcare, provided medical writing assistance, funded by AstraZeneca.

Funding
AstraZeneca funded this *post-hoc* analysis. The authors generated the hypotheses of this *post-hoc* analysis, Magnus Lindberg (of AstraZeneca) performed the analyses on the pooled data from the three AstraZeneca-sponsored phase III studies, and distributed the data outputs to the authors, who were responsible for the interpretation of the data.

Authors' contributions
CJ, GE, EB, HR, MS, ML and PO contributed to data interpretation, and conceiving, writing and revising the manuscript. ML was responsible for statistical analyses. CJ, the corresponding author, had full access to all the data in the study and had final responsibility for the decision to submit for publication. All authors read and approved the final manuscript.

Competing interests
C. Jenkins has received consultancy fees, travel and expense support from AstraZeneca for participation in a working group that performed analyses of databases that led to this paper; has received consultancy fees for advisory board and/or steering committee membership from AstraZeneca, GlaxoSmithKline, Boehringer Ingelheim, Novartis and Mundipharma; has received payment for delivering lectures from GlaxoSmithKline, Boehringer Ingelheim, AstraZeneca, Novartis and Mundipharma, and payment for the development of educational presentations from GlaxoSmithKline, Boehringer Ingelheim, AstraZeneca, Novartis, Mundipharma; and has also been paid an hourly rate for face-to-face individual consultations and for offering advice on regulatory issues for airways disease medications from GlaxoSmithKline, Boehringer Ingelheim, AstraZeneca and Novartis.
E. D. Bateman has received consulting fees from AstraZeneca for participation in a working group that performed analyses of databases that led to this paper; has received compensation for board membership from Almirall, AstraZeneca, Boehringer Ingelheim, GlaxoSmithKline, Merck, Novartis and Takeda; has received consultancy fees from ALK-Abelló, Almirall and Cephalon; has received or has grants pending from Actelion, Aeras, Almirall, AstraZeneca, Boehringer Ingelheim, GlaxoSmithKline, Roche/Genentech, Merck, Novartis, Takeda, TEVA and Cephalon; and has received payment for delivering lectures from AstraZeneca, Boehringer Ingelheim, Chiesi, GlaxoSmithKline, Novartis and Takeda, as well as from Novartis for the development of education presentations.
G. Eriksson was previously employed by AstraZeneca, from which he also received stock/stock options, and has thereafter received consultancy fees from ALK, Almirall, Novartis and Medicon Valley Inhalation Consortium.
H. K. Reddel has received consultancy fees from AstraZeneca for face-to-face meetings at which this manuscript and other studies were discussed; has received compensation for board membership from AstraZeneca, GlaxoSmithKline, Merck and Novartis; has received consultancy fees from AstraZeneca and Novartis; has received grants from GlaxoSmithKline and AstraZeneca; and has received payment from AstraZeneca, Boehringer Ingelheim, GlaxoSmithKline, Novartis, Mundipharma and Teva for delivering independent educational presentations.
M. R. Sears has consultant arrangements with AstraZeneca and Novartis, has received payment for lectures from AstraZeneca and Merck, and holds an AstraZeneca endowed chair in Respiratory Epidemiology.
M. Lindberg is an employee of AstraZeneca and owns stock/options in the company.
P. M. O'Byrne has received compensation for board membership from the Joint Oversight Board for a LABA safety study, and has received consultancy fees from AstraZeneca, GlaxoSmithKline, Merck, Boehringer and Novartis, and has received or has grants pending from AstraZeneca, Amgen, Genentech, Axikin, Novartis and Sanofi.

Consent for publication
Not applicable.

Author details
[1]Department of Thoracic Medicine, Concord Hospital and The George Institute for Global Health, PO Box M201Missenden Rd, Sydney, NSW 2050, Australia. [2]Department of Respiratory Medicine and Allergology, University Hospital, Lund, Sweden. [3]Division of Pulmonology, Department of Medicine, University of Cape Town, Cape Town, South Africa. [4]Clinical Management Group, Woolcock Institute of Medical Research, University of Sydney, Sydney, Australia. [5]Michael G DeGroote School of Medicine, Faculty of Health Sciences, McMaster University, Hamilton, Canada. [6]Biometrics and Information Sciences (B&I), AstraZeneca R&D, Mölndal, Sweden.

References
1. O'Byrne PM, Parameswaran K. Pharmacological management of mild or moderate persistent asthma. Lancet. 2006;368:794–803.
2. Sadatsafavi M, Lynd L, Marra C, Carleton B, Tan WC, Sullivan S, Fitzgerald JM. Direct health care costs associated with asthma in British Columbia. Can Respir J. 2010;17:74–80.
3. GINA Global strategy for asthma management and prevention. Updated 2015.
4. Bateman ED, Reddel HK, Eriksson G, Peterson S, Ostlund O, Sears MR, Jenkins C, Humbert M, Buhl R, Harrison TW, Quirce S, O'Byrne PM. Overall asthma control: the relationship between current control and future risk. J Allergy Clin Immunol. 2010;125:600–8. e6.
5. Greening AP, Ind PW, Northfield M, Shaw G. Added salmeterol versus higher-dose corticosteroid in asthma patients with symptoms on existing inhaled corticosteroid. Lancet. 1994;344:219–24.
6. Woolcock A, Lundback B, Ringdal N, Jacques LA. Comparison of addition of salmeterol to inhaled steroids with doubling of the dose of inhaled steroids. Am J Respir Crit Care Med. 1996;153:1481–8.
7. National Asthma Education and Prevention Program. Expert panel report 3 (EPR-3): guidelines for the diagnosis and management of asthma - summary report. J Allergy Clin Immunol. 2007;120:S94–S138.
8. Ait-Khaled N, Enarson D, Chen-Yuan C, Marks G and Bissell K. Management of Asthma: A Guide to the Essentials of Good Clinical Practice. Third edition. International Union Against Tuberculosis and Lung Disease); 2008. http://www.theunion.org/what-we-do/publications/english/pub_asthma-guide_eng.pdf.
9. Bateman ED, Harrison TW, Quirce S, Reddel HK, Buhl R, Humbert M, Jenkins CR, Peterson S, Ostlund O, O'Byrne PM, Sears MR, Eriksson GS. Overall asthma control achieved with budesonide/formoterol maintenance and reliever therapy for patients on different treatment steps. Respir Res. 2011;12:38.
10. Rabe KF, Pizzichini E, Stallberg B, Romero S, Balanzat AM, Atienza T, Lier PA, Jorup C. Budesonide/formoterol in a single inhaler for maintenance and relief in mild-to-moderate asthma: a randomized, double-blind trial. Chest. 2006;129:246–56.
11. Scicchitano R, Aalbers R, Ukena D, Manjra A, Fouquert L, Centanni S, Boulet LP, Naya IP, Hultquist C. Efficacy and safety of budesonide/formoterol single inhaler therapy versus a higher dose of budesonide in moderate to severe asthma. Curr Med Res Opin. 2004;20:1403–18.
12. O'Byrne PM, Bisgaard H, Godard PP, Pistolesi M, Palmqvist M, Zhu Y, Ekstrom T, Bateman ED. Budesonide/formoterol combination therapy as both maintenance and reliever medication in asthma. Am J Respir Crit Care Med. 2005;171:129–36.
13. Quanjer PH, Tammeling GJ, Cotes JE, Pedersen OF, Peslin R, Yernault JC. Lung volumes and forced ventilatory flows. Report working party standardization of lung function tests, European community for steel and coal. Official statement of the European Respiratory Society. Eur Respir J Suppl. 1993;16:5–40.
14. Reddel HK, Taylor DR, Bateman ED, Boulet LP, Boushey HA, Busse WW, Casale TB, Chanez P, Enright PL, Gibson PG, de Jongste JC, Kerstjens HA, Lazarus SC, Levy ML, O'Byrne PM, Partridge MR, Pavord ID, Sears MR, Sterk PJ, Stoloff SW, Sullivan SD, Szefler SJ, Thomas MD, Wenzel SE. An official American Thoracic Society/European Respiratory Society statement: asthma control and exacerbations: standardizing endpoints for clinical asthma trials and clinical practice. Am J Respir Crit Care Med. 2009;180:59–99.

15. Robertson CF, Rubinfeld AR, Bowes G. Pediatric asthma deaths in Victoria: the mild are at risk. Pediatr Pulmonol. 1992;13:95–100.
16. Royal College of Physicians 2014 Why asthma still kills. National Review of Asthma Deaths (NRAD). Report May 2014. (London
17. Abramson M J, Bailey M J, Couper F J, Driver J S, Drummer O H, Forbes A B, McNeil J J, Haydn Walters E and Victorian Asthma Mortality Study Group. Are asthma medications and management related to deaths from asthma? Am J Respir Crit Care Med. 2001;163:12–8.
18. Rabe KF, Adachi M, Lai CK, Soriano JB, Vermeire PA, Weiss KB, Weiss ST. Worldwide severity and control of asthma in children and adults: the global asthma insights and reality surveys. J Allergy Clin Immunol. 2004;114:40–7.
19. Bateman ED, Buhl R, O'Byrne PM, Humbert M, Reddel HK, Sears MR, Jenkins C, Harrison TW, Quirce S, Peterson S, Eriksson G. Development and validation of a novel risk score for asthma exacerbations: the risk score for exacerbations. J Allergy Clin Immunol. 2015;135:1457–64. e4.
20. Williams LK, Peterson EL, Wells K, Ahmedani BK, Kumar R, Burchard EG, Chowdhry VK, Favro D, Lanfear DE, Pladevall M. Quantifying the proportion of severe asthma exacerbations attributable to inhaled corticosteroid nonadherence. J Allergy Clin Immunol. 2011;128:1185–91. e2.
21. Patel M, Pilcher J, Pritchard A, Perrin K, Travers J, Shaw D, Holt S, Harwood M, Black P, Weatherall M, Beasley R. Efficacy and safety of maintenance and reliever combination budesonide-formoterol inhaler in patients with asthma at risk of severe exacerbations: a randomised controlled trial. Lancet Respir Med. 2013;1:32–42.
22. Barnes PJ. Scientific rationale for combination inhalers with a long-acting b2-agonists and corticosteroids. Eur Respir J. 2002;19:182–91.
23. Giembycz MA, Kaur M, Leigh R, Newton R. A holy grail of asthma management: toward understanding how long-acting β2-adrenoceptor agonists enhance the clinical efficacy of inhaled corticosteroids. Br J Pharmacol. 2008;153:1094–104.
24. O'Byrne PM, FitzGerald JM, Zhong N, Bateman E, Barnes PJ, Keen C, Almqvist A, Pemberton K, Jorup C, Ivanov S, Reddel HK. The SYGMA programme of phase 3 trials to evaluate the efficacy and safety of budesonide/formoterol given 'as needed' in mild asthma: study protocols for two randomised controlled trials. Trials. 2017;18:12.

4

Asthma control using fluticasone propionate/salmeterol in Asian and non-Asian populations: a post hoc analysis of the GOAL study

Jean Bousquet[1,2,3*], Neil Barnes[4,5], Michael Gibbs[4], Nadeem Gul[6], Susan A Tomkins[6], Xin Zhou[7], Young-Joo Cho[8], Hae-Sim Park[9], William Busse[10] and Nanshan Zhong[11]

Abstract

Background: To analyse the efficacy of fluticasone propionate (FP) alone and combined with salmeterol (SAL) in achieving guideline-defined asthma control in Asian patients.

Methods: A post hoc analysis of the GOAL study in which patients were stratified by prior-medication use into inhaled corticosteroid (ICS)-naïve (Stratum [S] 1), low-dose ICS (S2), and medium-dose ICS (S3), and randomised to receive FP/SAL or FP. Doses were stepped-up every 12 weeks until Totally Controlled asthma or maximum dose was reached (PhI) and then maintained until study end (PhII). The primary endpoint was the proportion of patients achieving Well-Controlled asthma during PhI. Additional endpoints included Total Control and adverse events. Asian and non-Asian patients were analysed separately.

Results: In Asian patients in PhI, 74% ($n = 87/118$) in S1 achieved Well-Controlled asthma with FP/SAL versus 74% ($n = 89/121$) with FP alone ($p = 0.839$); corresponding values were 76% ($n = 81/107$) versus 60% ($n = 62/104$; $p = 0.005$) in S2, and 58% ($n = 59/102$) versus 43% ($n = 41/95$; $p = 0.015$) in S3. More patients in all three strata achieved Totally Controlled asthma with FP/SAL versus FP alone. Control was achieved more rapidly and with lower ICS doses with FP/SAL versus FP. A high proportion of patients who achieved control during PhI maintained control during PhII. Similar trends were found in non-Asian patients. No new safety concerns were identified.

Conclusions: A greater proportion of Asian patients (S2 and S3, for Well-Controlled; all strata, for Totally Controlled) achieved guideline-defined asthma control with FP/SAL versus FP alone. High proportions of Asian patients in S1 achieved Well-Controlled asthma in both treatment groups.

Keywords: Asian patients, Asthma, Asthma control, Asthma treatment, Fluticasone propionate/salmeterol, ICS/LABA treatment

* Correspondence: jean.bousquet@orange.fr
[1]Fondation MACVIA-LR, Contre les Maladies Chroniques pour un Vieillissement Actif en Languedoc-Roussillon, European Innovation Partnership on Active and Healthy Ageing Reference Site, University of Montpellier, Montpellier, France
[2]INSERM, VIMA: Ageing and Chronic Diseases, Epidemiological and Public Health Approaches, U1168, Paris, France
Full list of author information is available at the end of the article

Background

In the past two decades, asthma guidelines have been revised to emphasise management based on the control of symptoms and exacerbations rather than classification of the patient by disease severity [1, 2]. The current Global Initiative for Asthma (GINA) guidelines describe the level of asthma symptom control as well-controlled, partly controlled and uncontrolled [1].

The Gaining Optimal Asthma controL (GOAL) study was the first large study to examine whether guideline-defined asthma control can be achieved in patients who were uncontrolled on either short-acting β2-agonist (SABA) alone or low- to medium-dose inhaled corticosteroid (ICS) [3]. GOAL was a 1-year, randomised, multinational trial which included 3,421 patients from 44 countries [3]. The study evaluated fluticasone propionate (FP) in combination with salmeterol (SAL) (FP/SAL) compared with FP alone, and demonstrated that guideline-defined asthma control could be achieved in the majority of patients [3].

The large size and multinational nature of GOAL allows for analysis of population subgroups, for example, by ethnicity. The relatively few clinical trials evaluating asthma control in Asian patients have demonstrated that effective control can be achieved with usual therapies of ICS alone or a combination of ICS/long-acting β_2-agonist (LABA) [4–6]. However, two large, population-based surveys in Asia have shown that good asthma control is not always achieved in this geographic area, despite the availability of effective treatments [7–9]. In the Asthma Insights and Reality in Asia-Pacific (AIRIAP) survey, a high proportion of patients had poorly-controlled asthma according to GINA criteria [7]. Approximately half of patients surveyed had experienced daytime or night-time asthma symptoms over the past month, and a similar proportion had required emergency care over the past year [7]. The REcognise Asthma and LInk to Symptoms and Experience (REALISE) Asia study reported uncontrolled asthma in half the patients surveyed and only partial control in a further one-third [9]. Two out of three patients missed work because of asthma, and even patients reported as having controlled asthma had experienced acute exacerbations during the previous year [8].

The underlying reasons for poor control in patients with asthma are unknown. Several studies have demonstrated that lung function measures in Asian populations are lower than those in Caucasian populations [10–13]. How this difference may impact on the level of asthma control that can be achieved with treatment in Asian patients is unknown. To help answer this question, we conducted a post hoc subgroup analysis of Asian patients in the GOAL study, using the composite asthma control criteria used in the original global population. The primary objective of this post hoc analysis was to evaluate the efficacy of FP/SAL compared with FP alone in achieving guideline-defined asthma control in Asian patients. Additionally, data from the non-Asian population are presented to provide a descriptive comparison with the results from the Asian population.

Methods

Study design

This was a post hoc subgroup analysis of the randomised, double-blind, parallel-group GOAL study (GSK identifier: SAM40027). The design and methodology of the GOAL study have been published in detail [3] (Additional file 1). Patients were recruited between December 2000 and December 2001 and stratified according to their medication use in the 6 months prior to screening. Stratum 1 included patients who were ICS-naïve, stratum 2 included patients who received low-dose ICS treatment (≤500 μg daily of beclomethasone dipropionate or equivalent), and stratum 3 included patients who received medium-dose ICS treatment (>500– ≤1000 μg daily of beclomethasone dipropionate or equivalent).

Patients were randomised (1:1) to receive either FP/SAL or FP, stratified by baseline therapy. The starting doses (taken twice daily) were FP/SAL 100/50 μg or FP 100 μg (patients in stratum 1 and stratum 2) or FP/SAL 250/50 μg or FP 250 μg (patients in stratum 3). The study was divided into two phases. In Phase I, doses were "stepped-up" every 12 weeks until either Total Control (as defined by the GINA and National Institutes of Health [NIH] Guidelines at the time of the original study [14]; Additional file 2: Table S1) was achieved or the maximum dose (FP/SAL 500/50 μg or FP 500 μg) was reached. Patients in stratum 1 and stratum 2 had up to three treatment steps (step 1: FP/SAL 100/50 μg or FP 100 μg; step 2: FP/SAL 250/50 μg or FP 250 μg; step 3: FP/SAL 500/50 μg or FP 500 μg) while patients in stratum 3 had up to two steps (step 1: FP/SAL 250/50 μg or FP 250 μg; step 2: FP/SAL 500/50 μg or FP 500 μg). In Phase II (reached either after achieving Total Control in Phase I or after 12 weeks on the maximum dose), patients remained on the dose that achieved Total Control or the maximum dose until the end of the 1-year double-blind study period. Patients who failed to achieve Total Control by the end of Phase II entered a 4-week, open-label phase during which they received oral prednisolone (0.5 mg/kg up to 60 mg per day for 10 days) and FP/SAL 500/50 μg twice daily.

Study population

Only patients who did not demonstrate Well-Controlled asthma for at least 2 weeks of the 4-week run-in period were eligible for inclusion in GOAL (Additional file 2: Table S1). For this post hoc subgroup analysis, the Asian population was defined as patients of Chinese, Japanese, Korean, Thai, Malay or

Filipino origin living in South East Asia (China, Japan, Hong Kong, Malaysia, Philippines, Singapore, South Korea, Taiwan, Thailand) during the study. The non-Asian population included all patients in the intent-to-treat (ITT) population who were not in the Asian subgroup (full inclusion criteria of the GOAL study can be found in the Additional file 1).

Study endpoints

The primary endpoint of the GOAL study and of this post hoc subgroup analysis was the proportion of patients achieving Well-Controlled asthma with FP/SAL compared with FP alone during Phase I. The proportion of patients achieving Total Control of asthma was also evaluated. Asthma control was defined according to composite measures based on the GINA/NIH criteria developed for the GOAL study [3, 14], as shown in Additional file 2: Table S1. Well-Controlled asthma and Total Control of asthma were achieved if the patient recorded 7 out of 8 consecutive assessment weeks with Well-Controlled asthma or Total Control of asthma, respectively. Additional endpoints included: the ICS dose at which Well-Controlled asthma and Total Control of asthma was achieved; the cumulative probabilities from analysis of time to achieve the first week of Well-Controlled asthma and Total Control of asthma; the maintenance of Well-Controlled asthma and Total Control of asthma status from Phase I until the end of Phase II; the stability of weekly control during Phase II; rate of exacerbations (requiring oral corticosteroids, hospitalisations or emergency visits); and morning predose clinic forced expiratory volume in 1 s (FEV_1) and asthma quality of life (QoL) as assessed using the Asthma Quality of Life Questionnaire (AQLQ) [15]. The incidence of adverse events (AEs) was also monitored.

Calculation of the sample size

Sample size calculations were performed for the original GOAL study [3]; however, as the current analysis was post hoc, no further sample size calculations were required and therefore all analyses are descriptive only, including the calculated p-values.

Statistical analysis

The ITT population, defined as all patients who were randomised and received at least one dose of a study drug, was used for all analyses. Using data from a Caucasian-only subpopulation (comprising approximately 90% of the non-Asian patients in the GOAL study), the primary endpoint was analysed and found to have little difference compared with the overall non-Asian population, so data from the non-Asian population are presented here.

The statistical analysis of the proportion of patients who achieved Well-Controlled asthma and Total Control of asthma was performed using logistic regression with covariates for baseline FEV_1, sex, age and treatment group. The analysis of the ICS dose at which Well-Controlled asthma and Total Control of asthma was first achieved was performed using proportional odds logistic regression on dose with the same covariates. The effects of treatment on exacerbation rates were determined using Poisson regression with generalised estimating equations with the same covariates (treatment differences were expressed as the ratio of FP/SAL over FP, with treatment ratios greater than 1 in favour of FP/SAL). Time to achieve Well-Controlled asthma and Total Control of asthma was assessed using inverse Kaplan–Meier plots with Log-Rank tests. The statistical analysis of mean change in clinic FEV_1 (L) was performed using analysis of covariance with covariates for baseline FEV_1, sex, age and treatment group (treatment differences were expressed as a difference of FP/SAL from placebo in FEV_1 [L], with positive treatment differences in favour of FP/SAL).

Analyses were completed using SAS 9.3 (Cary, NC, USA).

Results

Study population

A total of 5,068 patients were screened and 3,421 qualified for inclusion in the primary study [3]. Of these patients, 652 Asian patients and 2,764 non-Asian patients were randomised and treated and therefore included in this post hoc subgroup analysis (Fig. 1).

The demographics and baseline characteristics of the two populations were generally similar across the different strata and treatment groups (Table 1). However, compared with the Asian patients, non-Asian patients had a numerically greater mean height, weight and percent predicted pre-FEV_1 (Table 1). Patient race is shown in Additional file 3: Table S2.

Achievement of guideline-defined asthma control

Overall control

In Phase I, the same percentage of Asian patients in stratum 1 achieved Well-Controlled asthma with FP/SAL (74% [87/118]) and with FP alone (74% [89/121]) (odds ratio [OR]: 0.94; 95% confidence interval [95% CI]: 0.52, 1.70; $p = 0.839$). More Asian patients in stratum 2 and stratum 3 achieved Well-Controlled asthma with FP/SAL than with FP alone (stratum 2: 76% [81/107] vs 60% [62/104], respectively [OR: 2.44; 95% CI: 1.31, 4.56; $p = 0.005$]; stratum 3: 58% [59/102] vs 43% [41/95], respectively [OR: 2.08; 95% CI: 1.15, 3.76; $p = 0.015$]). For the non-Asian population, more patients in all three strata achieved Well-Controlled asthma with FP/SAL than with FP alone (stratum 1: 70% [296/421] vs 63%

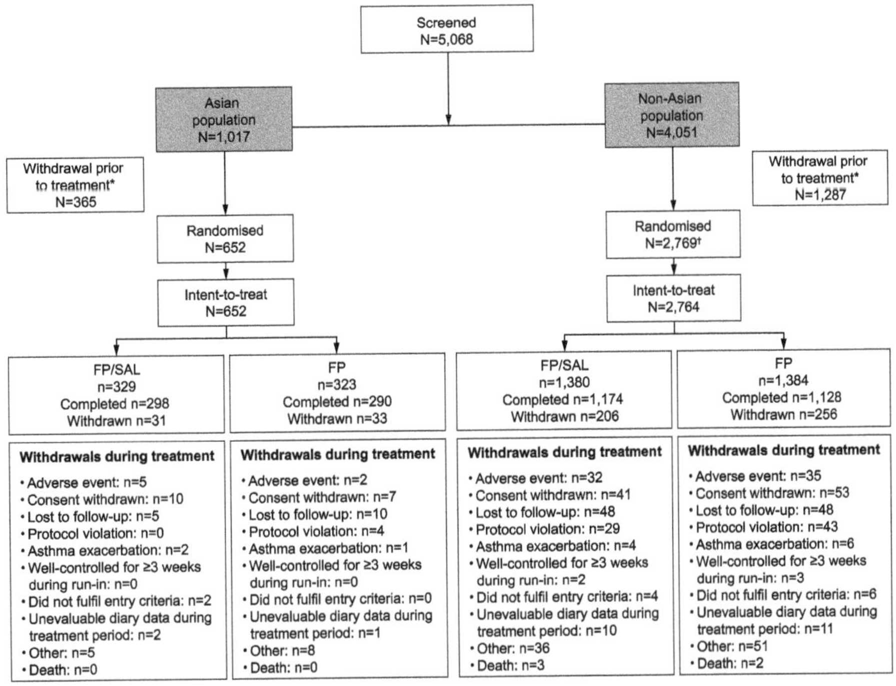

Fig. 1 Patient disposition. *Includes those who were classified as screen or run-in failures; †includes five patients who were excluded from the intent-to-treat population as they did not take a dose of the study drug. *FP* fluticasone propionate, *SAL* salmeterol

[267/423], respectively [OR: 1.41; 95% CI: 1.06, 1.88; $p = 0.020$]; stratum 2: 67% [319/476] vs 51% [240/473] [OR: 2.00; 95% CI: 1.53, 2.61; $p < 0.001$]; stratum 3: 49% [229/466] vs 31% [147/472] [OR: 2.19; 95% CI: 1.68, 2.87; $p < 0.001$]).

In Phase I, more patients in all three strata achieved Total Control of asthma with FP/SAL compared with FP alone in both the Asian and non-Asian populations. In Asian patients in stratum 1, Total Control was achieved in 42% (49/118) of patients with FP/SAL and 28% (34/121) with FP (OR: 1.77; 95% CI: 1.02, 3.08; $p = 0.043$), in stratum 2 this was achieved in 36% (39/107) versus 25% (26/104), respectively (OR: 1.86; 95% CI: 1.00, 3.43; $p = 0.049$), and in stratum 3 this was achieved in 26% (27/102) versus 6% (6/95), respectively (OR: 7.16; 95% CI: 2.65, 19.35; $p < 0.001$). In non-Asian patients in stratum 1, Total Control was achieved in 42% (176/421) of patients with FP/SAL and 32% (135/423) with FP (OR: 1.56; 95% CI: 1.18, 2.07; $p = 0.002$), in stratum 2 this was achieved in 32% (150/476) versus 19% (88/473), respectively (OR: 1.99; 95% CI: 1.47, 2.70; $p < 0.001$), and in stratum 3 this was achieved in 17% (79/466) versus 8% (37/472), respectively (OR: 2.42; 95% CI: 1.60, 3.67; $p < 0.001$).

ICS dose at which control was achieved

The study also evaluated control according to the ICS dose received. The proportion of Asian patients achieving Well-Controlled asthma and Total Control of asthma was higher with FP/SAL than with FP alone, when FP/SAL was administered at an ICS dose that was the same or lower than the ICS dose with FP alone (Fig. 2).

More patients (in stratum 1 and stratum 2) achieved Well-Controlled asthma using FP/SAL than FP alone in the Asian population receiving the lowest dose of ICS (FP 100 μg) in Phase I (Fig. 2a). Findings in the non-Asian population were similar (Fig. 2a). In the Asian population, the odds of achieving Well-Controlled asthma at the same or lower dose of ICS for FP/SAL versus FP alone in stratum 1 increased by 47% (OR: 1.47; 95% CI: 0.91, 2.38; $p = 0.119$) and more than doubled in stratum 2 (OR: 2.78; 95% CI: 1.64, 4.71; $p < 0.001$) and stratum 3 (OR: 2.38; 95% CI: 1.36, 4.14; $p = 0.002$). Findings of analyses by dose at which control was achieved in the non-Asian population were similar; the use of FP/SAL increased the odds of achieving Well-Controlled asthma compared with FP alone in stratum 1 (OR: 1.37; 95% CI: 1.07, 1.76; $p = 0.014$), stratum 2 (OR: 2.04; 95% CI: 1.61, 2.59; $p < 0.001$), and stratum 3 (OR: 2.20; 95% CI: 1.69, 2.85; $p < 0.001$).

Again, in the Asian population, when analysed by ICS dose at which control was achieved, Total Control of asthma was achieved by a greater proportion of patients using FP/SAL than FP alone (Fig. 2b). The use of FP/SAL increased the odds of achieving Total Control compared with FP alone (by ICS dose) in stratum 1 (OR: 1.66; 95% CI: 0.97, 2.84; $p = 0.062$), stratum 2 (OR: 1.90; 95% CI: 1.05, 3.46; $p = 0.035$), and stratum 3 (OR: 7.39;

Table 1 Patient demographics and baseline characteristics (ITT population)

	Asian population						Non-Asian population					
	S1		S2		S3		S1		S2		S3	
	FP/SAL	FP	FP/SAL	FP	FP/SAL	FP	FP/SAL	FP	FP/SAL	FP	FP/SAL	FP
	n = 120	n = 122	n = 107	n = 104	n = 102	n = 97	n = 428	n = 428	n = 478	n = 474	n = 474	n = 482
Age, mean (SD), years[a]	37.2 (14.4)	39.1 (14.4)	41.9 (15.4)	41.4 (13.5)	45.8 (14.3)	43.1 (12.4)	35.8 (16.0)	35.6 (15.8)	40.0 (16.6)	40.1 (17.2)	43.7 (16.2)	42.6 (16.3)
Female, n (%)[a]	67 (56)	75 (61)	62 (58)	61 (59)	53 (52)	63 (65)	245 (57)	241 (56)	278 (58)	288 (61)	276 (58)	279 (58)
Height, mean (SD), cm[a]	161.9 (9.5)	158.6 (8.8)	161.3 (8.9)	162.7 (8.8)	161.6 (9.5)	161.3 (7.9)	167.8 (9.8)	167.7 (10.1)	166.5 (10.2)	166.5 (10.2)	167.1 (10.1)	166.6 (10.3)
Weight, mean (SD), kg[a]	60.8 (12.9)	58.6 (11.7)	61.5 (11.3)	61.8 (11.1)	63.2 (14.0)	61.7 (10.6)	72.4 (17.6)	71.8 (17.9)	72.6 (16.7)	72.7 (17.9)	74.5 (16.5)	73.4 (16.4)
BMI, mean (SD)[a]	23.15 (4.57)	23.25 (3.94)	23.59 (3.69)	23.28 (3.41)	24.07 (4.33)	23.68 (3.37)	25.63 (5.72)	25.41 (5.73)	26.16 (5.52)	26.10 (5.56)	26.59 (5.09)	26.53 (5.46)
Mean FEV_1 at visit 2 (SD), L[b]	2.08 (0.69) *n = 118*	1.92 (0.68) *n = 121*	1.91 (0.64) *n = 107*	1.97 (0.58) *n = 104*	1.93 (0.75) *n = 102*	2.04 (0.68) *n = 95*	2.61 (0.88) *n = 421*	2.69 (0.82) *n = 423*	2.53 (0.82) *n = 476*	2.46 (0.82) *n = 473*	2.36 (0.81) *n = 466*	2.38 (0.79) *n = 472*
Mean % predicted[c] FEV_1 at visit 2 (SD), %[b]	68.6 (16.6) *n = 118*	67.6 (17.0) *n = 121*	66.7 (16.8) *n = 107*	67.0 (15.6) *n = 104*	67.3 (17.1) *n = 102*	71.1 (16.8) *n = 95*	78.8 (18.6) *n = 421*	81.8 (18.0) *n = 423*	80.4 (17.6) *n = 476*	79.3 (18.2) *n = 473*	76.2 (18.6) *n = 466*	77.1 (17.6) *n = 472*
Median pre-randomisation reversibility, (min., max.), %	21.4 (10.5, 95.2) *n = 91*	20.0 (9.0, 112.5) *n = 98*	25.0 (2.7, 124.7) *n = 87*	24.0 (11.1, 78.9) *n = 80*	25.3 (4.2, 92.0) *n = 63*	20.2 (8.3, 68.6) *n = 67*	23.8 (1.0, 95.7) *n = 318*	22.0 (2.5, 97.0) *n = 324*	21.4 (−0.6, 123.6) *n = 346*	21.6 (3.7, 111.5) *n = 346*	22.2 (−0.4, 115.3) *n = 356*	21.9 (3.1, 224.0) *n = 366*
Mean am PEF (SD), L/min	310.5 (76.3) *n = 120*	299.0 (72.7) *n = 122*	312.3 (92.3) *n = 107*	311.0 (70.9) *n = 104*	320.1 (84.2) *n = 102*	327.9 (90.5) *n = 97*	353.8 (92.9) *n = 427*	358.4 (93.8) *n = 427*	356.9 (98.0) *n = 478*	350.7 (96.5) *n = 474*	350.4 (100.8) *n = 473*	352.5 (97.0) *n = 482*
Mean % predicted[b] am PEF (SD), %	71.1 (14.1) *n = 120*	71.9 (14.4) *n = 122*	74.1 (18.4) *n = 107*	72.7 (15.9) *n = 104*	74.8 (14.4) *n = 102*	77.5 (17.2) *n = 97*	76.9 (14.5) *n = 427*	77.9 (14.1) *n = 427*	79.4 (15.3) *n = 478*	79.3 (16.2) *n = 474*	78.4 (16.2) *n = 473*	79.2 (16.0) *n = 482*
Mean daily rescue usage, (SD)	1.9 (1.6) *n = 120*	1.7 (1.3) *n = 122*	1.7 (1.3) *n = 107*	1.5 (1.1) *n = 103*	1.5 (1.5) *n = 102*	1.6 (1.4) *n = 97*	2.0 (1.7) *n = 426*	1.8 (1.5) *n = 428*	1.8 (1.5) *n = 478*	1.8 (1.5) *n = 473*	2.0 (1.4) *n = 473*	2.0 (1.4) *n = 482*
Median night-time awakenings, (min., max.)	0.5 (0, 3) *n = 120*	0.5 (0, 3) *n = 122*	0.2 (0, 3) *n = 107*	0.2 (0, 2) *n = 104*	0.2 (0, 2) *n = 102*	0.3 (0, 4) *n = 95*	0.4 (0, 4) *n = 425*	0.3 (0, 4) *n = 427*	0.2 (0, 3) *n = 476*	0.2 (0, 3) *n = 471*	0.3 (0, 4) *n = 471*	0.2 (0, 3) *n = 479*
Mean asthma symptom score, (SD)	1.9 (0.8) *n = 120*	1.7 (0.8) *n = 121*	1.7 (0.9) *n = 107*	1.6 (0.8) *n = 104*	1.6 (0.9) *n = 102*	1.8 (1.0) *n = 97*	1.8 (0.8) *n = 427*	1.7 (0.9) *n = 428*	1.8 (0.9) *n = 478*	1.8 (0.9) *n = 473*	2.0 (0.9) *n = 472*	1.9 (0.9) *n = 482*
Patients with atopy, n (%)[a]	54 (45)	46 (38)	54 (50)	59 (57)	62 (61)	46 (47)	259 (61)	253 (59)	298 (62)	278 (59)	300 (63)	290 (60)
Patients with unknown atopy, n (%)[a]	8 (7)	10 (8)	13 (12)	9 (9)	18 (18)	10 (10)	46 (11)	34 (8)	31 (6)	25 (5)	32 (7)	30 (6)

am morning, *BMI* body mass index, *FEV_1* forced expiratory volume in 1 s, *FP* fluticasone propionate, *FP/SAL* fluticasone propionate/salmeterol, *ICS* inhaled corticosteroids, *ITT* intent-to-treat, *max.* maximum, *min.* minimum, *PEF* peak expiratory flow, *S1* patients who were ICS naïve at study entry, *S2* patients who received low-dose ICS treatment prior to study entry, *S3* patients who received medium-dose ICS treatment prior to study entry, *SD* standard deviation

[a]Number of patients with data to analyse for this variable as in the column heading, apart from weight and BMI in the non-Asian/S2/FP cells, where *n* = 473 (italicised *n* = in other rows are the number of patients with data available for analysis in this variable); [b]pre-bronchodilator; [c]predicted values calculated from European Community for Coal and Steel (ECCS) values

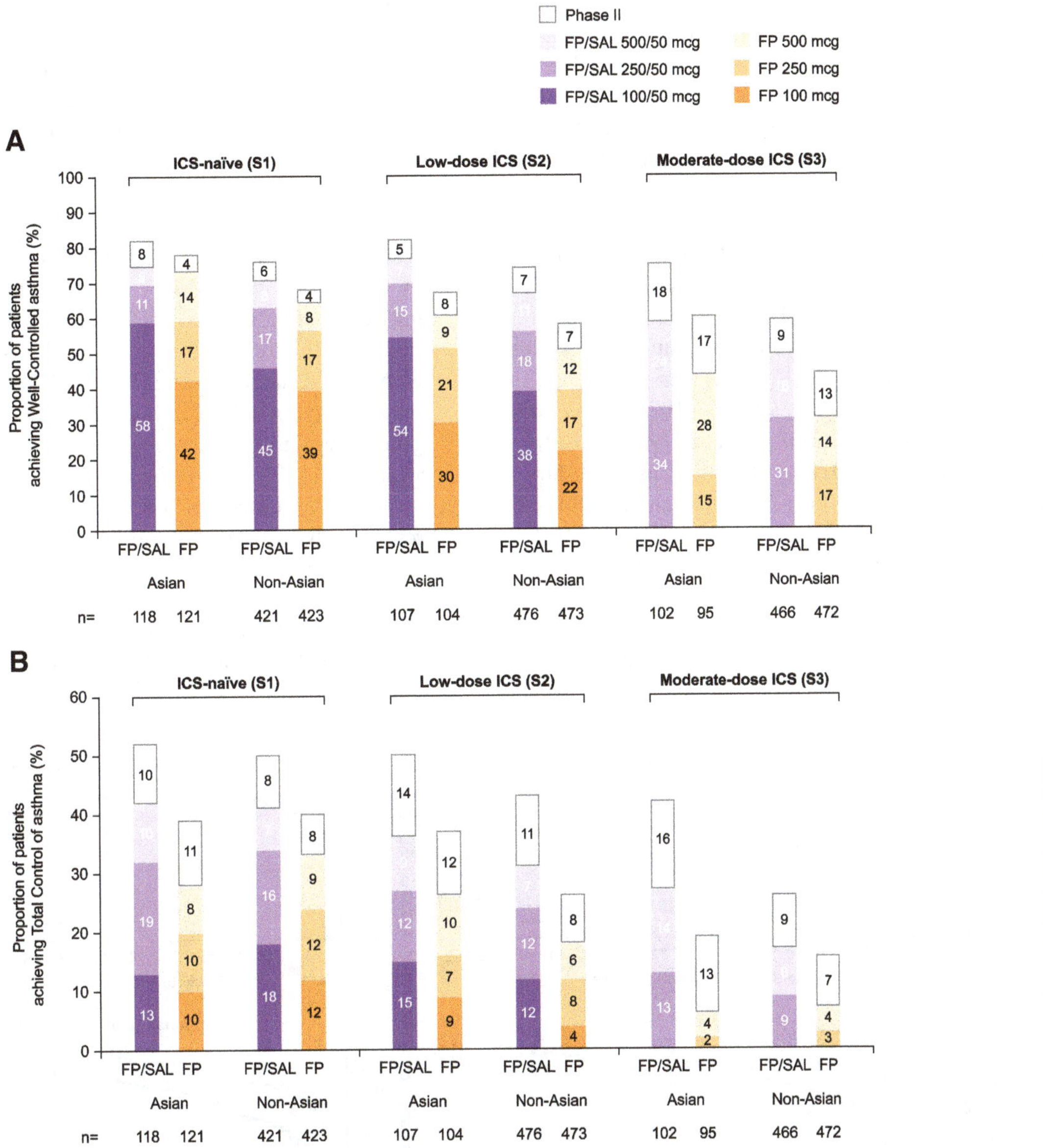

Fig. 2 Proportion of patients who achieved Well-Controlled* (**a**) and Total-Control of* (**b**) asthma. *Phase I data are presented by dose and Phase II data are overall proportions only. *FP* fluticasone propionate, *ICS* inhaled corticosteroid, *S1* patients who were ICS naïve at study entry, *S2* patients who received low-dose ICS treatment prior to study entry, *S3* patients who received medium-dose ICS treatment prior to study entry, *SAL* salmeterol

95% CI: 2.74, 19.92; $p < 0.001$). Findings in the non-Asian population were similar; the use of FP/SAL increased the odds of achieving Total Control compared with FP alone in stratum 1 (OR: 1.61; 95% CI: 1.22, 2.12; $p < 0.001$), stratum 2 (OR: 2.06; 95% CI: 1.53, 2.78; $p < 0.001$), and stratum 3 (OR: 2.46; 95% CI: 1.62, 3.72; $p < 0.001$).

Control in Phase II

During Phase II of the study, in which patients received a constant dose of medication, additional patients achieved Well-Controlled asthma and Total Control of asthma. The overall proportion of Asian patients achieving Well-Controlled asthma at the end of Phase II was higher with FP/SAL compared with FP alone: 82% (97/118) and 78% (94/121) in stratum 1, 80% (86/107) and 67% (70/104) in stratum 2, and 75% (77/102) and 60% (57/95) in stratum 3 (Fig. 2a). Corresponding values for Total Control of asthma with FP/SAL and FP, respectively, were 52% (61/118) and 39% (47/121) in stratum 1, 50% (54/107) and 37% (38/104) in stratum 2, and 42% (43/102) and 19% (18/95) in stratum 3 (Fig. 2b). A higher proportion of non-Asian patients also achieved control at the end of Phase II with FP/SAL versus FP alone (Fig. 2a and b).

Analysis of time to control

Analysis of time to control, defined as the time to achieve the first week of Well-Controlled asthma or the first week of Total Control, showed that patients in all groups achieved control more rapidly with FP/SAL than with FP alone, and the cumulative probability of achieving control by Week 52 was greater with FP/SAL than with FP alone (Fig. 3 and Fig. 4).

The cumulative probability of achieving the first week of Well-Controlled asthma by Week 52 with FP/SAL and FP alone, respectively, was 97% (n/N, where N = subgroup total, not the censored value used within the Kaplan–Meier analysis: 115/120) versus 92% (110/122) ($p = 0.064$) for stratum 1, 94% (98/107) versus 90% (92/104) ($p = 0.018$) for stratum 2, and 95% (96/102) versus 85% (79/97) ($p = 0.002$) for stratum 3 in the Asian population (Fig. 3). In the non-Asian population, corresponding values were 95% (392/428) versus 89% (361/428) ($p < 0.001$) for stratum 1, 91% (422/478) versus 87% (393/474) ($p < 0.001$) for stratum 2, and 84% (386/474) versus 77% (349/482) ($p < 0.001$) for stratum 3 (Fig. 3). The time point by which the cumulative probability reached 0.5 in the Asian population for Well-Controlled asthma was 1.3 weeks with FP/SAL versus 3.3 weeks with FP alone in stratum 1, 1.3 weeks versus 3.3 weeks in stratum 2, and 1.8 weeks versus 5.3 weeks in stratum 3. In the non-Asian population, corresponding values were 2.3 weeks versus 3.3 weeks in stratum 1, 1.3 weeks versus 7.3 weeks in stratum 2, and 4.3 weeks versus 10.3 weeks in stratum 3.

For Total Control of asthma, the cumulative probability of patients in the Asian stratum 1 population achieving their first week of control by Week 52 was numerically greater for the FP/SAL group compared with the FP alone group (68% [80/120] vs 58% [69/122], respectively, $p = 0.075$). It was higher in the FP/SAL group than the FP alone group for Asian patients in stratum 2 (71% [73/107] vs 55% [56/104], respectively, $p = 0.024$) and stratum 3 (65% [65/102] vs 47% [43/97], respectively, $p = 0.014$), and in all three strata in non-Asian patients (stratum 1: 77% [311/428] vs 67% [261/428], $p < 0.001$; stratum 2: 69% [311/478] vs 53% [232/474], $p < 0.001$; stratum 3: 55% [247/474] vs 43% [187/482]; $p < 0.001$) (Fig. 4). The time point by which the

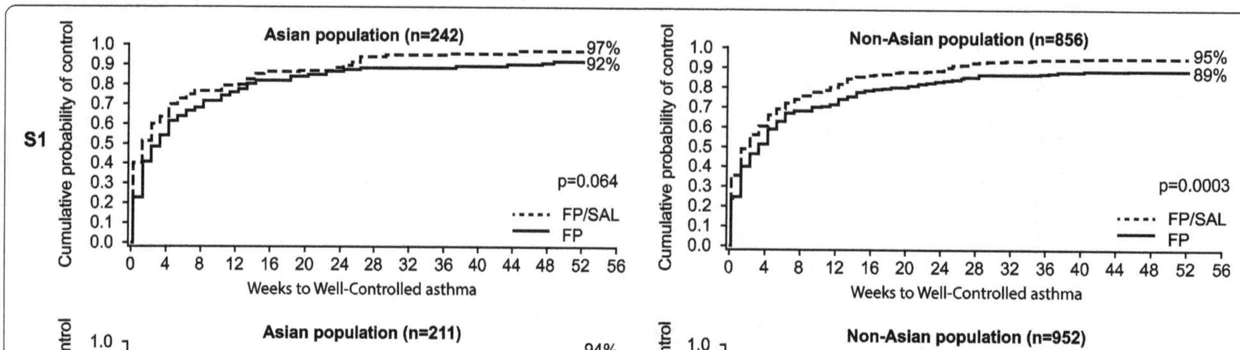

Fig. 3 Time to achieve Well-Controlled asthma in Asian and non-Asian patients (S1, S2 and S3), *FP* fluticasone propionate, *ICS* inhaled corticosteroids, *S1* patients who were ICS naïve at study entry, *S2* patients who received low-dose ICS treatment prior to study entry, *S3* patients who received medium-dose ICS treatment prior to study entry, *SAL* salmeterol

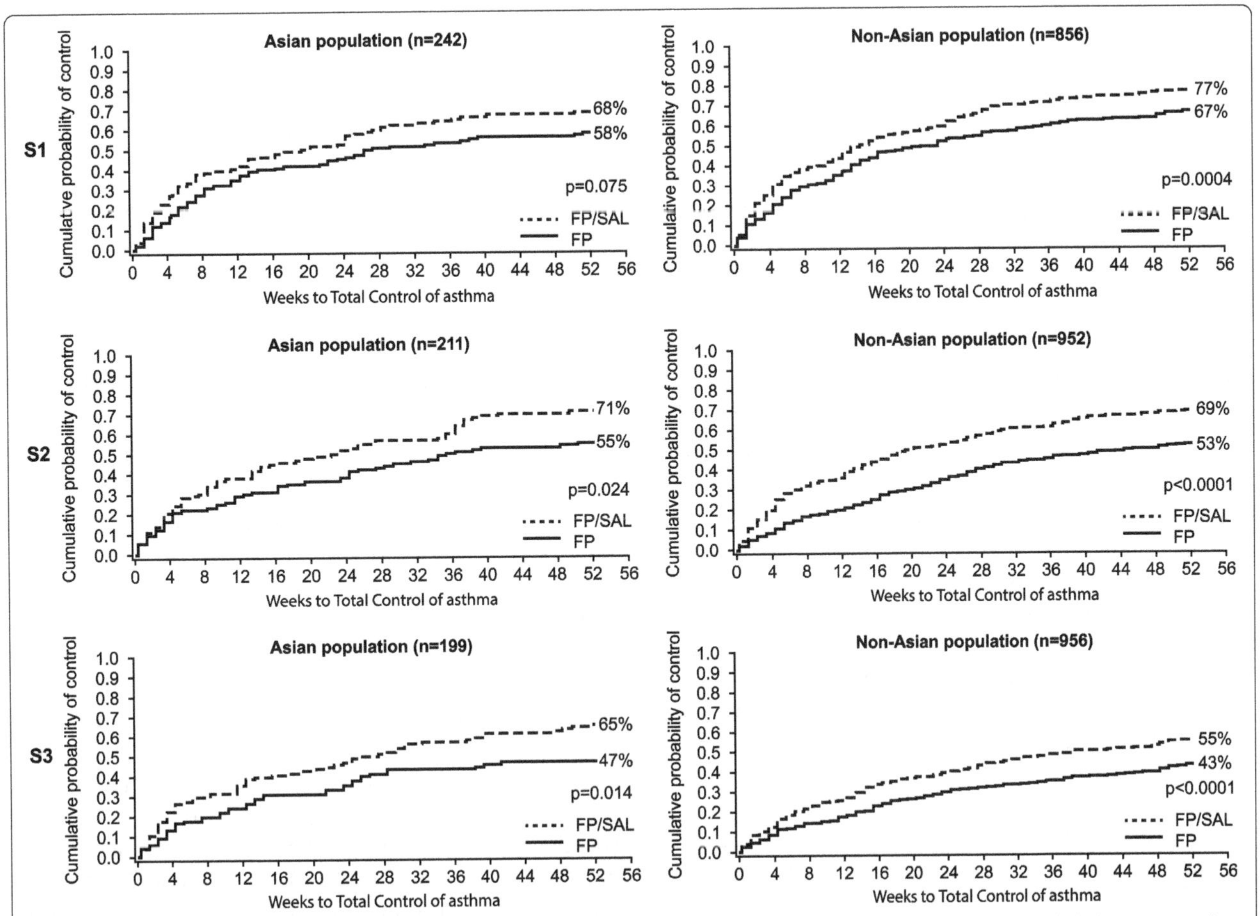

Fig. 4 Time to achieve Total-Control of asthma in Asian and non-Asian patients (S1, S2 and S3). *FP* fluticasone propionate, *ICS* inhaled corticosteroids, *S1* patients who were ICS naïve at study entry, *S2* patients who received low-dose ICS treatment prior to study entry, *S3* patients who received medium-dose ICS treatment prior to study entry, *SAL* salmeterol

cumulative probability reached 0.5 in the Asian population for Total Control of asthma was 19.3 weeks with FP/SAL versus 26.3 weeks with FP alone in stratum 1, and 23.3 weeks versus 35.3 weeks in stratum 2. In stratum 3, the first time point of control was achieved by 27.3 weeks with FP/SAL but was not reached with FP. In the non-Asian population, corresponding values were 14.3 weeks versus 23.3 weeks in stratum 1, 20.3 weeks versus 45.3 weeks in stratum 2, and 38.3 weeks versus not reached in stratum 3.

Stability of control

In the Asian population, the majority of patients who achieved Well-Controlled asthma or Total Control of asthma during Phase I (based on an 8-week assessment period) maintained control each week during Phase II (Fig. 5).

In stratum 1, of patients receiving FP/SAL who achieved Well-Controlled asthma during Phase 1 (8-week assessment period), 83% (72/87) had maintained control at the end of Phase II (8-week assessment period) compared with 80% (71/89) receiving FP alone. Corresponding values were 78% (63/81) and 82% (51/62) in stratum 2, and 86% (51/59) and 73% (30/41) in stratum 3 for FP/SAL and FP alone, respectively. For Total Control of asthma, the proportion of patients in the Asian population maintaining control during Phase II with FP/SAL and FP, respectively, were 73% (36/49) and 74% (25/34) in stratum 1, 64% (25/39) and 73% (19/26) in stratum 2, and 78% (21/27) and 83% (5/6) in stratum 3. In the non-Asian population, corresponding values for Well-Controlled asthma were 78% (232/296) and 76% (203/267) in stratum 1, 84% (269/319) and 73% (175/240) in stratum 2, and 75% (172/229) and 78% (115/147) in stratum 3. For Total Control of asthma in the non-Asian population, the proportion maintaining control with FP/SAL and FP, respectively, were 68% (119/176) and 74% (100/135) in stratum 1, 71% (107/150) and 59% (52/88) in stratum 2, and 67% (53/79) and 73% (27/37) in stratum 3. In the Asian population, for patients who did not achieve Well-Controlled asthma or Total Control of asthma in Phase I, a greater proportion of patients using FP/SAL compared with FP gained control in Phase II.

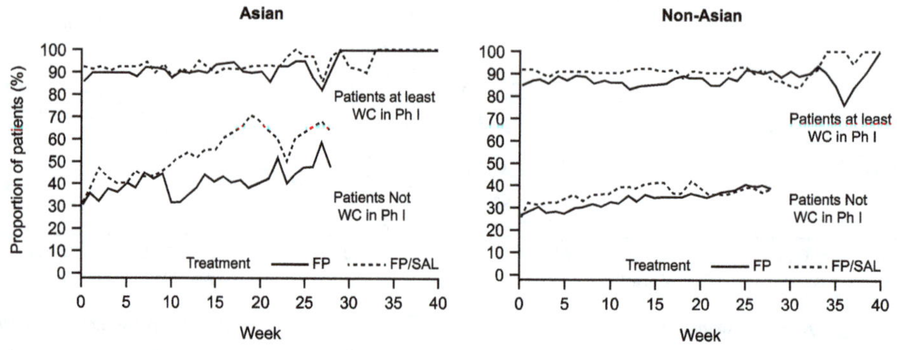

Fig. 5 Proportion of patients who achieved at least one week of Well-Controlled asthma during Phase II. Data pooled across all strata within a treatment. This analysis included Phase II treatment only (up to 40 weeks) and control was assessed at each individual week after Phase I. Phase I control status was based on an 8-week assessment period. *FP* fluticasone propionate, *Ph I* Phase I, *SAL* salmeterol, *WC* well controlled

Effects of treatments on exacerbations

As the number of exacerbations reported in the study was low, data were combined across all strata for this analysis. In the Asian population, the incidence of exacerbations over 52 weeks was 0.19 for FP/SAL ($n = 327$) and 0.24 for FP ($n = 320$); rate ratio 0.792 (95% CI: 0.508, 1.236) (Fig. 6). In the non-Asian population, the incidence of exacerbations was 0.12 for FP/SAL ($n = 1363$) and 0.18 for FP ($n = 1,368$); rate ratio 0.668 (95% CI: 0.529, 0.844) (Fig. 6).

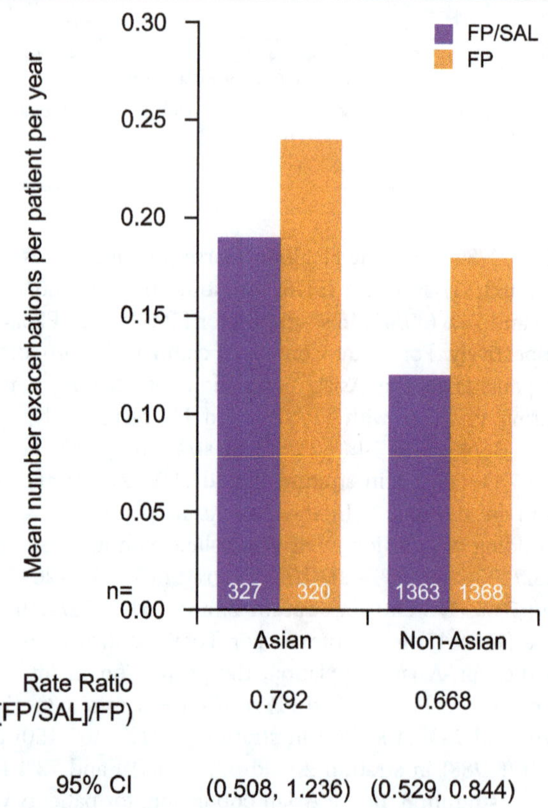

Fig. 6 Incidence of exacerbations over 52 weeks. *CI* confidence interval, *FP* fluticasone propionate, *FP/SAL* fluticasone propionate/salmeterol, *ICS* inhaled corticosteroids

Lung function (FEV_1)

At Week 52, the change in FEV_1 was greater with FP/SAL than with FP alone in both the Asian and non-Asian populations: the difference between treatments (FP/SAL minus FP) in adjusted mean change from baseline was 0.22 (95% CI: 0.11, 0.33) in stratum 1, 0.07 (−0.04, 0.18) in stratum 2, and 0.15 (0.04, 0.26) in stratum 3 for the Asian population, and 0.16 (0.10, 0.22) in stratum 1, 0.15 (0.09, 0.20) in stratum 2, and 0.15 (0.09, 0.20) in stratum 3 for the non-Asian population (Additional file 4: Figure S1).

Asthma QoL

Analysis of AQLQ scores by stratum was limited by few patients completing the questionnaire (in the Asian population, 121 patients treated with FP/SAL and 123 patients with FP alone; in the non-Asian population, 689 patients and 650 patients, respectively, completed the questionnaire); pooled data were therefore analysed. AQLQ scores improved with both FP/SAL and FP alone from baseline to Week 52, in both the Asian and non-Asian populations (Additional file 5: Figure S2).

Incidence of AEs

The overall incidence of AEs was similar in both treatment groups in both populations. In the Asian population, 192 out of 329 (58%) patients experienced AEs with FP/SAL and 185 out of 323 (57%) with FP alone (Additional file 6: Table S3). Corresponding values in the non-Asian population were 859 out of 1,380 (62%) with FP/SAL and 847 out of 1,384 (61%) with FP alone. The most common AEs reported in both treatment groups were upper respiratory tract infections (in 29–31% of the Asian population, and 9% of the non-Asian population) and nasopharyngitis (in 7–9% of the Asian population, and 14–15% of the non-Asian population) (Additional file 6: Table S3).

Discussion

This analysis indicated that guideline-defined control can be achieved and maintained in the majority of Asian patients with uncontrolled asthma across a range of severities. More patients in the strata previously receiving a low or medium dose of ICS (stratum 2 + stratum 3) achieved control with FP/SAL compared with FP alone, and did so more quickly and with a lower dose of ICS. For the stratum of patients who were uncontrolled on SABA-only treatment at study entry (stratum 1), there was no difference between the treatments for the primary endpoint of Well-Controlled asthma during the dose-escalation phase. However, there was an advantage for FP/SAL compared with FP alone for Total Control of asthma. This difference could be because Well-Controlled asthma is easier to achieve than Total Control, so treatment differences between FP and FP/SAL are more clearly visible when examining achievement of Total Control; however, the Asian population, although sizeable in this analysis, was too small to examine this observation further. Despite this, a high proportion of patients receiving SABA-only at entry did achieve control. This was accompanied by a noticeable improvement in lung function (0.22 L), as measured by FEV_1, over the 52 weeks.

During the maintenance phase, additional patients in the Asian population achieved control for both study measures of control compared with the dose-escalation phase. Furthermore, control during the maintenance phase was relatively stable. This benefit of sustained treatment was larger for Total Control than for Well-Controlled asthma across all strata and may reflect additional time required to improve airway inflammation in patients with asthma. Sustained treatment has previously been shown to improve airway hyper-responsiveness over 3 years [16], and it is established that airway hyper-responsiveness is associated with inflammatory markers, such as eosinophilia, in symptomatic patients [17].

As was observed in the total GOAL study population [3], maintaining treatment also had a clear benefit on health status in both the Asian and non-Asian populations studied in this analysis. Insufficient patients in each stratum of the Asian population completed the AQLQ to allow a by-stratum analysis, therefore, the AQLQ data were analysed across in the entire dataset (244 Asian patients in total). The analysis showed that Asian patients experienced a substantial improvement in health status such that the AQLQ score approached or exceeded the value of 6, suggesting that asthma no longer had a significant impact on QoL [18].

The incidence of exacerbations in the Asian patients was low and in keeping with the total study population as previously reported [3]. There was a significant improvement in FEV_1 for stratum 1 and stratum 3 (0.22 and 0.15 L, respectively), values very similar to those seen in the non-Asian population. The treatment difference for patients in stratum 2 was only 0.07 L.

The findings of the current analysis are in agreement with other studies exploring the efficacy of ICS/LABA combinations in improving asthma control in Asian patients. Although the multinational COSMOS study (1-year, randomised, parallel-group study investigating budesonide/formoterol vs FP/SAL) was conducted in a population that differed from the GOAL population (it included patients with a history of asthma exacerbations in the year prior to entry), a post hoc analysis of the COSMOS Asian population also demonstrated improved asthma control over a 1-year period with two ICS/LABA combinations [5]. Compared with baseline, both combinations provided clinically relevant improvements in asthma control (assessed using the five-item version of the Asthma Control Questionnaire [ACQ]), QoL (assessed using the AQLQ) and FEV_1 [5]. It should be noted, however, that the ACQ measured asthma control over a recall period of only 7 days, whereas control in the GOAL study was measured over 8-week periods. In another study, the efficacy of a different ICS/LABA combination (fluticasone furoate/vilanterol) was compared with that of FP alone in Asian patients in a 12-week, randomised trial [19]. This ICS/LABA combination provided significantly greater improvements in peak expiratory flow (PEF) compared with FP alone [19]. In a study in Korean patients treated with FP/SAL, the number of patients with Well-Controlled asthma, assessed by the AQLQ and the Asthma Control Test, increased from baseline and was accompanied by a clinically relevant improvement in QoL [20].

Although this is a post hoc analysis of a subgroup of patients from the original, much larger, population [3], it is reassuring to see that existing and well-established treatments are as effective in Asian patients as in a wider group of patients at achieving and maintaining comprehensive control of asthma, and that this is accompanied by additional outcome benefits.

Safety findings from the present analysis were also similar with the findings from the other studies, with the most common AEs reported with ICS/LABA combinations or ICS alone being upper respiratory tract infection (URTI) and nasopharyngitis [5, 19, 20]. A substantial difference was noted between Asian and non-Asian patients in the incidence of these AEs: ~30% of Asian patients experienced URTI compared with only 9% of non-Asian patients, whilst fewer Asian patients (8%) experienced nasopharyngitis than non-Asian patients (14%). Differences in patterns of antibiotic prescription in Asian and non-Asian countries may explain the difference in the incidence of URTI between the two populations, but could not account for the discrepancy in nasopharyngitis. An alternative explanation may simply be that different terms are used in the different countries included within the populations to describe the same symptoms.

This analysis suggests that, in Asian patients, baseline lung function may not be an accurate predictor of future asthma control. While asthma severity is related to FEV_1 [21] and ethnic differences in lung function (including FEV_1) have also been reported [10, 11], it is unclear how these different factors are linked. Lung function also varies with gender and age [11, 22], and so further research into the factors determining severity and differences in baseline physiology in Asians compared with non-Asians is required.

Strengths of this study included the large number of Asian patients within the analyses and the use of the guideline-defined composite endpoints of asthma control. A number of limitations should be taken into account when considering these findings. This was a post hoc subgroup analysis and was not designed to analyse treatment differences in asthma control within and between the Asian and non-Asian populations. The Asian subgroup population was also much smaller (N = 652) than the non-Asian subgroup population (N = 2,764), and, therefore, within and between subgroup comparisons must be interpreted with caution. This difference in sample size may have impacted some of the results. For example, in Asian patients who were ICS-naïve at baseline, there was no difference between FP/SAL and FP alone with regard to the proportion achieving Well-Controlled asthma, but a benefit of FP/SAL over FP alone was observed in this group for Total Control of asthma. In the corresponding group of non-Asian patients, a benefit for FP/SAL was seen for both endpoints. Patient numbers were too small to enable analyses by stratum for some outcomes (i.e. AQLQ); only pooled data were presented for these parameters. Although this Asian subgroup is one of the largest populations studied with regard to a composite score of asthma control, it was not large enough to conduct a by-stratum analysis of exacerbations, an important outcome for patients with asthma. Finally, the Asian patient population included in this analysis was heterogeneous as it included patients from several countries. This may limit generalisability to more homogeneous, single country populations.

Conclusions

The results of the GOAL study in Asian patients reflected those seen in the overall population [3]. In addition, the present analysis demonstrated similar trends in Asian compared with non-Asian patients. The post hoc subgroup analyses showed that guideline-defined asthma control, measured by a composite of clinically relevant endpoints, can be achieved and maintained with the combination of FP/SAL in a substantial proportion of Asian patients. Overall, FP/SAL was more effective at a lower dose of ICS than FP alone in achieving control and achieved control more quickly than FP alone.

Additional files

Additional file 1: Supplementary materials. Study oversight and study population.

Additional file 2: Table S1. Definitions of Total Control of asthma and Well-Controlled asthma, modified from the GINA/NIH Guidelines.

Additional file 3: Table S2. Patient race (ITT population).

Additional file 4: Figure S1. Lung function (FEV_1) at Phase II endpoint.

Additional file 5: Figure S2. Asthma quality of life questionnaire score (pooled data) in Asian and non-Asian patients, at baseline and after 52 weeks of treatment.

Additional file 6: Table S3. Summary of the most common adverse events (≥5%) in the Asian and non-Asian populations.

Abbreviations

ACQ: Asthma Control Questionnaire; AEs: Adverse events; AIRIAP: Asthma Insights and Reality in Asia-Pacific survey; am: Morning; AQLQ: Asthma Quality of Life Questionnaire; BMI: Body mass index; CI: Confidence interval; ECCS: European Community for Coal and Steel; FEV_1: Forced expiratory volume in 1 s; FP: Fluticasone propionate; GINA: Global Initiative for Asthma; GOAL: Gaining Optimal Asthma controL; ICS: Inhaled corticosteroid; ITT: Intent-to-treat; LABA: Long-acting β_2-agonist; max.: Maximum; min.: Minimum; NIH: National Institutes of Health; OR: Odds ratio; PEF: Peak expiratory flow; QoL: Quality of life; REALISE: REcognise Asthma and LInk to Symptoms and Experience study; S: Stratum; SABA: Short-acting β2-agonist; SAL: Salmeterol; SD: Standard deviation; URTI: Upper respiratory tract infection; WC: Well controlled

Acknowledgements

Editorial support (in the form of writing assistance, including development of the initial draft based on author input, assembling tables and figures, collating authors comments, grammatical editing and referencing) was provided by Gillian Groeger, PhD, of Fishawack Indicia Ltd, UK, and was funded by GlaxoSmithKline (GSK).

Funding

This study was funded by GSK (SAM40027). Employees of GSK were involved with the study design, data analysis and writing of the manuscript.

Authors' contributions

JB and WB contributed to the conception and design of the original GOAL study, and the data analysis and interpretation of these post hoc analyses. SAT and NB contributed to the data analysis and interpretation of these post hoc analyses. MG, NG, XZ, Y-JC, H-SP and NZ were involved in the acquisition of data and contributed to the data analysis and interpretation. MG, NB and NG also contributed to the conception and design of these post hoc analyses. All authors read and approved the final manuscript.

Competing interests

NB, MG, NG and SAT are employees of GSK and hold GSK stocks/shares.

JB reports personal fees from Almirall, AstraZeneca, Chiesi, GSK, Meda, Menarini, Merck, MSD, Novartis, Sanofi-Aventis, Takeda, Teva and Uriach, outside the submitted work.
WB reports personal fees from Novartis, GSK, Genentech, Roche, Pfizer, Merck, Boehringer Ingelheim, Sanofi, Gilead, Teva, Takeda, Aerocrine, Boston Scientific, personal fees from Circassia, ICON and AstraZeneca, outside the submitted work.
H-SP reports consultancy work with Novartis, clinical trial investigator for AstraZeneca, Sanofi-Aventis, GSK, Novartis, MSD and Mundipharma International.
Y-JC reports clinical trial investigator for AstraZeneca and Roche.
XZ and NZ declare no competing interests.

Consent for publication

Not applicable (no individual level patient data contained within this manuscript).

Author details

[1]Fondation MACVIA-LR, Contre les Maladies Chroniques pour un Vieillissement Actif en Languedoc-Roussillon, European Innovation Partnership on Active and Healthy Ageing Reference Site, University of Montpellier, Montpellier, France. [2]INSERM, VIMA: Ageing and Chronic Diseases, Epidemiological and Public Health Approaches, U1168, Paris, France. [3]UVSQ, UMR-S 1168, Université Versailles St-Quentin-en-Yvelines, Paris, France. [4]Global Respiratory Franchise, GSK House, Brentford, Middlesex, UK. [5]William Harvey Institute, Barts and the London School of Medicine and Dentistry, London, UK. [6]Quantitative Science, Clinical Statistics, GSK, Stockley Park, Middlesex, UK. [7]Shanghai First People's Hospital, Shanghai, China. [8]Ewha Womans University, School of Medicine, Seoul, South Korea. [9]Ajou University Medical Center, Suwon, South Korea. [10]University of Wisconsin, School of Medicine and Public Health, Madison, WI, USA. [11]State Key Laboratory of Respiratory Disease, Guangzhou Institute of Respiratory Disease, First Affiliated Hospital of Guangzhou Medical University, Guangzhou, China.

References

1. Global Initiative for Asthma (GINA). Global Strategy for Asthma Management and Prevention. 2016. Available from: http://www.ginasthma.org. Accessed 23 May 2016.
2. Pedersen S. From asthma severity to control: a shift in clinical practice. Prim Care Respir J. 2010;19:3–9.
3. Bateman ED, Boushey HA, Bousquet J, Busse WW, Clark TJ, Pauwels RA, et al. Can guideline-defined asthma control be achieved? The Gaining Optimal Asthma ControL study. Am J Respir Crit Care Med. 2004;170:836–44.
4. Liam CK, Pang YK, Chua KT. Satisfaction level and asthma control among Malaysian asthma patients on Symbicort Maintenance and Reliever Therapy (SMART) in the primary care setting (SMARTEST study). Asian Pac J Allergy Immunol. 2014;32:145–52.
5. Vogelmeier C, Naya I, Ekelund J. Budesonide/formoterol maintenance and reliever therapy in Asian patients (aged >/=16 years) with asthma: a sub-analysis of the COSMOS study. Clin Drug Investig. 2012;32:439–49.
6. Tan WC, Lamm CJ, Chen YZ, O'Byrne PM, Pedersen S, Busse WW, et al. Effectiveness of early budesonide intervention in Caucasian versus Asian patients with asthma: 3-year results of the START study. Respirology. 2006;11:767–75.
7. Lai CK, De Guia TS, Kim YY, Kuo SH, Mukhopadhyay A, Soriano JB, et al. Asthma control in the Asia-Pacific region: the asthma insights and reality in Asia-Pacific Study. J Allergy Clin Immunol. 2003;111:263–8.
8. Price D, David-Wang A, Cho SH, Ho JC, Jeong JW, Liam CK, et al. Time for a new language for asthma control: results from REALISE Asia. J Asthma Allergy. 2015;8:93–103.
9. Price D, Fletcher M, van der Molen T. Asthma control and management in 8,000 European patients: the REcognise Asthma and LInk to Symptoms and Experience (REALISE) survey. NPJ Prim Care Respir Med. 2014;24:14009.
10. Ching B, Horsfall PA. Lung volumes in normal Cantonese subjects: preliminary studies. Thorax. 1977;32:352–5.
11. Korotzer B, Ong S, Hansen JE. Ethnic differences in pulmonary function in healthy nonsmoking Asian-Americans and European-Americans. Am J Respir Crit Care Med. 2000;161:1101–8.
12. Oscherwitz M, Edlavitch SA, Baker TR, Jarboe T. Differences in pulmonary functions in various racial groups. Am J Epidemiol. 1972;96:319–27.
13. Seltzer CC, Siegelaub AB, Friedman GD, Collen MF. Differences in pulmonary function related to smoking habits and race. Am Rev Respir Dis. 1974;110: 598–608.
14. GINA/NIH. Global Strategy for Asthma Management and Prevention. 2002. Available from: http://www.ginasthma.org/local/uploads/files/GINAwr02.pdf. Accessed 22 Feb 2016.
15. Juniper EF, Guyatt GH, Epstein RS, Ferrie PJ, Jaeschke R, Hiller TK. Evaluation of impairment of health related quality of life in asthma: development of a questionnaire for use in clinical trials. Thorax. 1992;47:76–83.
16. Lundback B, Ronmark E, Lindberg A, Jonsson AC, Larsson LG, James M. Asthma control over 3 years in a real-life study. Respir Med. 2009;103:348–55.
17. Jansen DF, Rijcken B, Schouten JP, Kraan J, Weiss ST, Timens W, et al. The relationship of skin test positivity, high serum total IgE levels, and peripheral blood eosinophilia to symptomatic and asymptomatic airway hyperresponsiveness. Am J Respir Crit Care Med. 1999;159:924–31.
18. Bateman ED, Frith LF, Braunstein GL. Achieving guideline-based asthma control: does the patient benefit? Eur Respir J. 2002;20:588–95.
19. Lin J, Kang J, Lee SH, Wang C, Zhou X, Crawford J, et al. Fluticasone furoate/ vilanterol 200/25 mcg in Asian asthma patients: a randomized trial. Respir Med. 2015;109:44–53.
20. Jung KS, Uh ST, Lee YC, Shim JJ, Park SK, Williams AE, et al. Comparison of the clinical efficacy and safety of salmeterol/fluticasone propionate versus current care in the management of persistent asthma in Korea. Curr Med Res Opin. 2008;24:3571–82.
21. Haldar P, Pavord ID, Shaw DE, Berry MA, Thomas M, Brightling CE, et al. Cluster analysis and clinical asthma phenotypes. Am J Respir Crit Care Med. 2008;178:218–24.
22. McDonnell WF, Seal Jr E. Relationships between lung function and physical characteristics in young adult black and white males and females. Eur Respir J. 1991;4:279–89.

5

Arginase 1 deletion in myeloid cells affects the inflammatory response in allergic asthma, but not lung mechanics, in female mice

Roy H. E. Cloots[1], Selvakumari Sankaranarayanan[1], Matthew E. Poynter[3], Els Terwindt[1], Paul van Dijk[1], Wouter H. Lamers[1,2] and S. Eleonore Köhler[1*]

Abstract

Background: (Over-)expression of arginase may limit local availability of arginine for nitric oxide synthesis. We investigated the significance of arginase1 (ARG1) for the development of airway hyperresponsiveness (AHR) and lung inflammation in female mice with ovalbumin (OVA)-induced allergic asthma.

Methods: *Arg1* was ablated in the lung by crossing $Arg1^{fl/fl}$ and $Tie2Cre^{tg/-}$ mice. OVA sensitization and challenge were conducted, and AHR to methacholine was determined using the Flexivent system. Changes in gene expression, chemokine and cytokine secretion, plasma IgE, and lung histology were quantified using RT-qPCR, ELISA, and immunohistochemistry, respectively.

Results: *Arg1* ablation had no influence on the development of OVA-induced AHR, but attenuated OVA-induced increases in expression of *Arg2* and *Nos2, Slc7a1, Slc7a2,* and *Slc7a7* (arginine transporters), *Il4, Il5* and *Il13* (T_H2-type cytokines), *Ccl2* and *Ccl11* (chemokines), *Ifng* (T_H1-type cytokine), *Clca3* and *Muc5ac* (goblet cell markers), and OVA-specific IgE. Pulmonary IL-10 protein content increased, but IL-4, IL-5, IL-13, TNFα and IFNγ content, and lung histopathology, were not affected. *Arg1* elimination also decreased number and tightness of correlations between adaptive changes in lung function and inflammatory parameters in OVA/OVA-treated female mice. OVA/OVA-treated female mice mounted a higher OVA-IgE response than males, but the correlation between lung function and inflammation was lower. *Arg1*-deficient OVA/OVA-treated females differed from males in a more pronounced decline of arginine-metabolizing and -transporting genes, higher plasma arginine levels, a smaller OVA-specific IgE response, and no improvement of peripheral lung function.

Conclusion: Complete ablation of *Arg1* in the lung affects mRNA abundance of arginine-transporting and -metabolizing genes, and pro-inflammatory genes, but not methacholine responsiveness or accumulation of inflammatory cells.

Keywords: Arginase1, Airway hyperresponsiveness, Inflammation

* Correspondence: leo.koehler@maastrichtuniversity.nl
[1]Department of Anatomy & Embryology and NUTRIM School of Nutrition and Translational Research in Metabolism, Maastricht University, P.O. Box 616, 6200, MD, Maastricht, The Netherlands
Full list of author information is available at the end of the article

Background

Allergic asthma is a prevalent disease characterized by airway inflammation, hyperresponsiveness, and eventually remodeling. Development of allergic asthma starts upon binding of inhaled allergens to their complementary IgEs, which activates IgE receptor-bearing mast cells and basophils. These cells, in turn, activate an inflammatory cascade that causes lung infiltration with eosinophils, neutrophils, alternatively activated (M2) macrophages and (T_H2) lymphocytes. The inflammatory response is typically accompanied by mucus production, mucosal edema, and smooth-muscle hyperresponsiveness, which all contribute to the development of airway hyperresponsiveness (AHR) upon exposure to e.g. histamine and methacholine [1, 2]. Repeated episodes of allergic inflammation eventually lead to fibrosis and wall thickening in large and small airways ("airway remodeling").

Adult women suffer more often and more severely from asthma than men do (for a recent review, see: [3]). Female (BALB/c) mice develop a more severe airway inflammation with more myeloid dendritic cells, effector T cells, alternatively activated macrophages, eosinophils, and higher concentrations of IgE and cytokines than male mice in ovalbumin (OVA)-induced allergic asthma models [4–6]. Male (C57BL/6) [7, 8] and progesterone-treated female mice [9], on the other hand, develop stronger AHR due to the relaxing effect of estrogens on airway smooth muscle [8, 10, 11]. Taken together, these data reveal a sex difference in mice with respect to the respiratory and immune responses to allergens (for a recent review, see [12]).

Depending on the pro-inflammatory agent, alveolar macrophages can develop into classically activated (M1) macrophages, alternatively activated M2) macrophages, and intermediate forms [13]. Alternatively activated lung macrophages appear to be major players in the development of airway inflammation of OVA-sensitized and -challenged (OVA/OVA) mice, and are more prevalent in female than in male mice [14]. The *arginase1* (*Arg1*) gene is highly expressed in the cytoplasm of M2 macrophages [13, 15]. Accordingly, OVA-induced *Arg1* expression is present in cells with the morphological characteristics of macrophages [16, 17]. The prominence of ARG1-containing macrophages underlies the hypothesis that arginine availability plays a key role in the development and presentation of asthma [18–20].

Arginase and nitric oxide synthase (NOS) share, and compete for the substrate L-arginine. Since NO relaxes the smooth-muscle cells of the bronchi and blood vessels, insufficient NO production may underlie AHR [4]. A high concentration of NO, however, promotes inflammation, mucosal swelling, and mucus secretion in the lung [21, 22]. Although the NOS enzymes have a ~500-fold higher affinity for arginine than arginase, the V_{max} of arginase is ~1000-fold higher than that of NOS, which makes regional substrate depletion of arginine possible [21, 23]. Inhibition of arginine uptake into macrophages by ablation of the arginine transporter *Cat2* [24] and excess cationic proteins, such as eosinophil-derived major basic protein (MBP) [25], also inhibits NO production, whereas pharmacological inhibition of arginase activity attenuates AHR, *Arg1* expression, cell number in bronchoalveolar lavage fluid, and expression of the inflammatory markers IL-4, IL-5, IL-13, and NOS2 [26–29], and induces NO-mediated smooth-muscle relaxation [30]. Furthermore, supplementation of arginine mitigates the inflammatory airway response, increases arginase expression and activity, and elevates NOx levels [31, 32]. These findings suggest that arginase-mediated differences in substrate availability for NO synthesis may determine the clinical presentation of allergic asthma.

In an earlier study, we reported that *Arg1* ablation in macrophages improved peripheral lung function and decreased mRNA expression of arginine-metabolizing and -transporting genes in OVA/OVA-treated male C57Bl/6 mice, but had no effect on airway inflammation [33]. In a similar study with *Arg1$^{fl/fl}$/Tie2Cre$^{tg/-}$* mice, in which *Arg1* exons 7 and 8 instead of exon 4 were flanked by *loxP* sites, Barron et al. also reported the lack of an effect of *Arg1* elimination in myeloid cells on allergic lung inflammation, but found no effect on peripheral lung mechanics [34]. However, these authors did not differentiate between male and female mice. In the present study, we examined the role of ARG1 on lung function and inflammation in OVA/OVA-treated female *Arg1$^{fl/fl}$/Tie2Cre$^{tg/-}$* mice. We report that *Arg1* ablation in the lung of female C57Bl/6 mice did not protect peripheral lung mechanics, as in male mice, but did cause a smaller increase in the expression of L-arginine-metabolizing enzymes and transporters, and of inflammatory cytokines and chemokines.

Methods

Generation of transgenic mice and husbandry

All animal experiments were approved by the Committee for Animal Care and Use of Maastricht University (DEC2005-146). The generation of the transgenic mice was described before [33]. In brief: exon 4 of the mouse *Arg1* gene was flanked with *loxP* sites [33] and offspring were genotyped with primers *Arg1-F1* and *Arg1-R1* (Additional file 1: Table S1). To ablate the floxed *Arg1* allele (*Arg1^{fl}*) specifically in macrophages, *Arg1$^{fl/fl}$* mice were crossed with either LysM-Cre [35] or Tie2-Cre mice [36]. The resulting *Arg$^{fl/fl}$/LysM-Cre$^{tg/-}$* (Arg1-KO^{LysM}) mice and their *Arg$^{fl/fl}$/LysM-Cre$^{-/-}$* littermates (Arg1-Con) or *Arg$^{fl/fl}$/Tie2-Cre$^{tg/-}$* (Arg1- KO^{Tie2}) mice and *Arg$^{fl/fl}$/Tie2-Cre$^{-/-}$* littermates (Arg1-Con) were analyzed for the presence of the *LysM-Cre* or *Tie2-Cre* transgene by PCR using primer pairs *LysM-F* and *LysM-R* or *Tie2-F* and

Tie2-R, respectively (Additional file 1: Table S1). The Cre-excised *Arg1* allele (298 bp) was detected with the primers *Arg1-F2* (Additional file 1: Table S1) and *Arg1-R1*. Mice were kept with 2-3 animals per filter-top cage with wood shavings as bedding on a 12-h light/dark cycle, with standard chow and water ad libitum. Mice were checked daily for their well being by dedicated personnel of the animal facility.

Antigen sensitization and challenge

Antigen sensitization and challenge have been described before [33]. In brief, ten-week old female mice were injected intraperitoneally on days 0 and 14 with 10 µg of ovalbumin (OVA), grade V (Sigma-Aldrich, Zwijndrecht, The Netherlands) in the presence of 1 mg/mL of alum adjuvant (Imject Alum®, Thermo Scientific, Rockford, IL, USA). On days 21-27, mice were exposed daily for 30 min to 1% (*w*/*v*) aerosolized OVA in PBS. Lung function was assessed 12 h after the last challenge. Groups, each containing 2-3 Arg1-Con or Arg1-KO mice pretreated with PBS or OVA (in total 7-8 mice per genotype and treatment), were tested at 3-4 different occasions to correct for any "session" effects [37].

Airway hyperresponsiveness

Assessment of methacholine responsiveness was carried out as previously described [33]. Briefly, 7-8 mice per genotype and treatment were anesthetized with 80 mg/kg sodium pentobarbital and an additional 40 mg/kg 30 min later. An 18-gauge blunt needle was inserted into the trachea and connected to a mechanical small-animal ventilator (FlexiVent, Scireq, Montreal, Canada). Mice were ventilated at 200 breaths/min with a delivered tidal volume of 0.25 mL against a positive end-expiratory pressure (PEEP) of 3 cm H_2O applied by a water trap. Lungs were challenged by delivering successively 0, 3.1, 12.5 and 50 mg/mL aerosolized methacholine (Sigma) in PBS through the tracheal cannula using an ultrasonic nebulizer during 10 deep inhalations with a tidal volume of 0.8 mL. Following each methacholine challenge, the input impedance (Z_{rs}) of the respiratory system was measured. Parameters measured were: R_N, the Newtonian airflow resistance, mostly in the conducting pulmonary airways; H, "tissue elastance", or the elastic energy stored in tissues; G, "tissue resistance", or viscous dissipation of energy in respiratory tissues and airflow heterogeneity.

Plasma collection and analysis

After each experiment, blood was collected from the inferior caval vein of 7-8 mice per group in heparin-coated tubes, centrifuged 3 min at 5000*g, snap-frozen and stored at −80 °C as described previously [33]. Plasma OVA-specific IgE levels were determined by ELISA (MD Biosciences, M036005, Zürich, Switzerland). For the determination of plasma amino acids, 50 µL of plasma was added to 4 mg sulfosalicylic acid, vortexed, snap-frozen in liquid nitrogen and stored at −80 °C until use. Plasma amino-acid concentrations were measured as described [33].

Tissue isolation

Following euthanasia, the left lung was filled with 10% buffered formalin (Klinipath, Deventer, The Netherlands) for 10 min at a pressure of 20 cm H_2O and submersed overnight in 4% formaldehyde at room temperature prior to paraffin embedding. The right lung was snap frozen in liquid nitrogen, pulverized in a liquid-nitrogen-chilled mortar, and stored at −80 °C as described previously [33].

Immunostaining

Immunostaining was performed as described previously [33]. In brief, paraffin-embedded tissue was cut into 4 µm sections and stained with hematoxylin & eosin (H&E), reticulin, or Sirius red. Epitope retrieval was carried out by heating the slides for 5 min in 10 mM sodium citrate (pH 6 at room temperature (RT)) at 95 °C and cooling to RT for 30 min. Endogenous peroxidase was blocked with peroxidase block (DAKO, S2001, Enschede, the Netherlands) for 10 min at RT. Non-specific antibody binding was blocked with 10% normal goat serum for 30 min. After washing in PBS, slides were incubated with anti-ARG1 (Amsterdam Liver Center, AMS40.11.13), anti-myeloperoxidase (MPO; DAKO), or anti-major basic protein (MBP; kindly provided by Dr. James Lee, MT14.3.7, Mayo Clinic Scottsdale, AZ, USA) as described [33]. After washing, sections were incubated with a 1:200 diluted biotinylated rabbit anti-rat secondary antibody (DAKO) for 45 min at RT, washed, incubated with strepta-vidin/HRP (Vector) for 30 min at RT, and developed with 3,3′-diaminobenzidine (Sigma) for 10 min. Sections stained for ARG1 were incubated with an AP-labeled secondary antibody (DAKO) for 45 min, developed with nitroblue-tetrazolium and 5-bromo-4-chloro-3-indolyl phosphate (Roche, Almere, The Netherlands) dissolved in 50 mM MgSO4, 100 mM Tris·HCl (pH 9.5) for 30 min, and cover-slipped with an aqueous mounting medium (DAKO). To facilitate quantification, the immunostained slides were not counterstained.

Histological assessment

Lung inflammation was assessed on H&E-stained sections. MBP and MPO images were digitized with the Pannoramic slide scanner 250 (3DHistech, Budapest, Hungary), and counted using the Pannoramic viewer software application. Color deconvolution was adjusted to detect diaminobenzidine-stained cells. Only cells with a diameter between 10 and 15 µm were included.

Arginase-positive cells were counted manually in three different locations (peribronchiolar, perivenous and in the intervening parenchyma). The density of the counted cells was expressed per mm^2 tissue.

Milliplex assay

Tissue powder was homogenized in PBS, pH 7.6, in the presence of a proteinase inhibitor cocktail (Complete, Roche). Cytokines (CCL11 (eotaxin-1), IL-4, IL-5, IL-10, IL-13, TNFα, and IFNγ) were quantified using a Luminex ® xMAP® multiplex platform, combined with a customized Milliplex™ mouse chemokine/cytokine panel from Millipore™, as described previously [33].

RNA isolation and quantification

RNA purification and quantification was performed as described previously [33]. In brief, tissue powder was homogenized in Tri reagent (Sigma) with the Mini Bead-Beater (Biospec products, Bartlesville, OK, USA). To remove genomic DNA, RNA was precipitated with 2 M LiCl for at least 30 min at −20 °C. RNA integrity was checked by denaturing gel electrophoresis. RNA concentration was determined with a NanoDrop-ND-1000 spectrophotometer at 260 nm (Isogen Life Sciences, Wilmington, DE, USA). 400 ng of total RNA was transcribed using a first-strand synthesis kit (Roche). Quantitative PCR was performed in a Lightcycler 480 (Roche), using Lightcycler 480® SYBRgreen mastermix (Roche) and the following settings: denaturation: 30 s at 95 °C; annealing 30 s at 60 °C; elongation 30 s at 72 °C; 45 cycles; and a final elongation step for 5 min at 72 °C. If reverse transcriptase was omitted, no product was formed. Primary fluorescence data were quantified as described [33] and expressed relative to that of *18S* rRNA. Primer sequences are given in Additional file 1: Table S1.

Western blot

Western blot analysis was performed as described previously [33]. In brief, tissue powder was homogenized in RIPA buffer (25 mM Tris·HCl (pH 7.6), 150 mM NaCl, 1% NP-40, 1% Na-deoxycholate, 0.1% SDS, containing Complete® cocktail (Roche). Protein concentration was measured with the bicinchoninic-acid assay (Pierce, Rockford, IL, USA). Twenty-five µg protein was separated by SDS-PAGE, transferred onto 0.45 µm nitrocellulose membranes, using a wet transfer system (Biorad, Hercules, CA, USA). Equal loading of lanes was confirmed by Ponceau S staining, followed by a wash-step with TBS (50 mM Tris, 150 mM NaCl, pH 7.6) and blocking of non-specific binding with 5% skimmed milk in TBS/0.5% Tween-2. Rabbit anti-ARG1 antibody (1:200), followed by an HRP-conjugated swine anti-rabbit secondary antibody (DAKO) was used to visualize ARG1. Signal was developed with the Super Signal West Pico Substrate (Pierce) and quantified in a Fuji systems darkbox (Fuji Film Life Sciences, Tokyo, Japan).

Statistical analyses

Groups were compared using the Kruskal-Wallis test for PBS/OVA- versus OVA/OVA-treated, and Arg1-Con versus Arg1-KO^{Tie2} mice, as described previously [33]. If this nonparametric test indicated a difference, a multiple comparison of the groups was carried out. Values were considered as statistically significant if $P < 0.05$, and as indicating a trend if $P < 0.10$.

The bivariate two-tailed Pearson correlation coefficients between each of the lung-function parameters, mRNA and protein concentrations, histology quantification data and plasma amino-acid concentrations were determined after combining the data from the comparable PBS/OVA and OVA/OVA groups. In the Tables, *P*-values of the resulting correlation coefficients were color-coded, with red indicating a $P < 0.001$, orange $0.01 > P > 0.001$, and yellow $0.05 > P > 0.01$.

Results

Arg1 expression in the lungs of OVA-sensitized and -challenged mice with *Arg1*-deficient macrophages

Arg1-KO^{LysM} mice, Arg1- KO^{Tie2} mice, and their Arg1-Con littermates were either sensitized-and-challenged with ovalbumin (OVA/OVA), or mock-sensitized and then challenged with ovalbumin (PBS/OVA). As expected, we found no ARG1-positive cells in the lungs of PBS/OVA-treated mice, whereas the lungs of OVA/OVA-treated Arg1-Con mice contained many ARG1-positive cells (Fig. 1a). ARG1-positive cells were completely absent from the lungs of OVA/OVA-treated Arg1-KO^{Tie2}, whereas the number of ARG1-positive cells was reduced, but not eliminated, in the lungs of similarly treated Arg1-KO^{LysM} mice. Of note, we observed no appreciable ARG1 in the endothelial cells in PBS/OVA (Fig. 1a) or OVA/OVA-treated lung blood vessels (Fig. 1d). Furthermore, we did not observe any ARG1 protein or mRNA expression in the lungs of mice undergoing the PBS/OVA protocol, whereas a robust induction of ARG1 protein and mRNA expression was found in the lungs of Arg1-Con mice exposed to the OVA/OVA protocol (black columns in Figs. 1b and 2). Pulmonary *Arg1* mRNA and protein concentration in OVA/OVA-treated Arg1-KO^{Tie2} mice were reduced to 5 ± 2% and 2 ± 0.2%, respectively, and in OVA/OVA-treated Arg1-KO^{LysM} mice to 20 ± 8% and 19 ± 10%, respectively, of that found in similarly treated Arg1-Con littermates (Figs. 1b and 2, white columns). We also counted

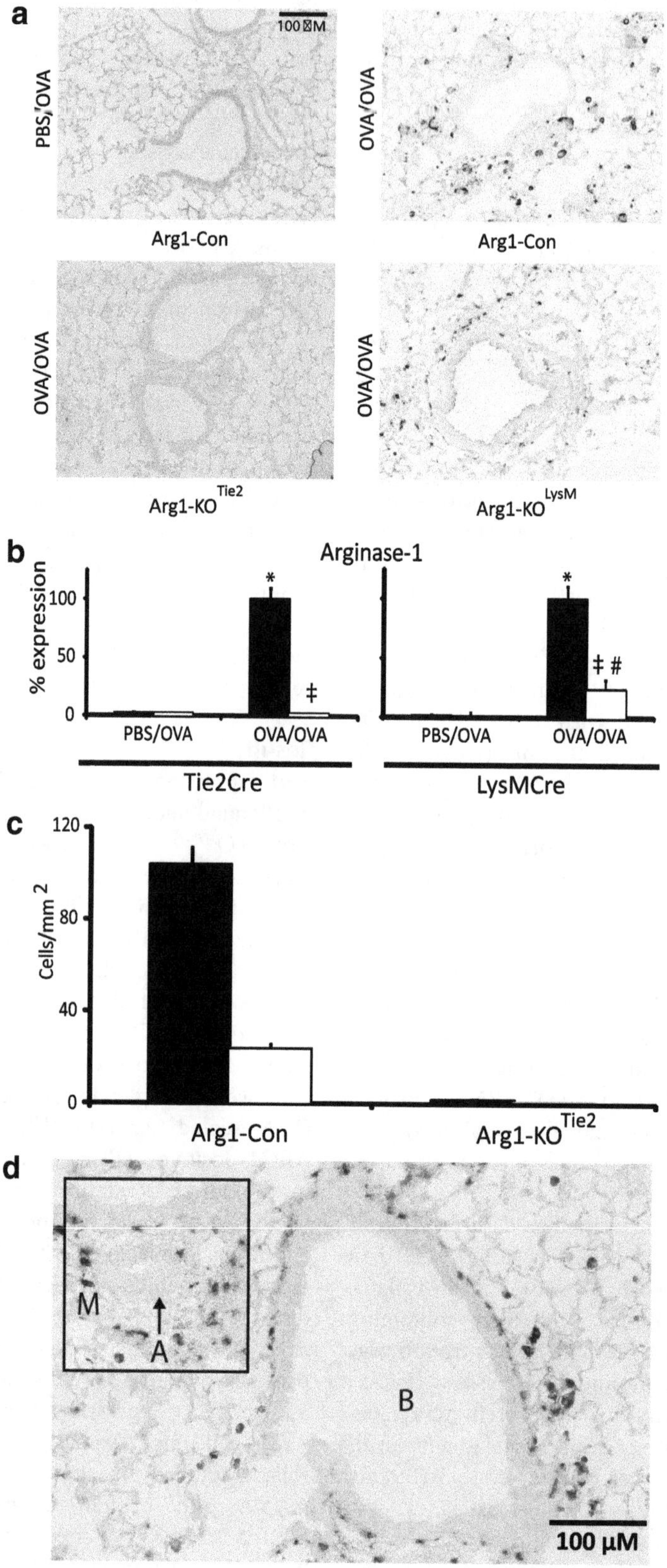

Fig. 1 (See legend on next page.)

(See figure on previous page.)

Fig. 1 Validation of *Arg1* ablation in lung of female $Arg1^{fl/fl}$ mice. **a** Lungs of PBS/OVA- and OVA/OVA-treated female control mice, respectively (top row), and of OVA/OVA-treated female Arg1-KO^{Tie2} and Arg1-KO^{LysM} mice, respectively (bottom row). Note the complete absence of ARG1-positive macrophages in Arg1-KO^{Tie2} mice and the reduction in Arg1-KO^{LysM} mice. **b** Reduction of ARG1 protein content in the lungs of OVA/OVA-treated Arg1-KO^{Tie2} and Arg1-KO^{LysM} mice (white bars) compared to the corresponding Arg1-Con^{LysM} or Arg1-Con^{Tie2} mice (black bars). Means ± SEM ($n = 8$ mice per group). **c** Number of ARG1-positive cells per mm^2 lung tissue. Cells were counted near bronchioles and arteries (black bars) and in the lung parenchyma (white bars). Means ± SEM are shown ($n = 8$ mice per group). **d** Detail of ARG1 protein content in OVA/OVA-treated control lung. The absence of ARG1 in arterial endothelium is noteworthy. Abbreviations: A = artery, and M = ARG1-positive macrophages. Significance symbols: *: $P < 0.001$ OVA/OVA vs. PBS/OVA Arg1-Con; #: $P < 0.001$ OVA/OVA vs. PBS/OVA Arg1-KO^{Lysm}; ‡: $P < 0.001$ OVA/OVA Arg1-KO^{Lysm} or Arg1-KO^{Tie2} vs. OVA/OVA Arg1-Con

ARG1-positive cells surrounding bronchioles and arteries, and in parenchyma of OVA/OVA-treated Arg1-Con and Arg1-KO ^{Tie2} mice, and found no ARG1-positive cells in lung tissue of Arg1-KO ^{Tie2} mice (Fig. 1c). From this finding, we conclude that the floxed 4th exon of *Arg1* was accessible to the Cre enzyme and that the reduction in *Arg1* expression was near complete in female Arg1-KO^{Tie2} mice (reduction to ~2%), whereas residual *Arg1* expression was present in female Arg1-KO^{LysM} mice (reduction to ~20%). Since Arg1-KO^{LysM} mice showed an incomplete elimination of *Arg1* expression and an intermediate phenotype, we limit the description of our study to Arg1-KO^{Tie2} mice and their Arg1-Con littermates.

Effect of *Arg1* deletion on arginine-metabolizing and -transporting genes in the lung

We investigated to what extent ablation of *Arg1* in the lung caused changes in the expression of arginine-metabolizing enzymes and arginine transporters. Figure 2 shows that the pulmonary mRNA abundance of *Arg1, Arg2, Nos2, Slc7a1, Slc7a2* and *Slc7a7* was induced by the OVA/OVA protocol compared to the PBS/OVA protocol. More importantly, the induction was consistently lower in Arg1-KO^{Tie2} than in Arg1-Con female mice subjected to the OVA/OVA protocol. As a result, OVA/OVA treatment no longer induced the expression of *Arg2, Nos2, Slc7a1, Slc7a2,* and *Slc7a7* in Arg1-KO^{Tie2} mice. These data clearly show that effective ablation of *Arg1* expression in macrophages suppressed the induction of arginine-metabolizing enzymes and arginine transporters in the lungs of OVA/OVA-treated female mice.

The effect of *Arg1* ablation on circulating amino acids

OVA/OVA treatment of female Arg1-Con mice caused a significant drop in the concentration of circulating arginine levels relative to their PBS/OVA-treated littermates (Additional file 1: Table S2). The decline was not seen in OVA/OVA-treated Arg1-KO^{Tie2} mice, implying an effect of ARG1. In both Arg1-KO^{Tie2} and Arg1-Con mice, OVA/OVA treatment also caused an increase in the plasma concentration of ornithine and a decline in that of glycine relative to the corresponding PBS/OVA-treated mice (Additional file 1: Table S2). As a result, the arginine bioavailability index (the ratio of arginine and ornithine *plus* lysine concentrations) decreased non-significantly to ~71% ($P = 0.369$) in OVA/OVA-treated Arg-Con, but remained unchanged in Arg1-KO^{Tie2} mice.

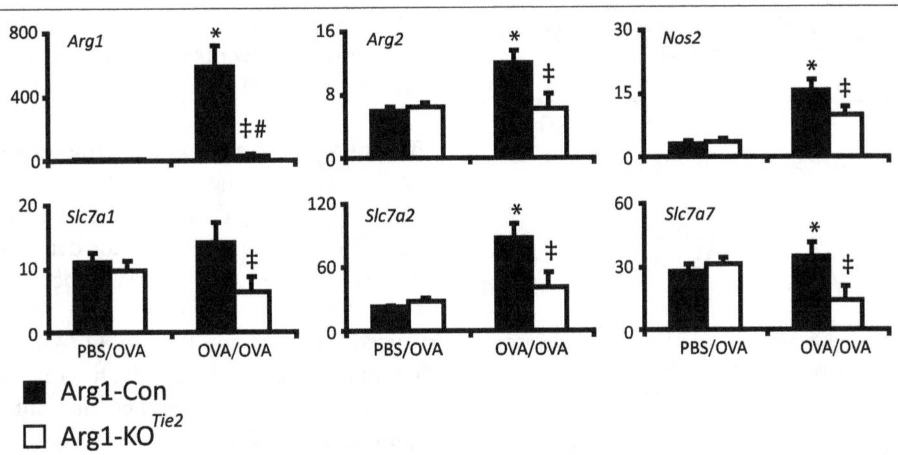

Fig. 2 Effect of *Arg1* ablation in the lung on the expression of arginine-metabolizing enzymes and arginine transporters. Black bars represent Arg1-Con mice and white bars Arg1-KO^{Tie2} mice. The specific treatment (PBS/OVA or OVA/OVA) is indicated below the columns. mRNA abundance (AU = number of mRNA copies normalized to 18S rRNA expression and multiplied by 10^4) of the arginine-metabolizing enzymes *Arg1, Arg2,* and *Nos2* and the arginine transporters *Slc7a1, Slc7a2* and *Slc7a7* is shown as mean ± SEM of 7-8 mice per group. Significance symbols: *: $P < 0.05$ OVA/OVA vs. PBS/OVA Arg1-Con; #: $P < 0.05$ OVA/OVA vs. PBS/OVA Arg1-KO^{Tie2}; ‡: $P < 0.05$ OVA/OVA Arg1-Con vs. Arg1-KO^{Tie2}

Ablation of *Arg1* in the lung has no effect on allergen-induced airway hyperresponsiveness

To address the question whether *Arg1* ablation in the lung affects respiratory mechanics, we measured methacholine responsiveness in PBS/OVA- and OVA/OVA-treated Arg1-KO^{Tie2} mice and their Arg1-Con littermates (Fig. 3). Compared to PBS/OVA treatment, OVA/OVA treatment increased airway resistance (R_N), tissue elastance (H), and tissue resistance (G) in female Arg1-Con and Arg1-KO^{Tie2} mice, without an effect of *Arg1* depletion. Collectively, these findings show that *Arg1* ablation in the lung did not affect AHR in female mice.

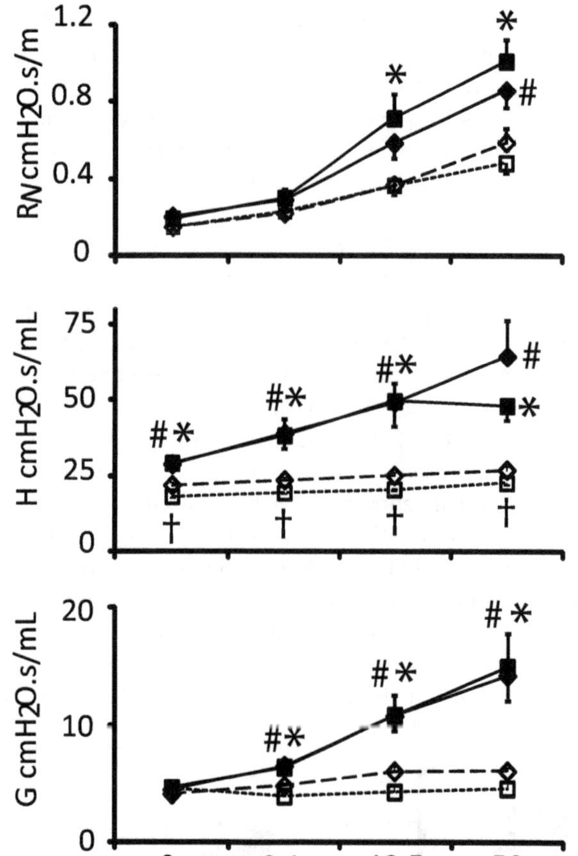

Fig. 3 Effect of *Arg1* ablation in the lung on lung function as measured with the FlexiVent. PBS/OVA-treated Arg1-Con mice are represented by open diamonds connected by dashed lines and PBS/OVA-treated Arg1-KO^{Tie2} mice by open squares connected by dotted lines. OVA/OVA-treated Arg1-Con mice are represented by filled diamonds and OVA/OVA treated Arg1-KO^{Tie2} mice by filled squares both connected by continuous lines. Airway resistance R_N, tissue elastance H, and tissue resistance G are shown in panels A, B, and C, respectively. Values on the X-axis indicate the concentrations of aerosolized methacholine. Means ± SEM ($n = 7$-8 mice per group). Significance symbols: #: $P < 0.01$ (OVA/OVA vs. PBS/OVA Arg1-Con); *: $P < 0.01$ (OVA/OVA Arg1-KO^{Tie2} vs. PBS/OVA Arg1-KO^{Tie2}); †: $P < 0.01$ (PBS/OVA Arg1-KO^{Tie2} vs. PBS/OVA Arg1-Con). Arg1-KO^{Tie2} and Arg1-Con mice did not differ in their response to OVA/OVA treatment

Ablation of *Arg1* in the lung affects mRNA abundance of inflammatory genes

We investigated whether *Arg1* ablation in the lung affected the expression of asthma-associated cytokines (Fig. 4). OVA/OVA treatment increased the abundance of *Il13, Il4, Il5, Ccl2, Ccl11 (Eotaxin-1),* and *Il10* mRNAs in Arg1-Con mice as expected, while the expression of *Tnfa* and *Ifng* remained unchanged. Furthermore, OVA/OVA treatment of Arg1-Con mice increased gene expression of respiratory epithelium-specific *Muc5ac* and *Clca3*. OVA/OVA-treated female Arg1-KO^{Tie2} mice differed from their OVA/OVA-treated Arg1-Con littermates by showing a significantly lower expression of the *Il13, Il4, Ccl2, Ccl11, Ifng, Muc5ac,* and *Clca3* mRNAs. These findings imply a direct relation between *Arg1* elimination in the lung and the decreased expression of inflammatory genes in the lungs of OVA/OVA-treated mice.

Arg1 ablation in the lung does not affect protein levels of cytokines and chemokines

To determine whether *Arg1* ablation in the lung had an effect on the protein concentration of pulmonary cytokines and chemokines, we measured IL-4, IL-5, IL-10, IL-13, CCL11, TNFα and IFNγ protein in extracts of whole-lung homogenates (Fig. 5). Compared to PBS/OVA-treated female mice, OVA/OVA-treated Arg1-Con and Arg1-KO^{Tie2} mice had increased concentrations of IL-5, CCL11 and TNFα in their lungs, whereas the concentration of IL-4, IL-13, and IFNγ was unchanged. IL-10 was lower in OVA/OVA- than in PBS/OVA-treated Arg1-Con mice and higher in OVA/OVA- treated Arg1-KO^{Tie2} mice than in similarly treated Arg1-Con mice. Apart from IL-10, no differences in cytokine and chemokine protein concentration were found between OVA/OVA-treated Arg1-Con and Arg1-KO^{Tie2} mice.

Effect of *Arg1* deletion on the immune response to OVA

We investigated whether the production of ovalbumin-specific IgE antibodies was affected by the ablation of *Arg1*. OVA-specific IgE was not detectable in plasma of PBS/OVA-treated mice. OVA-specific IgE levels in OVA/OVA-treated female Arg1-KO^{Tie2} mice were reduced to ~50% of that in OVA/OVA-treated Arg1-Con mice, but due to the high variance in plasma IgE concentrations this difference did not reach statistical significance ($P = 0.14$).

Effects of *Arg1* deletion in the lung on pulmonary inflammation

We investigated the effect of *Arg1* ablation on the OVA/OVA-induced inflammatory response in lung tissue

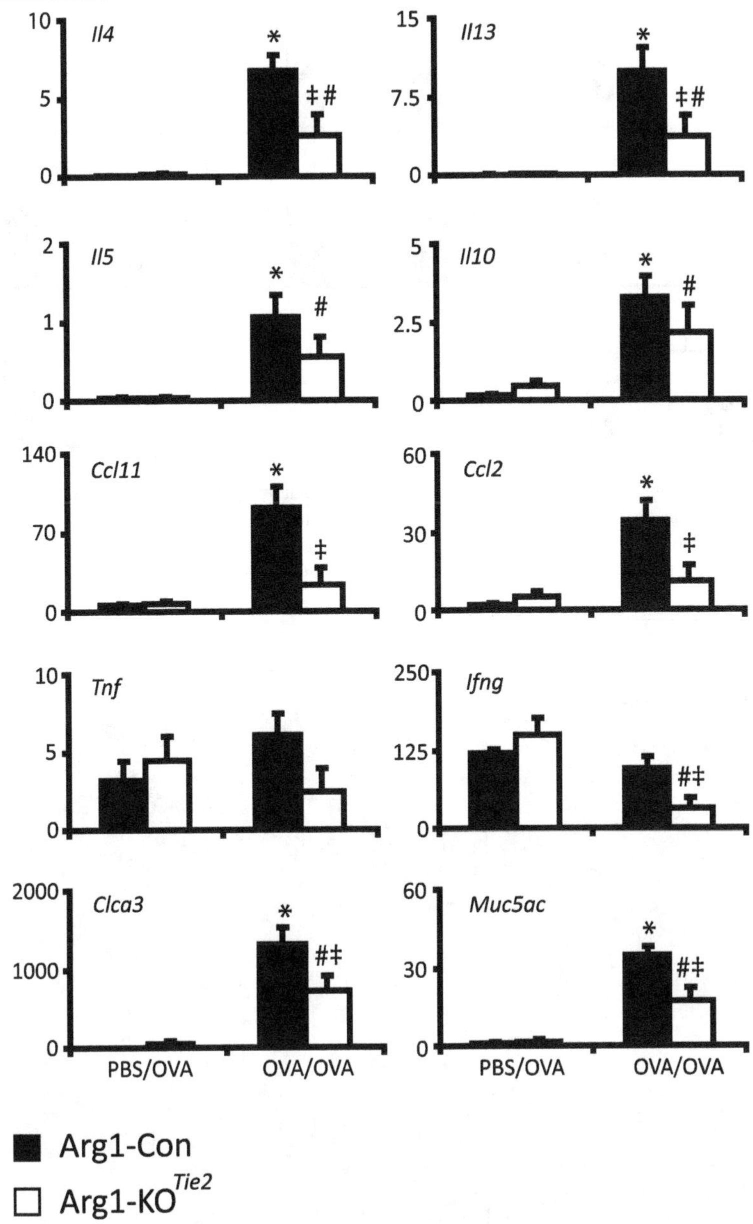

Fig. 4 Effect of *Arg1* ablation in the lung on the expression of inflammatory genes. Black bars represent Arg1-Con mice and white bars Arg1-KO^{Tie2} mice. mRNA abundance (AU = number of mRNA copies normalized to 18S rRNA expression and multiplied by 10^4) of the T_H2-related inflammatory genes *Il4, Il13, Il5* and *Ccl11*, the macrophage-chemotactic protein *Ccl2*, the anti-inflammatory gene *Il10*, the T_H1-related inflammatory genes *Tnfa* and *Ifng*, and the marker genes for the activation of bronchiolar epithelium *Muc5ac* and *Clca3* are shown as means ± SEM (n = 7-8 mice per group). Significance symbols: *: $P < 0.05$ (OVA/OVA vs. PBS/OVA Arg1-Con); #: $P < 0.05$ (OVA/OVA vs. PBS/OVA Arg1-KO^{Tie2}); ‡: $P < 0.05$ (OVA/OVA Arg1-KO^{Tie2} vs OVA/OVA Arg1-Con)

(Fig. 6). H&E-stained sections of lung tissue did not reveal any inflammatory cells in PBS/OVA-treated mice (Fig. 6A). This finding was confirmed by staining the same lungs for the presence of eosinophils and neutrophils using MBP and MPO as markers, respectively (Fig. 6A). As expected, many inflammatory cells were present in the lungs of OVA/OVA-treated mice, but their number was not different between female Arg1-KO^{Tie2} mice and their Arg1-Con littermates (Fig. 6B). To investigate whether there was a difference in lung remodeling between female Arg1-KO^{Tie2} mice and their Arg1-Con littermates, we stained slides for reticulin and collagen (Sirius red), but did not detect differences either (Fig. 7).

Comparison of responses to allergic asthma in female Arg1-Con and Arg1-KO^{Tie2} mice

To investigate whether the presence or absence of ARG1 activity affected the adaptive responses to OVA-induced

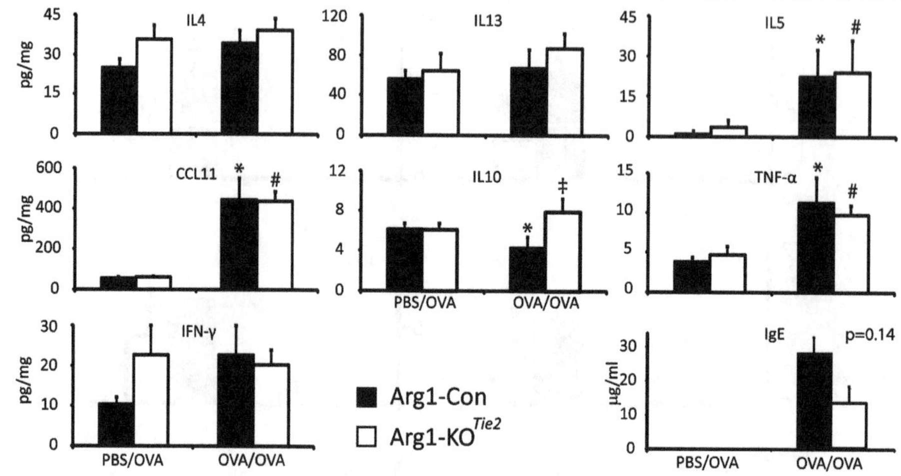

Fig. 5 Effect of *Arg1* ablation in the lung on the pulmonary concentration of inflammatory cytokines, chemokines, and OVA-specific IgE. Black bars represent Arg1-Con mice and white bars Arg1-KO^{Tie2} mice. Treatment of the mice (PBS/OVA or OVA/OVA) is indicated. The pulmonary concentrations of IL-4, IL-13, IL-5, CCL11, IL-10, TNFα and IFNγ (pg/mg total protein), and OVA-specific IgE (ng/mL) in plasma are shown as means ± SEM (n = 7-8 mice per group). Significance symbols: *: $P < 0.05$ (OVA/OVA vs. PBS/OVA Arg1-Con); #: $P < 0.05$ (OVA/OVA vs. PBS/OVA Arg1-KO^{Tie2}); ‡: $P < 0.05$ (OVA/OVA Arg1-KO^{Tie2} vs OVA/OVA Arg1-Con)

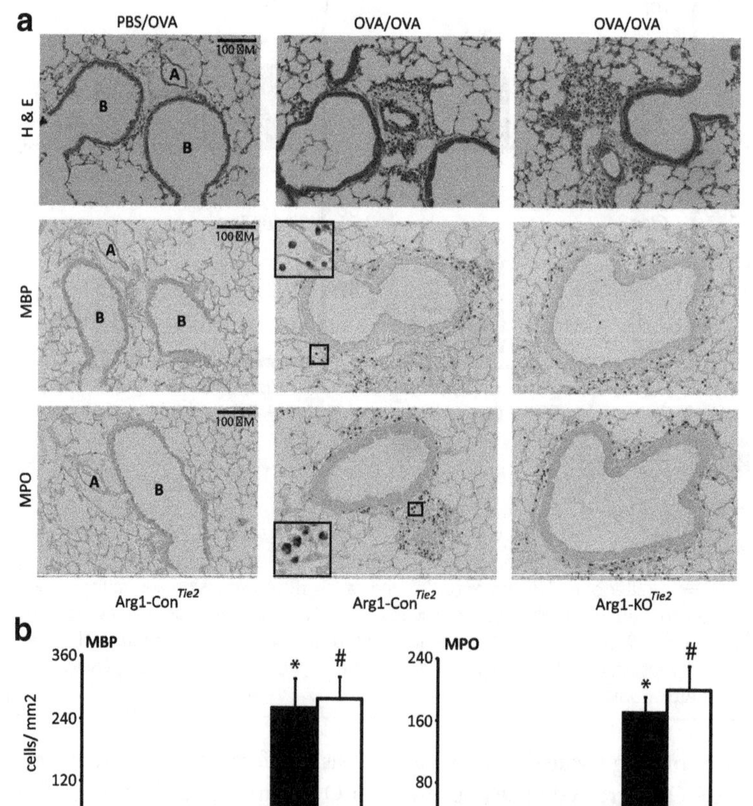

Fig. 6 Effect of *Arg1* ablation in the lung on the prevalence of inflammatory cells in the lungs. A: The left two columns show lungs of PBS/OVA- and OVA/OVA-treated Arg1-Con mice, while the right column shows lungs of OVA/OVA-treated Arg1-KO^{Tie2} mice. Top row: hematoxylin and eosin; middle row: MBP staining for eosinophils; bottom row: MPO staining for neutrophils. Bar: 100 μm. B: Quantification of the inflammatory cells in OVA/OVA-treated Arg1-Con (black bars) and Arg1-KO^{Tie2} (white bars) mice. All sections were stained simultaneously. Means and SEM of 7-8 mice per group are shown. *: $P < 0.05$ (OVA/OVA vs. PBS/OVA Arg1-Con); #: $P < 0.05$ (OVA/OVA vs. PBS/OVA Arg1-KO^{Tie2})

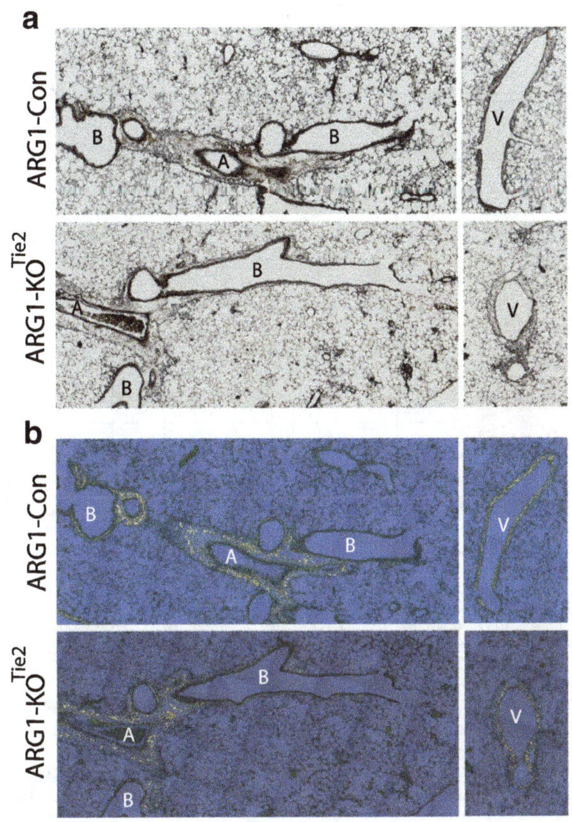

Fig. 7 Effect of *Arg1* ablation on lung remodeling. **a**: Bright-field images of reticulin-stained sections of OVA/OVA-treated female Arg1-Con and Arg1-KO^{Tie2} mice. **b**: Polarized-light images of Sirius red-stained sections of OVA/OVA-treated female Arg1-Con and Arg1-KO^{Tie2} mice to assess collagen content (serial sections of panel A). The left-sided panels show sections of periarterial areas and the right-handed panels sections of perivenous areas. Abbreviations: B = bronchiole, A = artery, and V = vein

asthma in a quantitatively similar way, we also investigated to what extent changes in lung-function parameters, mRNA and protein concentrations, histology quantitation and plasma amino-acid concentrations correlated in either Arg1-Con or Arg1-KO^{Tie2} mice (Fig. 8). Strikingly, lung-function parameters and mRNA concentrations in Arg1-Con females strongly corresponded within, but hardly between both categories. Noticeable exceptions were a correlation between the response of lung-function parameters H and G and the expression of *Il4* mRNA, and the near absence of a correlation between the response of the pro-inflammatory cytokines *Tnfa* and especially *Ifng*, and all other mRNAs measured. Female Arg1-KO^{Tie2} differed from Arg1-Con mice (Fig. 8) by a pronounced decrease in the tightness of the correspondence between the adaptive responses that were mounted. Striking examples were the loss of correspondence between the response of H and G, and *Il4* mRNA expression, and the loss of correspondence of the expression of the mRNAs of arginine transporters *Slc7a7* and *Slc7a1*, and that of all other mRNAs.

Discussion

Tie2Cre-dependent deletion of *Arg1* expression in myeloid cells prevented the expression of ARG1 in lung inflammatory cells of OVA/OVA-treated Arg1-KO^{Tie2} mice. Compared to female OVA/OVA-treated Arg1-Con mice, Arg1-KO^{Tie2} mice had lower OVA-specific IgE levels and a lower expression of arginine-metabolizing or -transporting genes (*Arg2, Nos2, Slc7a1, Slc7a2,* and *Slc7a7*), of cyto- and chemokine genes (*Il4, Il13, Il5, Ccl11, Ccl2,* and *Ifng*), and of epithelial marker genes (*Muc5ac* and *Clc3a*), but *Arg1* deficiency did not affect airway resistance (R_N), tissue elastance (H), or tissue resistance (G). Furthermore, the tightness of the correspondence between the adaptive responses that were mounted in OVA/OVA-treated female mice were strongly reduced if these mice were unable to express *Arg1* in their alveolar macrophages.

Efficacy of *Tie2Cre*-mediated *Arg1* ablation in allergically inflamed lungs

Tie2Cre mice excise *loxP*-flanked DNA in both endothelial and early hematopoietic progenitor cells [36, 38]. As in male mice [33] and in other studies [34, 36, 39, 40], *Tie2Cre*-mediated excision of *Arg1* resulted in a near-complete deletion of *Arg1* mRNA and protein expression in macrophages. A near-complete *Arg1* excision was also observed in peritoneal macrophages of Arg1-KO^{Tie2} mice [41]. Importantly, we did not observe ARG1 protein in the endothelium of the pulmonary blood vessels of PBS/OVA- or OVA/OVA-treated Arg1-Con mice (Fig. 1a,d), even after prolonged incubation with the alkaline-phosphatase substrate (up to 90 min). In support of this finding, most other studies found no or only minimal arginase1 protein in lung epithelium and smooth muscle [42–44], also after inducing allergic inflammation [45–47]. Based on these findings, we conclude that Arg1-KO^{Tie2} mice can be used for the ablation of *Arg1* in macrophages of allergically inflamed lungs.

The near 100% efficacy of *Tie2Cre*-mediated excision of *loxP*-flanked *Arg1^{fl}* sequences contrasts with the 70-80% efficacy *LysMCre*-mediated *Arg1^{fl}* excision found in the present study and in our earlier study in male Arg1-KO mice [33]. Other studies [35, 48–50] also report *LysMCre*-mediated target excision in only 50-80% of the target cells. Since the 20% remaining expression of *Arg1* in the lungs of OVA/OVA-treated Arg1-KO^{LysM} mediated an intermediate phenotype between OVA/OVA-treated Arg1-Con and Arg1-KO^{Tie2Cre} mice, we limited our description of the effects of pulmonary *Arg1* deficiency on allergic asthma to Arg1-KO^{Tie2Cre} mice.

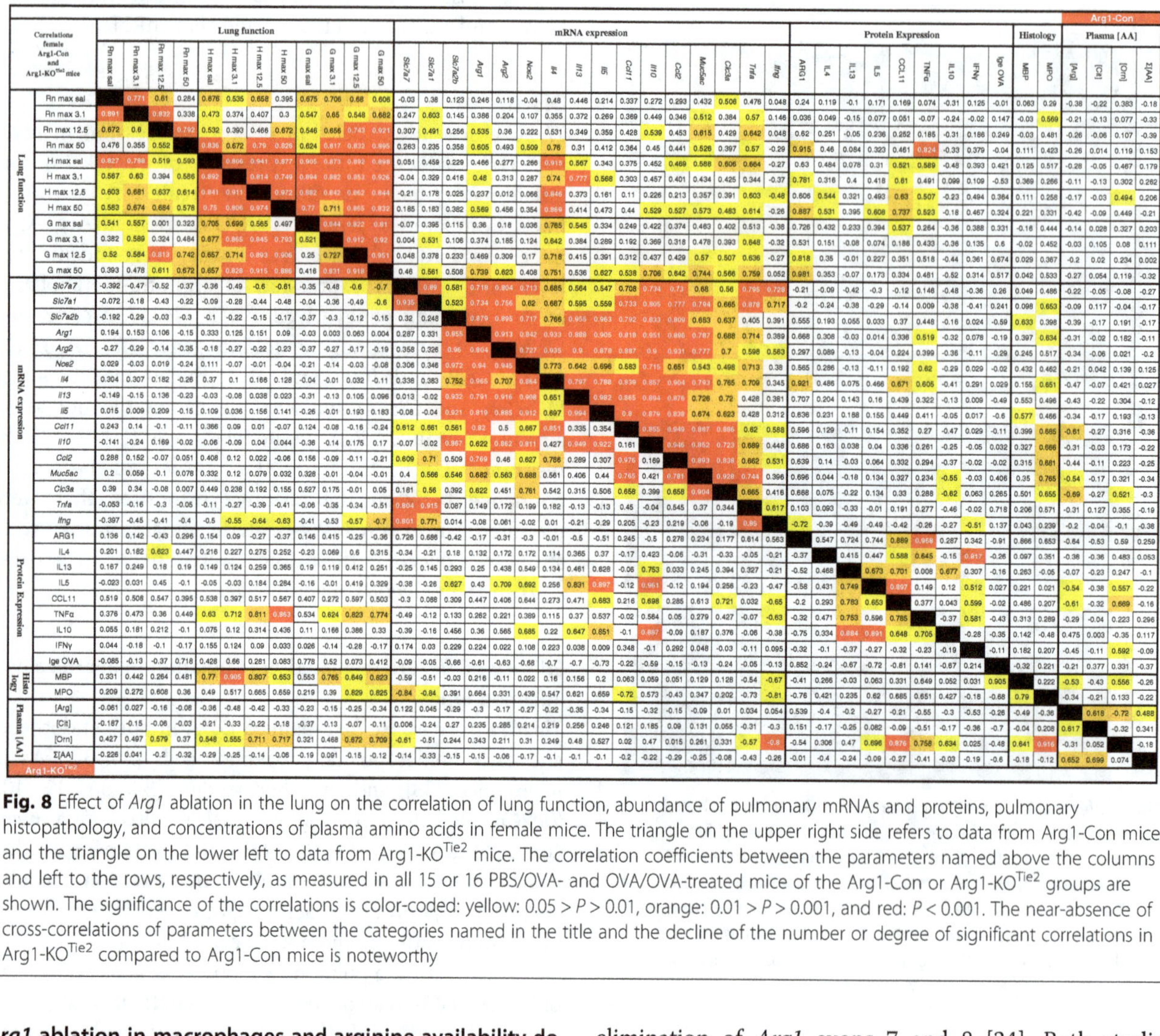

Fig. 8 Effect of *Arg1* ablation in the lung on the correlation of lung function, abundance of pulmonary mRNAs and proteins, pulmonary histopathology, and concentrations of plasma amino acids in female mice. The triangle on the upper right side refers to data from Arg1-Con mice and the triangle on the lower left to data from Arg1-KO^{Tie2} mice. The correlation coefficients between the parameters named above the columns and left to the rows, respectively, as measured in all 15 or 16 PBS/OVA- and OVA/OVA-treated mice of the Arg1-Con or Arg1-KO^{Tie2} groups are shown. The significance of the correlations is color-coded: yellow: $0.05 > P > 0.01$, orange: $0.01 > P > 0.001$, and red: $P < 0.001$. The near-absence of cross-correlations of parameters between the categories named in the title and the decline of the number or degree of significant correlations in Arg1-KO^{Tie2} compared to Arg1-Con mice is noteworthy

Arg1 ablation in macrophages and arginine availability do not affect lung biomechanics in allergically inflamed mouse lungs

Lung mechanics were measured using the forced-oscillation technique, which yields data on airway resistance (R_N) in the large airways, and on tissue elastance (H) and resistance (G) that reflect the function of the peripheral parts of the lung [51, 52]. Arg1-KO^{Tie2} and Arg1-Con mice did not differ in any of these parameters with or without OVA/OVA treatment. This finding in female mice contrasts with our earlier observation in male mice, in which *Arg1* deficiency in macrophages improved the peripheral lung mechanics parameters H and G [33]. Since the experiments in male and female mice were carried out concurrently with mice from the same litters, the difference cannot be attributed to a session effect. However, the present finding does agree with studies in which deficiency of *Arg1* in macrophages was mediated by bone-marrow transfer of constitutively *Arg1*-deficient stem cells [53] or *Tie2Cre*-mediated elimination of *Arg1* exons 7 and 8 [34]. Both studies tested, in addition to the OVA/OVA protocol, allergic inflammation in response to *Aspergillus fumigatus* and *Schistosoma mansoni* eggs in both C57BL/6 and BALB/c mice, but did not state whether the lung function tests were carried out in male and/or female mice.

The lack of an effect of *Arg1* deficiency on lung mechanics is in line with a smaller increase in the expression of arginine-metabolizing and -transporting genes upon OVA/OVA treatment (Fig. 2). Administration of pharmacological arginase inhibitors reduced AHR of allergen-induced asthma in both male and female mice. Whereas arginase inhibitors reduced lung inflammation in male mice [28, 29], they enhanced inflammation in female mice [26]. Because we observed no effect on AHR and a reduced inflammatory response in *Arg1*-deficient lungs, the effects of systemic inhibition of arginase-1 and -2 activities apparently differ from those of a deletion of *Arg1* from macrophages. Arginine analogues may exert additional effects, as NOS2 depletion or inhibition did not affect AHR, but that of NOS1- and -3 did [30, 54, 55].

The circulating concentration of L-arginine (Additional file 1: Table S2) was ~17% lower in OVA/OVA-treated Arg1-Con mice than in similarly treated Arg1-KO^{Tie2} mice, showing that *Arg1* expression in hematopoietic tissue had an impact on plasma arginine. Because the concentration of plasma ornithine increased and that of citrulline was unchanged, the plasma [Arg]/([Orn] + [Cit]) index decreased, in agreement with a recent report in female BALB/c mice [56]. Scott et al. [56] attributed an important role to lung arginase in the increase of plasma ornithine, but we observed a similar increase in plasma ornithine in mice with and without arginase1 in their lungs. Furthermore, we did not find an increase in plasma ornithine or a decrease in the arginine availability index in OVA/OVA-treated male Arg1-Con and Arg1-KO mice [33], even though methacholine responsiveness was decreased by *Arg1* deletion in male mice. The plasma [Arg]/([Orn] + [Lys]) index, which may reflect the availability of basic amino acids, only declined in OVA/OVA-treated female Arg1-KO mice. The question, therefore, is whether plasma arginine concentration or any plasma arginine availability index is important for respiratory function. Barron et al. [34] suggested that the enormous perfusion of the lung, which equals the cardiac output, assures that the supply of arginine from plasma to tissue cells is hardly impaired by local arginase activity. In addition, we have recently shown that citrulline rather than arginine is the more efficient extracellular source for intracellular arginine [57].

Arg1 ablation does not affect pro-inflammatory protein content in allergically inflamed lungs

OVA/OVA treatment of Arg1-KO mice resulted in a similar degree of lung infiltration with inflammatory cells as seen in Arg1-Con littermates, but *Il13, Il4, Il5, Ccl2, Ccl11, Ifng, Muc5ac,* and *Clca3* were expressed to a lesser extent in Arg1-KO ^{Tie2} than in Arg1-Con mice. Such a coordinated transcriptional response of genes probably reflects the activity of one or more common regulatory genes or proteins. However, as far as measured, changes in mRNA abundance of the chemo- and cytokines were not reflected in the corresponding protein concentrations in lung tissue (Fig. 8). This finding can be explained by the fact that cyto- and chemokines are secreted proteins, but inefficient translation of the mRNAs in Arg1-KO mice can also contribute, because posttranscriptional regulation of expression is a well-known feature of cyto- and chemokines [58]. In OVA/OVA-treated Arg1-Con males, we did observe a reasonable correspondence between mRNA and protein levels in 4 out of 8 combinations measured, but this correspondence disappeared in OVA/OVA-treated Arg1-KO male mice. The decline in circulating arginine concentration in OVA/OVA-treated males [33] was similar to that observed in females. Low circulating arginine concentrations are known to affect translation by inducing endoplasmic reticulum (ER) stress [59].

Comparison of the adaptive responses to OVA sensitization and challenge in male and female Arg1-Con mice

In a parallel study, we investigated the effects of *Arg1* ablation in the lung of genetically identical, similarly treated male mice [33]. Since the biology of female mice is underreported and since females are more often affected by allergic asthma than males [4–6, 60], we compared the adaptive responses of Arg1-Con mice in both sexes (Additional file 1: Table S3). The OVA-specific IgE concentration was ~3-fold higher in plasma of OVA/OVA-treated female than male mice. The sex difference in IgE accumulation is well-established [4]. *Arg1* deficiency did not reduce the induction of plasma IgE concentration in males, but tended to reduce it by ~2-fold in females. However, this reduction in plasma IgE did not modify the inflammatory response in OVA/OVA-treated *Arg1*-deficient lungs. OVA/OVA-treated BALB/c female mice further have higher lung concentrations of IL-4, IL-5, IL-10, IL-13, IFN-γ, and TNF-α protein [4, 6, 61] than male BALB/c mice, but we observed similar IL-4, IL-13, IL10, CCL11, TNFα, and IFNγ concentrations in OVA/OVA-treated male and female C57BL/6 mice. It is well-recognized that C57BL/6 and BALB/C mice differ in their response to OVA/OVA treatment [62, 63].

OVA/OVA-treated Arg1-Con females accumulated ~3-fold more *Arg1* mRNA than similarly treated males, without showing different numbers of arginase1-positive macrophages in the lung. As far as we are aware, a sex difference in macrophage *Arg1* mRNA and protein expression in OVA/OVA-treated mice has not yet been reported. Furthermore, the expression of *Il4, Il13* and, to a lesser extent, *Il5* was affected by *Arg1* deletion in female mice only, suggesting a sex difference in the expression of M2 cytokines in OVA/OVA-treated mice. In Coxsackie virus-induced myocarditis, the ~4-fold higher *Arg1* expression in macrophages of female over male mice was attributed to skewing of the macrophage polarization towards an M2 phenotype in females, and towards an M1 phenotype in males [64]. Depending on the inducing agent, alveolar macrophages can also develop an M1, M2, or even an intermediate phenotype [13]. These sex difference may arise because female steroid hormones promote alternative activation of macrophages, whereas testosterone inhibits the M2 phenotype [65, 66].

We also studied whether there were sex differences in the coordination of the responses to OVA/OVA treatment (Additional file 2: Figure S1). Adaptive changes in methacholine responsiveness and mRNA expression (except the M1-macrophage markers *Ifng* and, to a lesser extent, *Tnfa*) correlated more strongly within their category in females than in males, whereas, as already discussed, IL-4, IL-13, IL-5, CCL11, and TNFα protein concentrations correlated better with the corresponding mRNA concentrations and with lung function parameters H and G in males. These data imply that the respiratory responses to OVA/OVA treatment were less integrated with the inflammatory responses in female than in male mice.

Conclusion

Complete ablation of *Arg1* in the lung does not affect methacholine responsiveness or the invasion of inflammatory cells, but does change the gene-expression profile of these cells in OVA/OVA-treated female mice. Since the asthmatic responses in mice and humans show similar sex-related differences, and since ablation of *Arg1* did improve peripheral lung function in male mice only, we hypothesize that treatment of asthma by modulating arginase activity in the lung will primarily benefit male patients.

Additional files

Additional file 1: Tables S1-S3. Table S1. Primers pairs used in genotyping and quantitative PCR. **Table S2.** Amino-acid concentrations in venous plasma (μM ± SEM) of Arg1-Con and Arg1-KO^{Tie2Cre} mice *: $P < 0.05$ OVA/OVA vs. PBS/OVA Arg1-Con; #: $P < 0.05$ OVA/OVA vs. PBS/OVA Arg1-KO^{Tie2}. **Table S3.** Differences between male and female Arg1-Con mice after treatment with the OVA/OVA protocol.

Additional file 2: Figure S1. Correlation of lung-function, abundance of pulmonary mRNAs and proteins, pulmonary histopathology, and concentrations of plasma amino acids in wild-type male and female mice. The lower-left triangle refers to data obtained female and the upper-right triangle to data from male Arg1-Con mice. The numbers show the correlation coefficients between parameters indicated above and to the left of the columns and rows, respectively, as measured in all 15 or 16 male and female Arg1-Con mice studied, that is, both the PBS/OVA- and the OVA/OVA-treated groups. The significance of the correlations is color-coded according to the *P*-value of the correlation coefficient: yellow: $0.05 > P > 0.01$, orange: $0.01 > P > 0.001$, and red: $P < 0.001$. Note the difference in the degree of cross-correlations of parameters between the categories named in the title in males and females.

Abbreviations

AHR: airway hyperresponsiveness; ARG1, *Arg1*: arginase 1 protein or *gene*; Arg1-Con: *Arg$^{fl/fl}$/LysM-Cre$^{-/-}$* or *Arg$^{fl/fl}$/Tie2-Cre$^{-/-}$* control littermates; Arg1-KO^{LysM} or Arg1-KO^{Tie2} : *Arg$^{fl/fl}$/LysM-Cre$^{tg/-}$* or *Arg$^{fl/fl}$/Tie2-Cre$^{tg/-}$* tissue-specific knockout mice; *Arg2*: arginase 2 gene; *Cat2*: cationic amino acid transporter aka *Slc7a2*; *Ccl11*: C-C motif chemokine 11, aka *eotaxin-1*; *Ccl2*: C-C-motif chemokine ligand 2; *Clca3*: chloride channel accessory 3; G: tissue resistance; H: tissue elastance; H&E: hematoxylin & eosin; IFNγ, *Ifng*: interferon gamma; IgE: immunoglobulin E; IL10: interleukin 10; IL13: interleukin 13; IL4: interleukin 4; IL5: interleukin 5; MBP: major basic protein; MPO: myeloperoxidase; *Muc5ac*: mucin 5 ac; NOS2: nitric oxide synthase; OVA: ovalbumin; OVA/OVA: ovalbumin-sensitized and challenged; PBS/OVA: mock-sensitized and ovalbumin-challenged; R_N: Newtonian airflow resistance; RT: room temperature; *Slc7a1*: solute carrier family 7 member 1, aka as *Cat1*; *Slc7a2*: solute carrier family 7 member 2, aka as *Cat2*; *Slc7a7*: solute carrier family 7 member 7; TNFα, *Tfna*: tumour necrosis factor alpha

Acknowledgements
Not applicable

Funding
This study was supported by a grant from the Transnational University Limburg, the Netherlands, 31,962,140 T. The funding body had no role in the design of the study, data collection, analysis, interpretation, or writing of the manuscript.

Authors' contributions
RC and SS participated in the design of the study, data acquisition, statistical analysis, and drafting of the manuscript. MP participated in acquisition of the data and reviewing the drafted manuscript. ET and PvD participated in acquisition of the data and technical support. WL and EK conceived of the study, and participated in its design and coordination and helped to draft the manuscript. All authors read and approved the final manuscript.

Ethics approval
All animal experiments were approved by the Committee for Animal Care and Use of Maastricht University (DEC 2055-146).

Consent for publication
Not applicable

Competing interests
The authors declare that they have no competing interests.

Author details
Department of Anatomy & Embryology and NUTRIM School of Nutrition and Translational Research in Metabolism, Maastricht University, P.O. Box 616, 6200, MD, Maastricht, The Netherlands. [2]Tytgat Institute for Liver and Intestinal Research, Academic Medical Center, Amsterdam, The Netherlands. [3]Division of Pulmonary Disease and Critical Care, Department of Medicine, College of Medicine, University of Vermont, Burlington, VT, USA.

References
1. Bousquet J, Jeffery PK, Busse WW, Johnson M, Vignola AM. Asthma. From bronchoconstriction to airways inflammation and remodeling. Am J Respir Crit Care Med. 2000;161(5):1720–45.
2. Busse WW, Lemanske RF Jr. Asthma. N Engl J Med. 2001;344(5):350–62.
3. Sathish V, Martin YN, Prakash YS. Sex steroid signaling: implications for lung diseases. Pharmacol Ther. 2015;150:94–108.
4. Melgert BN, Postma DS, Kuipers I, Geerlings M, Luinge MA, van der Strate BW, Kerstjens HA, Timens W, Hylkema MN. Female mice are more susceptible to the development of allergic airway inflammation than male mice. Clin Exp Allergy. 2005;35(11):1496–503.
5. Riffo-Vasquez Y, Ligeiro de Oliveira AP, Page CP, Spina D, Tavares-de-Lima W. Role of sex hormones in allergic inflammation in mice. Clin Exp Allergy. 2007;37(3):459–70.
6. Blacquiere MJ, Hylkema MN, Postma DS, Geerlings M, Timens W, Melgert BN. Airway inflammation and remodeling in two mouse models of asthma: comparison of males and females. Int Arch Allergy Immunol. 2010;153(2):173–81.
7. Card JW, Carey MA, Bradbury JA, DeGraff LM, Morgan DL, Moorman MP, Flake GP, Zeldin DC. Gender differences in murine airway responsiveness and lipopolysaccharide-induced inflammation. J Immunol. 2006;177(1):621–30.

8. Matsubara S, Swasey CH, Loader JE, Dakhama A, Joetham A, Ohnishi H, Balhorn A, Miyahara N, Takeda K, Gelfand EW. Estrogen determines sex differences in airway responsiveness after allergen exposure. Am J Respir Cell Mol Biol. 2008;38(5):501–8.
9. Hellings PW, Vandekerckhove P, Claeys R, Billen J, Kasran A, Ceuppens JL. Progesterone increases airway eosinophilia and hyper-responsiveness in a murine model of allergic asthma. Clin Exp Allergy. 2003;33(10):1457–63.
10. Carey MA, Card JW, Bradbury JA, Moorman MP, Haykal-Coates N, Gavett SH, Graves JP, Walker VR, Flake GP, Voltz JW, et al. Spontaneous airway hyperresponsiveness in estrogen receptor-alpha-deficient mice. Am J Respir Crit Care Med. 2007;175(2):126–35.
11. Dimitropoulou C, Drakopanagiotakis F, Chatterjee A, Snead C, Catravas JD. Estrogen replacement therapy prevents airway dysfunction in a murine model of allergen-induced asthma. Lung. 2009;187(2):116–27.
12. Bosse Y. Endocrine regulation of airway contractility is overlooked. J Endocrinol. 2014;222(2):R61–73.
13. Katsura Y, Harada N, Harada S, Ishimori A, Makino F, Ito J, Kamachi F, Okumura K, Akiba H, Atsuta R, et al. Characteristics of alveolar macrophages from murine models of OVA-induced allergic airway inflammation and LPS-induced acute airway inflammation. Exp Lung Res. 2015;41(7):370–82.
14. Melgert BN, Oriss TB, Qi Z, Dixon-McCarthy B, Geerlings M, Hylkema MN, Ray A. Macrophages: regulators of sex differences in asthma? Am J Respir Cell Mol Biol. 2010;42(5):595–603.
15. Munder M. Arginase: an emerging key player in the mammalian immune system. Br J Pharmacol. 2009;158(3):638–51.
16. Zimmermann N, King NE, Laporte J, Yang M, Mishra A, Pope SM, Muntel EE, Witte DP, Pegg AA, Foster PS, et al. Dissection of experimental asthma with DNA microarray analysis identifies arginase in asthma pathogenesis. J Clin Invest. 2003;111(12):1863–74.
17. Takemoto K, Ogino K, Shibamori M, Gondo T, Hitomi Y, Takigawa T, Wang DH, Takaki J, Ichimura H, Fujikura Y, et al. Transiently, paralleled upregulation of arginase and nitric oxide synthase and the effect of both enzymes on the pathology of asthma. Am J Physiol Lung Cell Mol Physiol. 2007;293(6):L1419–26.
18. Morris CR, Poljakovic M, Lavrisha L, Machado L, Kuypers FA, Morris SM Jr. Decreased arginine bioavailability and increased serum arginase activity in asthma. Am J Respir Crit Care Med. 2004;170(2):148–53.
19. Mabalirajan U, Ahmad T, Leishangthem GD, Joseph DA, Dinda AK, Agrawal A, Ghosh B. Beneficial effects of high dose of L-arginine on airway hyperresponsiveness and airway inflammation in a murine model of asthma. J Allergy Clin Immunol. 2010;125(3):626–35.
20. Benson RC, Hardy KA, Morris CR. Arginase and arginine dysregulation in asthma. J Allergy (Cairo). 2011;2011:736319.
21. Akata K, Yatera K, Wang KY, Naito K, Ogoshi T, Noguchi S, Kido T, Toyohira Y, Shimokawa H, Yanagihara N, et al. Decreased bronchial Eosinophilic inflammation and mucus Hypersecretion in asthmatic mice lacking all nitric oxide Synthase Isoforms. Lung. 2016;194(1):121–4.
22. Naura AS, Zerfaoui M, Kim H, Abd Elmageed ZY, Rodriguez PC, Hans CP, Ju J, Errami Y, Park J, Ochoa AC, et al. Requirement for inducible nitric oxide synthase in chronic allergen exposure-induced pulmonary fibrosis but not inflammation. J Immunol. 2010;185(5):3076–85.
23. Bratt JM, Franzi LM, Linderholm AL, O'Roark EM, Kenyon NJ, Last JA. Arginase inhibition in airways from normal and nitric oxide synthase 2-knockout mice exposed to ovalbumin. Toxicol Appl Pharmacol. 2010;242(1):1–8.
24. Rothenberg ME, Doepker MP, Lewkowich IP, Chiaramonte MG, Stringer KF, Finkelman FD, MacLeod CL, Ellies LG, Zimmermann N. Cationic amino acid transporter 2 regulates inflammatory homeostasis in the lung. Proc Natl Acad Sci U S A. 2006;103(40):14895–900.
25. Hammermann R, Hirschmann J, Hey C, Mossner J, Folkerts G, Nijkamp FP, Wessler I, Racke K. Cationic proteins inhibit L-arginine uptake in rat alveolar macrophages and tracheal epithelial cells. Implications for nitric oxide synthesis. Am J Respir Cell Mol Biol. 1999;21(2):155–62.
26. Ckless K, Lampert A, Reiss J, Kasahara D, Poynter ME, Irvin CG, Lundblad LK, Norton R, van der Vliet A, Janssen-Heininger YM. Inhibition of arginase activity enhances inflammation in mice with allergic airway disease, in association with increases in protein S-nitrosylation and tyrosine nitration. J Immunol. 2008;181(6):4255–64.
27. North ML, Khanna N, Marsden PA, Grasemann H, Scott JA. Functionally important role for arginase 1 in the airway hyperresponsiveness of asthma. Am J Physiol Lung Cell Mol Physiol. 2009;296(6):L911–20.
28. Ogino K, Kubo M, Takahashi H, Zhang R, Zou Y, Fujikura Y. Anti-inflammatory effect of arginase inhibitor and corticosteroid on airway allergic reactions in a Dermatophogoides farinae-induced NC/Nga mouse model. Inflammation. 2013;36(1):141–51.
29. Takahashi N, Ogino K, Takemoto K, Hamanishi S, Wang DH, Takigawa T, Shibamori M, Ishiyama H, Fujikura Y. Direct inhibition of arginase attenuated airway allergic reactions and inflammation in a Dermatophagoides farinae-induced NC/Nga mouse model. Am J Physiol Lung Cell Mol Physiol. 2010; 299(1):L17–24.
30. Meurs H, McKay S, Maarsingh H, Hamer MA, Macic L, Molendijk N, Zaagsma J. Increased arginase activity underlies allergen induced deficiency of cNOS derived nitric oxide and airway hyperresponsiveness. Br J Pharmacol. 2002; 136(3):391–8.
31. Arikan-Ayyildiz Z, Karaman M, Tuncel T, Kiray M, Bagriyanik A, Yilmaz O, Uzuner N, Karaman O. Beneficial effects of arginase inhibition and inhaled L-arginine administration on airway histology in a murine model of chronic asthma. Allergol Immunopathol (Madr). 2014;42(4):316–23.
32. Zhang R, Kubo M, Murakami I, Setiawan H, Takemoto K, Inoue K, Fujikura Y, Ogino K. L-Arginine administration attenuates airway inflammation by altering l-arginine metabolism in an NC/Nga mouse model of asthma. J Clin Biochem Nutr. 2015;56(3):201–7.
33. Cloots RH, Sankaranarayanan S, de Theije CC, Poynter ME, Terwindt E, van Dijk P, Hakvoort TB, Lamers WH, Kohler SE. Ablation of Arg1 in hematopoietic cells improves respiratory function of lung parenchyma, but not that of larger airways or inflammation in asthmatic mice. Am J Physiol Lung Cell Mol Physiol. 2013;305(5):L364–76.
34. Barron L, Smith AM, El Kasmi KC, Qualls JE, Huang X, Cheever A, Borthwick LA, Wilson MS, Murray PJ, Wynn TA. Role of arginase 1 from myeloid cells in th2-dominated lung inflammation. PLoS One. 2013;8(4):e61961.
35. Clausen BE, Burkhardt C, Reith W, Renkawitz R, Forster I. Conditional gene targeting in macrophages and granulocytes using LysMcre mice. Transgenic Res. 1999;8(4):265–77.
36. Kisanuki YY, Hammer RE, Miyazaki J, Williams SC, Richardson JA, Yanagisawa M. Tie2-Cre transgenic mice: a new model for endothelial cell-lineage analysis in vivo. Dev Biol. 2001;230(2):230–42.
37. Ruijter JM, Thygesen HH, Schoneveld OJ, Das AT, Berkhout B, Lamers WH. Factor correction as a tool to eliminate between-session variation in replicate experiments: application to molecular biology and retrovirology. Retrovirology. 2006;3:2.
38. Schlaeger TM, Mikkola HK, Gekas C, Helgadottir HB, Orkin SH. Tie2Cre-mediated gene ablation defines the stem-cell leukemia gene (SCL/tal1)-dependent window during hematopoietic stem-cell development. Blood. 2005;105(10):3871–4.
39. Koni PA, Joshi SK, Temann UA, Olson D, Burkly L, Flavell RA. Conditional vascular cell adhesion molecule 1 deletion in mice: impaired lymphocyte migration to bone marrow. J Exp Med. 2001;193(6):741–54.
40. Hamada K, Sasaki T, Koni PA, Natsui M, Kishimoto H, Sasaki J, Yajima N, Horie Y, Hasegawa G, Naito M, et al. The PTEN/PI3K pathway governs normal vascular development and tumor angiogenesis. Genes Dev. 2005; 19(17):2054–65.
41. Van den Bossche J, Lamers WH, Koehler ES, Geuns JM, Alhonen L, Uimari A, Pirnes-Karhu S, Van Overmeire E, Morias Y, Brys L, et al. Pivotal advance: Arginase-1-independent polyamine production stimulates the expression of IL-4-induced alternatively activated macrophage markers while inhibiting LPS-induced expression of inflammatory genes. J Leukoc Biol. 2012;91(5): 685–99.
42. Lee J, Ryu H, Ferrante RJ, Morris SM Jr, Ratan RR. Translational control of inducible nitric oxide synthase expression by arginine can explain the arginine paradox. Proc Natl Acad Sci U S A. 2003;100(8):4843–8.
43. Choi S, Park C, Ahn M, Lee JH, Shin T. Immunohistochemical study of arginase 1 and 2 in various tissues of rats. Acta Histochem. 2012;114(5):487–94.
44. Hochstedler CM, Leidinger MR, Maher-Sturm MT, Gibson-Corley KN, Meyerholz DK. Immunohistochemical detection of arginase-I expression in formalin-fixed lung and other tissues. J Histotechnol. 2013;36(4):128–34.
45. Zeki AA, Bratt JM, Rabowsky M, Last JA, Kenyon NJ. Simvastatin inhibits goblet cell hyperplasia and lung arginase in a mouse model of allergic asthma: a novel treatment for airway remodeling? Transl Res. 2010;156(6): 335–49.
46. North ML, Amatullah H, Khanna N, Urch B, Grasemann H, Silverman F, Scott JA. Augmentation of arginase 1 expression by exposure to air pollution exacerbates the airways hyperresponsiveness in murine models of asthma. Respir Res. 2011;12:19.

47. Xu W, Ghosh S, Comhair SA, Asosingh K, Janocha AJ, Mavrakis DA, Bennett CD, Gruca LL, Graham BB, Queisser KA, et al. Increased mitochondrial arginine metabolism supports bioenergetics in asthma. J Clin Invest. 2016; 126(7):2465–81.
48. Gordy C, Pua H, Sempowski GD, He YW. Regulation of steady-state neutrophil homeostasis by macrophages. Blood. 2011;117(2):618–29.
49. Jakubzick C, Bogunovic M, Bonito AJ, Kuan EL, Merad M, Randolph GJ. Lymph-migrating, tissue-derived dendritic cells are minor constituents within steady-state lymph nodes. J Exp Med. 2008;205(12):2839–50.
50. Zhang Z, Zhang F, An P, Guo X, Shen Y, Tao Y, Wu Q, Zhang Y, Yu Y, Ning B, et al. Ferroportin1 deficiency in mouse macrophages impairs iron homeostasis and inflammatory responses. Blood. 2011;118(7):1912–22.
51. Bates JH, Rincon M, Irvin CG. Animal models of asthma. Am J Physiol Lung Cell Mol Physiol. 2009;297(3):L401–10.
52. Lundblad LK, Rinaldi LM, Poynter ME, Riesenfeld EP, Wu M, Aimi S, Barone LM, Bates JH, Irvin CG. Detrimental effects of albuterol on airway responsiveness requires airway inflammation and is independent of beta-receptor affinity in murine models of asthma. Respir Res. 2011;12:27.
53. Niese KA, Collier AR, Hajek AR, Cederbaum SD, O'Brien WE, Wills-Karp M, Rothenberg ME, Zimmermann N. Bone marrow cell derived arginase I is the major source of allergen-induced lung arginase but is not required for airway hyperresponsiveness, remodeling and lung inflammatory responses in mice. BMC Immunol. 2009;10:33.
54. Xiong Y, Karupiah G, Hogan SP, Foster PS, Ramsay AJ. Inhibition of allergic airway inflammation in mice lacking nitric oxide synthase 2. J Immunol. 1999;162(1):445–52.
55. Boer J, Duyvendak M, Schuurman FE, Pouw FM, Zaagsma J, Meurs H. Role of L-arginine in the deficiency of nitric oxide and airway hyperreactivity after the allergen-induced early asthmatic reaction in guinea-pigs. Br J Pharmacol. 1999;128(5):1114–20.
56. Scott JA, North ML, Rafii M, Huang H, Pencharz P, Grasemann H. Plasma arginine metabolites reflect airway dysfunction in a murine model of allergic airway inflammation. J Appl Physiol (1985). 2015;118(10):1229–33.
57. Wijnands KA, Vink H, Briede JJ, van Faassen EE, Lamers WH, Buurman WA, Poeze M. Citrulline a more suitable substrate than arginine to restore NO production and the microcirculation during endotoxemia. PLoS One. 2012; 7(5):e37439.
58. Rattenbacher B, Bohjanen PR. Evaluating posttranscriptional regulation of cytokine genes. Methods Mol Biol. 2012;820:71–89.
59. Marion V, Sankaranarayanan S, de Theije C, van Dijk P, Lindsey P, Lamers MC, Harding HP, Ron D, Lamers WH, Kohler SE. Arginine deficiency causes runting in the suckling period by selectively activating the stress kinase GCN2. J Biol Chem. 2011;286(11):8866–74.
60. Postma DS. Gender differences in asthma development and progression. Gend Med. 2007;4 Suppl B:S133–46.
61. Hayashi T, Adachi Y, Hasegawa K, Morimoto M. Less sensitivity for late airway inflammation in males than females in BALB/c mice. Scand J Immunol. 2003;57(6):562–7.
62. Takeda K, Haczku A, Lee JJ, Irvin CG, Gelfand EW. Strain dependence of airway hyperresponsiveness reflects differences in eosinophil localization in the lung. Am J Physiol Lung Cell Mol Physiol. 2001;281(2):L394–402.
63. Gueders MM, Paulissen G, Crahay C, Quesada-Calvo F, Hacha J, Van Hove C, Tournoy K, Louis R, Foidart JM, Noel A, et al. Mouse models of asthma: a comparison between C57BL/6 and BALB/c strains regarding bronchial responsiveness, inflammation, and cytokine production. Inflamm Res. 2009; 58(12):845–54.
64. Ahmad T, Mabalirajan U, Ghosh B, Agrawal A. Altered asymmetric dimethyl arginine metabolism in allergically inflamed mouse lungs. Am J Respir Cell Mol Biol. 2010;42(1):3–8.
65. Routley CE, Ashcroft GS. Effect of estrogen and progesterone on macrophage activation during wound healing. Wound Repair Regen. 2009; 17(1):42–50.
66. Frisancho-Kiss S, Coronado MJ, Frisancho JA, Lau VM, Rose NR, Klein SL, Fairweather D. Gonadectomy of male BALB/c mice increases Tim-3(+) alternatively activated M2 macrophages, Tim-3(+) T cells, Th2 cells and Treg in the heart during acute coxsackievirus-induced myocarditis. Brain Behav Immun. 2009;23(5):649–57.

6

Effects of treatment changes on asthma phenotype prevalence and airway neutrophil function

Collin R. Brooks[1*], Christine J. Van Dalen[1], Elizabeth Harding[1], Ian F. Hermans[2] and Jeroen Douwes[1]

Abstract

Background: Asthma inflammatory phenotypes are often defined by relative cell counts of airway eosinophils/neutrophils. However, the importance of neutrophilia remains unclear, as does the effect of ICS treatment on asthma phenotypes and airway neutrophil function. The purpose of this study was to assess asthma phenotype prevalence/characteristics in a community setting, and, in a nested preliminary study, determine how treatment changes affect phenotype stability and inflammation, with particular focus on airway neutrophils.

Methods: Fifty adult asthmatics and 39 non-asthmatics were assessed using questionnaires, skin prick tests, spirometry, exhaled nitric oxide (FENO) measurement, and sputum induction. Twenty-one asthmatics underwent further assessment following treatment optimisation ($n = 11$) or sub-optimisation ($n = 10$).

Results: Forty percent (20/50) had eosinophilic asthma (EA) and 8% had neutrophilic asthma. EA was associated with increased FENO, bronchodilator reversibility (BDR) and reduced lung function ($p < 0.05$). Following optimisation/sub-optimisation, the EA/NEA (non-eosinophilic asthma) phenotype changed in 11/21 (52%) asthmatics. In particular, fewer subjects had EA post treatment optimisation, but this was not statistically significant. However, a significant ($p < 0.05$) reduction in FENO, ACQ7 score, and BDR was observed after treatment optimisation, as well as an increase in FEV_1-% predicted ($p < 0.05$). It was also associated with reduced eosinophils ($p < 0.05$) and enhanced neutrophil phagocytosis ($p < 0.05$) in EA only, and enhanced neutrophil oxidative burst in both EA and NEA ($p < 0.05$).

Conclusions: In this community based population, non-eosinophilic asthma was common, less severe than EA, and at baseline most asthmatics showed no evidence of inflammation. In the nested change in treatment study, treatment optimisation was associated with reduced sputum eosinophils, improved symptoms and lung function, and enhanced neutrophil function, but a significant reduction in EA could not be demonstrated.

Keywords: Asthma, Inflammatory phenotype, Induced sputum, Neutrophils, Eosinophils

* Correspondence: C.R.Brooks@massey.ac.nz
[1]Centre for Public Health Research, Massey University Wellington Campus, Private Box 756, Wellington 6140, New Zealand
Full list of author information is available at the end of the article

Background

Airway inflammation is a defining feature of asthma, often associated with eosinophilic, TH2-mediated immunopathology [1]. However, asthma may occur in the absence of airway eosinophils in approximately 50% of cases [2]. Non-eosinophilic asthma (NEA) can be observed across the spectrum of severity, is associated with distinct pathological features [3] and appears less responsive to inhaled corticosteroids (ICS) [4]. Identification and further characterisation of inflammatory asthma phenotypes may therefore help guide asthma treatment and contribute to novel treatment options for corticosteroid resistant asthma.

Non-eosinophilic asthma may be the result of neutrophilic airway inflammation [2], associated with microbial and/or other irritant exposures. In support, some studies of NEA have reported increased sputum neutrophils, levels of neutrophil-associated mediators, and bacterial endotoxin [5–8]. However, other studies in adults and children have shown little evidence of neutrophilic inflammation in NEA [3, 4]. Neutrophilic asthma (NA) may therefore only be important in a proportion of NEA, and possibly only in some populations.

Initial studies suggested that inflammatory asthma phenotypes are stable [5, 9], although recent reports suggest that temporal changes may be common [10–12]. ICS treatment in particular may affect inflammatory phenotype through a reduction in sputum eosinophils and an increase in neutrophils [10]. Moreover, neutrophils may play a role in poorly controlled asthma, as observed in adults undergoing exacerbation [13]. Nonetheless, effects of asthma control and ICS treatment on inflammatory phenotypes are often not taken into account with most studies assessing airway inflammation only once, and mostly during periods of stable asthma. In addition, many studies have been conducted in hospital settings, in which asthma is likely to be treated with high ICS doses [9]. This may have led to an underestimation of the prevalence of EA in previous studies. Also, assessment of airway inflammation has often not involved methods such as flow cytometry [14], which allow improved definition of inflammatory mechanisms and assessment of the functional status of airway leukocytes, such as neutrophils. Whilst a previous study has suggested that airway neutrophil numbers increase with ICS treatment [10], the effects on airway neutrophil oxidative burst and phagocytosis (which may be associated with effective clearance of debris and dying cells in the airways) [15] has not previously been examined.

In this community based study, we assessed the prevalence and characteristics of inflammatory asthma phenotypes in a general adult population sample. In a preliminary study conducted in a subset of asthmatics, we also examined phenotype stability, and changes in clinical and inflammatory parameters including neutrophil numbers and function (using flow cytometry) following changes in treatment.

Methods

Study population

To obtain a reasonably representative sample of asthmatics we recruited 53 asthmatics and 44 non-asthmatics, aged 17–65, by newspaper advertisement and posters in general practice clinics. As is common for population-based asthma studies, asthmatics were defined on the basis of having both been diagnosed with asthma by a physician and having had wheeze in the last 12 months (with no additional criteria regarding bronchial hyperreactivity, asthma control or lung function results) [14, 16–18]. Non-asthmatics were defined as having had no previous or current asthma diagnosis, no history of wheeze or nocturnal cough in the last 12 months, and forced expiratory volume in 1 s (FEV_1) > 75% predicted. As respiratory infection is associated with airway neutrophilia, participants who had symptoms or evidence of either upper or lower respiratory infection within four weeks prior to assessment were asked to return at a later date. All participants underwent a respiratory health questionnaire and hypertonic saline sputum induction test. Asthma control status was based on asthma control questionnaire (ACQ) 7 score [19], and as the majority of asthmatics were using inhaled corticosteroids at the time of assessment, was used in preference to asthma severity (as advocated by the Global Initiative for Asthma) [20]. Eighty-nine subjects (91.8%) successfully produced sputum and were included in data analyses examining phenotype prevalence and characteristics (referred to in the remainder of this paper as the "prevalence study"). In a preliminary study of a subset of asthmatics we examined the effects of treatment alterations on phenotype stability, inflammation and neutrophil function, referred to as the "CIT (change in treatment) study" (Figure 1). The CIT study included "only" 27 asthmatics as many were uncomfortable with changing their ICS use/asthma control due to the risk of exacerbations. The study was approved by the Upper South A and Lower South Regional Ethics Committee, New Zealand. All subjects gave written informed consent. The CIT study has retrospective registration at the Australia and New Zealand Clinical Trials Registry (ANZCTR), number 12617001356358.

Change in treatment study

Twenty-seven randomly selected asthmatics (who stated at initial assessment that they were amenable to asthma treatment change) were included in the CIT study. Participants were interviewed and asked to record morning and evening peak expiratory flow (PEF) using a Vitalograph

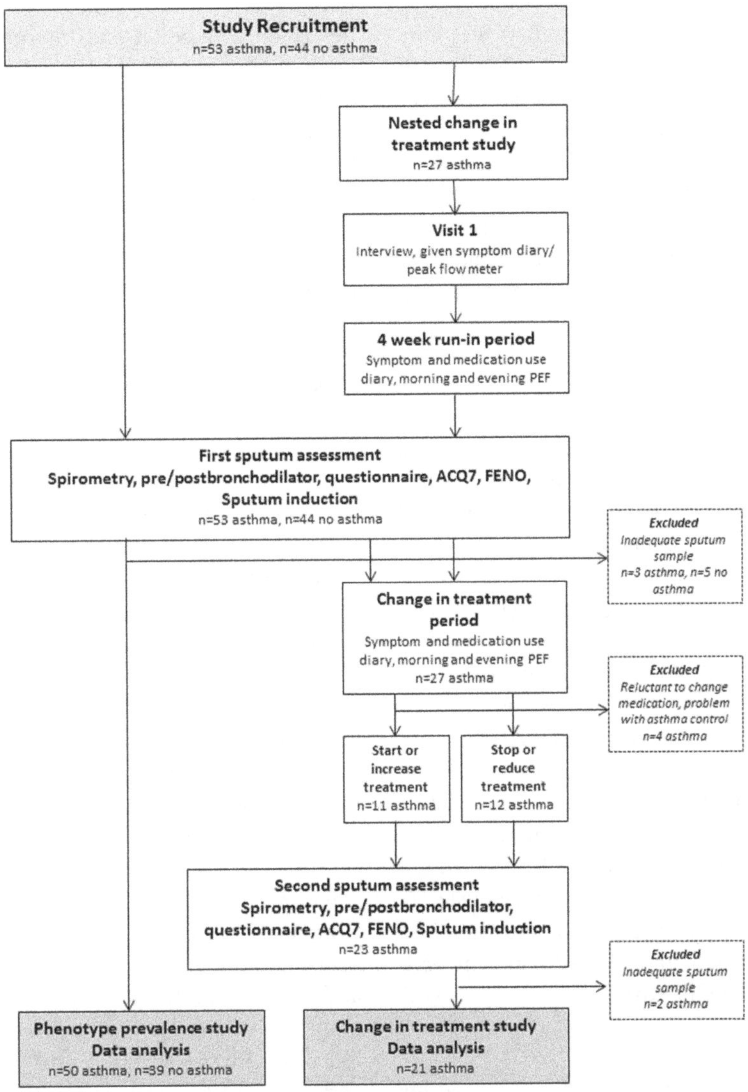

Fig. 1 Study plan flow chart. Recruitment of participants, and the assessments involved in the phenotype prevalence and change in treatment components of the study

asmaPLAN (Bucks, UK) peak flow meter, and symptoms and medication use over a 4 week 'run-in' period, after which they returned for assessment. Asthma control status was based on ACQ-7 score, PEF and symptom diary. Four subjects left the study as they were subsequently reluctant to change asthma treatment, or had difficulty maintaining asthma control. A change in treatment was made on an individual basis for the remaining 23 subjects by a clinician according to the National Asthma Education and Prevention Program (NAEPP) Expert Panel Report 3 (EPR 3) guidelines [21]. Subjects with adequately controlled asthma had their treatment sub-optimised to a reduced dose of ICS ($n = 6$) or to no ICS ($n = 6$). Subjects with inadequately controlled asthma had their treatment optimised, and either commenced ICS ($n = 5$) or increased ICS dose ($n = 6$). All participants used short-acting beta-agonists (SABA) as required. Changes in treatment (including long-acting beta-agonists (LABA)) for CIT participants are shown in Additional file 1: Table S1.

Subjects returned for a second assessment with a repeat of all previous tests after 4–6 weeks, similar to previous studies assessing the effects of change in treatment on asthma inflammatory phenotypes [10, 11] (Figure 1). Those undergoing treatment sub-optimisation followed a defined safety protocol (see Additional file 1) and asthma treatment was readjusted according to asthma control prior to discharge from the study. Two subjects undergoing treatment sub-optimisation were excluded from CIT study analyses as they were unable to provide an adequate sputum sample at the second assessment.

Clinical assessment

Skin prick testing (to determine atopy status) was conducted as described in Additional file 1. Spirometric measurements were conducted for all participants according to American Thoracic Society (ATS) criteria [22] using an EasyOne spirometer (NDD Medizintechnik AG, Zurich, Switzerland). NHANES III equations were used for lung function parameters. Exhaled nitric oxide (FENO) measurements were conducted at 50mls/s according to ATS/ERS guidelines [23] using a Hypair FENO analyser (Medisoft, Sorinnes, Belgium).

Sputum induction

Sputum induction using hypertonic saline and sample processing was conducted as described previously [6] (Additional file 1). Supernatants and cell suspensions were used for subsequent tests, including differential cell counts by light microscopy. Asthmatics with ≥2% eosinophils were classified as EA; those who also had ≥61% neutrophils were classified as mixed granulocytic asthma (MGA). Asthmatics with <2% eosinophils were classified as NEA; those who also had ≥61% neutrophils were classified neutrophilic asthma (NA) and those with <61% neutrophils as paucigranulocytic asthma (PGA) [5].

Measurement of sputum supernatant IL-8 and MMP-9 levels was conducted using sandwich ELISA, and bacterial endotoxin was measured using the Limulus amebocyte assay, as described previously [7]. Neutrophil elastase (NE) was measured as described previously [7] but was undetectable in >90% of samples, and therefore reported as undetected/detected. Endotoxin and NE were only measured in the CIT study.

Flow cytometry

For the CIT study, remaining sputum cells were used for flow cytometry according to the protocol described in Additional file 1. For neutrophil respiratory burst measurement (paired samples available for seven asthmatics), data were expressed as the percentage of dihydrorhodamine (DHR) 123 (Molecular Probes, Eugene, OR) positive neutrophils after phorbol 12-myristate 13-acetate (PMA, Sigma-Aldrich) stimulation minus negative control. For phagocytosis measurement (paired samples available for 16 asthmatics) data were presented as the percentage of opsonized Texas Red-labelled zymosan A microbeads (Molecular Probes) positive neutrophils after incubation at 37 °C minus percentage bead positive neutrophils in a background control sample. All cell aliquots were also washed and antibody labelled to identify neutrophils by flow cytometry as described previously [14].

Statistical analysis

Data analyses were performed using STATA version 11.0 (STATA Corp, College Station, TX, USA) and Prism 5 (Graphpad Software Inc., La Jolla, CA, USA). Data are described as median and interquartile ranges (IQR) unless otherwise stated. Univariate analyses were conducted using either student's t-test or Pearson's correlation (parametric data), or Mann-Whitney u-testing or Spearman's correlation (non-parametric data). For the prevalence study, asthmatics were grouped according to either the EA/PGA/NA/MGA or EA/NEA classifications described above to allow comparison with previous studies [2, 5, 10, 11]. For the CIT study, data were initially analysed separately for asthmatics undergoing an increase in treatment ($n = 11$) and asthmatics undergoing a decrease in treatment ($n = 10$). Subsequently, data were combined to increase power and allow comparison of the two visits for all CIT participants when considered as sub-optimised/optimised ($n = 21$). As it has been suggested that EA and NEA have distinct pathologies and response to ICS [3, 4], and that neutrophils may be particularly important in NEA [2], additional analyses were conducted to assess differences associated with CIT in asthmatics characterised as EA/NEA (EA defined as having 2% or greater sputum eosinophils at either assessment). Data were analysed using the paired t-test or Wilcoxon's matched pairs test as appropriate. Fisher's exact test was used for categorical data, and Kruskal-Wallis with Dunn's post-test analysis was used for multiple group comparison.

Results

Compared with non-asthmatics, asthmatics had higher sputum eosinophil relative cell counts ($p < 0.0001$) and FENO levels ($p = 0.01$), were more likely to be atopic ($p < 0.0001$), had greater bronchodilator reversibility (BDR; $p = 0.0007$), and lower FEV_1-% predicted and FEV_1/FVC (both $p < 0.005$) (Table 1). Forty percent of asthmatics were classified as EA and 60% NEA, of which 8% were NA and 52% were PGA; none were classified as MGA. EA was associated with reduced lung function, increased FENO and BDR, and poorer ACQ7 scores; (all $p < 0.05$) compared to PGA (Table 1) or all NEA (data not shown). Eosinophilia correlated with FENO ($r = 0.74$; $p < 0.0001$). With the exception of increased eosinophils in the EA group and increased neutrophils in the NA group (due to phenotype classification), few differences in inflammatory parameters between phenotypes were observed (Table 1). In asthmatics, airway neutrophils were correlated with IL-8 and MMP-9 ($p = 0.02$–0.002; data not shown), but no associations between neutrophils and clinical parameters such as FEV_1-% predicted, FEV_1/FVC, BDR or ACQ-7 score (all $p > 0.1$) were observed.

Following treatment optimisation in the nested preliminary CIT study, fewer asthmatics were classified as EA i.e. of the 11 subjects, EA prevalence reduced from 9

Table 1 Clinical characteristics and sputum sample inflammatory characteristics of all participants at baseline

	Neutrophilic asthma (NA)	Paucigranulocytic asthma (PGA)	Eosinophilic asthma (EA)	All asthma	No asthma
Number (% of asthma)	4 (8%)	26 (52%)	20 (40%)	50	39
Sex (female)	4 (100%)	17 (68%)	8 (40%)	30 (60%)	27 (69.2%)
Age	60.5 (40.5–64)	35 (26–47.5)	33.5 (27–43)	35.5 (27–51.8)	37 (27–47)
Atopy	3 (75%)	21 (80.8%)	20 (100%)	44 (88%)	16 (41%)[c]
ACQ7	0.86 (0.25–1.89)	0.57 (0.29–1.00)	1.14 (0.86–1.86)[a]	0.86 (0.43–1.57)	–
FEV1% predicted	92.70 (84.45–100.9)	94.30 (85.25–100.4)	87.25 (79.08–93.90)[a]	91.6 (83.5–98.5)	96.6 (90.5–105.5)[c]
FEV1/ FVC	0.72 (0.68–0.79)	0.79 (0.69–0.84)	0.69 (0.64–0.82)[a]	0.71 (0.65, 0.75)	0.83 (0.77–0.86)[c]
BDR	3.32 (−0.92–13.88)	4 (0–6.00)	13.97 (5.99–19.33)[a]	5.9 (2.06–13.75)	3.0 (1.0–5.0)[c]
FENO (ppb)	28.35 (18.43–86.5)	26.65 (18.63–48.5)	139.5 (95–195.6)[ab]	49.5 (22.4–134.5)	33 (27.3–38.5)[c]
ICS use (%)	4 (100%)	18 (72%)	16 (80%)	38 (76%)	–
TCC/ml	6.07 (0.8–6.12)	1.29 (0.73–2.39)	1.88 (1.2–2.84)	1.40 (0.92–2.84)	1.42 (0.90–2.05)
Viability %(non-squamous cells)	80.74 (69.44–88.24)	65.15 (58.39–74.33)	68.57 (57–81.3)	69.38 (59.5–76)	74.45 (57.5–83)
Sputum eosinophils %	0.12 (0–1.04)	0.47 (0–1.33)	5.8 (3.52–11.78)[ab]	1.358 (0.24–4.61)	0 (0–0.25)[c]
Total sputum eosinophils × 10^4 ml	1.48 (0–7.89)	0.65 (0–1.48)	12.31 (4.88–29.20)[a]	1.53 (0.37–8.81)	0 (0–0.32)[c]
Sputum neutrophils %	63.14 (61.46–67.47)[a]	24.24 (13.02–33.14)	26.90 (17.43–40.19)[b]	27 (17.21–42.82)	32.1 (19.27–45.43)
Total sputum neutrophils ×10^4 ml	390.5 (49.03–419.4)	31.27 (11.18–55.04)	48.75 (20.79–96.24)	33.94 (15.7–81.6)	47.51 (10.90–73.10)
Sputum macrophages %	32.37 (30.46–35.59)[a]	68.88 (56.07–77.08)[b]	62.25 (48.93–67.97)	63.95 (49.76–74.58)	60.49 (45.55–78.44)
Total sputum macrophages × 10^4 ml	185.2 (28.98–188.5)	90.14 (46.87–146.2)	109.7 (67.18–158.7)	96.80 (53.16–160.6)	80.94 (41.71–125.9)
Sputum lymphocytes%	2.36 (1.16–3.99)	1.47 (0.83–2.32)	2.61 (1.69–4.37)[a]	1.94 (0.98–3.14)	2.12 (1.25–3.45)
Total sputum lymphocytes × 10^4 ml	5.93 (1.39–18.09)	1.83 (0.72–2.92)	4.70 (2.24–8.96)[a]	2.37 (1.15–6.24)	3.15 (1.28–6.22)
Sputum IL-8 (ng/ml)	2.33 (1.47–3.39)	1.77 (1.01–3.08)	2.36 (1.52–3.39)	2.19 (1.26–3.18)	1.62 (1.66–2.33)
Sputum MMP-9	1595 (1084–2943)	528.9 (185.8–1040)	1063 (374–2126)	693.7 (374–1363)	736.7(334.5–1340)

The first three columns report the characteristics of the asthma phenotypes previously described.[5] No MGA phenotype was detected. NA and PGA combined make up the NEA phenotype described in Results [2]
BDR change in FEV1% predicted post bronchodilator. Median (IQR) or number (%)
Comparing EA, NA and PGA:
[a]Significantly different ($p < 0.05$) than PGA
[b]Significantly different ($p < 0.05$) than NA
Comparing asthma and no asthma:
[c]Significantly different ($p < 0.05$) than asthma

(82%) at first assessment to 6 (55%) at second assessment (Table 2), but this did not reach statistical significance. Correspondingly, following sub-optimisation we found a doubling of EA cases (from two to four i.e. 20% to 40%), more asthmatics with NA (i.e. a change of 3 (30%) from 0 (0%)), and lower levels of MMP-9 and NE (not IL-8), but none of these differences were statistically significant. Overall, 11/21 (52%) asthmatics changed phenotype during the course of the study. When combining those who were initially identified as undergoing sub-optimal treatment with those whose treatment was sub-optimised as part of the study we found that 13/21 (62%) were categorised as EA; this was lower than what was observed during optimised treatment (either as part of the initial assessment or as a result of optimisation) i.e. 8/21 (38.1%), but again this was not statistically significant (Table 2). Sputum bacterial endotoxin levels significantly decreased in the optimisation group (Table 2).

Treatment optimisation was associated with significantly lower BDR ($p = 0.002$), increase in FEV_1-% predicted ($p = 0.026$), and decrease in FENO ($p = 0.002$) and ACQ7 ($p = <0.0001$; Table 2). When the treatment groups were stratified on the basis of ≥2% eosinophils at either visit as EA/NEA (as it has been suggested that these phenotypes show different responses to ICS) [3, 4], significant lung function and clinical improvements were observed only in the subjects that had been identified as EA on at least one assessment during the CIT study (Fig. 2a-d). The exception to this was a decrease in ACQ7 in NEA with treatment optimisation. Also, there was a significant decrease in eosinophils in the treatment-optimised EA group (Fig. 2e, $p<0.05$) when compared with sub-optimal treatment.

Sputum neutrophils showed a significant increase in oxidative burst after PMA stimulation ($p < 0.05$) and a significant improvement in phagocytosis ($p < 0.05$) (Fig. 3a-b)

Table 2 Alterations in clinical/inflammatory characteristics and inflammatory phenotypes during changes in asthma treatment (CIT study)

	A) Start or increase ICS ($n = 11$)			B) Stop or decrease ICS ($n = 10$)			C) All ($n = 21$) when assessed during:		
	Visit 1 (suboptimal Rx)	Visit 2 (optimised Rx)	Δ	Visit 1 (optimised Rx)	Visit 2 (suboptimal Rx)	Δ	Suboptimal Rx	Optimised Rx	Δ
Female (%)	5 (45%)	–	–	7 (70%)	–	–	12 (57%)	–	–
Age	36 (33, 43)	–	–	44 (27, 56)	–	–	37.0 (31, 55)	–	–
Atopy	10 (91%)	–	–	10 (100%)	–	–	20 (95%)	–	–
ICS dose (μg, budesonide equiv.)	0 (0, 140)	1000 (800, 1000)	1000**	775 (500, 850)	0 (0, 500)	−775**	0 (0, 375)	800 (500, 1000)	800***
ACQ7	1.71 (1.14, 2.14)	0.71 (0.57, 1.07)	−1.00**	0.57 (0.54, 0.90)	1.22 (0.89, 1.82)	0.65**	1.71 (1.07, 2.07)	0.57 (0.57, 1.00)	−1.14***
FEV1% predicted	71.5 (68.2, 82.6)	79.3 (69.5, 82.4)	7.8	82.1 (76.2, 92.4)	85.5 (73.0, 90.9)	3.4	75.6 (69.6, 86.4)	79.3 (74.1, 85.8)	3.7*
FEV1/FVC	0.65 (0.63, 0.68)	0.71 (0.59, 0.78)	0.06	0.74 (0.65, 0.83)	0.73 (0.63, 0.83)	−0.01	0.67 (0.64, 0.76)	0.71 (0.65, 0.78)	0.04
BDR (post-bronchodilator reversibility)% change	15.4 (9.3, 21.8)	11.1 (8.0, 15.5)	−4.3**	5.0 (1, 8.6)	7.7 (1.8, 11.9)	2.7	11.4 (5.3, 16.2)	8.6 (3.9, 12.5)	−2.8**
FENO (ppb)	124 (87–188)	84 (25.6–110)	−40**	44.0 (21.0, 74.0)	62.0 (34.0, 98.0)	18*	89.0 (47.0, 165.5)	51.0 (23.8, 90.0)	−38**
EA (%)	9 (82%)	6 (55%)	−3 (−27%)	2 (20%)	4 (40%)	2 (20%)	13 (61.9%)	8 (38.1%)	−5 (−23.8%)
NEA (%) of which:	2 (18%)	5 (45%)	3 (27%)	8 (80%)	6 (60%)	−2 (−20%)	8 (38.1%)	13 (61.9%)	5 (23.8%)
NA (%)	1 (9%)	1 (9%)	0 (0%)	0 (0%)	3 (30%)	3 (30%)	4 (19.0%)	1 (4.8%)	−3 (−14.3%)
PGA (%)	1 (9%)	4 (36%)	3 (27%)	8 (80%)	3 (30%)	−5 (−50%)	4 (19.0%)	12 (57.1%)	8 (38.1%)
Sputum eosinophils %	6.9 (2.2, 17.2)	3.1 (0.9, 9.1)	−5.4	1.4 (0.6, 1.7)	0.9 (0, 7.4)	−0.5	4.4 (0.7, 15.3)	1.5 (0.8, 4.8)	−2.9
Sputum neutrophils %	27.4 (9.3, 43.7)	30.4 (17.4, 38.7)	3	38.0 (14.5, 45.1)	43.9 (18.9, 63.9)	5.9	35.8 (14, 53.9)	34.5 (17.3, 43.2)	−1.3
TCC/ml	2.33 (0.94, 3.08)	2.08 (1.80, 3.25)	−0.25	1.23 (0.95, 2.07)	0.89 (0.70, 1.47)	−0.34	1.26 (0.74, 2.44)	1.8 (1.17, 3.07)	−0.54
Viability % (non-squamous cells)	69.4 (56.6, 83.1)	78.8 (57.0, 84.4)	9.4	70.9 (63.5, 78.1)	80.2 (65.5, 86.9)	9.3	73.8 (60.3, 85.4)	76.0 (64.0, 81.7)	2.2
Sputum IL-8 (ng/ml)	2.19 (0.58, 2.53)	1.94 (1.19, 4.26)	−0.25	2.53 (1.35, 3.85)	2.05 (1.02, 3.39)	−0.48	2.19 (0.93, 3.11)	2.11 (1.28, 3.57)	−0.08
Sputum MMP-9	411 (259, 2490)	637 (421, 1289)	226	1160 (295, 1584)	1293 (326, 2003)	133	666 (277, 2042)	1094 (376, 1408)	428
NE detected (%)	1 (9%)	0 (0%)	−1 (−9%)	0 (0%)	3 (30%)	3 (30%)	4 (19%)	0 (0%)	−4 (−19%)
Endotoxin (EU/ml)	2027 (1172, 2342)	1235 (546, 1769)	−792*	2227 (720, 4087)	1879 (1477, 3054)	−348	1894 (1354, 2577)	1361 (559, 2650)	−533

ICS dose – average daily dose ICS over recording period in μg budesonide equivalent. Data expressed as number (percentage) or median (IQR). Δ difference between median values of paired groups. ***$p < 0.001$, ** $p < 0.01$, * $p < 0.05$ when compared with matched group

A and B represent the data derived from the assessments as described ($n = 11$ go from sub-optimised to optimised, n = 10 from optimised to sub-optimised). C represents the data from all 21 CIT participants when data are stratified according to their treatment status

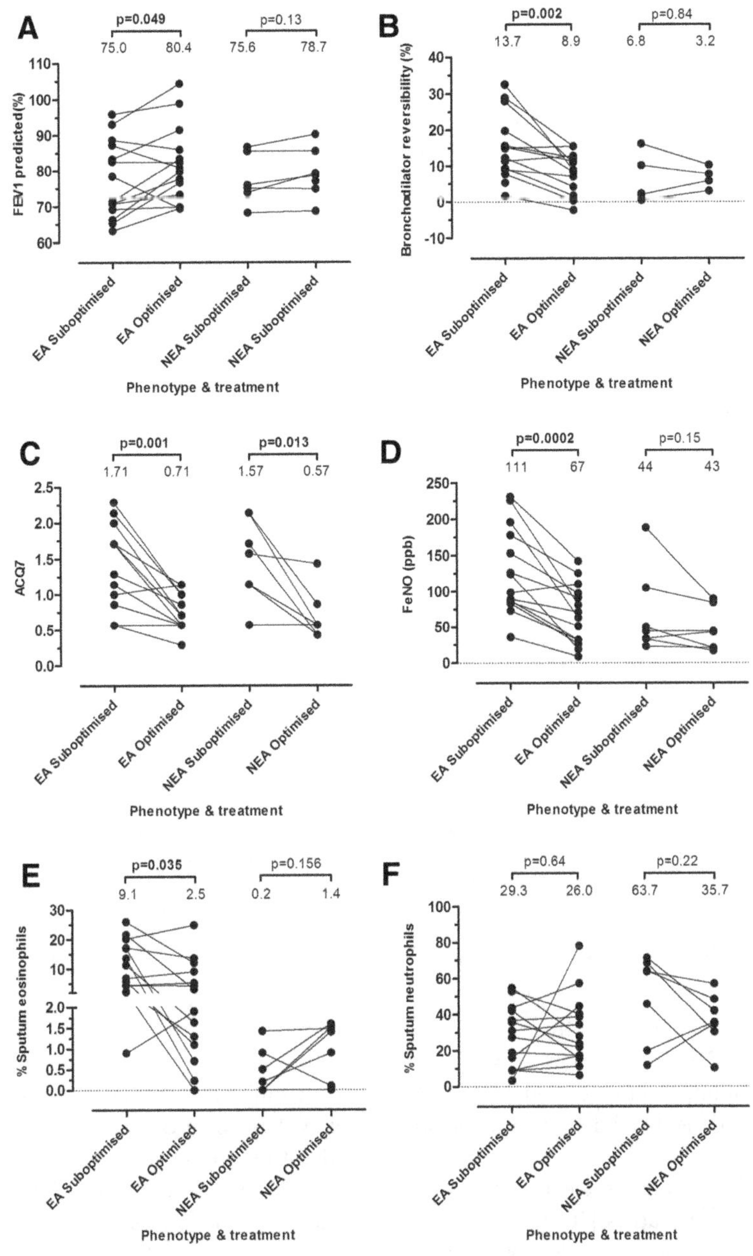

Fig. 2 Clinical and sputum sample inflammatory parameters for all CIT participants ($n = 21$). Data represent the assessment in which treatment was considered as sub-optimised or optimised. **a** – FEV1% predicted, **b**- change in FEV1% predicted post-bronchodilator (BDR), **c** – ACQ7, **d**- exhaled NO levels, **e** – change in % sputum eosinophils, **f**-change in % sputum neutrophils. Median data values are expressed at the top of each group

with optimised treatment. When phagocytosis was compared between EA/NEA groups, a significant increase ($p < 0.05$) in phagocytosis with optimised treatment was only observed in sputum neutrophils from the EA group (Figure 3c). As a loss of neutrophils was observed during in vitro stimulation, we compared this between sub-optimised and optimised treatment, but no significant difference was found (data not shown).

Discussion

In this community based study of adult asthmatics, in cross-sectional assessment the dominant asthma phenotypes were EA (40%) and PGA (52%). EA was associated with increased airway obstruction, ACQ7 score and BDR. In the nested CIT study, alteration in asthma treatment resulted in more than half of the asthmatics changing phenotype; in particular, sub-optimisation of treatment was associated with a non-significant increased prevalence

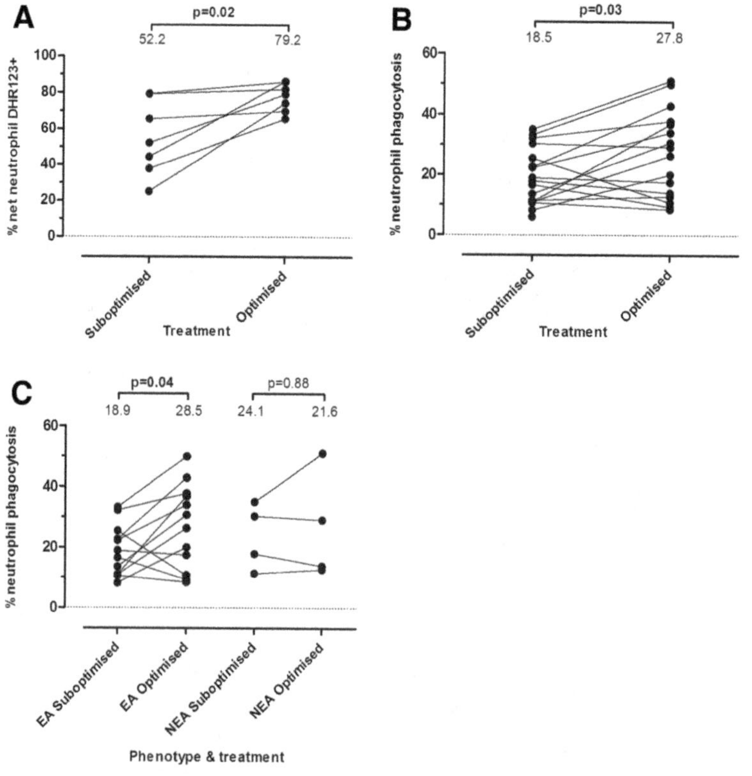

Fig. 3 Sputum neutrophil functional parameters (as assessed using flow cytometry). Data represent CIT participants who produced an adequate sample for neutrophil oxidative burst ($n = 7$) or phagocytosis measurement ($n = 16$) at both visits. Groups are stratified on the basis of treatment status (sub-optimised or optimised). **a** – change in % sputum neutrophils undergoing oxidative burst after stimulation with PMA, **b** – change in % sputum neutrophils that are capable of phagocytosing fluorescent zymosan beads in culture at 37 °C, **c**- change in % sputum neutrophils that are capable of phagocytosing fluorescent zymosan beads in culture at 37 °C when stratified into EA/NEA. Median values are expressed at the top of each group

of EA and NA, whilst optimisation of treatment was associated with an increase in PGA. Treatment optimisation was associated with clinical improvement, reduced eosinophil numbers and increased neutrophil function, statistically significant only in EA.

In our sample of adult asthmatics we found NA in only 8%, consistent with other studies [10, 11]. However, some previous studies have reported that NA is common [5, 13]. We speculate that the higher prevalence of the neutrophilic phenotype found in such studies may be in part due to specific environmental exposures associated with particular occupations or heavy industry [24–26]. Furthermore, NA has previously been reported in association with aging [5, 27]. In agreement, we observed NA only in older individuals, with 3/4 asthmatics classified as NA at any assessment being >60 yrs. of age. Also, consistent with others [28, 29] we found significantly lower FEV_1, FEV_1/FEV, and higher ACQ7 scores and BDR in EA.

PGA (which made up the majority of NEA) was associated with significantly higher eosinophil percentages than non-asthmatics despite levels being below the 2% cut-off used to define EA. Therefore, PGA - as defined in this and other studies - may not necessarily be indicative of different asthma pathology, but may represent a less evident form of EA, overlapping phenotypes [30], or be due to treatment effect (discussed further below).

Whilst some studies have shown that NEA is relatively stable over time [5], 52% of asthmatics in our study altered phenotype following changes in treatment. Similar findings have been previously reported. For example, Hancox et al. found that NEA/EA changes occurred in 50 to 100% of adult asthmatics ($n = 54$) in response to changes in ICS therapy [11]. Similar findings have also been described in children [12]. ICS use may therefore contribute to misclassification of NEA, as it may reduce sputum eosinophil numbers below the commonly used cut-point of 2%. Our findings, although not reaching statistical significance, thus support previous suggestions that inflammatory phenotype classification based upon a single assessment may not be valid for all asthmatics [31].

Although some previous reports have shown ICS to be less effective in NEA compared with EA [4, 32, 33], we observed improvements in ACQ7 score in the NEA group with optimised treatment. Other studies have also shown that symptoms improve in NEA with ICS treatment, although EA remains associated with a better response [10, 11]. As noted above, it is possible that some NEA subjects have a degree of ICS-responsiveness, but have undetectable (in sputum) eosinophilic inflammation. Alternatively, ICS may act through suppression of non-TH2 mediated pathways in NEA, such as epithelial cytokine production [34].

ICS use has previously been associated with an increase in sputum neutrophils and neutrophil survival [10], possibly via impairment of apoptosis [35]. We saw no significant changes in airway neutrophil percentages with treatment alterations. However, 33% (3/9) of individuals with PGA changed to NA after a *reduction* in ICS dose. This contrasts with previous findings suggesting that asthma exacerbations after tapered ICS withdrawal are associated with eosinophilic inflammation [36, 37]. However, one previous report suggested that sudden ICS withdrawal, as conducted in our study, may result in neutrophilic exacerbations [38]. It is therefore possible that the nature of airway inflammation post-ICS withdrawal may be dependent upon the kinetics of withdrawal.

We observed that neutrophil function (oxidative burst and phagocytosis) was enhanced with treatment optimisation, with the greatest effect observed in EA. Although earlier asthma studies have investigated sputum phagocyte function [39, 40], we believe that this is the first study assessing neutrophil function in response to changes in asthma treatment. The association between improved neutrophil function and treatment optimisation is intriguing. It is possible that improved neutrophil phagocytosis may be one of the mechanisms by which asthma treatment leads to a reduction in eosinophilic inflammation, possibly through improved efferocytosis [15]. Alternatively, improved neutrophil function may have affected the airway microbiome [41] as suggested by significantly reduced bacterial endotoxin (a strong pro-inflammatory agent) levels (Table 2). It is also possible that impairment of neutrophil apoptosis (described above) may have altered neutrophil maturation status, leading to the altered functional phenotype observed. However, larger longitudinal investigations are required to confirm these findings and more comprehensively determine the effect of medication on neutrophil function; in particular, whether the functional changes observed are directly relevant to the improvement of asthma symptoms, whether treatment leads to alteration of peripheral neutrophil function (blood samples were not available for assessment in the current study) or if treatment is indirectly affecting neutrophil function through modulation of other cell populations, such as macrophages or eosinophils. Also, although not addressed here, there is a possibility that the hypertonic saline challenge or sputum sample processing procedure may directly result in altered or activated neutrophil phenotype. Previous studies have reported increased expression of the activation markers CD11b and CD66 on sputum neutrophils when compared with blood or broncho-alveolar lavage neutrophils [42, 43], but it is not clear if this is due to the airway environment or sampling procedure. However, in the current study, as all samples were processed in the same manner, it is unlikely that the observed differences could be due to either saline challenge or sputum processing.

There were some limitations to this study. Firstly, although asthmatics reported a doctor's diagnosis of asthma and recent symptoms, as we did not use objective tests (such as bronchodilator reversibility or airway hyperreactivity) to confirm asthma diagnosis, it is possible that some misclassification may have occurred. However, we consider that any bias introduced as result will be minimal given that this approach, which has been used in many previous studies [14, 16–18, 26], generally compares well with more clinical definitions of asthma [16, 17]. Also, in some cases it has been shown to be better than more objective measures such as airway hyperreactivity [18]. Indeed, there are a number of issues with objective testing for confirmation of asthma diagnosis in a community based setting, particularly given the inherently variable nature of the condition, and when the majority of asthmatics are not treatment naïve (76% of asthmatics in the current study were using ICS at the time of assessment). This (amongst other reasons) has led to recent recommendations that asthma be considered on the basis of symptoms rather than pathophysiology [44]. Secondly, as the majority of asthmatics were undergoing ICS therapy, and there were safety concerns about total ICS withdrawal in some cases in the CIT study, it is possible that ICS treatment may be "cloaking" physiological responses, as well as eosinophilic inflammation. Thirdly, the relatively large number of cells required to investigate cell function meant that only samples with larger cell yields could be assessed. For this reason, respiratory burst was assessed in relatively few samples ($n = 7$ for respiratory burst and 16 for phagocytosis assessment). This may have resulted in selection bias. However, our data suggest that there is no significant difference between sputum total cell count between asthmatics and non-asthmatics, and therefore this is unlikely to be a major issue. Fourthly, treatment changes were limited to a 4–6 week period (similar to previous studies [10, 11] and varied somewhat among CIT study participants as asthma management was considered on a case-by-case basis i.e. subjects did not receive a uniform reduction or increase in ICS dose (Additional file 1: Table S1), and in cases in which participants were using combined ICS/LABA inhalers, LABA was also altered. All participants were also using SABA as required. This may have led to some variation in the effect on (particularly eosinophilic) inflammation and/or asthma control, as there are reports that some SABA (in particular terbutaline) may have a permissive effect on airway inflammation, and their use may be associated with an increase in airway eosinophils [45]. However, the evidence for this is mixed, and may not be the case for all SABA [46, 47]. Fifthly, the asthmatics studied were recruited from the general population, and as such had varying levels of asthma control and severity at assessment which makes the interpretation of the results more difficult. Finally, the relatively small number of participants included in the CIT study (due to the reluctance of some study participants to undergo CIT) may have led to non-significant findings in terms of inflammatory phenotype changes. Despite the latter two limitations, the trends observed (i.e. increased EA with suboptimised treatment, reduced eosinophils, improvement in asthma control and increased NEA with optimised treatment) were generally similar to those previously described in studies in which ICS was withdrawn or added to asthma therapy [10, 11].

Conclusions

In this sample of adult asthmatics, NEA was common and associated with less severe disease, with only a small proportion of NEA demonstrating evidence of neutrophilic inflammation. This study also showed that treatment optimisation was associated with reduced sputum eosinophils, improved symptoms and lung function, and enhanced neutrophil function, but a significant reduction in EA could not be demonstrated.

Abbreviations

ACQ: Asthma control questionnaire; BDR: Bronchodilator reversibility; CIT: Change in treatment; DHR: Dihydrorhodamine; EA: Eosinophilic asthma; FENO: Fractional exhaled nitric oxide; FEV_1: Forced expiratory volume in 1 s; FVC: Forced vital capacity; ICS: Inhaled corticosteroid; LABA: Long acting β2-agonist; MGA: Mixed granulocytic asthma; NA: Neutrophilic asthma; NE: Neutrophil elastase; NEA: Non-eosinophilic asthma; PEF: Peak expiratory flow; PGA: Paucigranulocytic asthma; PMA: Phorbol 12-myristate 13-acetate; SABA: Short acting β2- agonist

Acknowledgements

Not applicable.

Funding

Funding was provided by the Asthma and Respiratory Foundation of New Zealand, Health Research Council of New Zealand, and the Royal Society of New Zealand Marsden Fund. These bodies played no part in in the design of the study or collection, analysis, interpretation of data or writing of this manuscript.

Authors' contributions

Conception and design of study: CVD, CB, IH, JD; Data collection: CVD, EH, CRB; Analysis and interpretation of data: CRB, CVD; Drafting and revision of manuscript: CB, CVD, EH, IH, JD; All authors read and approved the final manuscript.

Consent for publication

Not applicable.

Competing interests

The authors declare that they have no competing interests.

Author details

[1]Centre for Public Health Research, Massey University Wellington Campus, Private Box 756, Wellington 6140, New Zealand. [2]Malaghan Institute of Medical Research, Wellington, New Zealand.

References

1. Barnes PJ. Immunology of asthma and chronic obstructive pulmonary disease. Nat Rev Immunol. 2008;8:183–92.
2. Douwes J, Gibson P, Pekkanen J, Pearce N. Non-eosinophilic asthma: importance and possible mechanisms. Thorax. 2002;57:643–8.
3. Wenzel SE, Schwartz LB, Langmack EL, et al. Evidence that severe asthma can be divided pathologically into two inflammatory subtypes with distinct physiologic and clinical characteristics. Am J Respir Crit Care Med. 1999;160:1001–8.
4. Berry M, Morgan A, Shaw DE, et al. Pathological features and inhaled corticosteroid response of eosinophilic and non-eosinophilic asthma. Thorax. 2007;62:1043–9.
5. Simpson JL, Scott R, Boyle MJ, Gibson PG. Inflammatory subtypes in asthma: assessment and identification using induced sputum. Respirology. 2006;11:54–61.
6. Gibson PG, Simpson JL, Saltos N. Heterogeneity of airway inflammation in persistent asthma: evidence of neutrophilic inflammation and increased sputum interleukin-8. Chest. 2001;119:1329–36.
7. Simpson JL, Grissell TV, Douwes J, Scott RJ, Boyle MJ, Gibson PG. Innate immune activation in neutrophilic asthma and bronchiectasis. Thorax. 2007;62:211–8.
8. Jatakanon A, Uasuf C, Maziak W, Lim S, Chung KF, Barnes PJ. Neutrophilic inflammation in severe persistent asthma. Am J Respir Crit Care Med. 1999; 160:1532–9.
9. Simpson JL, McElduff P, Gibson PG. Assessment and reproducibility of non-eosinophilic asthma using induced sputum. Respiration. 2010;79:147–51.
10. Cowan DC, Cowan JO, Palmay R, Williamson A, Taylor DR. Effects of steroid therapy on inflammatory cell subtypes in asthma. Thorax. 2010;65:384–90.
11. Hancox RJ, Cowan DC, Aldridge RE, et al. Asthma phenotypes: consistency of classification using induced sputum. Respirology. 2012;17:461–6.
12. Fleming L, Tsartsali L, Wilson N, Regamey N, Bush A. Sputum inflammatory phenotypes are not stable in children with asthma. Thorax. 2012;67:675–81.
13. Wang F, He XY, Baines KJ, et al. Different inflammatory phenotypes in adults and children with acute asthma. Eur Respir J. 2011;38:567–74.
14. Brooks CR, van Dalen CJ, Hermans IF, Douwes J. Identifying leukocyte populations in fresh and cryopreserved sputum using flow cytometry. Cytometry B Clin Cytom. 2013;84:104–13.
15. Donnelly LE, Barnes PJ. Defective phagocytosis in airways disease. Chest. 2012;141:1055–62.
16. Pekkanen J, Pearce N. Defining asthma in epidemiological studies. Eur Respir J. 1999;14:951–7.
17. Bai J, Peat JK, Berry G, Marks GB, Woolcock AJ. Questionnaire items that predict asthma and other respiratory conditions in adults. Chest. 1998; 114:1343–8.
18. Jenkins MA, Clarke JR, Carlin JB, et al. Validation of questionnaire and bronchial hyperresponsiveness against respiratory physician assessment in the diagnosis of asthma. Int J Epidemiol. 1996;25:609–16.
19. Juniper EF, Bousquet J, Abetz L, Bateman ED. Identifying 'well-controlled' and 'not well-controlled' asthma using the asthma control questionnaire. Respir Med. 2006;100:616–21.

20. Global Initiative for Asthma. Global strategy for asthma management and prevention report, 2011 update. http://ginasthma.org.
21. NAEPP. National Asthma Education and Prevention Program Expert Panel: Guidelines for the Diagnosis and Management of Asthma. 2007; http://www.nhlbi.nih.gov/guidelines/asthma/asthsumm.pdf.
22. ATS. Standardization of Spirometry, 1994 update. American Thoracic Society. Am J Respir Crit Care Med. 1995;152:1107–36.
23. ATS/ERS. ATS/ERS recommendations for standardized procedures for the online and offline measurement of exhaled lower respiratory nitric oxide and nasal nitric oxide, 2005. Am J Respir Crit Care Med. 2005;171:912–30.
24. Jung KS, Park HS. Evidence for neutrophil activation in occupational asthma. Respirology. 1999;4:303–6.
25. Adelroth E, Hedlund U, Blomberg A, et al. Airway inflammation in iron ore miners exposed to dust and diesel exhaust. Eur Respir J. 2006;27:714–9.
26. Bosson J, Pourazar J, Forsberg B, Adelroth E, Sandstrom T, Blomberg A. Ozone enhances the airway inflammation initiated by diesel exhaust. Respir Med. 2007;101:1140–6.
27. Brooks CR, Gibson PG, Douwes J, Van Dalen CJ, Simpson JL. Relationship between airway neutrophilia and aging in asthmatics and non-asthmatics. Respirology. 2013;18:857–65.
28. Louis R, Lau LC, Bron AO, Roldaan AC, Radermecker M, Djukanovic R. The relationship between airways inflammation and asthma severity. Am J Respir Crit Care Med. 2000;161:9–16.
29. Woodruff PG, Khashayar R, Lazarus SC, et al. Relationship between airway inflammation, hyperresponsiveness, and obstruction in asthma. J Allergy Clin Immunol. 2001;108:753–8.
30. Wenzel SE. Asthma phenotypes: the evolution from clinical to molecular approaches. Nature Med. 2012;18:716–25.
31. Wark P. Airway inflammation in asthma, a single measurement is not enough. Respirology. 2012;17:393–4.
32. Pavord ID, Brightling CE, Woltmann G, Wardlaw AJ. Non-eosinophilic corticosteroid unresponsive asthma. Lancet. 1999;353:2213–4.
33. Green RH, Brightling CE, Woltmann G, Parker D, Wardlaw AJ, Pavord ID. Analysis of induced sputum in adults with asthma: identification of subgroup with isolated sputum neutrophilia and poor response to inhaled corticosteroids. Thorax. 2002;57:875–9.
34. Ek A, Larsson K, Siljerud S, Palmberg L. Fluticasone and budesonide inhibit cytokine release in human lung epithelial cells and alveolar macrophages. Allergy. 1999;54:691–9.
35. Cox G. Glucocorticoid treatment inhibits apoptosis in human neutrophils. Separation of survival and activation outcomes. J Immunol. 1995;154:4719–25.
36. Jatakanon A, Lim S, Barnes PJ. Changes in sputum eosinophils predict loss of asthma control. Am J Respir Crit Care Med. 2000;161:64–72.
37. In't Veen JC, Smits HH, Hiemstra PS, Zwinderman AE, Sterk PJ, Bel EH. Lung function and sputum characteristics of patients with severe asthma during an induced exacerbation by double-blind steroid withdrawal. Am J Respir Crit Care Med. 1999;160:93–9.
38. Maneechotesuwan K, Essilfie-Quaye S, Kharitonov SA, Adcock IM, Barnes PJ. Loss of control of asthma following inhaled corticosteroid withdrawal is associated with increased sputum interleukin-8 and neutrophils. Chest. 2007;132:98–105.
39. Alexis NE, Soukup J, Nierkens S, Becker S. Association between airway hyperreactivity and bronchial macrophage dysfunction in individuals with mild asthma. Am J Physiol Lung Cell Mol Physiol. 2001;280:L369–75.
40. Simpson JL, Gibson PG, Yang IA, et al. Impaired macrophage phagocytosis in non-eosinophilic asthma. Clin Exp Allergy. 2013;43:29–35.
41. Huang YJ, Lynch SV. The emerging relationship between the airway microbiota and chronic respiratory disease: clinical implications. Expert Rev Respir Med. 2011;5:809–21.
42. Alexis N, Soukup J, Ghio A, Becker S. Sputum phagocytes from healthy individuals are functional and activated: a flow cytometric comparison with cells in bronchoalveolar lavage and peripheral blood. Clin Immunol. 2000;97:21–32.
43. Tak T, Hilvering B, Tesselaar K, Koenderman L. Similar activation state of neutrophils in sputum of asthma patients irrespective of sputum eosinophilia. Clin Exp Immunol. 2015;182:204–12.
44. Pavord ID, Beasley R, Agusti A, et al. After asthma: redefining airways diseases. Lancet. 2017;6736:30879–6. (epublished ahead of print)
45. Aldridge RE, Hancox RJ, Taylor DR, et al. Effects of terbutline and budesonide on sputum cells and bronchial hyperresponsiveness in asthma. Am J Resp Crit Care Med. 2000;161:1459–64.
46. Cianchetti S, Bacci E, Ruocco L, et al. Salbutamol pretreatment does not change eosinophil percentage and eosinophil cationic protein concentration in hypertonic saline-induced sputum in asthmatic subjects. Clin Exp Allergy. 1999;29:712–8.
47. Evans DW, Salome CM, King GG, et al. Effect of regular inhaled salbutamol on airway responsiveness and airway inflammation in rhinitic non-asthmatic subjects. Thorax. 1997;52:136–42.

7

Association between risk of asthma and gene polymorphisms in CHI3L1 and CHIA

Yanting Zhu, Xin Yan, Cui Zhai, Lan Yang and Manxiang Li*

Abstract

Background: Previous studies have indicated that chitinase 3-like 1 (CHI3L1) gene rs4950928 polymorphism and acidic mammalian chitinase (AMCase or CHIA) gene rs10494132 polymorphism are associated with the risk of asthma. However, the results are inconsistent because of small sample size and varied ethnicity and age in studies. Therefore, a systematic meta-analysis was important to clarify the effect of CHI3L1 rs4950928 polymorphism and CHIA rs10494132 variant on asthma risk.

Methods: An electronic literature search was conducted to identify all the eligible studies. Odds ratios (ORs) with 95% confidence intervals (CIs) were calculated and sensitivity analysis as well as publication bias were assessed to investigate the associations. All statistical analyses were performed using STATA 12.0.

Results: Eight published articles with 10 case-control studies were included, 5 studies were of CHI3L1 rs4950928 polymorphism and another 5 studies involved CHIA rs10494132 polymorphism. Overall, no significant association was found between CHI3L1 polymorphism and asthma susceptibility. After stratified according to ethnicity, CHI3L1 rs4950928 variant was associated with decreased asthma risk in Caucasians (GG + GC vs. CC: OR = 0.621, 95% CI = 0.484–0.797, $P = 0.000$; GC vs. CC: OR = 0.612, 95% CI = 0.470–0.796, $P = 0.000$; G vs. C: OR = 0.696, 95% CI = 0.567–0.856, $P = 0.001$). When stratified population by age, there was no association in children under all genetic models. As for CHIA rs10494132 polymorphism, no evidence of association between CHIA rs10494132 polymorphism and asthma risk was identified. Furthermore, subgroup analysis by ethnicity revealed a positive correlation between CHIA rs10494132 polymorphism and asthma risk among Asians (TT vs. TC + CC: OR = 1.476, 95% CI = 1.071–2.032, $P = 0.017$; T vs. C: OR = 1.326, 95% CI = 1.024–1.717, $P = 0.032$). Additionally, in the subgroup analysis conducted according to age, CHIA rs10494132 variant was also found to be associated with the increased risk of asthma in children (TT vs. TC + CC: OR = 1.472, 95% CI = 1.067–2.030, $P = 0.019$; T vs. C: OR = 1.320, 95% CI = 1.016–1.713, $P = 0.037$).

Conclusions: The G allele of CHI3L1 rs4950928 might be a protective factor against the development of asthma. However, the rs10494132 polymorphism of CHIA might be a risk factor for asthma.

Keywords: Asthma, Gene polymorphism, CHI3L1, CHIA, Meta-analysis

* Correspondence: manxiangli@hotmail.com
Department of Respiratory Medicine, The First Affiliated Hospital of Xi'an Jiaotong University, No.277, West Yanta Road, Xi'an 710061, Shaanxi, People's Republic of China

Background

Asthma is a chronic inflammatory respiratory disease that is characterized by airway hyper-reactivity to some environmental stimuli, reversible airway obstruction, and gradually appeared airway structural remodeling [1]. Although the exact etiology of asthma remains uncertain, it has become evident that a combination of genetic predisposition and environmental exposures plays a vital role in pathogenesis of asthma [2–4]. Recently, with numerous advances in genetic research, many genetic variants regulating the expression of proteins involved in the development of asthma have been found to be related to susceptibility to this disease, including interleukin-17F (IL-17F), toll-like receptor 4 (TLR4), and the genes encoding chitinase 3–like 1 (CHI3L1) and acidic mammalian chitinase (AMCase or CHIA) [5–8].

Chitin is an abundant, naturally occurring polysaccharide functioning as a major structural polymer in many lower life forms as well as an important nutritional source for many organisms, which triggers allergies or asthma attacks in people [9–11]. The chitinase family has three members: two of which are the true chitinases—acidic mammalian chitinase and chitotriosidase (CHIT); the other is the structurally related chitinase-like protein YKL-40 [12–14]. It has been reported that chitinase and chitinase-like proteins are highly expressed in lungs and serum of asthma patients [12], which are also found to regulate TH2 immune response and mediate airway inflammation and airway remodeling in mouse asthmatic models [15, 16]. YKL-40 is encoded by the chitinase 3-like 1 gene (CHI3L1), which is 10 exons long and is located on chromosome 1q31-q32 [17]. Genetic studies have demonstrated that the variants of CHI3L1 may contribute to the pathogenesis of asthma [7, 18]. A Genome-wide Association Study (GWAS) has identified that the rs4950928 polymorphism in the CHI3L1 gene is associated with the risk of asthma, circulating YKL-40 level and pulmonary function [18]. The gene for CHIA is present on chromosome 1q13.1–21.3 and contains 12 exons [13]. Recent genetic study has described that several CHIA polymorphisms is related to asthma risk in a German pediatric population [19].

Although several genetic studies have reported the correlation between CHI3L1 rs4950928 polymorphism or CHIA rs10494132 variant and the risk of asthma [7, 8, 18, 20], these results were controversial and inconclusive since they are performed in an individual medical center with small sample size and in different ethnicities. Therefore, it is important to perform a meta-analysis of all eligible studies to clarify the effects of CHI3L1 rs4950928 polymorphism and CHIA rs10494132 variant on risk of asthma.

Methods

Literature search strategy

The systematic electronic databases of PubMed, Embase, Web of Science, China National Knowledge Infrastructure (CNKI) and Wanfang Database were comprehensively searched for all the eligible studies published up to May 2017 using the search terms: ("chitinase 3–like 1" or "CHI3L1"), ("single nucleotide polymorphism" or "SNP" or "polymorphism" or "variation" or "mutation") and ("asthma" or "asthmatic") or ("acidic mammalian chitinase" or "CHIA"), ("single nucleotide polymorphism" or "SNP" or "polymorphism" or "variation" or "mutation") and ("asthma" or "asthmatic"). Besides, the reference lists of all selected articles were manually searched for further potentially eligible articles. No restrictions with regard to language, population, publication date, or type of report were imposed; and unpublished data were excluded.

Inclusion and exclusion criteria

All the potential studies were independently selected by two reviewers (Yanting Zhu and Xin Yan) according to the following inclusion and exclusion criteria. Inclusion criteria in this meta-analysis were: (1) studies that were using a case-control design; (2) studies that evaluated the correlation between CHI3L1 rs4950928 polymorphism or CHIA rs10494132 polymorphism and risk of asthma; (3) studies that provided sufficient data on the genotypic and allelic distributions of CHI3L1 rs4950928 polymorphism or CHIA rs10494132 polymorphism for estimating the odds ratios (ORs) and its corresponding 95% confidence intervals (CIs). Exclusion criteria were as follow: (1) studies without the control groups; (2) studies with no available data reported; (3) studies with inappropriate article types (reviews, case reports, letters, or abstracts); (4) studies with duplicated data. For overlapping studies, the largest or most recent publication was selected.

Data extraction

The information of each eligible study was independently extracted by two investigators (Cui Zhai and Lan Yang). The following data were extracted: first author, year of publication, country, ethnicity, age, number of cases and controls, genotyping method and genotype distribution in cases and controls. Discrepancies were resolved by discussion or additional assessment by a third author (Manxiang Li), and consensus was achieved on each item.

Subgroup criteria

Subgroup analyses were performed according to the ethnicity and age. Ethnicity is determined by the descent of all the subjects in each eligible study. For CHI3L1 rs4950928 polymorphism, three studies of European descent from European countries Sweden, Germany and

USA, were enrolled and belonged to Caucasian ethnicity. One study of Asian descent came from China, which belonged to Asian ethnicity. Another study of African descent from Mauritius belonged to African ethnicity. As for CHIA rs10494132 polymorphism, three studies of Asian descent, belonged to Asian ethnicity, came from China and were enrolled in this study. Another two studies of European descent came from North India and belonged to Caucasian ethnicity. As depicted in Table 1, for CHI3L1 rs4950928 polymorphism, three studies with an age of 0–16 years were considered as children group. One study with a range of 18–72 years was adults group. Another study range from 7 to 74 was mixture group. As for CHIA rs10494132 polymorphism, two studies range from 5 to 14 years were considered as children group. Another two studies with a range of 18–49 years were adults group. Asthma and genetic susceptibility are different in 0–4 years compared to early school age and high school students. However, we could not perform subgroup analysis in children group according to different stages (preschool age, early school age and high school age) duo to insufficiency of relevant studies in literature. Gender is also an important factor for the heterogeneity. While, it was impossible to perform subgroup analysis according to gender since original data in the eligible studies were insufficient.

Statistical analysis

This meta-analysis was performed using STATA version 12.0 software (Stata Corporation, College Station, Texas, USA). The Hardy-Weinberg equilibrium (HWE) for the genotype frequencies was evaluated only in controls using Chi-squared test to check whether samples in eligible studies were from a large population in HWE and whether the sample bias existed. Samples in cases may show departure from HWE since the biases existed in case groups, such as age, the ratio of gender and so on. $P < 0.05$ was considered statistically significant in HWE testing. The between-study heterogeneity was assessed by Chi-square-based Q test and I^2 statistics. The random-effect model was adopted for analysis, if there was statistical heterogeneity ($P < 0.10$). Otherwise, the fixed-effect model was applied for analysis as the pooling method. The pooled ORs and its corresponding 95%CIs were calculated to evaluate the associations of CHI3L1 rs4950928 polymorphism and CHIA rs10494132 polymorphism with asthma risk under five genetic models: recessive model (CHI3L1 rs4950928: GG vs. GC + CC; CHIA rs10494132: TT vs. TC + CC); dominant model (CHI3L1 rs4950928: GG + GC vs. CC; CHIA rs10494132: TT + TC vs. CC); codominant model (CHI3L1 rs4950928: GC vs. CC; CHIA rs10494132: TC vs. CC); homozygote model (CHI3L1 rs4950928: GG vs. CC; CHIA rs10494132: TT vs. CC); allele model (CHI3L1 rs4950928: G vs. C; rs10494132: T vs. C). Z-test was performed to assess the significance of the pooled ORs, and $P < 0.05$ considered statistically significant. Publication bias was assessed by Begg's test and Egger's test and $P < 0.05$ was considered significant publication bias.

Results

Study characteristics

The literature retrieval process was presented in Fig. 1. In total, 363 articles were identified through the initial search of databases. After a systematical literature search based on the inclusion criteria, 10 case-control studies from 8 published articles containing 1858 cases and 1778 controls were identified for this meta-analysis to investigate the relations of CHI3L1 and CHIA variants with asthma risk [7, 8, 18, 20–24]. Among the selected studies, 5 studies in 4 eligible publications [7, 18, 20, 21] were conducted for evaluating CHI3L1 rs4950928 polymorphism with a total

Table 1 Main characteristics of all eligible studies in this meta-analysis

Author	Year	Country	Ethnicity	Age group	Cases	Controls	Genotyping method
rs4950928							
Li [21]	2015	China	Asian	Children	316	297	Mass Array
James [7]	2016	Sweden	Caucasian	Adults	111	57	TaqMan
Ober [18]	2008	USA	Caucasian	Children	344	294	TaqMan
Ober [18]	2008	USA	Caucasian	Mixed	99	197	TaqMan
Ramphul [20]	2015	Mauritius	African	Children	192	189	TaqMan
rs10494132							
Chatterjee [8]	2008	India	Caucasian	Adults	270	292	EMSAs
Chatterjee [8]	2008	India	Caucasian	Adults	150	101	EMSAs
Huang [23]	2013	China	Asian	Children	158	198	Mass Array
Chen [22]	2014	China	Asian	Adults	150	101	Mass Array
Shao [24]	2017	China	Asian	Children	68	52	Mass Array

NA Not available, *EMSAs* Electrophoretic mobility shift assays

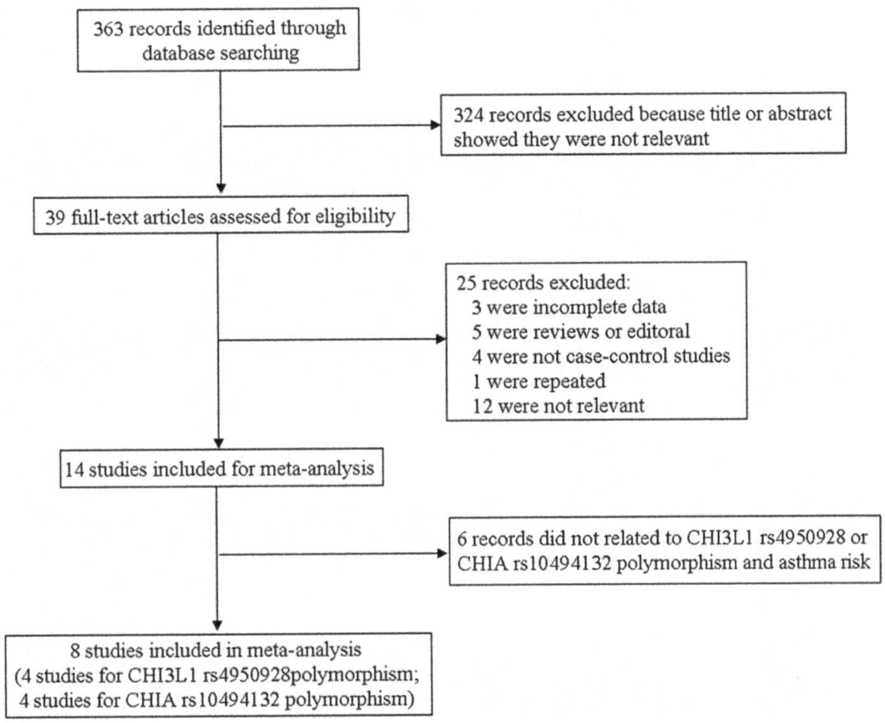

Fig. 1 Flowchart of study selection procedure

of 1062 cases and 1034 controls enrolled; 5 studies containing 796 cases and 744 controls were performed for investigating CHIA rs10494132 polymorphism in 4 published articles [8, 22–24]. The main characteristics of each study were shown in Table 1. For CHI3L1 rs4950928 polymorphism, 3 studies [7, 18] were carried out among Caucasians, 1 study [21] was conducted in Asians and another one [20] was conducted in African subjects in terms of ethnicity. 3 studies on the CHI3L1 rs4950928 polymorphism were conducted in children [18, 20, 21]. Only 1 study was performed in adults [7] and the rest was performed in mixture [18]. As for CHIA rs10494132 polymorphism, there were 3 studies [22–24] of Asian ethnicity and 2 studies [8] of Caucasian ethnicity. 3 studies [8, 23, 24] were performed in children and the rest [8, 22] were conducted in adults. Genotype distributions and HWE examination results were exhibited in Table 2. The genotypes of CHI3L1 rs4950928 polymorphism in the control groups were in agreement with HWE ($P > 0.05$). As for CHIA rs10494132 polymorphism, HWE deviation existed in control of 1 eligible study [24].

Meta-analysis and subgroup analysis

The genetic effects of CHI3L1 rs4950928 polymorphism and CHIA rs10494132 variant on asthma risk were presented in Table 3.

For CHI3L1 rs4950928 polymorphism, there was no statistically significant association observed under the following genetic models: recessive model (GG vs. GC + CC: OR = 0.946, 95% CI = 0.626–1.428, P = 0.791); dominant model (GG + GC vs. CC: OR = 0.917, 95% CI = 0.767–1.097, P = 0.342); codominant model (GC vs. CC: OR = 0.915, 95% CI = 0.759–1.103, P = 0.351); homozygote model (GG vs. CC: OR = 0.889, 95% CI = 0.588–1.346, P = 0.579) and allele model (G vs. C: OR = 0.933, 95% CI = 0.802–1.058, P = 0.369). After categorizing

Table 2 Distributions of CHI3L1 rs4950928 and CHIA rs10494132 polymorphisms among asthmatic patients and controls

Study	Cases			Controls			*P* for HWE
rs4950928	GG	GC	CC	GG	GC	CC	
Li [21]	13	111	192	9	71	217	0.288
James [7]	8	34	69	3	14	40	0.254
Ober [18]	17	100	227	24	120	150	1.000
Ober [18]	5	25	69	7	80	111	0.103
Ramphul [20]	6	64	122	5	63	121	0.339
rs10494132	TT	TC	CC	TT	TC	CC	
Chatterjee [8]	150	85	30	166	97	24	0.075
Chatterjee [8]	91	43	14	55	38	6	0.868
Huang [23]	130	26	2	138	50	10	0.063
Chen [22]	91	43	16	55	38	8	0.691
Shao [24]	30	22	16	23	17	12	0.023

HWE Hardy- Weinberg equilibrium

Table 3 Meta-analysis of CHI3L1 rs4950928 and CHIA rs10494132 polymorphisms and asthma

Subgroup	Genetic model	Genotype/ Allele	Type of model	Heterogeneity		Test of Association		
				I^2	P_{het}	OR	95% CI	P_{meta}
rs4950928								
Overall	Recessive model	GG vs. GC + CC	F	0.00%	0.430	0.946	0.626–1.428	0.791
	Dominant model	GG + GC vs. CC	R	86.70%	0.000	0.917	0.767–1.097	0.342
	Codominant model	GC vs. CC	R	85.80%	0.000	0.915	0.759–1.103	0.351
	Homozygote model	GG vs. CC	F	39.10%	0.160	0.889	0.588–1.346	0.579
	Allele model	G vs. C	R	84.90%	0.000	0.933	0.802–1.085	0.369
Caucasians	Recessive model	GG vs. GC + CC	F	21.40%	0.128	0.794	0.475–1.327	0.378
	Dominant model	GG + GC vs. CC	R	70.20%	0.035	0.621	0.484–0.797	0.000
	Codominant model	GC vs. CC	R	65.70%	0.054	0.612	0.470–0.796	0.000
	Homozygote model	GGvs. CC	F	40.40%	0.187	0.675	0.402–1.134	0.138
	Allele model	G vs. C	R	68.70%	0.041	0.696	0.567–0.856	0.001
Children	Recessive model	GG vs. GC + CC	F	28.00%	0.249	0.844	0.529-1.346	0.476
	Dominant model	GG + GC vs. CC	R	91.90%	0.000	0.955	0.782–1.166	0.651
	Codominant model	GC + CC	R	90.90%	0.000	0.970	0.788-1.196	0.777
	Homozygote model	GG vs. CC	R	64.00%	0.062	0.797	0.499-1.275	0.345
	Allele model	G vs. C	R	91.30%	0.000	0.946	0.799–1.120	0.522
rs10494132								
Overall	Recessive model	TT vs. TC + CC	F	35.80%	0.182	1.212	0.981–1.497	0.075
	Dominant model	TT + TC vs. CC	F	21.80%	0.276	0.857	0.597–1.230	0.403
	Codominant model	TC vs. CC	F	0.00%	0.455	0.748	0.504–1.109	0.149
	Homozygote model	TT vs. CC	F	24.70%	0.257	0.916	0.630–1.331	0.646
	Allele model	T vs. C	R	57.90%	0.050	1.094	0.924–1.297	0.298
Asians	Recessive model	TT vs. TC + CC	F	29.80%	0.240	1.476	1.071–2.032	0.017
	Dominant model	TT + TC vs. CC	F	48.10%	0.145	1.125	0.654–1.933	0.671
	Codominant model	TC vs. CC	F	24.60%	0.266	0.926	0.507–1.691	0.802
	Homozygote model	TT vs. CC	F	48.90%	0.141	1.249	0.709-2.199	0.441
	Allele model	T vs. C	R	64.00%	0.062	1.326	1.024–1.717	0.032
Children	Recessive model	TT vs. TC + CC	F	30.60%	0.263	1.472	1.067–2.030	0.019
	Dominant model	TT + TC vs. CC	F	53.00%	0.119	1.101	0.629–1.927	0.737
	Codominant model	TC vs. CC	F	34.70%	0.216	0.903	0.485–1.681	0.748
	Homozygote model	TT vs. CC	F	53.30%	0.117	1.217	0.679–2.184	0.510
	Allele model	T vs. C	R	64.90%	0.058	1.320	1.016–1.713	0.037

OR Odds ratio, *CI* Confidence interval, P_{het} *P*-value of heterogeneity test, P_{meta} P-value of pooled effect, *R* Random effect model, *F* Fixed effect model

included studies into different subgroups according to the ethnicity of study population, results indicated that CHI3L1 rs4950928 variant was associated with decreased asthma risk among Caucasians under the dominant model (GG + GC vs. CC: OR = 0.621, 95% CI = 0.484–0.797, P = 0.000), the codominant model (GC vs. CC: OR = 0.612, 95% CI = 0.470–0.796, P = 0.000) and the allele model (G vs. C: OR = 0.696, 95% CI = 0.567–0.856, P = 0.001) (Fig. 2). While, no increased or reduced risk of asthma was examined among Caucasians under other genetic models (recessive model, GG vs. GC + CC: OR = 0.794, 95% CI = 0.475–1.327, P = 0.378 and homozygote model, GG vs. CC: OR = 0.675, 95% CI = 0.402–1.134, P = 0.138). No subgroup analysis was performed in Asians and Africans due to only 1 study included in Asians and Africans. When stratified population by age, no statistically significant association was found in children under all genetic models. We could not perform analysis in adults since only one study was included.

As for CHIA rs10494132 polymorphism, results based on all included studies provided no evidence of association between CHIA rs10494132 polymorphism and asthma

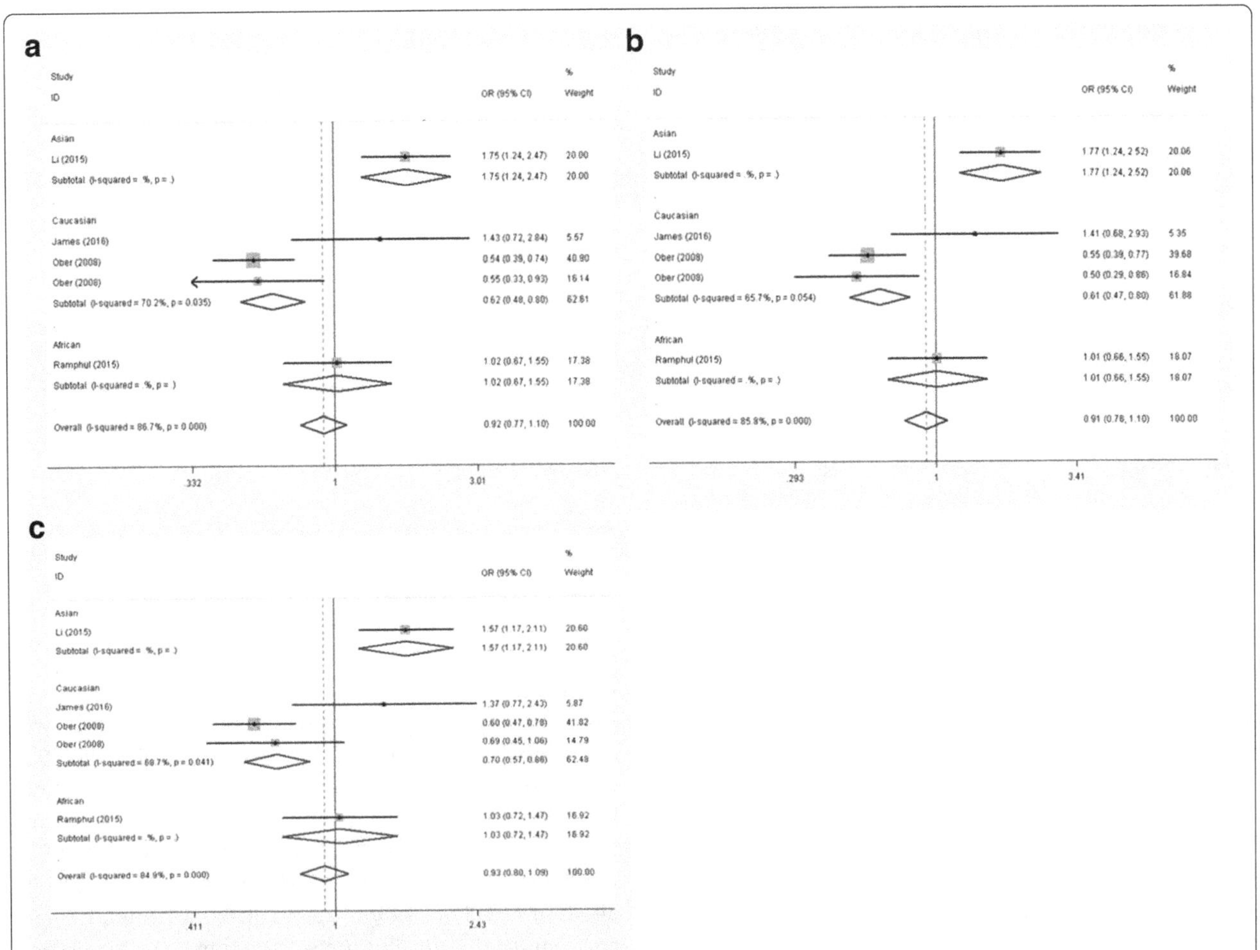

Fig. 2 Forest plot of the association between CHI3L1 rs4950928 polymorphism and asthma risk by ethnicity stratification under (**a**) the dominant model (GG + GC vs. CC), (**b**) the codominant model (GC vs. CC) and (**c**) the allele model (G vs. C)

risk in any genetic models in the overall population (recessive model, TT vs. TC + CC: OR = 1.212, 95% CI = 0.981–1.497, $P = 0.075$; dominant model, TT + TC vs. CC: OR = 0.857, 95% CI = 0.597–1.230, $P = 0.403$; codominant model, TC vs. CC: OR = 0.748, 95% CI = 0.504–1.109, $P = 0.149$; homozygote model, TT vs. CC: OR = 0.916, 95% CI = 0.630–1.331, $P = 0.646$ and allele model, T vs. C: OR = 1.094, 95% CI = 0.924–1.297, $P = 0.298$). In the subgroup analysis done on the basis of ethnicity, a positive correlation was found between CHIA rs10494132 polymorphism and asthma risk among Asians under the recessive model (TT vs. TC + CC: OR = 1.476, 95% CI = 1.071–2.032, $P = 0.017$) and the allele model (T vs. C: OR = 1.326, 95% CI = 1.024–1.717, $P = 0.032$) (Fig. 3). However, no significant association was observed under other genetic models (dominant model, TT + TC vs. CC: OR = 1.125, 95% CI = 0.654–1.933, $P = 0.671$; codominant model, TC vs. CC: OR = 0.926, 95% CI = 0.507–1.691, $P = 0.802$ and homozygote model, TT vs. CC: OR = 1.249, 95% CI = 0.709–2.199, $P = 0.441$). No subgroup analysis was performed in Caucasians due to limited studies included. Additionally, in the subgroup analysis conducted according to age, CHIA rs10494132 variant was also found to be associated with the increased risk of asthma in children under the recessive model (TT vs. TC + CC: OR = 1.472, 95% CI = 1.067–2.030, $P = 0.019$) and the allele model (T vs. C: OR = 1.320, 95% CI = 1.016–1.713, $P = 0.037$) (Fig. 4). While, no increased or reduced risk of asthma was detected in children under other genetic models (dominant model, TT + TC vs. CC: OR = 1.101, 95% CI = 0.629–1.927, $P = 0.737$; codominant model, TC vs. CC: OR = 0.903, 95% CI = 0.485–1.681, $P = 0.748$ and homozygote model, TT vs. CC: OR = 1.217, 95% CI = 0.679–2.184, $P = 0.510$). We could not perform subgroup analysis in adult group duo to insufficiency of relevant studies included.

Sensitivity analysis

In order to examine the stability of the pooled ORs, sensitivity analysis was performed by sequentially deleting one study at a time in all of the genetic models. For CHI3L1 rs4950928 and CHIA rs10494132 polymorphisms, the

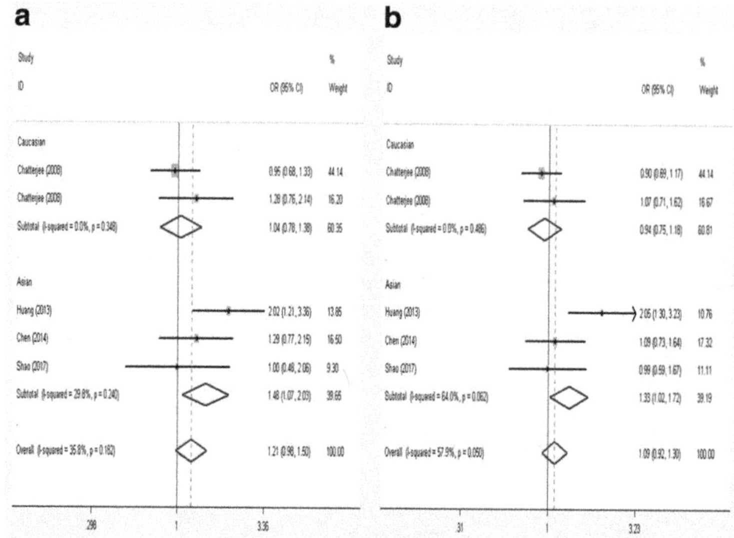

Fig. 3 Forest plot of the association between CHIA rs10494132 polymorphism and asthma risk stratified by ethnicity under (**a**) the recessive model (TT vs. TC + CC) and (**b**) the allele model (T vs. C)

corresponding pooled ORs did not impact in all genetic models, indicating that the results of this meta-analysis were stable.

Publication bias

Publication bias was evaluated by Begg's funnel plot and Egger's regression test. All the shapes of the funnel plots were found to be symmetrical (Fig. 5), indicating that there was no significant publication bias for the associations of CHI3L1 rs4950928 polymorphism and CHIA rs10494132 polymorphism in all the genetic models (all $P > 0.05$) (Table 4).

Discussion

In the present study, our results indicated that there was no significant association between CHI3L1 rs4950928 polymorphism and asthma susceptibility in overall analyses. However, following subgroup analysis by ethnicity, there was a protective effect of CHI3L1 rs4950928 polymorphism on asthma risk in Caucasians. The G allele of CHI3L1 rs4950928 might be a protective factor against the development of asthma. As for association between CHIA rs10494132 polymorphism and asthma risk, no evidence was found in the overall population, while a significantly increased risk of

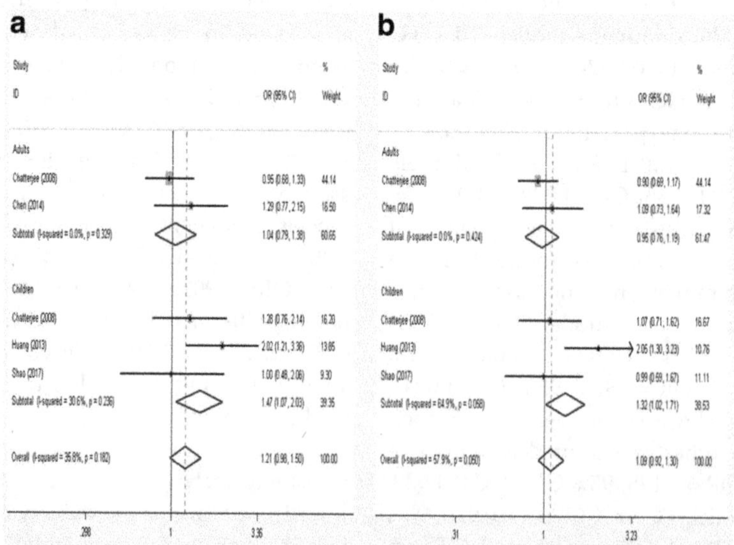

Fig. 4 Forest plot of the association between CHIA rs10494132 polymorphism and asthma risk by age stratification under (**a**) the recessive model (TT vs. TC + CC) and (**b**) the allele model (T vs. C)

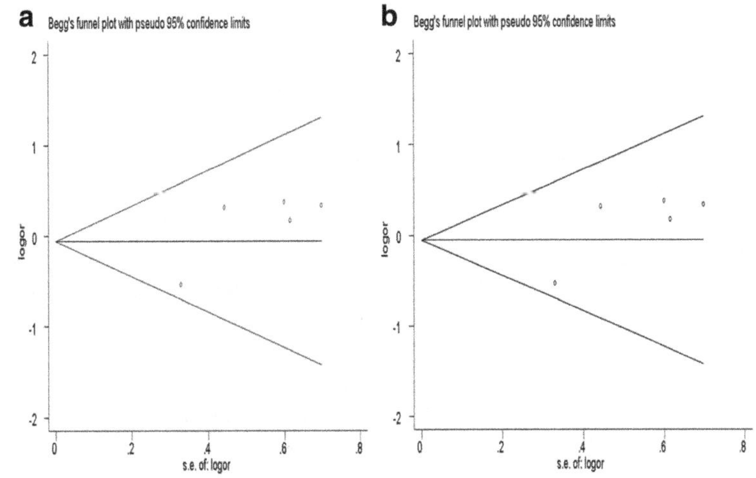

Fig. 5 Begg's funnel plots of publication bias for the association between CHI3L1 rs4950928 (**a**) and CHIA rs10494132 (**b**) polymorphisms and asthma risk under the recessive models (GG vs. GC + CC; TT vs. TC + CC)

asthma was found in Asians as well as in children of all ethnicities.

The gene CHI3L1, 10 exons long and located on chromosome 1q31-q32, codes for the chitinase-like protein YKL-40, which is a 40 kDa protein produced by cells in the airway mucosa, such as monocytes, macrophages and neutrophils [10, 17, 25]. YKL-40 binds with ubiquitously expressed chitin, but unlike chitinases CHIT1 and CHIA, which lacks measurable enzymatic chitinase activity [10]. Studies have shown that serum YKL-40 level is increased in patients with asthma and correlated with asthma severity, thickness of the subepithelial basement membrane, and pulmonary function, indicating that serum YKL-40 is an inflammatory biomarker associated with disease activity and mortality in asthmatic patients [12, 26]. Further study has shown that YKL-40 regulates TH2 immune response promoting airway inflammation in asthmatic mouse models as well as actives Akt, Erk, and p38 signaling pathway to promote human bronchial smooth muscle cell proliferation and migration, suggesting that YKL-40 is associated with the pathogenesis of asthma [27]. In addition, Genetic studies have demonstrated that the polymorphic variants of CHI3L1 gene contribute to the pathogenesis of asthma through influencing on airway inflammation and airway remodeling in the asthmatic patients [15, 26]. Recently, the relationship between CHI3L1 rs4950928 polymorphism and susceptibility to asthma was increasingly investigated [7, 18, 20, 21]. A Genome-wide Association Study (GWAS) reported by Ober et al. identified that the G allele of CHI3L1 rs4950928 is protective against asthma in three populations of European ancestry with mild

Table 4 Results of publication bias test

Subgroup	Genetic model	Genotype/ Allele	Begg's test		Egger's test	
			z value	*P* value	t value	*P* value
rs4950928						
Overall	Recessive model	GG vs. GC + CC	0.000	1.000	2.450	0.092
	Dominant model	GG + GC vs. CC	0.490	0.624	0.180	0.866
	Codominant model	GCvs.CC	0.490	0.624	0.060	0.958
	Homozygote model	GG vs. CC	0.980	0.327	1.880	0.157
	Allele model	Gvs.C	0.490	0.624	0.440	0.690
rs10494132						
Overall	Recessive model	TTvs. TC + CC	0.240	0.806	0.770	0.500
	Dominant model	TT + TCvs. CC	0.980	0.327	1.750	0.178
	Codominant model	TCvs. CC	0.490	0.624	1.050	0.373
	Homozygote model	TT vs. CC	1.470	0.142	2.200	0.116
	Allele model	T vs. C	0.490	0.624	1.200	0.317

asthma [18]. Another study have demonstrated that an association between CHI3L1 rs4950928 polymorphism and asthma is found, although the risk allele was opposite of that reported by Ober [21]. In contrast, additional publications have shown no significant association between genetic variation in the CHI3L1 rs4950928 and asthma risk [7, 20]. To date, the effect of genetic variation in CHI3L1 on asthma risk has not been fully addressed. Therefore, our meta-analysis provided a more statistical estimation demonstrating the relationship between CHI3L1 rs4950928 polymorphism and risk of asthma.

Our meta-analysis synthesized a total of 1062 cases and 1034 controls from 5 eligible studies to analyze the association between CHI3L1 rs4950928 polymorphism and asthma risk. The pooled results indicated no significant association between CHI3L1 rs4950928 polymorphism and asthma susceptibility. After stratified population by ethnicity, analysis indicated that the G allele of CHI3L1 rs4950928 had a reduced risk for asthma in Caucasians. No subgroup analysis was performed in Asians and Africans due to only 1 study included in Asians and Africans. When stratified population by age, the results remained non-significant in children. We could not perform analysis in adults since only one study was included.

The gene for CHIA is present on chromosome 1q13.1–21.3 and produces acid mammalian chitinase, which is a 50 kDa acid-stable protein [13]. Study has observed that serum CHIA level is overexpressed in ovalbumin-induced mouse model of asthma [16]. In addition, inhibition of CHIA expression reduced TH2-dependent airway inflammation, bronchial hyper-reactivity, and eosinophil counts in these asthma mouse model [16]. In humans, the expression of CHIA is strongly upregulated in lungs of asthmatic patients [16]. Furthermore, the CHIA enzyme has been found to be a downstream protein of interleukin-13, a cytokine implicated in the effect of human asthma [16]. Therefore, the CHIA enzyme has been suggested to be a positive mediator involved in the pathogenesis of asthma. Whereas, conflicting findings regarding its physiological role in asthma have reported that CHIA can inhibit chitin-induced allergic innate immune response in a mouse model by inhibiting eosinophil and basophil recruitment to the lungs [28]. Recently, one genetic study has described exonic CHIA polymorphisms are associated with bronchial asthma in a German pediatric population, indicating that exonic CHIA gene may be under the control of regulatory regions [19]. One promoter SNP, rs10494132, has been reported to be associated with pediatric asthma in Chinese population [23]. However, another three studies has demonstrated that no relationship between CHIA rs10494132 variation and risk of asthma is found [8, 22, 24]. Here we have performed meta-analysis to examine its association with asthma risk.

In this meta-analysis, 796 cases and 744 controls in 4 published articles were included. Results suggested that there was no significant relationship between CHIA rs10494132 polymorphism and asthma susceptibility. When population was stratified based on ethnicity, a positive correlation between CHIA rs10494132 polymorphism and asthma risk was found in Asians. No subgroup analysis was performed in Caucasians due to limited studies included. Moreover, in the subgroup analysis conducted according to age, CHIA rs10494132 variant was also found to be associated with the increased risk of asthma in children. We could not perform subgroup analysis in adult group duo to insufficiency of relevant studies included.

There are several limitations in this meta-analysis. Firstly, sample size in this meta-analysis was small, which might result in bias of the results when evaluating the association of CHI3L1 and CHIA gene polymorphisms with susceptibility to asthma. Secondly, the original data in some studies was lacking, which might limit sufficient statistical power to evaluate the potential effects of gene-gene and gene-environment interactions on the development of asthma. Thirdly, significant between-study heterogeneity was found in some pooled analyses. The exact sources of heterogeneity by meta-regression analysis were unable to further identify because of limited relevant data provided. Subgroup analysis was further performed based on ethnicity and age. However, heterogeneity was not resolved, indicating that other potentially relevant factors such as gender, genotyping method, phenotype of the disease may account for the heterogeneity. Fourthly, asthma is a heterogeneous disease with various genotypes and phenotypes. Although a genetic basis for asthma is undeniable, only a small proportion of heritability can be explained by the previously identified genetic polymorphisms associated with asthma because of the variability of the clinical phenotype. At last, only published studies were retrieved in the meta-analysis and possible publication bias might exist, despite no statistically significant publication bias was detected by Begg's test or Egger's test.

Conclusion

In conclusion, the present meta-analysis demonstrates that there was no significant association between CHI3L1 rs4950928 polymorphism and asthma susceptibility in overall analyses. However, following subgroup analysis by ethnicity, there was a protective effect of CHI3L1 rs4950928 polymorphism on asthma risk in Caucasians. The G allele of CHI3L1 rs4950928 might be a protective factor against the development of asthma. As for association between CHIA rs10494132 polymorphism and asthma risk, no evidence was found in the overall population, while a significantly increased risk of asthma was found in Asians as well as in children of all ethnicities.

Abbreviations

AMCase or CHIA: Acidic mammalian chitinase; CHI3L1: Chitinase 3–like 1; CHIT: Chitotriosidase; CI: Confidence interval; CNKI: China National Knowledge Infrastructure; GWAS: Genome-wide Association Study; HWE: Hardy-Weinberg equilibrium; IL-17F: Interleukin-17F; OR: Odds ratio; TLR4: Toll-like receptor 4

Acknowledgements

None.

Funding

This study was supported by the National Natural Science Foundation of China (Grant No. 81330002 and No. 81670051), a government funding in China. The grants are provided to cover the costs of the study. The funding agency had no role in study design, data collection and interpretation, analysis, or manuscript writing.

Authors' contributions

YZ: study protocol, literature search, data abstraction for meta-analysis, formulation of protocol, writing manuscript. XY, CZ and LY: literature search, data abstraction for meta-analysis. ML: study protocol, third reviewer of data abstraction, supervision of data abstraction, preparation of manuscript, submission for publication. All authors read and approved the final manuscript.

Consent for publication

Not applicable.

Competing interests

Authors declare no financial affiliations or conflicts of interest in submitting the study for publication.

References

1. Mims JW. Asthma: definitions and pathophysiology. International forum of allergy & rhinology. 2015; 5 Suppl 1: S2-S6.
2. Von Linstow ML, Porsbjerg C, Ulrik CS, Nepper-Christensen S, Backer V. Prevalence and predictors of atopy among young Danish adults. Clin Exp Allergy. 2002;32:520–5.
3. Thomsen SF, Ferreira MA, Kyvik KO, Fenger M, Backer V. A quantitative genetic analysis of intermediate asthma phenotypes. Allergy. 2009;64:427–30.
4. Wills-Karp M, Ewart SL. Time to draw breath: asthma-susceptibility genes are identified. Nat Rev Genet. 2004;5:376–87.
5. Du J, Han JC, Zhang YJ, Qi GB, Li HB, Zhang YJ, et al. Single-nucleotide polymorphisms of IL-17 gene are associated with asthma susceptibility in an Asian population. Med Sci. 2016;22:780–7.
6. Li S, Xie X, Song Y, Jiang H, Wu X, Su X, et al. Association of TLR4 (896A/G and 1196C/T) gene polymorphisms with asthma risk: a meta-analysis. Med Sci Monit. 2015;21:3591–9.
7. James AJ, Reinius LE, Verhoek M, Gomes A, Kupczyk M, Hammar U, et al. Increased YKL-40 and Chitotriosidase in asthma and chronic obstructive pulmonary disease. Am J Respir Crit Care Med. 2016;193:131–42.
8. Chatterjee R, Batra J, Das S, Sharma SK, Ghosh B. Genetic association of acidic mammalian chitinase with atopic asthma and serum total IgE levels. J Allergy Clin Immunol. 2008;122:202–8. 8.e1-7
9. Bussink AP, Speijer D, Aerts JM, Boot RG. Evolution of mammalian chitinase(–like) members of family 18 glycosyl hydrolases. Genetics. 2007; 177:959–70.
10. Lee CG, Da Silva CA, Lee JY, Hartl D, Elias JA. Chitin regulation of immune responses: an old molecule with new roles. Curr Opin Immunol. 2008;20:684–9.
11. Wills-Karp M, Karp CL. Chitin checking–novel insights into asthma. N Engl J Med. 2004;351:1455–7.
12. Chupp GL, Lee CG, Jarjour N, Shim YM, Holm CT, He S, et al. A chitinase-like protein in the lung and circulation of patients with severe asthma. N Engl J Med. 2007;357:2016–27.
13. Boot RG, Blommaart EF. Swart E, Ghauharali-van der Vlugt K, Bijl N, Moe C, et al. identification of a novel acidic mammalian chitinase distinct from chitotriosidase. J Biol Chem. 2001;276:6770–8.
14. Renkema GH, Boot RG, Muijsers AO, Donker-Koopman WE, Aerts JM. Purification and characterization of human chitotriosidase, a novel member of the chitinase family of proteins. J Biol Chem. 1995;270:2198–202.
15. Elias JA, Homer RJ, Hamid Q, Lee CG. Chitinases and chitinase-like proteins in T(H)2 inflammation and asthma. J Allergy Clin Immunol. 2005;116:497 500.
16. Zhu Z, Zheng T, Homer RJ, Kim YK, Chen NY, Cohn L, et al. Acidic mammalian chitinase in asthmatic Th2 inflammation and IL-13 pathway activation. Science (New York, NY). 2004;304:1678–82.
17. Ober C, Chupp GL. The chitinase and chitinase-like proteins: a review of genetic and functional studies in asthma and immune-mediated diseases. Curr Opin Allergy Clin Immunol. 2009;9:401–8.
18. Ober C, Tan Z, Sun Y, Possick JD, Pan L, Nicolae R, et al. Effect of variation in CHI3L1 on serum YKL-40 level, risk of asthma, and lung function. N Engl J Med. 2008;358:1682–91.
19. Bierbaum S, Nickel R, Koch A, Lau S, Deichmann KA, Wahn U, et al. Polymorphisms and haplotypes of acid mammalian chitinase are associated with bronchial asthma. Am J Respir Crit Care Med. 2005;172:1505–9.
20. Ramphul K, Hua L, Bao YX, Li JY, Liu QH, Ji RX, et al. Identification of IL13 C1923T as a single nucleotide polymorphism for asthma in children from Mauritius. Pediatr Allergy Immunol Pulmonol. 2015;28:92–5.
21. Ji-Ming LI, Xiao-Li SHEN, Hui XIE, Xing-Dong WU, Tong SHEN, Ye WANG. Association between CHI3L1 SNPs and susceptibility to childhood asthma. Chin J Contemp Pediatr. 2015;17(2):144–8.
22. Min CHEN, Xuanna ZHAO, Yingying LIU, Zhengni GAO, Dan HUANG, Shengming LIU. Correlation between CHI3L1 polymorphism and serum YL-40 and bronchial asthma. J Jilin University (Medicine Edition). 2014; 40(5):1058–63.
23. Xiang HUANG, Chunlei YUAN, Tao ZHOU, Yaling LUO. Genetic variants of CHIA and CHI3L1 gene are associated with childhood asthma of Han nationality. Chinese J Immunol. 2013;29:706–9.
24. SHAO Yawang, ZHENG Han, GOU Hongping, DONG Xiangyu. Correlation of CHI3L1 gene polymorphism with airway remodeling and inflammation in children with bronchial asthma. J Hainan Med College. 2017;23(8):1092-4.
25. Park JA, Drazen JM, Tschumperlin DJ. The chitinase-like protein YKL-40 is secreted by airway epithelial cells at base line and in response to compressive mechanical stress. J Biol Chem. 2010;285:29817–25.
26. Gomez JL, Crisafi GM, Holm CT, Meyers DA, Hawkins GA, Bleecker ER, et al. Genetic variation in chitinase 3-like 1 (CHI3L1) contributes to asthma severity and airway expression of YKL-40. J Allergy Clin Immunol. 2015; 136:51–8. e10
27. Bara I, Ozier A, Girodet PO, Carvalho G, Cattiaux J, Begueret H, et al. Role of YKL-40 in bronchial smooth muscle remodeling in asthma. Am J Respir Crit Care Med. 2012;185:715–22.
28. Reese TALH, Tager AM, et al. Chitin induces accumulation in tissue of innate immune cells associated with allergy. Nature. 2007;447:92–6.

8

Gene expression analysis in asthma using a targeted multiplex array

Christopher D. Pascoe[1,4,9*], Ma'en Obeidat[1,4], Bryna A. Arsenault[1,4], Yunlong Nie[1,4], Stephanie Warner[1,4], Dorota Stefanowicz[1,4], Samuel J. Wadsworth[1,4], Jeremy A. Hirota[8], S. Jasemine Yang[1,4], Delbert R. Dorscheid[1,4], Chris Carlsten[1,2,3,4,5], Tillie L. Hackett[1,4,6], Chun Y. Seow[1,4,7] and Peter D. Paré[1,2,4]

Abstract

Background: Gene expression changes in the structural cells of the airways are thought to play a role in the development of asthma and airway hyperresponsiveness. This includes changes to smooth muscle contractile machinery and epithelial barrier integrity genes. We used a targeted gene expression arrays to identify changes in the expression and co-expression of genes important in asthma pathology.

Methods: RNA was isolated from the airways of donor lungs from 12 patients with asthma (8 fatal) and 12 non-asthmatics controls and analyzed using a multiplexed, hypothesis-directed platform to detect differences in gene expression. Genes were grouped according to their role in airway dysfunction: airway smooth muscle contraction, cytoskeleton structure and regulation, epithelial barrier function, innate and adaptive immunity, fibrosis and remodeling, and epigenetics.

Results: Differential gene expression and gene co-expression analyses were used to identify disease associated changes in the airways of asthmatics. There was significantly decreased abundance of integrin beta 6 and Ras-Related C3 Botulinum Toxin Substrate 1 (RAC1) in the airways of asthmatics, genes which are known to play an important role in barrier function. Significantly elevated levels of Collagen Type 1 Alpha 1 (COL1A1) and COL3A1 which have been shown to modulate cell proliferation and inflammation, were found in asthmatic airways. Additionally, we identified patterns of differentially co-expressed genes related to pathways involved in virus recognition and regulation of interferon production. 7 of 8 pairs of differentially co-expressed genes were found to contain CCCTC-binding factor (CTCF) motifs in their upstream promoters.

Conclusions: Changes in the abundance of genes involved in cell-cell and cell-matrix interactions could play an important role in regulating inflammation and remodeling in asthma. Additionally, our results suggest that alterations to the binding site of the transcriptional regulator CTCF could drive changes in gene expression in asthmatic airways. Several asthma susceptibility loci are known to contain CTCF motifs and so understanding the role of this transcription factor may expand our understanding of asthma pathophysiology and therapeutic options.

Keywords: Asthma, Co-expression, Nanostring, Extracellular matrix, CTCF, Smooth muscle, Remodeling, Epithelium, Targeted expression

* Correspondence: cpascoe@chrim.ca
[1]UBC Institute for Heart Lung Health, St. Paul's Hospital, 1081 Burrard St, Vancouver, BC, Canada
[4]University of British Columbia Centre for Heart Lung Innovation, St. Paul's Hospital, 1081 Burrard St, Vancouver, BC, Canada
Full list of author information is available at the end of the article

Background

Asthma is a chronic inflammatory disease of the airways, characterized by symptoms of breathlessness, wheezing and cough, associated with variable airflow limitation and airway hyperresponsiveness (AHR). Asthma is also characterized by airway remodeling which includes goblet cell metaplasia, epithelial damage, subepithelial fibrosis, basement membrane thickening, and increased airway smooth muscle (ASM) mass [1]. The pathogenesis of asthma is believed to involve an interaction between the innate and adaptive immune systems [2], and phenotypic changes within the epithelial-mesenchymal trophic unit [3]. Genetic and genomic analyses have been used to discover the molecular mechanisms underlying these phenotypic changes. Large genome-wide association studies (GWAS) have reproducibly identified single nucleotide polymorphisms (SNPs) in or near genes predominantly expressed in the airway epithelium and immune cells as susceptibility factors for asthma. The specific genes include gasdermin B (*GSDMB*) [4], interleukin 33 (*IL33*), and thymic stromal lymphopoietin (*TSLP*) [5]. Another candidate gene *ADAM33*, expressed in ASM, has been shown to be associated with asthma in linkage analysis [6]. Genetic variants associated with susceptibility for asthma may exert their effect by altering gene expression levels; indeed many of the SNPs associated with asthma and AHR have been shown to be expression quantitative trait loci (eQTL) in lung tissue, epithelial and blood cells, and altered protein expression of some of these genes has been found in cells and tissue from asthmatic individuals [7].

In this hypothesis driven study we used a reproducible multiplexed technology (Nanostring®) to quantify the expression of 334 genes potentially involved in phenotypic changes in asthmatic airways. This technology is highly sensitive, reproducible, and is suitable for archived tissue specimens as it is insensitive to RNA degradation [8]. We hypothesized that changes in the expression patterns of genes involved in ASM contraction, the cytoskeleton, epithelial barrier function, innate/adaptive immunity, fibrosis and remodeling, and epigenetics would be present in the airway tissue of asthmatics compared to non-asthmatics. Our results suggest that alterations in the expression of genes involved in cell-cell and cell-matrix interactions may contribute to the pathogenesis of asthma, particularly severe asthma. The identification of altered gene co-expression networks may identify changes in transcriptional regulation that could be pathogenic and missed with commonly used analyses for differential expression.

Methods

Additional description of methods is provided in the online supplement.

Subject selection and RNA isolation

Human lungs were donated with consent from the IIAM and used with approval from the University of British Columbia and St. Paul's Hospital ethics committee. Diagnosis of asthma was determined through patient medical history and asthma medication usage as determined by family interview. Non-asthma donor deaths were primarily due to head trauma while 8 of the 12 donors with asthma died during exacerbations of their asthma. The other four donors with asthma died due to other, accidental causes (eg. head trauma). Subject demographics can be seen in Table 1 with full subject characteristics found in Additional file 1: Table S1. After surgical removal the lungs were flushed with Custodiol HTK solution (Odyssey Pharmaceuticals, East Hanover, NJ, USA) and transported on ice by plane. The time between harvesting and arrival at the University of British Columbia was 15–20 h. Tissues from the lungs have been used in previous studies [9–11]. Inflated frozen lungs were processed into tissue cores for sectioning on a crytostat. A total of twenty 10 μm thick sections per core were cut and stored at −80 °C until RNA was isolated. Sections 1, 5, 10, 15 and 20 were stained with hematoxylin and eosin (H&E) for morphometric measurements. For the remaining 15 sections, airways and a small amount of surrounding parenchyma were macroscopically dissected using a scalpel (Fisher Scientific® No. 11) for RNA isolation. Samples were only used if the airways seen on the first section were continuous for the 20 sequential sections. Large vessels were avoided. Sample airway is seen in Fig. 1. RNA was isolated using the Qiagen® RNeasy Mini Kit according to manufacturers protocol.

Characterization of airway dimensions

Measurements of ASM, epithelial, collagen, and total wall area in addition to basement membrane thickness were measured to quantify the degree of airway remodeling. The five sections stained with H&E (Fig. 2) from each core were digitally scanned and airway wall compartments were quantified using the Aperio® system (Leica Biosystems, Germany). ASM area, epithelial area and total airway wall area were quantified using a point counting method, where a grid of 4000 points was overlaid onto each airway of interest and the points falling on the area of interest were counted (Image Pro Plus ®, Media Cybernetics, Maryland). The measurements for all airways were normalized to the internal perimeter (Pi) of the airway and averaged across all the sections for each subject. The Pi was measured by tracing along the luminal side of the epithelium. For the measurement of basement membrane thickness and collagen area, two additional sections were cut from each core (same as used for RNA isolation and other measurements) to stain with Masson's trichrome (basement membrane) and Picrosirius red (collagen). To

Table 1 Patient demographics. Ages not significantly different

	Non-asthmatic (*n* = 12)	Asthmatic (n = 12)
Median Age (Range)	21 (4–63)	17.5 (8–36)
Male Sex – # (%)	6 (50)	7 (58.3)
Average Weight - kg (±SEM)	75.7 (7.5)	68.8 (6.4)
Inhaled Corticosteroids – # (%)	0 (0)	6 (50)
Smoking - # (%)	2 (16.7)	4 (33.3)
End of life steroids - # (%)	4 (33.3)	8 (66.7)
Fatal Asthma - # (%)		8 (66.7)

quantify the basement membrane thickness, a random series of line segments was placed over each image and the thickness of the basement membrane was measured at the points where any line segment crossed the basement membrane. All thickness measurements were made perpendicular to the epithelium. A minimum of 40 measurements were made for each airway. For the measurement of collagen content, Picrosirius red stained slides were visualized under polarized light where the Picrosirius red stain shows birefringence. The collagen appears red on a black background and the amount of collagen was quantified using color segmentation in Image Pro Plus®. All measurements were carried out in a blinded manner.

Gene expression analysis

Expression of mRNA for the 334 candidate genes and 12 housekeeping genes was measured with the Nanostring® system using a custom codeset panel. The most stable housekeeping genes were selected by measuring 12 common housekeeping genes. By comparing the % Coefficient of variation (%CV) across the 12 housekeeping genes we were able to determine that the 5 most stable genes for data normalization were: RNA Polymerase R2A (POLR2A), TATA box binding protein (TBP), Ribosomal Protein L19 (RPL19), Guanine nucleotide-binding protein subunit beta-2-like 1 (GNB2L1), and β-Glucuronidase (GUSB). These 5 genes were also selected because they spanned a range of counts from low (average 198 counts for GUSB) to high (average 22,486 counts for RPL19). Data were normalized in accordance with Nanostring® guidelines. See Additional file 1: Table S2 in the online supplement for a complete list of genes in the panel.

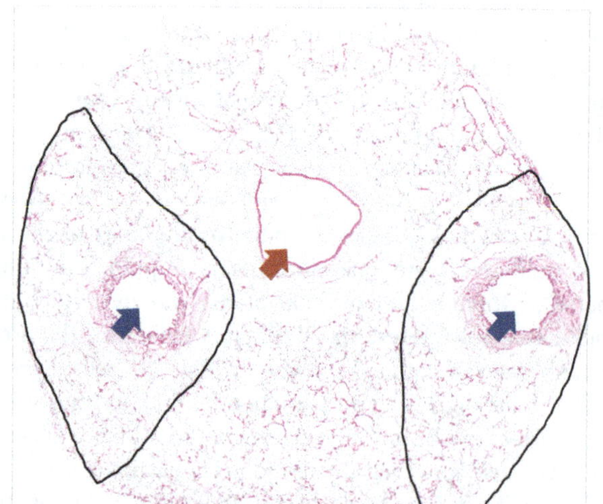

Fig. 1 Section of a frozen human lung core cut at 10 μm thickness. Blue arrows indicate airways. Red arrow indicates a blood vessel. The black lines show the outline of the tissue taken for isolation of total airway RNA. Scale bar = 5 mm

Candidate gene selection

We selected the candidate genes based on a priori hypotheses and grouped them based on their function and potential role in the pathogenesis of asthma and/or AHR. These are: ASM contraction and relaxation, structure and regulation of the cytoskeleton, epithelial barrier function, innate and adaptive immunity, fibrosis and remodeling and epigenetics. The rationale for the choice of groups of genes is provided below and the list of the genes by category is in Additional file 1: Table S2

1) **The contraction and relaxation of ASM and its regulation**; MYH11, MLCK, SM-22 and actin have been previously examined in the context of asthma [12]. Many of the genes in the contractile machinery group were taken from the Kyoto Encyclopedia of Genes and Genomes (KEGG) pathway for vascular smooth muscle contraction. Additionally, work by Sieck et al. [13] led to the selection of CD38 and other calcium handling proteins that have been shown to be expressed in cultured ASM cells. Genes within this pathway are involved in either contraction or relaxation of smooth muscle and so have the potential to play a role in AHR in asthma.
2) **The structure and regulation of the cytoskeleton**; genes within the cytoskeletal group were selected based on previous work by Gunst et al. [14]. Genes in this group have been shown to be important in transmitting ASM force to the external environment at adherens junctions, in maintaining the actin filament lattice or or regulating ASM stiffness independent of force generation [15].
3) **Epithelial barrier function**; a number of observations suggest that the airway epithelium is disrupted in asthma and that this may in part result from altered repair mechanisms [16]. Disrupted features include detachment of columnar ciliated cells, the presence of epithelial cell aggregates (Creola bodies) in sputum, decreased expression of epithelial cell-cell junction proteins (E-cadherin, ZO-

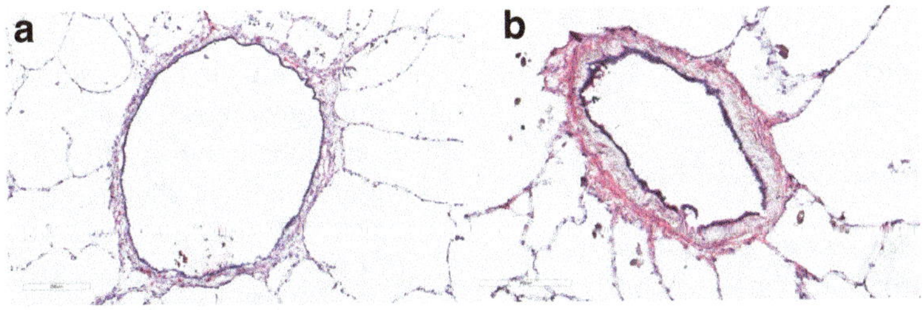

Fig. 2 Comparison of non-asthmatic airway (**a**) and asthmatic airway (**b**). Airways are stained using hematoxylin and eosin (H&E) to highlight remodeling changes within the airways. Scale bar is 200 μm

1, protocadherin-1) and increased expression of epithelial repair markers (TGF-β, EGFR and CD44), mucins, and altered expression of repair-associated fucosylated glycoproteins [17]. A defective epithelial barrier may have important consequences in asthma as it is thought to lead to increased accessibility of allergens to immune and structural cells within the mucosal and submucosal spaces.

4) **Innate/Adaptive immunity**; innate immune receptors and related mediators have been implicated in the pathogenesis of asthma (e.g. IL-33, TSLP, and ST2) [18]. Furthermore, it has been demonstrated that antiviral immune responses are compromised in airway epithelial cells from asthmatics [19]. Intrinsic differences in innate immune responses in airway epithelial cells may therefore contribute to disease development and exacerbations in response to environmental exposures including allergens, viruses, and air pollution [20]. We therefore determined the expression patterns of all Toll-like receptors (TLRs), Nod-like receptors (NLRs), and Rig-like receptors (RLRs) and related mediators to provide a comprehensive screen of these candidate genes in asthmatic and non-asthmatic airway wall samples.
5) **Fibrosis and remodeling**; the role of the myocardin pathway in proliferation of ASM cells [21] led to the selection of genes in this pathway. In addition, we interrogated members of the Notch family as these genes are integral to airway development and differentiation [22] and may play important roles in asthma. ECM proteins are altered in the airways of asthmatics and as such, we included a number of genes that code for ECM components thought to be involved in the remodeling of asthmatic airways. In vivo work has shown a role for matrix metalloproteinases (MMPs) in the development of airway inflammation and hyperresponsiveness [23].
6) **Epigenetics**; as a first line of contact with the external environment, the airway epithelium is an attractive target for epigenetic research. Alterations in DNA methylation and histone modifications have been reported in the airway epithelium of asthmatic subjects [24], however many of the mediators involved have not been studied. We targeted the histone acetyltransferases KAT2A, CREBBP, and EP300 as they are responsible for acetylating lysine 18 on histone 3 which is up regulated in asthmatic epithelial cells [24]. We also focused on AURKA, PRMT5, SUV39H1, and HDAC10 which have been identified to be potentially involved in the pathogenesis of asthma based on preliminary data from an array analysis of epigenetic modifying enzymes (58). A number of genes chosen for this study were previously found to be differentially methylated in preliminary (PTK7, BCL3, DNMT3b, and PTPRO) [25] and final (CRIP1, STAT5A, FGFR1, S100A2, ITGA2, EGR4, EID1, and IGSF4C) analyses of DNA methylation in asthmatic airway epithelial cells [26].

Additional genes were added to the list given their reproducible association in asthma GWAS and observation that the SNP's in these genes act as eQTLs.

Data and statistical analyses

Final Nanostring results were filtered to keep only genes that had an average count of at least 30. Normalized mRNA expression values were compared between asthmatic and non-asthmatic subjects using a linear model with a negative binomial distribution controlling for age, sex, and inhaled corticosteroid use. Differential gene expression data are presented as volcano plots as well as in a summary table showing the top differentially regulated genes. The level of expression of each transcript is not completely independent since there was strong co-expression between the 344 genes. To account for this, we employed the Matrix Spectral Decomposition analysis of Nyholt and Li et al. [27, 28] to identify the effective number of independent genes. This lead to the multiple comparison correction shown in Table 2 that is based on an effective n of 31. Adjusted p-values will be listed as p.adj and genes with a nominal unadjusted $p < 0.05$ will be listed as p.unadj.

Table 2 Significant differentially expressed genes after *p*-value correction

Gene name	Symbol	Fold change	Counts (Asthma)	Counts (Non-Asthma)	Adjusted *p*-value (p.adj)
Integrin Beta 6	ITGB6	−1.51	367.4 ± 27.9	475.3 ± 46.4	0.002
Collagen Type 1 Alpha 1	COL1A1	1.92	1344.4 ± 222.0	735.8 ± 172.1	0.01
Collagen Type 3 Alpha 1	COL3A1	1.84	5324.3 ± 1517.9	3321.1 ± 321.3	0.03

In addition to the analysis of differential gene expression, we performed an analysis of differential co-expression in our data set using the analysis package CoXpress for R. Differential co-expression analysis identifies pairs of genes that are differentially co-expressed i.e. have opposite correlation patterns in cases vs. controls or show correlations in one condition only. Genes that were differentially co-expressed were entered into WebGestalt for pathway enrichment analysis and are presented in table form. Network analyst was used to understand the protein-protein interaction network [PMID: 25,950,236} of all nominally significant genes (p.unadj < 0.05). Data are plotted using GraphPad version 5.04 (La Jolla California USA).

Results

Airway characteristics

The total number of airways analyzed was 52 in asthmatic and 53 in non-asthmatic subjects; with an average of 4.3 airways per subject ($p > 0.05$, asthmatic vs. non-asthmatic). The average internal perimeter (Pi) of asthmatic subjects was 5.1 ± 1.5 mm (geometric mean 4.0 ± 1.7 mm) and in non-asthmatic subjects was 5.3 ± 1.5 mm (geometric mean 4.9 ± 1.3 mm) (p > 0.05 for both arithmetic and geometric mean). Airway wall area per unit length of Pi was significantly greater in asthmatics (0.22 ± 0.024 mm^2/mm) than in non-asthmatics (0.13 ± 0.019 mm^2/mm, $p < 0.01$). There was also an increase in the ASM area per unit Pi (0.018 ± 0.0024 mm^2/mm vs. 0.011 ± 0.0015 mm^2/mm, $p < 0.05$) and in basement membrane thickness (6.9 ± 0.81 mm vs. 3.9 ± 0.73 mm, $p < 0.01$) in asthmatics versus non-asthmatics. There was no significant difference in the area of epithelium or collagen per unit Pi between donor groups ($p > 0.05$). Side by side comparison of asthmatic and non-asthmatic airway can be seen in Fig. 2.

Differential gene expression analysis

Gene expression changes in all genes are summarized in Fig. 3 with the candidate gene hypothesis categories plotted in Fig. 4. In total there were 51 genes differentially expressed based on a threshold *p*-value of $p < 0.05$ and three genes that were significant after p-value correction (Table 2, p.adj). In brief, there were three genes whose significance reached the adjusted p-value cutoff, Collagen Type 1 Alpha 1 (*COL1A1*), *COL3A1*, and integrin beta 6 (*ITGB6*). The gene for *COL1A1* was the most significantly up-regulated gene (1.83-fold increase, p.adj = 0.01) and integrin beta 6 (*ITGB6*) was the most significantly down-regulated gene (1.29-fold decrease, p.adj = 0.002) (Additional file 1: Table S2). COL1A1 expression was positively associated with the amount of collagen in the airway in asthmatics and non-asthmatics (Collagen/

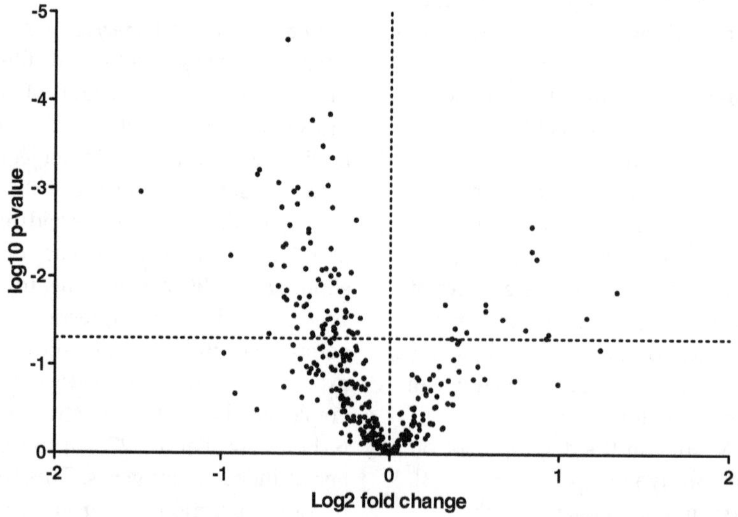

Fig. 3 Volcano plot summarizing the results of the gene expression analysis. Dotted vertical line indicates fold difference of zero. Fold differences greater than zero (positive) indicate increased gene expressed in asthmatics compared to non-asthmatics. Dotted horizontal line indicates significance at nominal *p*-value of 0.05

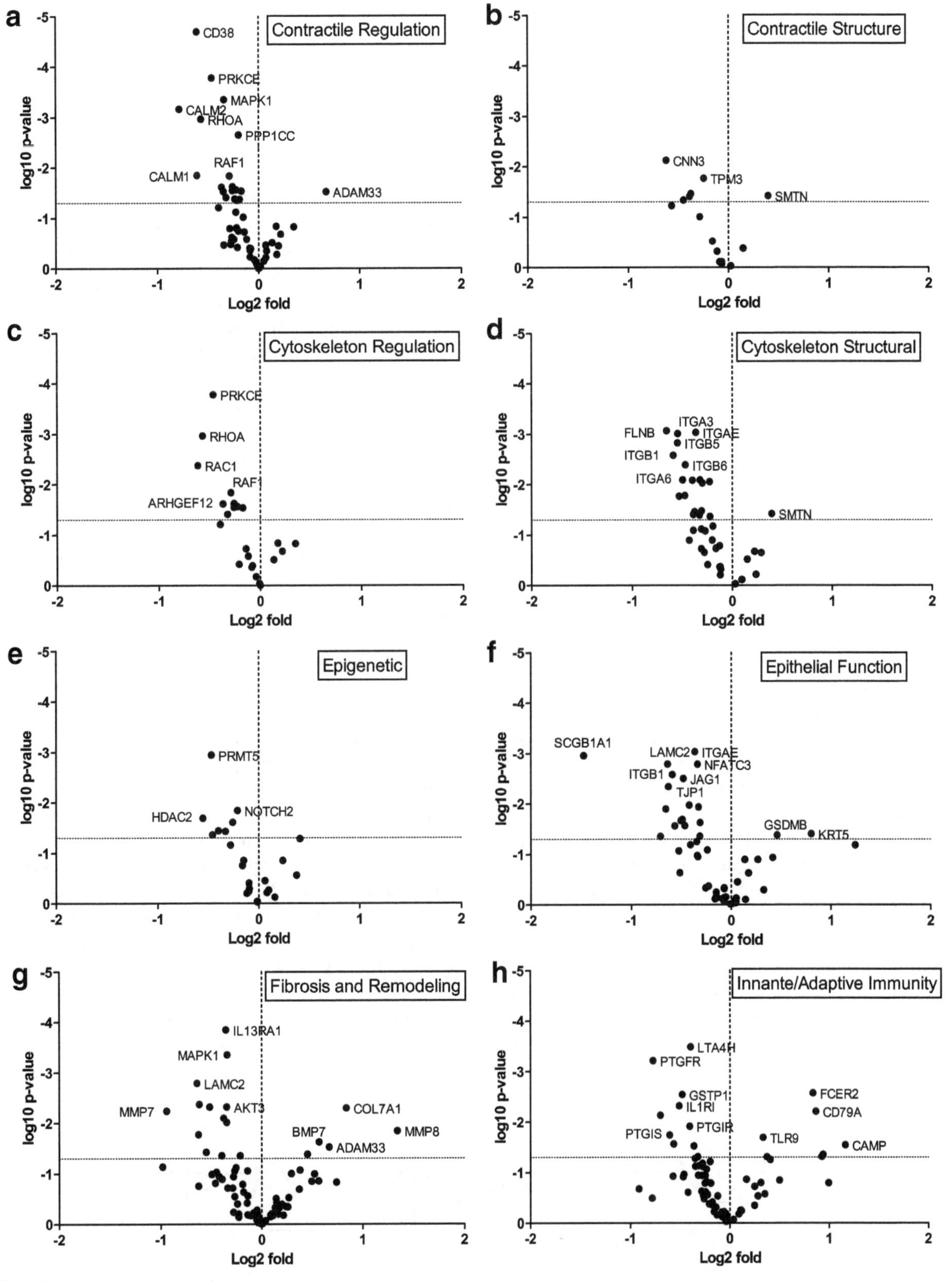

Fig. 4 (See legend on next page.)

(See figure on previous page.)
Fig. 4 Volcano plots summarizing the results of gene expression for each hypothesis group. Genes involved in (**a**) Contractile regulation, (**b**) Structure of the contractile apparatus, (**c**) Cytoskeletal regulation, (**d**) Structure of the cytoskeleton, (**e**) Epigenetic control, (**f**) Epithelial function, (**g**) Fibrosis and remodeling, (**h**) Innate and adaptive immunity. Some genes fall into more than one category and so are plotted in applicable categories. Dotted vertical line indicates fold differences of zero, dotted horizontal lines indicates significance at nominal *p*-value of 0.05

Pi, $R^2 = 0.2221$ and 0.2182 for asthma and non-asthma respectively, $p < 0.01$) and the thickness of the basement membrane in both groups combined ($R^2 = 0.1313$, $p = 0.01$). COL3A1 expression was positively associated with ASM/Pi ($R^2 = 0.2089$, $p = 0.02$) and Collagen/Pi ($R^2 = 0.2083$, $p = 0.03$) in asthma. ITGB6 expression was negatively associated with basement membrane thickness in asthma ($R^2 = 0.1801$, $p = 0.04$) and negatively associated with Epithelial area/Pi in both groups combined ($R^2 = 0.1158$, $p = 0.02$). There was an association between ITGB6 expression and Collagen/Pi in asthma that did not quite reach significance. ($R^2 = 0.144$, $p = 0.06$). In each hypothesis group there were a number of differentially expressed genes that did not reach significance after *p*-value adjustment, these included: contractile apparatus structure – Smoothelin (1.40 fold increase, p.unadj = 0.01); regulation of contraction – CD38 (1.66 fold decrease, p.unadj =0.003); cytoskeletal structure – ITGB6 (see above); cytoskeletal regulation – RAC1 (1.60 fold decrease, p.unadj =0.002); epigenetic regulation – PRMT5 (1.52 fold decrease, p.unadj =0.03); epithelial function – LAMC2 (1.59 fold decrease, p.unadj =0.006); fibrosis and remodeling – COL1A1 (see above); innate and adaptive immunity – PTGFR (2.18 fold decrease, p.unadj =0.004). The counts, *p*-values, and adjusted *p*-values for all significant genes can be seen in Additional file 1: Table S2. Of the 12 genes identified in GWAS or linkage analysis, only *ADAM33* (1.56-fold increase, p.unadj =0.0057) was up-regulated. There were no pathways significantly enriched in the differentially up or down-regulated genes.

Using Network Analyst, we identified a minimum protein-protein interaction network and key nodes from our nominally differentially expressed genes (Fig. 5). Green nodes indicate down-regulated genes, red nodes indicate up-regulated nodes (both relative to non-asthmatics), and grey nodes indicate first order interactions. This network highlights a number of key nodes in our data set including: Mitogen-Activated Protein Kinase 1 (MAPK1, degree = 24), c-FOS (degree = 22, and Calmodulin 3 (CALM3, degree = 21). Using this network, we were able to identify pathways significantly associated with up and down-regulated nodes (Table 3). These included key pathways in collagen degradation and remodeling and alterations to cell-cell communication.

Differential co-expression analysis

We identified groups of genes that were differentially co-expressed between asthmatics and non-asthmatics. In this analysis, genes are clustered together based on how their expression values correlate with each other. The analysis was performed twice with the comparison group being the non-asthmatics or asthmatics in the different analyses. Clusters of genes that are significantly co-expressed in one condition and not in the other are said to be differentially co-expressed. Figure 5 shows an example; expression of genes in cluster 11 changes from subject to subject in asthmatics (left) and non-asthmatics (right). Each line represents one gene in the group. Genes in cluster 11 follow a similar pattern of expression in asthmatics ($p < 0.001$) but not in non-asthmatics ($p = 0.32$). The rest of these figures can be seen in Additional file 1: Fig. S3 and S4.

In non-asthmatics, there were 3 groups of genes that were differentially co-expressed compared to asthmatics. These clusters (10, 35, and 53) had an average co-expression correlation coefficient of 0.772 ($p < 0.0001$) in non-asthmatics and 0.223 ($p > 0.05$) in asthmatics. The genes in these groupings are summarized in Additional file 1: Table S3. We performed pathways analysis on each group of genes with Webgestalt. These results are shown in Table 4. There were no pathways that were significantly

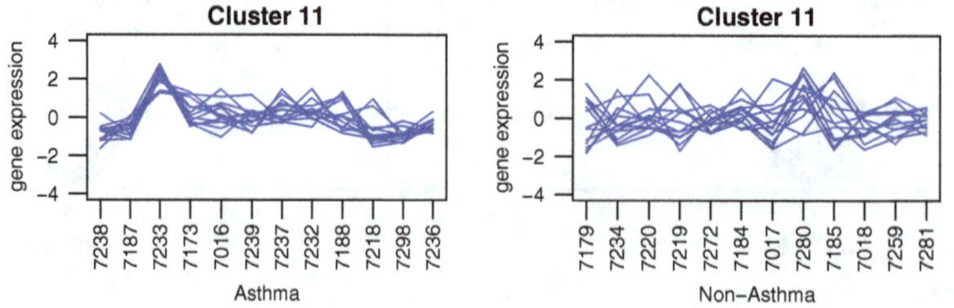

Fig. 5 Example of co-expression plots. Each line represents one gene in the cluster. Subjects are indicated along the x-axis, log expression values on the y-axis. *P*-values are for the significance of the co-expression in each group

Table 3 Pathways significantly associated with protein-protein interaction nodes

Pathway name	Hits/Total	FDR
Up-Regulated Pathways		
Degradation of Collagen	4/61	0.003
Extracellular Matrix Organization	5/157	0.003
Degradation of Extracellular Matrix	4/77	0.004
Assembly of Collagen Fibrills and Other Multimeric Structures	3/54	0.04
Collagen Biosynthesis and Modifying Enzymes	3/62	0.04
Down-regulated pathways		
Integrin Cell Surface Interactions	6/85	0.0007
Signal Transduction	17/1690	0.004
Cell-Cell Communication	6/143	0.004
Platelet Activation, Signaling, and Aggregation	7/220	0.004
TGF-beta Receptor Signaling in EMT	3/17	0.009
Hemostatis	9/511	0.01
Signaling by TGF-beta Receptor Complex	4/70	0.02
Sema4D Induced Cell Migration and Growth-Cone Collapse	3/29	0.03
Sema4D in Semaphorin Signaling	3/34	0.04
Fc-gamma Receptor Dependent Phagocytosis	4/86	0.04

enriched for genes differentially co-expressed in non-asthmatics. Further analysis identified specific gene pairs from cluster 10 that were both significantly positively correlated in non-asthmatics and significantly negatively correlated in asthmatics (Table 5). These included: chitinase 3-like 1(*CHI3L1*) and *GSDMB* ($R = 0.760$ and $R = -0.707$); *CHI3L1* and histone deacetylase 10 (*HDAC10*) ($R = 0.731$ and $R = -0.676$); *HDAC10* and thymocyte antigen 1 (*THY1* or *CD90*) ($R = 0.727$ and $R = -0.596$); and indoleamine 2,3-dioxygenase 1 (*IDO1*) and nuclear factor of activated T-cells, cytoplasmic 2 (*NFATC2*) ($R = 0.659$ and $R = -0.604$), in non-asthmatics and asthmatics respectively. All showed significant but opposite direction of correlation ($p < 0.05$ Fig. 6).

In asthmatic samples there were 6 clusters of genes that were found to be differentially co-expressed. These clusters had an average correlation coefficient of 0.728 ($p < 0.0001$) in asthmatics and 0.169 ($p > 0.05$) in non-asthmatics. The genes in these 6 clusters are summarized in Additional file 1: Table S3. Each of the clusters was also analyzed with Webgestalt (Table 4). In brief, asthmatic co-expressed genes were significantly enriched in pathways for cytoplasmic virus pattern recognition signaling ($p = 3.0 \times 10^{-4}$), positive, and negative regulation of type 1 interferon production ($p = 3.9 \times 10^{-3}$, and $p = 2.0 \times 10^{-3}$ respectively). Within the cluster of genes that were differentially co-expressed, there were 4 pairs

Table 4 Pathways enriched in differentially co-expressed genes. *p*-value comes from using list of 334 genes as background

Cluster #	# Genes in Cluster	# Genes From Cluster in Pathway	Biological Process	*p*-value
Coexpressed in Non-asthmatics				
10	25	3	Regulation of Cell-Cell Adhesion Involved in Gastrulation	2.0×10^{-1}
		13	Regulation of Multicellular Organismal Development	2.0×10^{-1}
		8	Regulation of Cell Adhesion	2.0×10^{-1}
53	6	4	Cell Migration	4.0×10^{-1}
		4	Locomotion	5.7×10^{-1}
		4	Localization of Cell	4.0×10^{-1}
Coexpressed in Asthmatics				
16	6	3	**Cytoplasmic Pattern Recognition Receptor Signaling Pathway in Response to Virus**	**3.0×10^{-4}**
		3	**Positive Regulation of Type 1 Interferon Production**	**3.9×10^{-3}**
		3	**Negative Regulation of Type 1 Interferon Production**	**2.0×10^{-3}**
20	6	4	Activation of MAPK Activity	6.9×10^{-2}
		4	Peptidyl-Tyrosine Phosphorylation	7.9×10^{-2}
		3	Eicosanoind Biosynthetic Pathway	7.9×10^{-2}
11	9	3	Odontogenesis	4.2×10^{-1}
17	7	4	Response to Bacterium	3.9×10^{-1}

Bolded pathways highlight those that reached statistical significance in the co-expression data set

Table 5 Pairs of differentially co-expressed genes

Gene 1	Gene 2	Asthma R	*p*-value	Non-Asthma R	*p*-value
LAMB2	MMP9	0.727	0.007	−0.686	0.013
BPIFA1	DDX58	0.814	0.001	−0.646	0.023
BMP2	NFATC2	0.707	0.010	−0.660	0.020
GNAS	NFATC2	0.665	0.018	−0.798	0.002
CHI3L1	GSDMB	−0.707	0.010	0.760	0.004
CHI3L1	HDAC10	−0.676	0.016	0.731	0.007
HDAC10	THY1	−0.596	0.041	0.727	0.007
IDO1	NFATC2	−0.604	0.037	0.659	0.0198

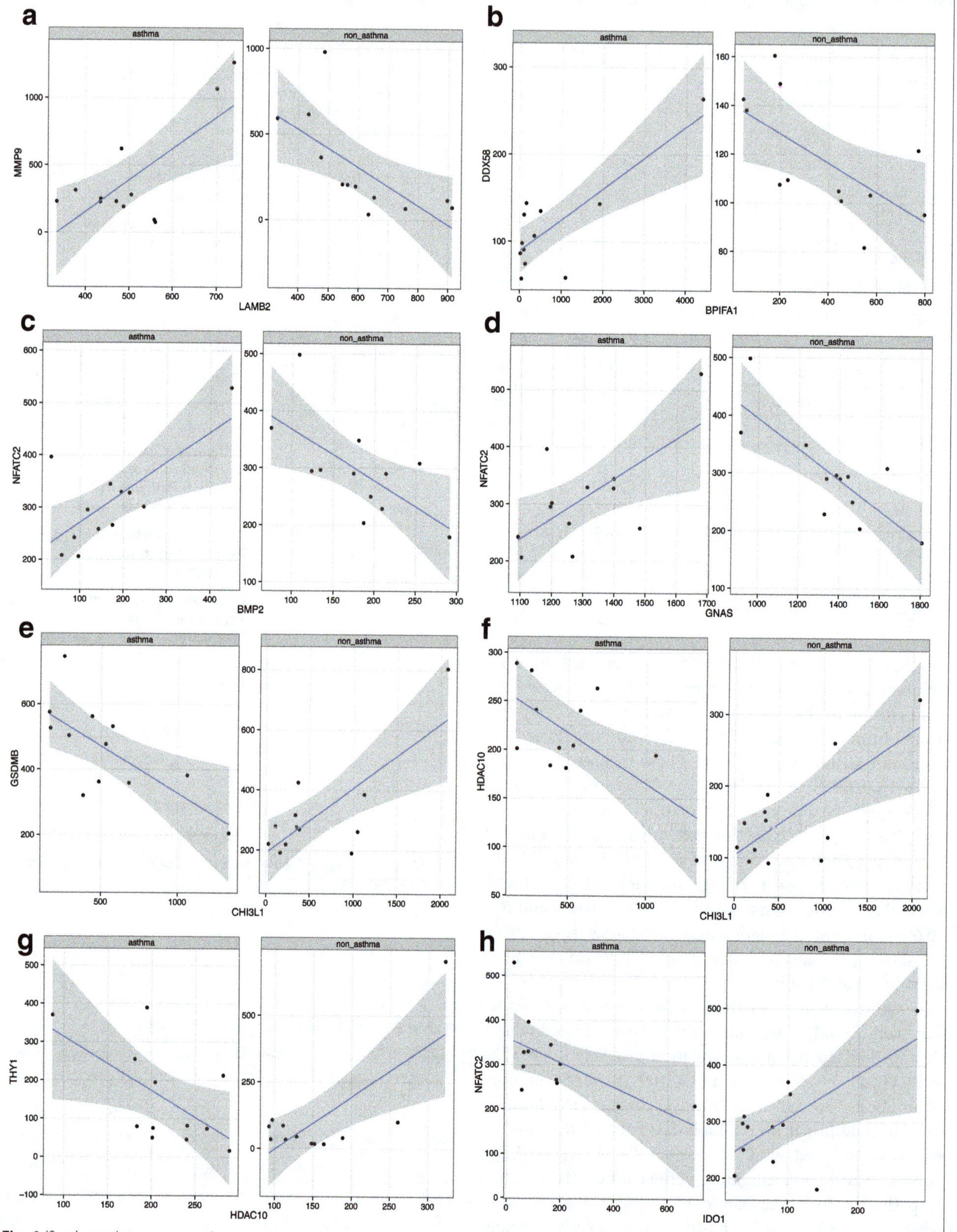

Fig. 6 (See legend on next page.)

(See figure on previous page.)
Fig. 6 Individual correlation plots for the pairs of differentially co-expressed genes in asthmatics and non-asthmatics. **a** LAMB2 vs. MMP9, (**b**) BPIFA1 vs. DDX58, (**c**) BMP2 vs. NFACT2, (**d**) GNAS vs. NFACT2, (**e**) CHI3L1 vs. GSDMB, (F) CHI3L1 vs. HDAC10, (G) HDAC10 vs. THY1, (F) IDO1 vs. NFATC2. Each point represents a sample and the values on the axes are gene counts. Lines of best fit are plotted with the 95% confidence interval (grey shaded area) for each correlation. Each of the correlations is significant ($p < 0.05$) and the direction indicates a positive or negative correlation

of genes whose expression were positively and significantly correlated in asthmatics but negatively and significantly correlated in non-asthmatics (Table 5). In brief: laminin B2 (*LAMB2*) and matrix metallopeptidase 9 (*MMP9*) (R = 0.727 and $R = -0.686$); BPI fold containing family A (BPFIA1) and DEAD box polypeptide 58 (*DDX58* or *RIG-1*, retinoic acid inducible gene 1 protein) ($R = 0.814$ and $R = -0.646$); bone morphogenetic protein 2 (*BMP2*) and *NFATC2* ($R = 0.707$ and $R = -0.660$); and G-protein alpha stimulating (*GNAS*) and *NFATC2* ($R = 0.665$ and $R = -0.798$), in asthmatics and non-asthmatic respectively. All were significantly correlated but in opposite directions ($p < 0.05$, Fig. 6).

All eight pairs of differentially co-expressed genes (Table 5) were entered into the ENCODE ChIP-SEQ significance tool. All but one of the genes (*IDO1*) from the pairs was regulated by the transcriptional repressor CCCTC-binding factor or CTCF. Since only 47% of the candidate genes have a CTCF binding site this represents a significant enrichment ($p = 0.0035$, Chi-squared test).

Discussion

In this study the Nanostring® platform was used to quantify the airway expression of candidate genes hypothesized to be important in the pathophysiology of asthma. mRNA was obtained from the airways of asthmatic (mainly fatal asthmatics) and non-asthmatic donor lungs and measures of airway remodeling were made on the sampled airways. Candidate genes were grouped into the following categories: ASM contraction, the cytoskeleton, epithelial barrier function, innate/adaptive immunity, fibrosis/remodeling, and epigenetics. 51 genes (15%) were nominally differentially expressed (p.unadj <0.05) in asthmatic airway tissue and included many genes important in cell-cell and cell-matrix interactions (COL1A1, COL3A1, ITGB6, LAMC2, RAC1). Of the 51 genes differentially expressed based on a nominal *p*-value, only 3 were significant following multiple comparison correction (ITGB6, COL1A1, COL3A1).

Cell-cell junctions are altered in the airway epithelium of asthmatics [29] and this may result in greater permeability of the epithelial layer and ultimately hypersensitivity of the ASM to agonist challenge [30]. The most significant differentially expressed gene in the data set was ITGB6. ITGB6 rapidly accumulates following injury to the epithelial layer and is considered to be important for normal wound healing [31]. In the mouse loss of ITGB6 causes an increase in the number of B-cells and T-cells around the airways, an increase in IL-4 production, and airway hyperresponsivenss in naïve mice without allergen challenge [31]. Additionally, influenza virus has been shown to interact with ITGB6 to cause epithelial cell death and collagen deposition in a TGF-ß dependent manner [32]. Another gene with lower abundance in asthmatics that did not meet the adjusted *p*-value cut off was RAC1. RAC1 has been shown to be important in the formation of tight junctions in an EGFR dependent manner [33], specifically by regulating tight junction protein 1 (or zona occluden 1) [34] which was also lower in abundance in the asthmatic samples. Changes in these genes could also affect epithelial-mesenchymal transition (EMT) [35], cytoskeletal stability, actin filament assembly/disassembly, cell stiffness and/or cell migration [36]. In addition, a protein-protein interaction network highlighted that down-regulated genes were enriched in pathways for cell-cell communication and integrin cell surface interactions.

The most significantly up-regulated gene in asthmatic samples was *COL1A1* which codes for the alpha chain in type 1 collagen. Collagen 1 is the major type of collagen in basement membrane and a major protein found in remodeled airways. Collagen 1 is important in airway remodeling [37], in particular thickening of the subepithelial space which is associated with worsening of asthma symptoms [38]. Collagen type 3 was also significantly elevated in asthmatic subjects and is also significantly elevated in the basement membrane of asthmatic subjects [39]. Type 1 and 3 collagen have both been associated with worsening lung function in a horse model of asthma [40]. Beyond the ability of collagens to affect distensibility of the airways, collagen 1 has been shown to stimulate ASM to produce MMP1 [41] and proliferate, in conjunction with FAK [42]. Collagen 1 and 3 expression has also been shown to be unaffected by corticosteroid usage in severe asthmatics [43] and collagen 1 and 3 contribute to the loss of the anti-mitotic effect of corticosteroids [44]. Enrichment of pathways involved in collagen remodeling was seen in our network analysis and highlights the importance of understanding fibrosis as it relates to fiber production, degradation, and organization and how this impacts normal cell function.

ADAM33 has been described in candidate gene studies to be associated with asthma [6] and was significantly elevated in asthmatic airways. *ADAM33* has been implicated in smooth muscle development, cell-cell connections, and cell proliferation and differentiation [45]. Over-expression of *ADAM33* in asthmatic airways has been described [46] and may be an important determinant of disease progression. There is evidence that ADAM33 can stimulate angiogenesis ex vivo and in vivo and by this mechanisms may contribute to airway remodeling [47]. Furthermore, ADAM33 family member TACE/ADAM17 can mediate release of TNF-α and fracktalkine (or CX3CL1) from the cell membrane [48, 49] and ADAM9 may mediate the release of growth factor HB-EGF [50]. If ADAM33 has a similar capacity for cytokine or growth factor cleavage this could make it a major contributor to airway remodeling in asthma.

Other genes in the 5 most differentially up or down regulated genes that were nominaly significant include: Cyclic ADP Ribose (CD38), Interleukin 13 Receptor Alpha 1 (IL13RA1), Prostaglandin F Receptor (PTGFR), Heat Shock Protein Beta 1 (HSPB1), and Interferon Induced with Helicase C Domain 1 (IFIH1). CD38 is a protein that generates the second messenger cADPR to cause calcium release. Recent work has explored the role of CD38 in asthma and has suggested that increased CD38 expression causes hypercontractility in ASM cells from asthmatics [51] although in our samples we saw no CD38 staining in the ASM layer (Additional file 1: Fig. S1 and S2). Additionally, CD38 deficient mice have reduced AHR following ovalbumin challenge [52]. Decreased IL13RA1 expression is surprising in the context of asthma but this could be due to a compensatory response to continued eosinophilia and IL13/IL4 exposure in the lung [53]. Prostaglandin's can be both pro and anti inflammatory but there is little research on the role of prostaglandin F in the context of asthma. HSPB1 (or heat shock protein 27) is a chaperone protein that has been implicated in cellular differentiation, apoptosis, and smooth muscle contraction [54]. Up-regulation of the gene could contribute to ASM hypercontractility in asthma but further work investigating the phosphorylation state and activity of HSP27 in asthma is needed to answer this question. IFIH1, also known as MDA5, is a DEAD box double stranded (ds) RNA helicases that can detect intracellular viral dsRNA and lead to the production of interferons [55]. MDA5 and TLR3 signaling have been shown to be deficient in bronchial epithelial cells from asthmatic subjects [56] and this could be responsible for the defective epithelial release of interferon I and III in response to rhino virus infection [57, 58].

Co-expression of genes does not imply interaction between their proteins but instead may suggest similarities in their regulation by transcription factors or epigenetic mechanisms [59]. Co-expression analyses can reveal changes in the regulation of gene expression [60] and have been used to identify epigenetic changes that affect gene co-expression in cancer [61]. In our study, genes that were differentially co-expressed between asthmatics and non-asthmatics were significantly enriched for pathways involved in virus recognition and regulation of interferon production (Table 4). The genes enriched in these pathways were from cluster 16 and were RIG-I (*DDX58*), RIG-1-like receptor 3 (*DHX58*), and interferon induced with helicase C domain 1 (*IFIH1*). This finding suggests that a central molecular mechanism may regulate diverse antiviral immune molecules in response to viral infections that may trigger asthma exacerbations and/or pathogenesis [62]. IFIH1, as discussed earlier, was also differentially expressed.

One of the most intriguing results was the identification of a single transcriptional repressor, CTCF, that controls the expression of all but one of the differentially co-expressed pairs of genes. CTCF influences gene expression through chromatin modifications [63] resulting in insulation of the target regions [64]. CTCF is an architectural protein that mediates inter- and intra-chromosomal interactions at distant genomic sites, and regulates three-dimensional genome architecture [63]. There are examples of CTCF silencing one gene while activating another [63]. Specific to asthma, differential expression at the *ZPBP2/GSDMB/ORMDL3* locus was identified resulting from allele-specific chromatin remodeling mediated by CTCF [65]. A SNP in *ZPBP2* created a CTCF binding site resulting in increased expression of ZPBP2 but diminished expression of *GSDMB* and *ORMDL3* [65]. Additionally, CTCF is highly sensitive to DNA methylation at CTCF binding sites [63]; changes to the methylome can have direct effects on the regulation of CTCF target genes. CTCF could play a crucial role in controlling the many gene expression changes observed in the airways of asthmatics and is worthy of more intense research that is beyond the scope of this paper.

There are several limitations of this study. Firstly, the use of whole airway RNA rather than RNA from specific cell types precludes us from conclusively identifying the site of gene expression. Secondly, the majority of the asthmatic patients were fatal asthmatics and experienced hypoxia and treatment with steroids during their fatal attack which can affect mRNA expression in tissues taken for research purposes. We addressed this by controlling for steroid use in our analysis of differential gene expression. Additionally, the use of more severe asthmatics may mean that these results are not generalizable to asthmatics as a whole. But considering severe asthmatic populations have the most hospital visits and are most at risk for exacerbations, we believe our results provide significant insight into the genes that are altered in fatal disease. Finally, the relatively small sample size limits our ability to detect differences in gene expression less than ~1.5 fold on average, although this also means that the changes we see are likely to be real. Procurement of donor lungs is time consuming and costly so increasing the number of patients for this study was not feasible, however future studies in asthmatic biopsies or cell culture experiments could confirm these results with the ability for much larger sample size. A limited number of donors with non-fatal asthma ($n = 4$) means we were unable to test for differences between these two groups of donors (fatal vs. non-fatal).

Conclusion

This study identifies changes in the expression and co-expression of genes thought to be important in asthma and AHR. Specifically, we identified altered abundance of genes involved in cell-cell and cell-matrix connections as well as those involved in the immune response and cell homeostasis. We also identified changes in the co-expression of genes involved in virus recognition and interferon production. The transcription factor CTCF could be an important regulator of the asthmatic phenotype and warrants further investigation. Future work should focus on elucidating the potential mechanisms behind altered CTCF binding as it relates to asthma pathophysiology.

Additional file

Additional file 1: Supplementary Methods – Methods describing selection of house keeping genes and immunohistochemical staining procedure. Supplementary Tables – Tables containing clinical demographics for subjects, average counts, fold change, and *p*-value for all genes studied, and all differentially co-expressed genes. Supplementary Figures and Legends – Figures showing sample immunohistochemical staining for proteins of significantly altered genes, co-expression plots.

Abbreviations

%CV: Percent coefficient of variation; ADAM17: ADAM metallopeptidase domain 17; ADAM33: ADAM metallopeptidase domain 33; ADAM9: ADAM metallopeptidase domain 9; AHR: Airway hyperresponsiveness; ASM: Airway smooth muscle; AURKA: Aurora kinase A; BCL3: B-Cell CLL/lymphoma 3; BMP2: Bone morphogenetic protein 2; BPIFA1: BPI fold containing family A member 1; cADPR: Cyclic ADP Ribose; CD38: Cluster of differentiation 38; CD44: Cluster of differentiation 44; CHI3L1: Chitinase 3-like; COL1A1: Collagen Type 1 Alpha 1; COL3A1: Collagen Type 3 Alpha 1; CREBBP: CREB binding protein; CRIP1: Cysteine rich protein 1; CTCF: CCCTC-binding factor; CX3CL1: Fracktalkine; DDX58: DExD/H-box helicase 58; DNA: Deoxyribonuleic acid; DNMT3b: DNA methyltransferase 3 Beta; ECM: Extracellular matrix; EGFR: Epidermal growth factor receptor; EGR4: Early growth response 4; EID1: EP300 interacting inhibitor of differentiation 1; EMT: Epithelial-mesenchymal transition; EP300: E1A binding protein P300; eQTL: Expression quantitative trait loci; FAK: Focal adhesion kinase; FGFR1: Fibroblast growth factor receptor 1; GNAS: Adenylate cyclase-stimulating G alpha protein; GNB2L1: Guanine nucleotide-binding protein subunit Beta-2-Like 1; GSDMB: Gasdermin B; GUSB: β-Glucuronidase; GWAS: Genome wide association study; H&E: Hemoatoxylin and eosin; HB-EGF: Heparin-binding EGF-like growth factor; HDAC10: Histone deacetylase 10; HSPB1: Heat shock protein 27; IDO1: Indoleamine 2,3-dioxygenase 1; IFIH1: Interferon induced with helicase C domain 1; IGSF4C: Immunoglobulin superfamily member 4C; IIAM: International Institute of the Advancement of Medicine; IL-13: Interleukin-13; IL33: Interleukin-33; IL4: Interleukin-4; ITGA2: Integrin subunit Alpha 2; ITGB6: Integrin subunit Beta 6; KAT2A: Lysine acetyltransferase 2A; KEGG: Kyoto encyclopedia of genes and genomes; LAMB2: Laminin subunit Beta 2; LAMC2: Laminin subunit Gamma 2; MDA5: Melanoma differentiation-associated protein 5; MLCK: Myosin light chain kinase; MMP1: Matrix metallopeptidase 1; MMP9: Matrix metallopeptidase 9; MYH11: Myosin heavy chain 11; NFATC2: Nuclear factor of activated T-cells, cytoplasmic 2; NLR: Nod-like receptor; ORMDL3: ORMDL sphingolipid biosynthesis regulator 3; Pi: Internal perimeter of the airway; POLR2A: RNA polymerase R2A; PRMT5: Protein arginine methyltransferase 5; PTGFR: Prostaglandin F receptor; PTK7: Protein tyrosine kinase 7; PTPRO: Protein tyrosine phosphatase, receptor type O; RAC1: Ras-related C3 botulinum toxin substrate 1; RIG-1: Retinoic acid inducible gene 1; RLR: Rig-like receptor; RNA: Ribonucleic acid; RPL19: Ribosomal protein L19; S100A2: S100 calcium binding protein A2; SEM: Standard error of the mean; SM-22: Smooth muscle protein 22-alpha/transgelin; SNP: Single nucleotide polymorphism; ST-2: Suppression of tumorigenicity 2; STAT5A: Signal transducer and activator of transcription 5A; SUV39H1: Suppressor of variegation 3–9 homolog 1; TACE: Tumor necrosis factor-α-converting enzyme; TBP: TATA box binding protein; TGF-β: Transforming growth factor Beta 1; THY1: Thymocyte antigen 1; TLR: Toll-like receptors; TNF- α: Tumor necoris factor alpha; TSLP: Thymic stromal lymphopoietin; ZO-1: Zona occludens-1; ZPBP2: Zona pellucida binding protein 2

Acknowledgements

Lu Wang PhD for her assistance in collection of histological images.

Funding

Research was funded by the Canadian Institute for Health Research (CIHR) and no role in the design, collection, analysis, or interpretation of data and results, and did not contribute to the writing of the manuscript.

Authors' contributions

CDP, PDP, and CYS contributed to the experimental design and setup. CDP, PDP, CYS, SW, DS, SW, JAH, SJY, DRD, CC, and TLH all contributed to the design of the gene expression panel. CDP, MO, YN, PDP, and CYS contributed to data analysis. TLH collected and inflated lung samples. CDP and BAA collected data for remodeling and protein expression. CDP, PDP, and MO drafted manuscript. CDP, PDP, MO, CC, TLH, JAH, DRD, SW, DS, and SW edited and revised manuscript. All authors have read and approved the final version of this manuscript.

Consent for publication

Not applicable.

Competing interests

The authors declare that they have no competing interests.

Author details

[1]UBC Institute for Heart Lung Health, St. Paul's Hospital, 1081 Burrard St, Vancouver, BC, Canada. [2]UBC Department of Medicine, Division of Respirology, University of British Columbia, Vancouver, BC, Canada. [3]UBC Chan-Yeung Centre for Occupational and Environmental Respiratory Disease, Gordon & Leslie Diamond Health Care Centre, Vancouver General Hospital, 2775 Laurel Street, 7th floor, Vancouver, BC, Canada. [4]University of British Columbia Centre for Heart Lung Innovation, St. Paul's Hospital, 1081 Burrard St, Vancouver, BC, Canada. [5]UBC School of Population and Public Health, University of British Columbia, Vancouver, BC, Canada. [6]UBC Department of

Anesthesiology, Pharmacology and Therapeutics, University of British Columbia, Vancouver, BC, Canada. [7]UBC Department of Pathology and Laboratory Medicine, University of British Columbia, Vancouver, BC, Canada. [8]Division of Respirology, Department of Medicine, McMaster University, Hamilton, ON, Canada. [9]Children's Hospital Research Institute of Manitoba, 513-715 McDermot Avenue, Winnipeg, MB R3E 3P4, Canada.

References

1. James AL, Elliot JG, Jones RL, Carroll ML, Mauad T, Bai TR, et al. Airway smooth muscle hypertrophy and hyperplasia in asthma. Am J Respir Crit Care Med. 2012;185:1058–64.
2. Barnes PJ. Inhaled Glucocorticoids for asthma. N Engl J Med. 1995; 332:868–75.
3. Holgate ST, Holloway J, Wilson S, Bucchieri F, Puddicombe S, Davies DE. Epithelial–Mesenchymal communication in the pathogenesis of chronic asthma. Proc Am Thorac Soc. 2004;1:93–8.
4. Tulah AS, Holloway JW, Sayers I. Defining the contribution of SNPs identified in asthma GWAS to clinical variables in asthmatic children. BMC Med Genet. 2013;14:100.
5. Torgerson DG, Ampleford EJ, Chiu GY, Gauderman WJ, Gignoux CR, Graves PE, et al. Meta-analysis of genome-wide association studies of asthma in ethnically diverse north American populations. Nat Genet. 2011;43:887–92.
6. van Eerdewegh P, Little RD, Dupuis J, del Mastro RG, Falls K, Simon J, et al. Association of the ADAM33 gene with asthma and bronchial hyperresponsiveness. Nature. 2002;418:426.
7. Hao K, Bosse Y, Nickle DC, Pare PD, Postma DS, Laviolette M, et al. Lung eQTLs to help reveal the molecular underpinnings of asthma. PLoS Genet. 2012;8:e1003029.
8. Veldman-Jones MH, Brant R, Rooney C, Geh C, Emery H, Harbron CG, et al. Evaluating robustness and sensitivity of the NanoString technologies nCounter platform to enable multiplexed gene expression analysis of clinical samples. Cancer Res. 2015;75:2587–93.
9. Chin LY, Bosse Y, Pascoe CD, Hackett TL, Seow CY, Pare PD. Mechanical properties of asthmatic airway smooth muscle. Eur Respir J. 2012;40:45–54.
10. Hackett T-L, Warner SM, Stefanowicz D, Shaheen F, Pechkovsky DV, Murray LA, et al. Induction of epithelial-mesenchymal transition in primary airway epithelial cells from patients with asthma by transforming growth factor-beta1. Am J Respir Crit Care Med. 2009;180:122–33.
11. Hirota JA, Hirota SA, Warner SM, Stefanowicz D, Shaheen F, Beck PL, et al. The airway epithelium nucleotide-binding domain and leucine-rich repeat protein 3 inflammasome is activated by urban particulate matter. J Allergy Clin Immunol. 2012;129:1116–25. e6
12. Woodruff PG, Dolganov GM, Ferrando RE, Donnelly S, Hays SR, Solberg OD, et al. Hyperplasia of smooth muscle in mild to moderate asthma without changes in cell size or gene expression. Am J Respir Crit Care Med. 2004;169:1001–6.
13. Sieck GC, White TA, Thompson MA, Pabelick CM, Wylam ME, Prakash YS. Regulation of store-operated Ca2+ entry by CD38 in human airway smooth muscle. Am J Physiol - Lung Cell Mol Physiol. 2008; 294:L378–85.
14. Gunst SJ, Zhang W. Actin cytoskeletal dynamics in smooth muscle: a new paradigm for the regulation of smooth muscle contraction. Am J Physiol - Cell Physiol. 2008;295:C576–87.
15. Lan B, Wang L, Zhang J, Pascoe CD, Norris BA, Liu JC-Y, et al. Rho-kinase mediated cytoskeletal stiffness in skinned smooth muscle. J Appl Physiol Bethesda Md. 1985;2013 https://doi.org/10.1152/japplphysiol.00654.2013.
16. Allahverdian S, Harada N, Singhera GK, Knight DA, Dorscheid DR. Secretion of IL-13 by airway epithelial cells enhances epithelial repair via HB-EGF. Am J Respir Cell Mol Biol. 2008;38:153–60.
17. Dorscheid DR, Wojcik KR, Yule K, White SR. Role of cell surface glycosylation in mediating repair of human airway epithelial cell monolayers. Am J Physiol Lung Cell Mol Physiol. 2001;281:L982–92.
18. Moffatt MF, Gut IG, Demenais F, Strachan DP, Bouzigon E, Heath S, et al. A large-scale, consortium-based genomewide association study of asthma. N Engl J Med. 2010;363:1211–21.
19. Xu J, Singhera GK, Dorscheid DR. Expression of surfactant protein D in airways of asthmatics and interleukin-13 modulation of surfactant protein D in human models of airway epithelium. Respir Res. 2015;16:26.
20. Hirota JA, Gold MJ, Hiebert PR, Parkinson LG, Wee T, Smith D, et al. The nucleotide-binding domain, leucine-rich repeat protein 3 inflammasome/IL-1 receptor I axis mediates innate, but not adaptive, immune responses after exposure to particulate matter under 10 μm. Am J Respir Cell Mol Biol. 2015;52:96–105.
21. Wang D-Z, Olson EN. Control of smooth muscle development by the myocardin family of transcriptional coactivators. Curr Opin Genet Dev. 2004; 14:558.
22. Tsao P-N, Vasconcelos M, Izvolsky KI, Qian J, Lu J, Cardoso WV. Notch signaling controls the balance of ciliated and secretory cell fates in developing airways. Dev Camb Engl. 2009;136:2297–307.
23. Kumagai K, Ohno I, Okada S, Ohkawara Y, Suzuki K, Shinya T, et al. Inhibition of matrix metalloproteinases prevents allergen-induced airway inflammation in a murine model of asthma. J Immunol Baltim Md 1950. 1999;162:4212–9.
24. Stefanowicz D, Lee JY, Lee K, Shaheen F, Koo H-K, Booth S, et al. Elevated H3K18 acetylation in airway epithelial cells of asthmatic subjects. Respir Res. 2015;16:95.
25. Stefanowicz D. Profiling the epigenetic landscape of the airway epithelium in asthma. 2014. https://circle.ubc.ca/handle/2429/47071. Accessed 2 Oct 2015.
26. Stefanowicz D, Hackett T-L, Garmaroudi FS, Günther OP, Neumann S, Sutanto EN, et al. DNA methylation profiles of airway epithelial cells and PBMCs from healthy, atopic and asthmatic children. PLoS One. 2012;7: e44213.
27. Nyholt DR. A simple correction for multiple testing for single-nucleotide polymorphisms in linkage disequilibrium with each other. Am J Hum Genet. 2004;74:765–9.
28. Li J, Ji L. Adjusting multiple testing in multilocus analyses using the eigenvalues of a correlation matrix. Heredity. 2005;95:221–7.
29. de Boer WI, Sharma HS, Baelemans SMI, Hoogsteden HC, Lambrecht BN, Braunstahl GJ. Altered expression of epithelial junctional proteins in atopic asthma: possible role in inflammation. Can J Physiol Pharmacol. 2008;86:105–12.
30. Barnes PJ, Cuss FM, Palmer JB. The effect of airway epithelium on smooth muscle contractility in bovine trachea. Br J Pharmacol. 1985; 86:685–91.
31. Huang XZ, Wu JF, Cass D, Erle DJ, Corry D, Young SG, et al. Inactivation of the integrin beta 6 subunit gene reveals a role of epithelial integrins in regulating inflammation in the lung and skin. J Cell Biol. 1996;133:921–8.
32. Jolly L, Stavrou A, Vanderstoken G, Meliopoulos VA, Habgood A, Tatler AL, et al. Influenza promotes collagen deposition via αvβ6 Integrin-mediated transforming growth factor β activation. J Biol Chem. 2014;289:35246–63.
33. Terakado M, Gon Y, Sekiyama A, Takeshita I, Kozu Y, Matsumoto K, et al. The Rac1/JNK pathway is critical for EGFR-dependent barrier formation in human airway epithelial cells. Am J Physiol Lung Cell Mol Physiol. 2011;300:L56–63.
34. Jou T-S, Schneeberger EE, Nelson WJ. Structural and functional regulation of tight junctions by RhoA and Rac1 small GTPases. J Cell Biol. 1998;142:101–15.
35. Hackett T-L. Epithelial-mesenchymal transition in the pathophysiology of airway remodelling in asthma. Curr Opin Allergy Clin Immunol. 2012;12:53–9.
36. Parsons JT, Horwitz AR, Schwartz MA. Cell adhesion: integrating cytoskeletal dynamics and cellular tension. Nat Rev Mol Cell Biol. 2010;11:633–43.
37. Liesker JJ, Hacken NHT, Zeinstra-Smith M, Rutgers SR, Postma DS, Timens W. Reticular basement membrane in asthma and COPD: similar thickness, yet different composition. Int J Chron Obstruct Pulmon Dis. 2009;4:127–35.
38. Chetta A, Foresi A, Del Donno M, Bertorelli G, Pesci A, Olivieri D. Airways remodeling is a distinctive feature of asthma and is related to severity of disease. Chest. 1997;111:852–7.
39. Wilson JW, Li X. The measurement of reticular basement membrane and submucosal collagen in the asthmatic airway. Clin Exp Allergy. 1997;27:363–71.
40. Setlakwe EL, Lemos KR, Lavoie-Lamoureux A, Duguay J-D, Lavoie J-P. Airway collagen and elastic fiber content correlates with lung function in equine heaves. Am J Physiol - Lung Cell Mol Physiol. 2014;307:L252–60.
41. Rogers NK, Clements D, Dongre A, Harrison TW, Shaw D, Johnson SR. Extra-cellular matrix proteins induce matrix Metalloproteinase-1 (MMP-1) activity and increase airway smooth muscle contraction in asthma. PLoS One. 2014; 9:e90565.

42. Dekkers BGJ, Spanjer AIR, van der Schuyt RD, Kuik WJ, Zaagsma J, Meurs H. Focal adhesion Kinase regulates collagen I–induced airway smooth muscle phenotype switching. J Pharmacol Exp Ther. 2013;346:86–95.
43. Chakir J, Shannon J, Molet S, Fukakusa M, Elias J, Laviolette M, et al. Airway remodeling-associated mediators in moderate to severe asthma: effect of steroids on TGF-β, IL-11, IL-17, and type I and type III collagen expression. J Allergy Clin Immunol. 2003;111:1293–8.
44. Bonacci JV, Schuliga M, Harris T, Stewart AG. Collagen impairs glucocorticoid actions in airway smooth muscle through integrin signalling. Br J Pharmacol. 2006;149:365–73.
45. Shapiro SD, Owen CA. ADAM-33 surfaces as an asthma gene. N Engl J Med. 2002;347:936–8.
46. Foley SC, Mogas AK, Olivenstein R, Fiset PO, Chakir J, Bourbeau J, et al. Increased expression of ADAM33 and ADAM8 with disease progression in asthma. J Allergy Clin Immunol. 2007;119:863–71.
47. Puxeddu I, Pang YY, Harvey A, Haitchi HM, Nicholas B, Yoshisue H, et al. The soluble form of a disintegrin and metalloprotease 33 promotes angiogenesis: implications for airway remodeling in asthma. J Allergy Clin Immunol. 2008;121:1400–6. 1406.e1–4
48. Black RA. Tumor necrosis factor-α converting enzyme. Int J Biochem Cell Biol. 2002;34:1–5.
49. Garton KJ, Gough PJ, Blobel CP, Murphy G, Greaves DR, Dempsey PJ, et al. Tumor necrosis factor-α-converting enzyme (ADAM17) mediates the cleavage and shedding of Fractalkine (CX3CL1). J Biol Chem. 2001;276: 37993–8001.
50. Izumi Y, Hirata M, Hasuwa H, Iwamoto R, Umata T, Miyado K, et al. A metalloprotease-disintegrin, MDC9/meltrin-gamma/ADAM9 and PKCdelta are involved in TPA-induced ectodomain shedding of membrane-anchored heparin-binding EGF-like growth factor. EMBO J. 1998;17:7260–72.
51. Jude JA, Dileepan M, Panettieri RA, Walseth TF, Kannan MS. Altered CD38/ cyclic ADP-ribose Signaling contributes to the asthmatic phenotype. J Allergy. 2012;2012:289468.
52. Deshpande DA, White TA, Guedes AGP, Milla C, Walseth TF, Lund FE, et al. Altered airway responsiveness in CD38-deficient mice. Am J Respir Cell Mol Biol. 2005;32:149–56.
53. Myrtek D, Knoll M, Matthiesen T, Krause S, Lohrmann J, Schillinger D, et al. Expression of interleukin-13 receptor alpha 1-subunit on peripheral blood eosinophils is regulated by cytokines. Immunology. 2004;112:597–604.
54. Salinthone S, Tyagi M, Gerthoffer WT. Small heat shock proteins in smooth muscle. Pharmacol Ther. 2008;119:44–54.
55. Reikine S, Nguyen JB, Modis Y. Pattern recognition and Signaling mechanisms of RIG-I and MDA5. Front Immunol. 2014;5 https://doi.org/10.3389/fimmu.2014.00342.
56. Parsons KS, Hsu AC, Wark PAB. TLR3 and MDA5 signalling, although not expression, is impaired in asthmatic epithelial cells in response to rhinovirus infection. Clin Exp Allergy J Br Soc Allergy Clin Immunol. 2014;44:91–101.
57. Wark PAB, Johnston SL, Bucchieri F, Powell R, Puddicombe S, Laza-Stanca V, et al. Asthmatic bronchial epithelial cells have a deficient innate immune response to infection with rhinovirus. J Exp Med. 2005;201:937–47.
58. Contoli M, Message SD, Laza-Stanca V, Edwards MR, Wark PAB, Bartlett NW, et al. Role of deficient type III interferon-lambda production in asthma exacerbations. Nat Med. 2006;12:1023–6.
59. Hsu C-L, Juan H-F, Huang H-C. Functional analysis and characterization of differential Coexpression networks. Sci Rep. 2015;5:13295.
60. de la Fuente A. From "differential expression" to "differential networking" – identification of dysfunctional regulatory networks in diseases. Trends Genet. 2010;26:326–33.
61. Ii M, Yamamoto H, Taniguchi H, Adachi Y, Nakazawa M, Ohashi H, et al. Co-expression of laminin β3 and γ2 chains and epigenetic inactivation of laminin α3 chain in gastric cancer. Int J Oncol. 2011;39:593–9.
62. Porritt RA, Hertzog PJ. Dynamic control of type I IFN signalling by an integrated network of negative regulators. Trends Immunol. 2015;36:150–60.
63. Ong C-T, Corces VG. CTCF: an architectural protein bridging genome topology and function. Nat Rev Genet. 2014;15:234–46.
64. Mishiro T, Ishihara K, Hino S, Tsutsumi S, Aburatani H, Shirahige K, et al. Architectural roles of multiple chromatin insulators at the human apolipoprotein gene cluster. EMBO J. 2009;28:1234–45.
65. Verlaan DJ, Berlivet S, Hunninghake GM, Madore A-M, Larivière M, Moussette S, et al. Allele-specific chromatin Remodeling in the ZPBP2/ GSDMB/ORMDL3 locus associated with the risk of asthma and autoimmune disease. Am J Hum Genet. 2009;85:377–93.

9

Effects of endogenous sex hormones on lung function and symptom control in adolescents with asthma

Mark D. DeBoer[1], Brenda R. Phillips[2], David T. Mauger[2], Joe Zein[3], Serpil C. Erzurum[3], Anne M. Fitzpatrick[4], Benjamin M. Gaston[5], Ross Myers[5], Kristie R. Ross[5], James Chmiel[5], Min Jie Lee[4], John V. Fahy[6], Michael Peters[6], Ngoc P. Ly[6], Sally E. Wenzel[7], Merritt L. Fajt[7], Fernando Holguin[7], Wendy C. Moore[8], Stephen P. Peters[8], Deborah Meyers[8], Eugene R. Bleecker[8], Mario Castro[9], Andrea M. Coverstone[9], Leonard B. Bacharier[9], Nizar N. Jarjour[10], Ronald L. Sorkness[10], Sima Ramratnam[10], Anne-Marie Irani[11], Elliot Israel[12], Bruce Levy[12], Wanda Phipatanakul[12], Jonathan M. Gaffin[12] and W. Gerald Teague[1*]

Abstract

Background: Although pre-puberty asthma is more prevalent in males, after puberty through middle-age, asthma is more prevalent in females. The surge of sex hormones with puberty might explain this gender switch.

Methods: To examine the effects of sex hormones on lung function and symptoms with puberty, Tanner stage was assessed in 187 children 6–18 years of age (59% severe) enrolled in the NIH/NHLBI Severe Asthma Research Program (SARP). The effects of circulating sex hormones ($n = 68$; testosterone, dehydroepiandrosterone sulfate (DHEA-S), estrogen, and progesterone) on lung function and 4 week symptom control (ACQ6) in cross-section were tested by linear regression.

Results: From pre–/early to late puberty, lung function did not change significantly but ACQ6 scores improved in males with severe asthma. By contrast females had lower post-BD FEV_1% and FVC% and worse ACQ6 scores with late puberty assessed by breast development. In males log DHEA-S levels, which increased by Tanner stage, associated positively with pre- and post-BD FEV_1%, pre-BD FVC %, and negatively (improved) with ACQ6. Patients treated with high-dose inhaled corticosteroids had similar levels of circulating DHEA-S. In females, estradiol levels increased by Tanner stage, and associated negatively with pre-BD FEV_1% and FVC %.

Conclusions: These results support beneficial effects of androgens on lung function and symptom control and weak deleterious effects of estradiol on lung function in children with asthma. Longitudinal data are necessary to confirm these cross-sectional findings and to further elucidate hormonal mechanisms informing sex differences in asthma features with puberty.

Keywords: Asthma, Sex hormones, Testosterone, Estradiol, Puberty, Lung function

* Correspondence: wgt2p@virginia.edu; WGT2P@hscmail.mcc.virginia.edu
[1]University of Virginia School of Medicine, Charlottesville, VA 22908, USA
Full list of author information is available at the end of the article

Background

The prevalence of current asthma in the U.S. is higher in children than in adults, and from pre-school to age 14 years is greater in boys than it is in girls [1]. Both asthma severity and hospitalizations start to decrease in late childhood and remain relatively low into young adulthood [2, 3]. After age 18 years, in young men, current asthma prevalence is lower than in childhood; in young women although lower than in childhood, current asthma prevalence is higher than it is in young men, and remains higher in women through middle-age [1]. Surges in endogenous sex hormones across adolescence could affect the "gender switch" in asthma status [2]. For example, DHEA-S, a circulating androgen that increases with puberty, inhibits human airway smooth muscle and airway fibroblast proliferation [4, 5] and may influence airway epithelial-to-mesenchymal transition [6]. Testosterone promotes airway smooth muscle relaxation [7]. In women both with and without asthma, FEV_1% peaks at the end of the luteal phase to the beginning of menstruation, and then decreases when circulating estrogen and progesterone decrease [8]. Accordingly, the fall in circulating estrogen and progesterone from the luteal to the follicular phase of the menstrual cycle is accompanied by a reduction in lymphocyte β_2 adrenoceptor density [9] and increased bronchial responsiveness in women with asthma [10]. Recent studies of dysanapsis (differential growth of airway caliber and lung volume) in healthy subjects suggest that, by adulthood, women develop more small airways resistance than do men [11]. Thus these studies support interdependent effects of sex and endogenous sex hormones on lung growth, and airways responsiveness that likely inform asthma status from puberty to middle-age.

Puberty is a dynamic process regulated by hormonal signals from the central nervous system that results in sexual maturation. Assessment of the stage of pubertal maturation is different in boys than girls [12]. In boys, androgen production gradually increases both from testes producing testosterone and the adrenal glands producing weaker androgens—ultimately leading to pubarche. Girls experience increases in the production of estrogen from the ovaries (driving thelarche and ultimately menarche) and androgens such as androstenedione and DHEA-S from the adrenal glands (driving pubarche in girls) [13]. In children studies of pubertal maturation and asthma status furthermore may be affected by corticosteroid treatment [14]. The primary purpose of the current studies was to do a cross-sectional analysis of the effects of pubertal maturation and sex hormone levels on asthma features in a sample of children enrolled in SARP. We found important differences in phenotypic features according to sex and pubertal stage. In boys higher DHEA-S levels positively associated with greater FEV_1% predicted and improved 4 week symptoms, whereas in girls, breast development, signifying estradiol effects, weakly associated with lower lung function.

Methods

Severe asthma research program

Details of the SARP III network, recruitment targets, enrollment and characterization procedures, and the longitudinal protocol have been previously published [15, 16]. Active tobacco smokers were excluded. Participants maintained medications for asthma as prescribed by their care provider. Study procedures were approved by the IRB at each institution and an independent Data Safety Monitoring Board (Additional file 1: Figure S1). All subjects provided written informed consent and/or assent. The study is listed on ClinicalTrials.gov.

Criteria for enrollment

Enrollees met criteria for current asthma based on responsiveness to β-agonist (≥12% increase in FEV_1 from baseline post-albuterol) and/or positive methacholine bronchoprovocation. Severe asthma was defined according to the ERS/ATS consensus definition [17]. Children whose asthma required treatment with high-dose inhaled corticosteroids (≥440 mcg of fluticasone equivalents per day for children 6–11 years of age; ≥880 mcg fluticasone equivalents per day ≥12 years of age) plus a second controller and/or systemic corticosteroids to maintain asthma control or which was uncontrolled despite these medications were assigned to the severe sub-group. Medications at this level were required for at least 6 of the previous 12 months and the 3 months prior to enrollment for participants to qualify for the severe sub-group. Those who did not meet criteria for severe asthma were assigned to the non-severe sub-group.

Characterization

Characterization procedures extended from the SARP I and II protocols [18–20] for SARP III included detailed history and physical examination, vital signs, height, weight, characterization questionnaires, assessment of four-week symptom control (asthma control questionnaire; ACQ6 [21]), and spirometry with maximal β-agonist reversibility testing (dose escalation protocol at 180 mcg albuterol increments up to 720 mcg).

Blood was drawn during the visit but not with systematic timing related to the timing of the spirometry. Pubertal stage was determined by study coordinators and investigators certified a priori to enrollment by a pediatric endocrinologist (MDD) with the method of Marshall and Tanner [12]. To identify central (CNS) puberty, Tanner stage for males was based on pubic hair and for females breast development. Females were also separated into pre–/early adrenarche and mid–/late adrenarche based on Tanner stages of pubic hair.

Spirometry, maximum bronchodilator challenge and methacholine challenge were performed by study coordinators certified after standard training and completion of an examination administered by the SARP III Data Coordinating Center on ATS-compatible equipment. Quality analysis of lung function tests and validation of results was accomplished by inspection of randomly sampled flow volume plots by a central over-reader. Population reference standards adjusted for age, height, and sex were from the Global Lung Initiative (GLI) [22].

Sex hormone assays

Sex hormone and SHBG levels were analyzed at the University of Virginia Center for Research in the Reproduction Ligand Core Laboratory. Estradiol levels were assessed with Calbiotech ELISA and all other metabolites were assessed using the Siemens Immulite 2000. Free testosterone was calculated from total testosterone and SHBG as previously described [23]. The lower limit of detection for assays were: testosterone 20 ng/dL; DHEAS 15 μg/dL; progesterone 0.20 ng/mL; and SHBG 10 nmol/L. For the purpose of mathematical analyses, individuals with measurements below the limit of detection were counted as having a value just below the lower limit of detection. Intra-/inter-assay coefficients of variation (CVs, %) were as follows: estradiol 6.3/8.1, testosterone 4.4/7.5, DHEAS 5.4/6.5, progesterone 4.4/7.8, and SHBG 2.7/5.2.

Data analysis

The analysis was restricted to enrollees with complete data sets with regards to Tanner stage and lung function. Because of natural variation in recruitment, mid-Tanner stages were relatively under-represented (Table 1). To examine the effects of pubertal maturation, participants were assigned to sub-groups including those with pre-/early puberty (Tanner 1–2) and mid-late puberty (Tanner 3–5).

Categorical data are presented as count and percentage, and continuous data as means ± standard deviations. Comparisons of differences by pubertal stage between males and females (both adrenarche and breast development) was performed by testing the stage by sex interaction term in a simple regression model. PC_{20} was evaluated on a log base 2 scale, with two zero values replaced by 0.016, or half of the minimum non-zero value. Univariable linear regression was used to evaluate relationships between measures of lung function or ACQ6 and individual 5-level Tanner stage. Multivariable linear regression tested associations of clinical outcomes (lung function and ACQ6) with sex hormone levels (for males, testosterone and DHEA-S; for females, estradiol, progesterone, free testosterone and DHEAS) as co-variates. With a backward selection method, hormones that were not significantly associated with the outcome were removed in steps and only significant associations were reported. These analyses were then further stratified based on BMI ≥85th percentile and < 85th percentile. *P*-values are unadjusted in these exploratory post hoc analyses.

Results

Sample features

The sample included 116 males and 71 females (Table 1). There were no significant differences between males and females with regard to age, racial/ ethnic background, asthma severity, or corticosteroid treatment. There were 110 severe and 77 non-severe participants in the analytic cohort. Of these, 74 severe- and 30 non-severe participants had an ACQ < 1.0 as an estimate of poor control (67% and 39%, respectively) [24]. Overall the sample was enriched in African Americans and severe asthma, with a high proportion with atopic sensitization. Among males, 84 (63%) were in pre-/early puberty and 32 (28%) in mid-/late puberty by Tanner stages of pubic hair development. Among females, 32 (45%) were in pre-/early puberty and 39 (56%) in mid-/late puberty by Tanner stages of breast development. 37 females (52%) were in pre-/early- and 34 (47%) in mid-/late adrenarche by Tanner stages of pubic hair. Adolescent females discordant for breast and pubic hair stages of development included 6 wherein pubic hair stage exceeded breast stage, and 1 wherein breast stage exceeded pubic hair (Additional file 1: Table S1).

Differences in sex hormones with puberty

68 children in the sample had circulating sex hormones measured (45 males, 23 females). From pre-/early to mid-/late puberty, testosterone increased in males, and estradiol increased in females (Additional file 1: Figure S2A and B). Likewise with puberty DHEA-S increased in males and DHEA-S, progesterone, and free testosterone increased in females (results not shown).

Differences in lung function with puberty

For males, there was a tendency for lung function and the maximum bronchodilator response to improve with pubertal maturation, but these differences were not statistically significant (Table 2). By contrast in females, both the post-bronchodilator FEV_1% and FVC % were significantly lower (by 8.9% and 9.1% respectively, $p = 0.01$ each) from pre-/early to mid-/late puberty as determined by breast development. In an analysis limited to severe females alone ($n = 44$), the lower FEV_1 (%) from early to late puberty remained significant. Similarly, the differences by pubertal maturation remained when participants were stratified by overweight/obesity status (Additional file 1: Table S2-A-1 and S2-A-2). These differences by Tanner stage are attributable to breast and not pubic hair development, supporting a likely estradiol effect.

Table 1 SARP III Pediatric sample features compared by sex

	Males ($n = 116$)	Females ($n = 71$)		P value
Age, years, mean (± sd)	11.3 (± 2.7)	11.8 (± 3.1)		0.21
Age of asthma diagnosis	3.1 (± 2.7)	3.1 (± 2.7)		0.90
Years since onset of asthma symptoms (asthma duration)	9.0 (± 3.2)	9.4(± 3.5)		0.50
BMI percentile	76.9 (± 26.5)	73.5 (± 27.1)		0.40
Race/ethnicity, n (%)				
White non-Hispanic	28 (24)	26 (37)		0.26
African American non-Hispanic	51 (44)	26 (37)		
Hispanic	17 (15)	11 (15)		
Other	20 (17)	8 (11)		
Asthma severity, n (%)				
Severe	66 (57)	44 (62)		0.49
Not severe	50 (43)	27 (38)		
Systemic Corticosteroid Treatment (current)	11 (9)	5 (7)		0.56
Systemic Corticosteroid Treatment (past 3 mos)	7 (6)	3 (4)		0.59
High-Dose Inhaled Corticosteroids	82 (71)	50 (70)		0.97
Low-Medium-Dose Inhaled Corticosteroids	23 (20)	14 (20)		0.99
Montelukast (during last 12 months) n(%)	71 (60)	54 (76)		0.03
Long-acting beta agonist	86 (74)	49 (69)		0.45
Atopic sensitization				
At Least One Positive Specific IgE (of 15 tests)	106 (93)	64 (91)		0.70
Number of Positive Specific IgEs (of 15 tests). Mean (± sd)	7.0 (4.3)	7.0 (4.9)		0.95
History of atopic dermatitis. n(%)	74 (64)	44 (62)		0.80
Tanner stage, n (%)	Males	Females		
	Pubic hair	Breast development	Pubic hair	
I	67 (58)	14 (20)	24 (34)	
II	17 (15)	18 (25)	13 (18)	
III	8 (7)	16 (23)	8 (11)	
IV	7 (6)	9 (13)	13 (18)	
V	17 (15)	14 (20)	13 (18)	

Differences in ACQ6 with puberty

With regards to four week symptom control (Table 3), with males ($n = 116$) the ACQ6 was not significantly different from pre–/early to mid–/late puberty, whereas in females ($n = 71$) the ACQ6 was higher (worse) with puberty assessed by breast bud ($p < 0.05$) and by pubic hair development ($p < 0.05$). In males with severe but not non-severe asthma, the ACQ6 was lower (improved) with pubertal maturation, whereas the ACQ6 was higher with pubertal stage in females with both severe ($n = 44$) and non-severe ($n = 37$) asthma ($p < 0.05$ for both). Again, the differences by pubertal maturation remained when participants were stratified by overweight/obesity status (Additional file 1: Table S2-B-1 and S2-B-2).

Multi-variable linear regression of lung function and ACQ6 with sex hormones

Males

For males in the sample 6–18 years of age, lung function associated positively with log DHEA-S values (Table 4). The pre-bronchodilator FEV_1% ($\beta = 8.05$; $p = 0.01$), post-BD FEV_1% ($\beta = 8.82$, $p = 0.008$), and pre-BD FVC % ($\beta = 8.33$, $p = 0.01$) had strongly positive β coefficients. The ACQ6 had a negative β coefficient with higher log DHEA-S values ($\beta = -0.59$, $p = 0.007$), indicating 4 week symptom improvement. These associations were driven largely by participant who were overweight/obese (Additional file 1: Table S3-A-1 and S3-A-2). The final model predicting ACQ6 included negative β coefficients for both log DHEA-S and testosterone, as well as the interaction of log DHEA-S with

Table 2 Lung function by sex and pubertal stage in children 6–18 years with asthma

	Males Tanner stages of pubic hair†				Females Tanner stages of breast development†				Females Tanner stages of pubic hair†			
	1–2 $n = 84$	3–5 $n = 32$	Ratio 3–5:1–2	Δ 3–5:1–2	1–2 $n = 32$	3–5 $n = 39$	Ratio 3–5:1–2	Δ 3–5:1–2	1–2 $n = 37$	3–5 $n = 34$	Ratio 3–5:1–2	Δ 3–5:1–2
Pre-BD FEV1 (%)	89.4 ± 18.5	89.1 ± 16.4	1.00	− 0.3	93.9 ± 13.0	87.2 ± 14.9	0.93	−6.8	90.4 ± 15.2	90.1 ± 13.7	1.00	− 0.3
Max Post-BD FEV1 (%)	103.5 ± 19.3	105.7 ± 10.2	1.02	2.2	109.4 ± 13.1	100.5 ± 13.1	0.92	− 8.9*	106.0 ± 14.4	102.9 ± 13.0	0.97	− 3.1
BD Resp. (% FEV_1 change)	17.3 ± 16.6	21.8 ± 20.8	1.26	4.5	17.2 ± 10.7	17.2 ± 17.5	1.00	−0.0	19.1 ± 17.1	15.2 ± 11.5	0.80	−3.9
Absolute BD Resp. (net FEV_1 change)	14.1 ± 10.3	16.7 ± 11.7	1.18	2.5	15.5 ± 8.3	13.4 ± 9.2	0.86	−2.1	15.7 ± 9.7	12.9 ± 7.6	0.82	−2.8
Pre-BD FVC (%)	101.4 ± 15.9	106.4 ± 16.0	1.05	5.0	106.3 ± 11.6	100.5 ± 12.9	0.94	−5.9*	102.9 ± 13.5	103.3 ± 11.8	1.01	0.4
Max Post-BD FVC (%)	109.2 ± 17.6	112.5 ± 13.8	1.03	3.3	113.8 ± 12.9	104.8 ± 13.7	0.92	−9.0*	110.4 ± 14.9	107.2 ± 13.0	0.97	− 3.2
Pre-BD FEV1/FVC (%)	87.3 ± 10.7	83.5 ± 11.6	0.96	−3.8	87.9 ± 8.4	86.3 ± 10.9	0.98	−1.5	87.2 ± 9.9	86.8 ± 9.9	1.00	−0.4
Max Post-BD FEV1/FVC (%)	94.9 ± 8.8	94.9 ± 7.4	1.00	0.0	97.2 ± 7.6	96.4 ± 8.2	0.99	−0.8	97.1 ± 7.8	96.4 ± 8.1	0.99	− 0.6
PC20 (log 2)	0.3 ± 1.9 $n = 35$	1.0 ± 3.0 $n = 10$	3.57	0.7	−0.7 ± 3.6 $n = 7$	0.0 ± 2.4 $n = 15$	− 0.05	0.7	− 0.3 ± 3.3 $n = 10$	−0.1 ± 2.4 $n = 12$	0.47	0.2

† Cross sectional, based on enrollment examination; * $p < 0.05$ Tanner Stage 1–2 versus Tanner Stage 3–5

Table 3 ACQ6 by sex, pubertal stage, and asthma severity in children 6–18 years of age

	Males				Females				Females			
	Tanner stages of pubic hair†				Tanner stages of breast development†				Tanner stages of pubic hair†			
	1–2 $n = 84$	3–5 $n = 32$	Ratio 3–5:1–2	Δ 3–5:1–2	1–2 $n = 32$	3–5 $n = 39$	Ratio 3–5:1–2	Δ 3–5:1–2	1–2 $n = 37$	3–5 $n = 34$	Ratio 3–5:1–2	Δ 3–5:1–2
ACQ6	1.2 ± 0.9	0.8 ± 0.7	0.70	−0.4	1.0 ± 0.8 $n = 32$	1.3 ± 1.0 $n = 39$	1.30	0.3*	1.1 ± 0.9 $n = 37$	1.3 ± 1.0 $n = 34$	1.24	0.3*
Severe												
ACQ6	1.5 ± 0.9 $n = 49$	0.9 ± 0.6 $n = 17$	0.63	−0.6*	1.1 ± 1.0 $n = 18$	1.3 ± 1.0 $n = 26$	1.18	0.2*	1.1 ± 1.0 $n = 21$	1.4 ±1.0 $n = 23$	1.22	0.3*
Non-severe												
ACQ6	0.8 ± 0.7 $n = 35$	0.7 ± 0.9 $n = 15$	0.94	−0.0	0.9 (0.6), $n = 14$	1.4 (1.1), $n = 13$	1.50	0.5*	1.0 (0.7), $n = 16$	1.3 (1.0), $n = 11$	1.25	0.3*

$^*p < 0.05$, Tanner Stage I-II compared to Tanner Stage III-V

Table 4 Linear regression analysis of lung function and ACQ6 by sex hormone levels in males 6–18 years with asthma

Outcome variable	Covariate remaining in the model*	Beta coefficient	Covariate p value	R squared	P value of the model
Pre-BD FEV_1 (%)	Log (DHEA-S)	9.285	0.011	0.168	0.011
Post-BD FEV_1 (%)	Log (DHEA-S)	9.527	0.006	0.160	0.006
Pre-BD FVC (%)	log (DHEA-S)	9.121	0.007	0.157	0.007
ACQ6	Log (DHEA-S)	−0.008	0.019	0.214	0.018
	Testosterone	−0.005	0.031		
	log (DHEA-S) *Testosterone #	0.003	0.05		

*Results reflect final results of a model that started with testosterone and DHEA-S. Covariates that were not significantly associated with the outcome in this model were then removed by backward selection and model was re-run with remaining variables. # A log (DHEA-S) * testosterone interaction was found and included in the final model

testosterone, an association not present when the cohort was stratified by overweight/obesity status. Circulating DHEA-S levels in males did not vary significantly when compared according to treatment with high-dose versus medium-dose inhaled corticosteroids (Additional file 1: Figure S3).

Females

For females 6–18 years of age, androgens associated positively, but estrogens negatively with lung function (Table 5). Free testosterone had a positive association with post-BD FEV_1% ($\beta = 3.99$, $p = 0.04$). In contrast, estradiol had negative β coefficients for pre-BD FEV_1% ($\beta = -0.47$, $p = 0.03$), post-BD FEV_1% ($\beta = -0.62$, $p = 0.0009$), pre-BD FVC % ($\beta = -0.36$, $p = 0.04$), and post-BD FVC % ($\beta = -0.33$, $p = 0.03$). These associations were not significant in either group when stratified by overweight/obesity status (Additional file 1: Table S3-B-1 and S3-B-2). For the ACQ6, only log DHEA-S had a significant association, it varied positively ($\beta = 0.49$, $p = 0.05$) and the correlation was relatively weak. ACQ6 was not associated with age (Additional file 1: Table S4).

Discussion

In children enriched in severe asthma enrolled in the NIH/NHLBI SARP III study ($n = 187$), there were important differences in lung function and four-week symptom control between males and females with pubertal maturation. In males, lung function was not different and symptom control improved when comparing those in early vs. late puberty, whereas in females lung function and symptom control were worse. Circulating sex hormones changed with puberty; in males greater androgen levels associated with better lung function and ACQ6, while in females greater circulating estrogens had a weak but significant negative association with lung function. These results support the general hypothesis that with pubertal maturation asthma severity is likely to improve in males but worsen in females [2]. Furthermore our data suggest a beneficial effect of endogenous androgens on lung function growth and ACQ6 in males in later puberty; and that endogenous estrogens may have weak deleterious effects on lung function growth in girls.

A beneficial effect of androgens is suggested by the presence of fewer asthma symptoms in late Tanner stage males with severe asthma. In females the presence of more asthma symptoms in late adolescence either reinforces the benefit of androgens (given an absence of significant androgens in females) or supports a negative role for estradiol. These integrated, Tanner-stage-based measurements of the effect of sex hormones over time are complemented by the association between DHEA-S and fewer asthma symptoms (lower ACQ6) and higher pre- and post-albuterol FEV1% observed in boys. Given that GLI-based normal ranges of lung function are age-specific these maturational and hormone-associated measures appear to be present beyond the expected changes in lung function based on age alone. Furthermore, we did not note associations between ACQ6 and age in either boys or girls. Note that it is unlikely that the level of corticosteroid therapy

Table 5 Multi-variable regression analysis of lung function and ACQ6 by sex hormone levels in females 6–18 years with asthma

Outcome variable	Covariate remaining in the model*	Beta coefficient	Covariate p value	R squared	P value of the model
Pre-BD FEV_1 (%)	Estradiol	−0.457	0.028	0.209	0.028
Post-BD FEV_1 (%)	Estradiol	−0.454	0.005	0.320	0.005
Pre-BD FVC (%)	Estradiol	−0.351	0.025	0.217	0.025
Post-BD FVC (%)	Estradiol	−0.322	0.015	0.249	0.015
ACQ6	log (DHEA-S)	0.006	0.048	0.173	0.048

*Results reflect final results of a model that started with log (DHEA-S), estradiol, progesterone, and free testosterone as covariates. Covariates that were not significantly associated with the outcome in this model were then removed by backward selection and model was re-run with remaining variables

caused the male/female discordance we observed because the males and females did not differ with regard to oral or inhaled corticosteroid dosing (Table 1). Furthermore treatment with high-dose corticosteroids did not suppress DHEA-S levels in males. Although the testosterone increase is quantitatively orders of magnitude greater than that of DHEA-S with puberty [25, 26], DHEA-S levels in our analysis were more strongly associated with better lung function and improved ACQ6 than was testosterone.

Of note, androgen receptors are expressed in bronchial smooth muscle tissue, and testosterone relaxes contracted airway smooth muscle, suggesting a beneficial effect of androgens on airway smooth muscle tone [7]. Additionally, DHEA-S inhibits human airway smooth muscle and airway fibroblast proliferation [5], and may influence airway epithelial-to-mesenchymal transition [6], suggesting that androgens may prevent adverse airway remodeling seen in severe asthma. Together, these affects could be associated with the lower asthma symptom scores we observed in association with increased DHEA-S and with late adolescence. Indeed a trial of androgen administration provided early data regarding safety and improved ACQ [27]. We noted associations between DHEA-S and lung function that were present in overweight/obese but not normal weight. This differential effect by weight status, which was seen only in boys, is of unclear significance and requires further investigation.

In females, subtle but significant discordance between loss of lung function observed in association with late puberty assessed by breast staging relative to pubic hair staging suggests that estrogen, which drives breast development, may be the main factor affecting lung function. Only females have a surge of estrogen or progesterone during puberty, and breast development is exclusively associated with this surge [28]. In our study the number of females with discordant pubertal examinations was small, whereas adrenal androgen effects confounded all assessments. We also cannot exclude an adverse effect of progesterone. For example, the effects of pregnancy on lung function may be either both estrogen and progesterone-dependent, and both hormones have been hypothesized to play roles in the worsening of lung function [2].

These results likewise support disparate changes in lung growth between males and females with puberty that bear on the remarkable decline in hospitalizations and asthma severity seen in young adults [3]. Asthma prevalence appears to decline more in males than it does in females by the second decade of life [1], a result which might be explained by disparate trends in airway growth due to sex hormones. Young adult females exhibit a "dysanaptic" pattern of airway growth which supports a pattern of anatomically "fixed" airflow limitation [11]. With regards to airway hyperreactivity, we found that the level of methacholine responsiveness actually fell in both males and females with Tanner stage, a finding differs from the results of Tantisera et al. [29] wherein females had increased methacholine responsiveness. The difference between the two studies may be due to sample differences, wherein the SARP III cohort is relatively enriched with African Americans and children with severe asthma.

It should also be noted that other hormonal changes during puberty could also affect lung function, including an increase in the degree of insulin resistance [30]—which itself is associated with increased risk of asthma in adults [31] and adolescent girls [32]—and elevations in stress hormones, including cortisol [33]—with such stress systems further associated with asthma risk [34]. While temporally related (i.e., during puberty), the processes of insulin resistance and stress response go beyond sex hormone regulation alone [30, 33]. Unfortunately, the timing of our blood collection was not specifically in the early morning (thus not as helpful to assess cortisol regulation) or with fasting status (for assessing insulin resistance), and thus we were not able to assess how these processes may have interacted with changes in sex hormones. Nevertheless, because we were able to assess relationships between measured levels of sex steroids and outcomes important to asthma severity, our findings suggest a direct role for sex steroids themselves.

This cross-sectional analysis of the effects of puberty on asthma features is exploratory and intended primarily to identify specific hypotheses to be tested with longitudinal measurements. We would point out that the veracity of the results is limited by the cross-sectional analytic approach, and the relative paucity of children who were in the mid-Tanner stages (III/IV) at the time of enrollment and our lack of knowledge for most female participants of whether central puberty or adrenarche began first. We lacked data on some participant characteristics, including depression status—which could affect stress response [34]—and the fraction of excreted nitrosoxide (FeNO)—which would have permitted assessment of the relationship between hormone levels with activity of Th2-high airway inflammation.

Conclusions

These results impact understanding of the differences in asthma features with pubertal maturation and the potential for new treatment. The androgen surge with puberty is likely to confer protective effects on lung growth in both males and females whereas estrogens may well have deleterious effects in females extending into adult development. A trial of weak androgen therapy in adolescent children with low androgen levels and poorly-controlled asthma could be considered to improve lung function. These data may help to explain the gender switch observed in asthma incidence during adolescence and likewise inform lung growth and asthma severity with subsequent maturation into adulthood.

Abbreviations

ACQ6: Asthma control questionnaire 6 item scale; DHEA-S: Dehydroepiandrostenedione sulfate; FEV_1%: Forced expired volume in one second percent predicted; FVC %: Forced expired vital capacity % predicted; NIH/NHLBI: National Institutes of Health/National Heart Lung Blood Institute; SARP: Severe Asthma Research Program

Acknowledgments

The authors wish to acknowledge the children and their parents who participated in the SARP III study, as well as the hard work of the site-based study coordinators and regulatory personnel, the oversight of the members of the Data Safety and Monitoring Board, and the diligent efforts of the NIH/NHLBI project officers and staff who administered the protocol.
SARP Principal/Co-Principal Investigators.
Eugene R. Bleecker, PI, Wake Forest University, U10 HL109164.
Mario Castro, PI, Washington University, U10 HL109257.
John V. Fahy, PI, University of California San Francisco, U10 HL109146.
Elliot Israel and Bruce Levy, Co-PI's, Brigham and Women's Hospital, U10 HL109172.
Benjamin Gaston, PI, Rainbow Babies and Children's Hospital Virginia-Cleveland Consortium, U10 HL109250.
Serpil Erzurum, Co-PI, Cleveland Clinic, Virginia-Cleveland Consortium, U10 HL109250.
W. Gerald Teague, Co-PI, Univ. of Virginia, Virginia-Cleveland Consortium, U10 HL109250.
Nizar N. Jarjour, PI, University of Wisconsin, U10 HL109168.
Sally E. Wenzel, PI, University of Pittsburgh, U10 HL109152.
David T. Mauger, PI, DCC, Penn State University, U10 HL109086-04.

Funding

This work was supported by the following grants: U10 HL109164, U10 HL109257, U10 HL109146, U10 HL109172, U10 HL109250, U10 HL109250, U10 HL109250, U10 HL109168, U10 HL109152, U10 HL109086–04.

Authors' contributions

BMG, MDD, WGT, BRP, ERB, MC, JVF, EI, BL, SCE, NNJ, SEW, and DTM devised the present study and/or the data analysis. BMG, WGT, ERB, MC, JVF, EI, BL, SCE, NNJ, SEW, AMF, RM, KRR, JC, MJL, MP, NPL, MLF, FH, WCM, SPP, DM, AMC, LBB, RLS, SR, AMI, WP and JMG were involved in participant recruitment and/or assessment. BRP performed the statistical analysis. MDD, BMG drafted the preliminary manuscript and WGT drafted the final version. All authors read and approved the final manuscript.

Competing interests

There are no conflicts of interest with the study sponsors (NIH/NHLBI) or any commercial entity in the study design, the collection, analysis, and interpretation of the data, the writing of the report, and the decision to submit the paper for publication. The authors submit they will declare potential conflicts of interests per BMC Pulmonary Medicine publication policies.

Author details

[1]University of Virginia School of Medicine, Charlottesville, VA 22908, USA. [2]Pennsylvania State University School of Medicine, Hershey, USA. [3]Lerner Research Institute, Cleveland Clinic Foundation, Cleveland, USA. [4]Emory University School of Medicine, Atlanta, USA. [5]Rainbow Babies and Children's Hospital, Cleveland, USA. [6]San Francisco School of Medicine, University of California, San Francisco, USA. [7]University of Pittsburgh School of Medicine, Pittsburgh, USA. [8]Wake Forest University School of Medicine, Winston-Salem, USA. [9]Washington University School of Medicine, St. Louis, USA. [10]University of Wisconsin School of Medicine, Madison, USA. [11]Virginia Commonwealth University School of Medicine, Richmond, USA. [12]Harvard University School of Medicine, Boston, USA.

References

1. National Center for Environmental Health, Division of Environmental Hazards and Health Effects, Centers for Disease Control and Prevention, Asthma Surveillance Data. www.cdc.gov/asthma/asthmadata.htm. Accessed 1 Feb 2018.
2. Zein JG, Erzurum SC. Asthma is Different in Women. Curr Allergy Asthma Rep. 2015;15(6):28.
3. Zein JG, Udeh BL, Teague WG, Koroukian SM, Schlitz NK, Bleecker ER, et al. Impact of age and sex on outcomes and hospital cost of acute asthma in the United States, 2011-2012. PLoS One. 2016;11(6):e0157301.
4. Koziol-White CJ, Goncharova EA, Cao G, Johnson M, Krymskaya VP, Panettieri RA. DHEA-S inhibits human neutrophil and human airway smooth muscle migration. Biochim Biophys Acta. 2012;1822(10):1638–42.
5. Mendoza-Milla C, Valero Jiménez A, Rangel C, Lozano A, Morales V, Becerril C, et al. Dehydroepiandrosterone has strong antifibrotic effects and is decreased in idiopathic pulmonary fibrosis. Eur Respir J. 2013;42(5):1309–21.
6. Xu L, Xiang X, Ji X, Wang W, Luo M, Luo S, et al. Effects and mechanism of dehydroepiandrosterone on epithelial-mesenchymal transition in bronchial epithelial cells. Exp Lung Res. 2014;40(5):211–21.
7. Kouloumenta V, Hatziefthimiou A, Paraskeva E, Gourgoulianis K, Molyvdas PA. Non-genomic effect of testosterone on airway smooth muscle. Br J Pharmacol. 2006;149(8):1083–91.
8. Farha S, Asosingh K, Laskowski D, Hammel J, Dweik RA, Wiedemann HP, Erzurum SC. Effects of the menstrual cycle on lung function variables in women with asthma. Am J Respir Crit Care Med. 2009;180:304–10.
9. Wheeldon NM, Newnham DM, Coutie WJ, Peters A, McDevitt DG, Lipworth BJ. Influence of sex-steroid hormones on the regulation of lymphocyte β_2 adrenoceptors during the menstrual cycle. Br J Clin Pharmacol. 1994;37:583–8.
10. Tan KS, McFarlane LC, Lipworth BJ. Loss of normal cyclical β_2 adrenoceptor regulation and increased premenstrual responsiveness to adenosine monophosphate in stable female asthmatic patients. Thorax. 1997;52(7):608–11.
11. Sheel AW, Dominelli PB, Molgat-Seon Y. Revisiting dysanapsis: sex-based differences in airways and the mechanics of breathing during exercise. Exp Physiol. 2016;101(2):213–8.
12. Marshall WA, Tanner JM. Variations in the pattern of pubertal changes in girls. Arch Dis Childhood. 1969;44:291–303.
13. Mouritsen A, Søeborg T, Hagen CP, Mieritz MG, Johannsen TH, Frederiksen H, Andersson AM, Juul A. Longitudinal changes in serum concentrations of adrenal androgen metabolites and their ratios by LC-MS/MS in healthy boys and girls. Clin Chim Acta. 2015;450:370–5.
14. Dorsey MJ, Cohen LE, Phipatanakul W, Denufrio D, Schneider LC. Assessment of adrenal suppression in children with asthma treated with inhaled corticosteroids: use of dehydroepiandrosterone sulfate as a screening test. Ann Allergy Asthma Immunol. 2006;97(2):182–6.
15. Denlinger L, Ramratnam S, Ross K, Phillips BR, Bhakta NR, Cardet JC, Castro M, Peters SP, Phipatanakul W, Aujla S, Bacharier LB, Bleecker ER, Comhair SAA, Coverstone A, DeBoer M, Erzurum SC, Fain SB, Fajt M, Fitzpatrick AM, Gaffin J, Gaston B, Hastie AT, Hawkins GA, Holguin F, Irani AM, Israel E, Levy BD, Ly N, Meyers DA, Moore WC, Myers R, Peters MC, Schiebler ML, Sorkness RL, Teague WG, Wenzel SE, Mauger DT, Fahy JV, Inflammatory JNN. Co-morbid features of patients with severe asthma and frequent exacerbations. Am J Respir Crit Care Med. 2017;195:302–13.
16. Phipatanakul W, Mauger DT, Sorkness RL, Gaffin JM, Holguin F, Woodruff PG, Ly NP, Bacharier LB, Bhakta NR, Moore WC, Bleecker ER, Hastie AT, Meyers DA, Castro M, Fahy J, Fitzpatrick A, Gaston BM, Jarjour NN, Levy BD, Peters SP, Teague WG, Fajt M, Wenzel SE, Erzurum SC, Israel E. The severe asthma research program. Effects of age and disease severity on systemic corticosteroid responses in asthma. In press. Am J Respir Crit Care Med. 2017;195(11):1439–48.
17. Chung KF, Wenzel SE, Brozek JL, Bush A, Castro M, Sterk P, Adcock IM, Bateman E, Bel E, Bleecker E, Boulet LP, Brightling C, Chanez P, Dahlen SE, Djukanovic R, Frey U, Gaga M, Gibson P, Hamid Q, Jarjour N, Mauad T, Sorkness R, Teague WG, International ERS. ATS consensus definition, mechanisms, evaluation and treatment of severe asthma. Eur Respir J. 2014;43(2):343–73.
18. Moore WC, Bleecker ER, Curran-Everett D, Erzurum SC, Ameredes BT, Bacharier L, et al. Characterization of the severe asthma phenotype by the National Heart, Lung, and Blood Institute's severe asthma research program. J Allergy Clin Immunol. 2007;119(2):405–13.
19. Moore WC, Meyers DA, Wenzel SE, Teague WG, Li H, Li X, et al. Identification of asthma phenotypes using cluster analysis in the severe asthma research program. Am J Respir Crit Care Med. 2010;181(4):315–23.
20. Fitzpatrick AM, Teague WG, Meyers DA, Peters SP, Li X, Li H, et al. Heterogeneity of severe asthma in childhood: confirmation by cluster analysis of children in the National Institutes of Health/National Heart, Lung,

and Blood Institute Severe Asthma Research Program. J Allergy Clin Immunol. 2011;127(2):382–9. e381–313
21. Juniper EF, Svensson K, Mork A, Stahl E. Measurement properties and interpretation of three shortened versions of the asthma control questionnaire. Respir Med. 2005;99:553–8.
22. Quanjer PH, Stanojevic S, Cole TJ, Baur X, Hall GL, Culver BH, Enright PL, Hankinson JL, Ip MSM, Zheng J, Stocks J. Multi-ethic reference values for spirometry for the 3-95 year age range: the global lung function 2012 equations. Eur Respir J. 2012;40.1324–43.
23. Vermeulen A, Verdonck L, Kaufman JM. A critical evaluation of simple methods for the estimation of free testosterone in serum. J Clin Endocrinol Metab. 1999;84(10):3666–72.
24. Juniper EF, Bousquet J, Abetz L, Bateman ED, Committee G. Identifying 'well-controlled' and 'not well-controlled' asthma using the asthma control questionnaire. Respir Med. 2006;100:616–21.
25. Chen F, Knecht K, Birzin E, Fisher J, Wilkinson H, Mojena M, et al. Direct agonist/antagonist functions of dehydroepiandrosterone. Endocrinology. 2005;146(11):4568–76.
26. Gao W, Bohl CE, Dalton JT. Chemistry and structural biology of androgen receptor. Chem Rev. 2005;105(9):3352–70.
27. Wenzel SE, Robinson CB, Leonard JM, Panettieri RA. Nebulized dehydroepiandrosterone-3-sulfate improves asthma control in the moderate-to-severe asthma results of a 6-week, randomized, double-blind, placebo-controlled study. Allergy Asthma Proc. 2010;31(6):461–71.
28. Palmert MR, Dunkel L. Clinical practice. Delayed puberty. N Engl J Med. 2012;366(5):443–53.
29. Tantisira KG, Colvin R, Tonascia J, Strunk RC, Weiss ST, Fuhlbrigge AL, et al. Airway responsiveness in mild to moderate childhood asthma: sex influences on the natural history. Am J Respir Crit Care Med. 2008;178(4):325–31.
30. Goran MI, Gower BA. Longitudinal study on pubertal insulin resistance. Diabetes. 2001;50:2444–50.
31. Thuesen BH, Husemoen LL, Hersoug LG, Pisinger C, Linneberg A. Insulin resistance as a predictor of incident asthma-like symptoms in adults. Clin Exp Allergy. 2009;39:700–7.
32. Kozyrskyj AL, Zeng Y, Saurek-Aleksandrovska N, Sellers EA, Ramsey CD, Becker AB. Insulin resistance, puberty, and nonatopic asthma in adolescent girls. Am J Respir Crit Care Med. 2014;190:474–7.
33. Gunnar MR, Wewerka S, Frenn K, Long JD, Griggs C. Developmental changes in hypothalamus-pituitary-adrenal activity over the transition to adolescence: normative changes and associations with puberty. Dev Psychopathol. 2009;21:69–85.
34. Bahreinian S, Ball GD, Vander Leek TK, Colman I, McNeil BJ, Becker AB, Kozyrskyj AL. Allostatic load biomarkers and asthma in adolescents. Am J Respir Crit Care Med. 2013;187:144–52.

10

Prevalence of asthma among the adult general population of five Middle Eastern countries

Hesham Tarraf[1], Omur Aydin[2], Dilsad Mungan[2], Mohammad Albader[3], Bassam Mahboub[4,5], Adam Doble[6], Aaicha Lahlou[7], Luqman Tariq[8], Fayaz Aziz[8] and Abdelkader El Hasnaoui[8*]

Abstract

Background: Asthma is a common chronic respiratory disease leading to morbidity, mortality and impaired quality of life worldwide. Information on asthma prevalence in the Middle East is fragmented and relatively out-dated. The SNAPSHOT program was conducted to obtain updated information.

Methods: SNAPSHOT is a cross-sectional epidemiological program carried out in five Middle Eastern countries (Egypt, Turkey, Kuwait, Saudi Arabia, and the United Arab Emirates, the latter three grouped into a Gulf cluster) to collect data on asthma, allergic rhinitis, benign prostatic hyperplasia and bipolar disorder. The survey was carried out by telephone in a random sample of the adult general population with quotas defined according to country demographics. The analysis presented in this paper focuses on asthma. Subjects were screened for asthma based on criteria from the global Asthma Insights and Reality studies. Current prevalence (last 12 months) was estimated. Multivariate logistic regression analyses were used to investigate risk factors related to asthma and the association with allergic rhinitis and other co-morbidities. Quality of life was assessed using the three-level EQ-5D questionnaire.

Results: 2124 out of the 33,486 subjects enrolled in the SNAPSHOT program fulfilled the criteria for asthma. The adjusted prevalence of asthma ranged from 4.4% [95% CI: 4.0–4.8%] in Turkey, to 6.7% [95% CI: 6.2–7.2%] in Egypt and 7.6% [95% CI: 7.1–8.0%] in the Gulf cluster. Prevalence was higher ($p < 0.0001$) in women than men and increased with age ($p < 0.0001$). Co-morbidities occurred more frequently in asthma subjects compared to the non-asthma population (38% vs. 15% $p < 0.0001$). Subjects with asthma reported a lower ($p < 0.0001$) EQ-VAS score (68.2 ± 22.9) compared to the general population (78.1 ± 17.5). The risk factors associated with asthma were age, gender, country, and certain co-morbidities, namely respiratory, cardiovascular, gastrointestinal, nervous, and neurological diseases.

Conclusion: The observed adjusted prevalence of asthma in the Middle East ranges from 4.4% to 7.6%, which is comparatively lower than the reported prevalence in Europe and North America. Asthma has a negative impact on quality of life, and is associated with high levels of co-morbid diseases, indicating a need for physicians to check for co-morbidities and ensure they are managed correctly in all asthma patients.

Keywords: Asthma, Prevalence, Middle East, SNAPSHOT, Quality of life, Co-morbidity

* Correspondence: abdelkader.a.el-hasnaoui@gsk.com
[8]GlaxoSmithKline, PO Box 50199, Dubai, United Arab Emirates
Full list of author information is available at the end of the article

Background

Asthma is one of the most common chronic respiratory diseases and is a major public health issue globally, affecting people of all ages, genders and ethnicities. It is estimated that the number of people with asthma worldwide may be as high as 334 million according to a report from the Global Asthma Network published in 2014 [1]. Prevalence has been shown to vary widely both between countries and within countries, and has been steadily increasing alongside that of allergy, as modern lifestyles are adopted and communities become more urbanised, a trend that is predicted to continue over the next two decades [2]. For those people affected by the disease, it can be a cause of major disability and impact greatly on quality of life [1, 2].

Asthma prevalence has been widely studied globally. However, many of the studies focus on the childhood prevalence of the disease, notably the International Study of Asthma and Allergies in Childhood (ISAAC) studies [3, 4]. In adults, three large, international, epidemiological projects assessing the prevalence of asthma have been conducted to date: the European Community Respiratory Health Survey (ECRHS) [5]; the World Health Survey (WHS) [6]; and the Global Allergy and Asthma Network of Excellence (GA2LEN) study in Europe [7]. Additional studies have estimated the prevalence and management of asthma in specific geographical areas such as the Asthma Insights and Reality (AIR) surveys [8], all of which utilise similar methodology and have now been carried out in a number of Middle Eastern countries including Turkey [9] and the Gulf [10]. However, to improve the understanding of asthma prevalence worldwide, further international studies are needed and require use of a consistent case definition for asthma and identical study methodologies. This would allow cross country comparison of data and provide a benchmark for future studies.

Despite the magnitude of the disease, data on the epidemiology and disease burden of asthma in the Middle East region are scarce. Local observational studies investigating the current prevalence of asthma in adults have been conducted, but few studies provide prevalence estimates at a multinational level using a standardised methodology and the data is relatively out-dated as the majority of the studies were completed prior to 2010. In Turkey, the published prevalence ranges from 2.11% - 8.35% [9, 11–15]. In the United Arab Emirates (UAE) the reported prevalence ranges from 2.79% - 8% [14, 16, 17] and in Saudi Arabia, a national household survey was carried out in 2013 which reported an asthma prevalence of 4.05% [18]. In the North African countries, the most recent data are from the AIR Maghreb (AIRMAG) study carried out between 2008 and 2009 [19], which investigated asthma prevalence in Algeria, Morocco and Tunisia. Earlier data (2002–2003) is available from the WHS survey [14]. In these countries, the reported prevalence rates ranged from 2.79% to 3.89%. In Egypt many studies on asthma have been performed in the paediatric age groups but very few addressed the adult population and were not representative of the whole country [20].

In some areas, there is limited regional information available. In addition, results from the existing studies rely on a variety of methodologies used to capture the information, the different population sources and variety of sampling methods, the different modes of interview, and the lack of a common case definition for asthma, and differing interpretation of symptoms in different countries all limit the ability to compare the data. Hence, there is a need to provide up to date information on the prevalence of asthma in Middle Eastern countries. To address this, we have conducted a large, cross-sectional, population-based study as part of the SNAPSHOT program, using a standardised methodology in five countries in the region, to investigate the current prevalence of asthma in the adult population.

Methods

The SNAPSHOT program

SNAPSHOT is a cross-sectional, observational, population-based program, comprising multiple studies, conducted in a random sample of the general population of five countries (Egypt, Kuwait, Saudi Arabia, Turkey, and the UAE). The objective of the SNAPSHOT program was to provide an omnibus approach to collect data simultaneously about multiple diseases using a standardised methodology. The program provides updated epidemiological data on the prevalence, burden of disease, quality of life and healthcare resource use related to four chronic diseases in the participating countries, namely: asthma, allergic rhinitis, bipolar disorder and benign prostatic hyperplasia (BPH). The selection of these diseases was based on the need to respond to emerging health technology assessment (HTA) requirements. The detailed study methodology is the subject of a separate manuscript [21].

The program was carried out by computer-assisted personal interviewing (CAPI) conducted over the telephone and the information collected via web-based electronic data capture. Interviews were proposed in Arabic, English or Turkish using translated validated questionnaires and conducted by trained staff of local specialised Contract Research Organisations (CROs); Omega (Turkey) for interviews in Turkey and Infomine Healthcare Research (Egypt) for interviews in the Arabic-speaking countries. Data management and analyses were performed by MS Health (Morocco).

The SNAPSHOT sample

The SNAPSHOT population was generated using a random stratified sampling method. Enrolment began in July

2014. A target sample of 10,000 subjects from the adult general population of Turkey and Egypt and 15,000 for the Gulf cluster (comprised of Kuwait, Saudi Arabia and the UAE) was defined based on the demographic structure of the country in terms of age and gender, to enable the estimate of prevalence and disease burden with a satisfactory precision. In the Gulf cluster, the target sample size could not be reached despite extensive efforts to accelerate subject enrolment. Therefore, it was decided to stop recruitment in February 2016. The combined number of interviews conducted to date in Saudi Arabia, Kuwait and UAE showed that the program objectives could be achieved from a sample size perspective. The database was locked on 11th April 2016.

Subject enrolment

Telephone numbers (landline and mobile) were generated in blocks using an assisted random-digit dialling procedure. Each number was dialled up to fifteen times on different days and times including weekends and evenings until contact was established. After fifteen attempts, outcomes were categorised as contact, unattributed, out-of-service, fax, or unreachable. In order to optimise response rates, successive blocks of numbers were defined and the release of a new block could only occur once the previous block had been completed. This process was repeated until the target number for each country / cluster was achieved.

If telephone contact was established, the interviewer first assessed the eligibility of the telephone number (business numbers were ineligible). For eligible numbers, the interviewer determined the respondent's age, gender and region of residence. All subjects ≥18 years of age who had been residing in the country for over 6 months were eligible, unless the pre-specified strata for age, gender and region was filled. If the subject was ineligible, this was documented and the phone call terminated. If the subject was eligible, the interview began. If the respondent agreed to continue the interview but asked to be called back later, up to ten attempts were made after which this was classified as a call-back failure and considered a refusal. Subject flow through the recruitment process is shown in Fig. 1. The overall response rate was 50.9%. At a country level it varied by a factor of almost two, from 35.3% in Kuwait, 40.0% in UAE and 40.6% in Saudi Arabia to 58.9% and 67.4% in Turkey and Egypt respectively.

Conduct of the interview

Standardised general information was provided at the start of the interview, specifying that participation was voluntary, confidential and anonymous. Verbal consent to participate was collected by the interviewee and recorded in the CAPI system and the interviewee was then invited to respond to a first questionnaire, screening for the four diseases of interest and to document social and demographic characteristics, as well as the presence of co-morbidities. If the interviewee did not want to answer, the contact was considered as a refusal and the interview terminated. If a subject screened positive for at least one of the four diseases, a second disease-specific questionnaire was administered to collect additional information on burden of disease, disease management and healthcare resource utilisation. In cases where respondents fulfilled the screening criteria for more than

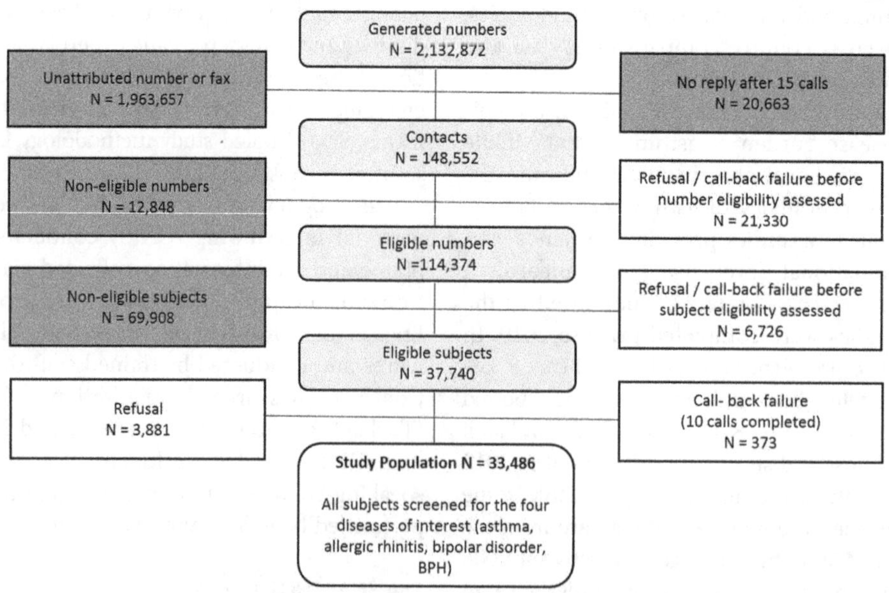

Fig. 1 Subject flow through the recruitment process. The grey boxes indicate excluded numbers or subjects, and the white boxes the groups of potentially eligible numbers or subjects taken into account in the calculation of the response rate

one disease, they were randomised by the CAPI system to respond to only one of the disease-specific questionnaires, in order to limit the duration of the interview. For all subjects the interview ended with the EuroQoL five-dimension questionnaire (EQ-5D), a measure of health status which captures the impact of a disease on physical, mental, and social functioning [22, 23]. All questionnaires were used in validated English, Turkish or Arabic translations; the translated versions are available on request. The full interview was conducted in one telephone call.

Case definition for asthma

Subjects were considered to have asthma if they fulfilled the screening criteria shown in Table 1, which were based on the criteria used in the global AIR studies [8]. A positive answer to any of the latter three questions (Q3-Q5) led to classification of the interviewee as a subject with asthma. It is important to note that the criteria were designed to collect information on the current prevalence (last 12 months) and not the lifetime prevalence of the disease.

Data collected for this analysis

This analysis focuses solely on asthma and aims to provide estimates of the current prevalence of asthma in the areas studied. Socio-demographic data were collected to describe the characteristics of the overall study population, including gender and age distribution, marital status, educational level, employment status, health system coverage, body mass index (BMI), the presence of co-morbidities and smoking status. If a respondent was a current or former smoker, they were asked to provide the duration and extent of exposure. Additionally, the type and frequency of co-morbidities were investigated and risk factors related to asthma identified. As part of the screening questionnaire, subjects were also screened for allergic rhinitis using the Score for Allergic Rhinitis (SFAR) questionnaire [24] and asked about any family history of this disease to identify asthma subjects who had co-morbid allergic rhinitis or a family history of allergic rhinitis. All subjects were also asked to complete the EQ-5D-3L questionnaire to measure quality of life, a generic questionnaire to measure health status. The questionnaire consists of five dimensions (mobility, self-care, usual activities, pain / discomfort, anxiety / depression) each of which can take one of three responses (no problems / moderate problems / extreme problems) and a visual analogue rating scale (EQ-VAS) [22]. Asthma prevalence data were collected using the case definition described and the prevalence by age, gender, country and region was assessed.

Table 1 Screening Criteria for Asthma. A positive answer to any of the latter three questions (Q3-Q5) led to classification of the interviewee as a subject with asthma

Screening Criteria for Asthma	
Q1 Have you been told by your doctor that you suffer from asthma?	□ No □ Yes
Q2 Have you had one of the following symptoms: wheezing, nocturnal coughing, chest tightness, or breathless ness in the last 12 months	□ No □ Yes
Q3. Have you had an asthma attack in the last 12 months?	□ No □ Yes
Q4. Have you used asthma medications in the last 12 months?	□ No □ Yes
Q5. Have you used Ventolin or inhaled bronchodilators or short acting β agonist in the last 12 months?	□ No □ Yes
If yes, what is the daily frequency of use?	□ Once □ Repeated

Statistical analysis

The data presented here are for the screening population of 33,486 subjects who accepted to participate in the study, completed all screening questionnaires and thus constituted the screening population. Prevalence was adjusted for age and gender by weighting each subject to take into account the actual structure of age and gender in the national population for each country [25]. This adjustment also took into account the additional weight given to men over the age of 50 which was necessary to enable the prevalence of BPH to be estimated accurately.

Data are presented as proportions and means with standard deviations (SD), or medians with interquartile ranges (IQR). 95% confidence intervals (95% CI) were calculated for binomial data. Associations between categorical variables were estimated using the χ^2 test and the Cochran–Mantel–Haenszel test as appropriate. Two-sided tests were used in all cases and a probability threshold of 0.05 was considered significant. Multivariate regression analysis was performed to identify risk factors associated with asthma. In a first step, variables were evaluated independently in a univariate analysis. All variables with a P value < 0.20 [26] in the univariate analysis were entered into the multiple logistic regression analysis in which variables were retained in the model using a backward stepwise selection to determine the variables associated with an increased risk of asthma at the probability level of 0.05. In addition, variables hypothesised to have clinical relevance but not found to be significant at 0.20 were maintained (e.g. age). A final multivariate analysis was conducted to generate odds ratios. Multivariate regression analysis was also performed to assess the relationship between co-morbidities and asthma independent of age, gender and country and the relationship between allergic rhinitis and asthma. All statistical analyses were performed using SAS® Version 9.4 (SAS, Cary, USA).

Results

Study sample

A total of 33,486 subjects agreed to participate in the screening questionnaire and constituted the screening population. This population was distributed between Egypt (10,014), Turkey (10,000) and the Gulf cluster (13,472). Overall, approximately 60% of respondents were men and 40% women (sex ratio: 1.41; 19,610 were men). The majority were aged between 18 and 35 (47.7%; $n = 15,959$). Just over half of the remaining respondents were between 35 and 50 years of age (29.6%; $n = 9921$) and the rest were aged 50 or above (22.7%; $n = 7606$). Selected demographics of the screening population are shown in Table 2. These data highlight that the majority of the screening population are non-smokers (65%) and either overweight or obese (54%).

Current prevalence of asthma

Of the subjects enrolled in the study 2124 fulfilled the case definition for asthma and were defined as the asthma population. Overall, the adjusted prevalence of asthma in the adult general population over 18 years of age in the countries studied was 6.4% [95% CI: 6.1–6.6%]. This ranged from 4.4% in Turkey, to 6.7% in Egypt and 7.6% in the Gulf cluster (Table 3). After adjusting for age and gender there is little difference between the crude and adjusted prevalence. The adjusted prevalence by country in the Gulf cluster was 9.5% [95% CI: 8.1–10.9%] in Kuwait, 4.9% [95% CI 4.2–6.6%] in the UAE, and 8.3 [95% CI 7.7–8.9%] in Saudi Arabia.

The current prevalence of asthma was significantly higher in women compared to men across all countries and the cluster of countries studied ($p < 0.0001$). Age is also an important factor; the current prevalence of asthma increased significantly with age ($p < 0.0001$). These results are presented in Table 3. Further analysis of the age and gender split by country showed that for each country or cluster of countries the observed prevalence of asthma was higher in women than in men across every age group studied (data not shown).

Current asthma prevalence was also investigated by region across the countries studied and these results are shown in Fig. 2. In Egypt, the highest prevalence was documented in Greater Cairo / North Egypt, and the Canal/other region followed by Upper Egypt ($p < 0.0096$). In the Gulf cluster, there was a significant difference in prevalence across the countries and regions studied ($p < 0.0001$). In Saudi Arabia, the central region reported a prevalence of 10.5% which is significantly higher than the coastal regions in the east and west which reported a prevalence of 6.5% and 7.0% respectively. The prevalence in Kuwait was comparatively high compared to most other regions in the Gulf cluster although the reported prevalence in western Kuwait (10.6%) was in line with that seen in central Saudi Arabia. The prevalence in the UAE was slightly lower than the rest of the Gulf cluster but consistent across the country. In Turkey, there was no significant difference in prevalence across the regions studied ($p = 0.36$).

Asthma and smoking status

There was no statistical difference ($p = 0.99$) in the percentage of respondents who smoked between the asthma population (66.5%) and the non-asthma population (66.3%). Among current or former smokers, there was no statistical difference ($p = 0.08$) in the number of pack-years for the asthma population (18.9 ± 23.0) compared to the non-asthma population (17.3 ± 20.4).

Risk factors for asthma

The following variables were tested in a univariate analysis looking at potential risk factors for asthma: marital status, employment status, BMI, smoking status, co-morbidities yes/no, age, gender and country (Egypt, Kuwait, Saudi Arabia, Turkey, UAE). Those variables found to be significant at 0.2 were entered into the multivariate analysis. The variable smoking status was not found to be significant. However, to further explore a potential association between smoking and asthma this variable was maintained in the multivariate analysis. The results of a multivariate regression analysis show a significant association between living in Kuwait or Saudi Arabia and having asthma (odds ratio (OR) 1.8 and 1.4 respectively) compared to living in Egypt ($p < 0.0001$). In addition, a significant association ($p < 0.0001$) was observed between asthma and obesity (OR 1.5), smoking (OR 1.4), and the presence of co-morbidities (OR 3.1). These results are shown in Fig. 3.

History of co-morbidities and the impact on the asthma population

The number of subjects that reported suffering from a chronic health condition was significantly higher ($p < 0.0001$) in the asthma population (38.4%) compared to the non-asthma population (15.4%). The following variables were tested in a univariate analysis looking at the relationship between co-morbidities and asthma: cardiovascular disease, nervous disease, neurological disease, respiratory disease, gastrointestinal disease, renal disease, rheumatological disease, endocrine disease (diabetes), malignancy disease, immunological disease and adjusted for age, gender and country (Egypt, Kuwait, Saudi Arabia, Turkey, UAE). Those found to be significant at 0.20 were entered into a multivariate analysis to investigate the relationship

Table 2 Demographics of the screening population

Demographic	Criteria	Egypt $N = 10{,}014$	Gulf cluster $N = 13{,}472$	Turkey $N = 10{,}000$
Gender *n* (%)	Count	10,014	13,472	10,000
	Men	5747 (57.4)	8524 (63.3)	5339 (53.4)
	Women	4267 (42.6)	4948 (36.7)	4661 (46.6)
Age *n* (%)	Count	10,014	13,472	10,000
	18–34 years	4978 (49.7)	7055 (52.4)	3926 (39.3)
	35–49 years	2453 (24.5)	4745 (35.2)	2723 (27.2)
	≥ 50 years	2583 (25.8)	1672 (12.4)	3351 (33.5)
Marital Status *n* (%)	Count	9814	13,013	9522
	Married	7357 (75.0)	9000 (69.2)	7054 (74.1)
	Living as unmarried couple	3 (0.03)	4 (0.03)	6 (0.06)
	Separated/divorced	160 (1.6)	325 (2.5)	130 (1.4)
	Widowed	362 (3.7)	206 (0.02)	390 (4.1)
	Single/never married	1932 (19.7)	3478 (26.7)	1942 (20.4)
Education level *n* (%)	Count	9755	12,877	9079
	No high school	2767 (28.4)	1789 (13.9)	5245 (57.8)
	Some high school	236 (2.4)	283 (1.2)	156 (1.7)
	High school graduate	2291 (23.5)	3501 (27.2)	1842 (20.3)
	Technical post-secondary	1386 (14.2)	834 (6.5)	306 (3.4)
	Some college	434 (4.5)	757 (5.9)	430 (4.8)
	College graduate	2267 (23.2)	4837 (37.5)	1040 (11.5)
	Post graduate degree	374 (3.8)	876 (6.8)	60 (0.7)
Employment Status *n* (%)	Count	9735	12,834	9721
	Employed (full or part time)	5592 (57.4)	8732 (68.0)	4299 (44.2)
	Unemployed	447 (4.6)	584 (4.6)	1243 (12.8)
	Retired and not working	579 (6.0)	291 (2.3)	1462 (15.0)
	Student	524 (5.4)	738 (0.06)	340 (3.5)
	Homemaker	2545 (26.1)	2466 (19.2)	2370 (24.4)
	Disabled or too ill to work	48 (0.5)	23 (0.2)	7 (0.07)
Yearly Household Income *n* (%)	Count	9.596	12,555	9125
	< minimum wage	3465 (36.1)	1616 (12.9)	1427 (15.6)
	Minimum wage	4110 (42.8)	8917 (71.0)	3023 (33.1)
	2 × minimum wage	1277 (13.3)	1243 (9.9)	4276 (46.9)
	> 2 times minimum wage	744 (7.8)	779 (6.2)	399 (4.4)
Smoking *n* (%)	Count	9814	13,014	9784
	Non-smoker	6513 (66.4)	9176 (70.5)	5942 (60.7)
	Current/former smoker	3301 (33.6)	3838 (29.5)	3842 (39.3)
BMI *n* (%)	Count	9338	12,156	9028
	Underweight	230 (2.5)	469 (3.9)	271 (3.0)
	Normal weight	3060 (32.8)	4605 (37.9)	3826 (42.4)
	Overweight	3253 (34.8)	4333 (35.6)	3299 (36.5)
	Obese	2795 (29.9)	2749 (22.6)	1632 (18.1)

Demographics of the screening population ($N = 33{,}486$) by country and cluster. BMI = body mass index

Table 3 Current prevalence of asthma

Variable		Egypt N = 10,014	Gulf cluster N = 13,472	Turkey N = 10,000
Number of Cases		676	1003	445
Crude Prevalence (%)		6.8	7.5	4.5
Adjusted Prevalence (%)		6.7	7.6	4.4
Adjusted 95% CI		[6.2–7.2]	[7.1–8]	[4.0–4.8]
Gender (%) [95% CI]	Men	5.5 [4.9–6.1]	6.2 [5.7–6.7]	2.9 [2.4–3.3]
	Women	8.4 [7.6–9.3]	9.6 [8.7–10.4]	6.3 [5.6–7]
	P value (CMH test)	$p < 0.0001$		
Age (%) [95% CI]	18–34	5.5 [4.8–6.1]	7.0 [6.4–7.6]	2.6 [2.1–3.1]
	35–49	7.7 [6.7–8.8]	7.7 [7–8.5]	4.0 [3.3–4.8]
	≥ 50	8.3 [7.3–9.4]	8.7 [7.3–10.0]	7.0 [6.1–7.8]
	P value (CMH test)	$p < 0.0001$		

Current prevalence (%) of asthma by country and cluster, adjusted by age and gender as required. CMH: Cochran Mantel-Haenszel; 95% CI = 95% Confidence Interval

between each of the co-morbidities and the risk of asthma, independent of age, gender and country. The results show that the co-morbidity with the highest impact is respiratory disease (OR 44.6). Detailed investigation into the conditions classified under the co-morbidity 'respiratory disease' revealed that this refers primarily to chronic obstructive pulmonary disease (COPD). This was followed by neurological disease (OR 2.5), cardiovascular disease (OR 2.1), gastrointestinal disease (OR 1.8) and nervous disease (OR 1.5). These results are presented in Fig. 4.

A large number of subjects with asthma (482) were found to have co-morbid allergic rhinitis and 271 subjects reported having a family history of the disease, although they did not have allergic rhinitis themselves. A multivariate regression analysis looking specifically at the relationship between allergic rhinitis and asthma, adjusted for age, gender and country showed a strong association ($p < 0.0001$) between the two diseases (OR 6.4; 95% CI 5.7–7.2). In case of a family history of allergic rhinitis in subjects without allergic rhinitis themselves a weaker association with asthma was observed (OR 1.7; 95% CI 1.0–3.0).

Impact of asthma on quality of life

Overall, subjects with asthma reported a significantly lower ($p < 0.0001$) mean EQ-5D-3L utility score (0.74 ± 0.34) than the general population (0.90 ± 0.21). This relationship was observed for all participating countries or cluster of countries. A similar observation was made for the mean EQ-VAS scores (68.2 ± 22.9 in subjects with asthma; 78.1 ± 17.5 in the general population $p < 0.0001$). The overall impact and the country-level results are presented in Fig. 5.

Discussion

Omnibus programs such as SNAPSHOT represent a powerful approach for generating standardised epidemiological data on important health indicators such as prevalence. In particular, the use of a common methodology to collect the data enables pertinent comparisons to be made between countries and between diseases. Although setting up multidimensional studies such as this on a large scale is time- and resource- consuming, once the data acquisition system has been validated it would be relatively straightforward to implement the same program in further groups of countries.

In this program the overall response rate was 50.9%. The SNAPSHOT program was conducted in a random selection of the general population using telephone interview. In this context, a high level of refusal is common since people often do no do not respond to such calls requesting information, from which they receive no immediate benefit. However, the combination of refusals and call-back failures, and the inclusion of subjects prior to confirmation of eligibility criteria in the response rate calculation, reflects a conservative approach. If we assume that the distribution of eligible/non-eligible subjects is identical for respondents and non-respondents, then the response rate could be estimated as 56.5%. Further exclusion of call-back failures from the calculation would have yielded a response rate of 70.6%. If this non-conservative response rate is used then the response rate for the SNAPSHOT program is within the range of that observed in AIR studies elsewhere, such as Europe (80%) [27], and the Maghreb [19].

The primary objective of this study was to estimate the prevalence of asthma in five countries in the Middle East (Egypt, Turkey Kuwait, Saudi Arabia, and the UAE).

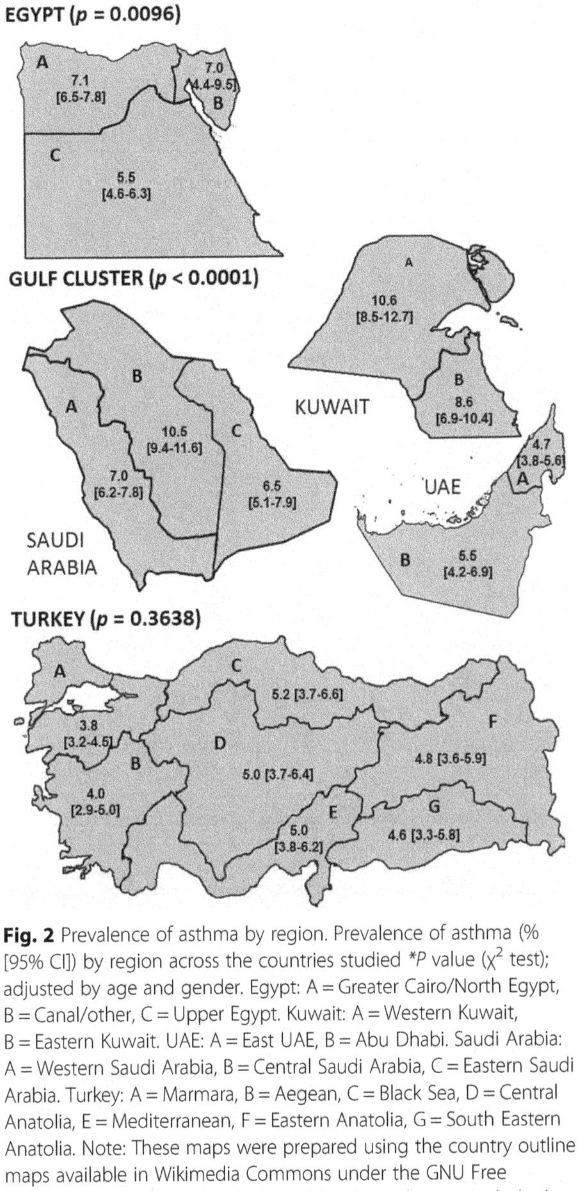

Fig. 2 Prevalence of asthma by region. Prevalence of asthma (% [95% CI]) by region across the countries studied **P* value (χ^2 test); adjusted by age and gender. Egypt: A = Greater Cairo/North Egypt, B = Canal/other, C = Upper Egypt. Kuwait: A = Western Kuwait, B = Eastern Kuwait. UAE: A = East UAE, B = Abu Dhabi. Saudi Arabia: A = Western Saudi Arabia, B = Central Saudi Arabia, C = Eastern Saudi Arabia. Turkey: A = Marmara, B = Aegean, C = Black Sea, D = Central Anatolia, E = Mediterranean, F = Eastern Anatolia, G = South Eastern Anatolia. Note: These maps were prepared using the country outline maps available in Wikimedia Commons under the GNU Free Documentation License and adapted by the authors to include the prevalence data

The overall current prevalence of asthma in the adult general population over 18 years of age in these countries was 6.4%. This ranged from 4.4% in Turkey, to 6. 7% in Egypt and 7.6% in the Gulf Cluster.

The global AIR studies have been conducted in many countries, and although these studies use the same questionnaire, a very broad range of prevalence estimates has been observed in the different studies conducted (ranging from 1% in Ecuador to 15% in Singapore) [28]. Comparison of the reported prevalence of asthma in these Middle Eastern countries with data obtained through the AIR studies demonstrates that the prevalence of asthma in the participating countries is low compared with the United Kingdom but slightly higher than some other European countries such as Germany [27], and considerably higher than countries in Asia such as China and Malaysia [29].

Comparison with published epidemiological data on the prevalence of asthma in the Middle East is difficult, since the criteria used to define asthma vary between studies and the methodologies are not consistent. For example, the studies use different case definitions for asthma; different populations, different modes of interview; or different age cut-offs for inclusion. This has led to a range of prevalence estimates being reported. One of the objectives of the SNAPSHOT program was to use a consistent case definition and study methodology across all countries included, to overcome this issue and enable comparison of the results.

To gain a better understanding of previously published asthma prevalence data in the region, a literature review was performed. This review focused on general population studies which investigated asthma prevalence in the Middle East and North Africa region. In line with the parameters of the SNAPSHOT study, the search was limited to population-based, observational studies that focused on the current prevalence of asthma in adults. The search was restricted to articles that were in English, available via PubMed, and were published between January 1st 2000 and December 31st 2015 [9, 11–19]. The findings, together with the results from the SNAPSHOT study (denoted by a red star), are depicted in Fig. 6. The reported prevalence of asthma in Turkey and the UAE is within the range of the published literature and there are no published studies that fulfil the specified inclusion criteria in Egypt and Kuwait. A higher prevalence of asthma was observed in Saudi Arabia compared to the previously published data. This could be due to methodological differences between the studies, (the interviews in the previous study had been conducted face-to-face which tends to yield lower prevalence estimates than telephone or postal questionnaires), although a real increase in prevalence over time cannot be excluded, perhaps linked to the increasing urbanisation of the country [30].

Whilst the prevalence of asthma in Turkey reported here is within the range reported by comparable studies in the country, the prevalence reported in Turkey was generally lower than in Egypt or the Gulf cluster, the reported prevalence in the 18–34 age group was particularly low at 2.6%. There are few published studies that have investigated asthma prevalence by age in Turkey, and none using equivalent methodology to SNAPSHOT. However, a study carried out in the city of Samsun reported the prevalence by asthma diagnosis as 1.0% in the 15–29 age group and 2.6% in the 30–49 age group, and by use of medication as 1.0% and 1.8% in these

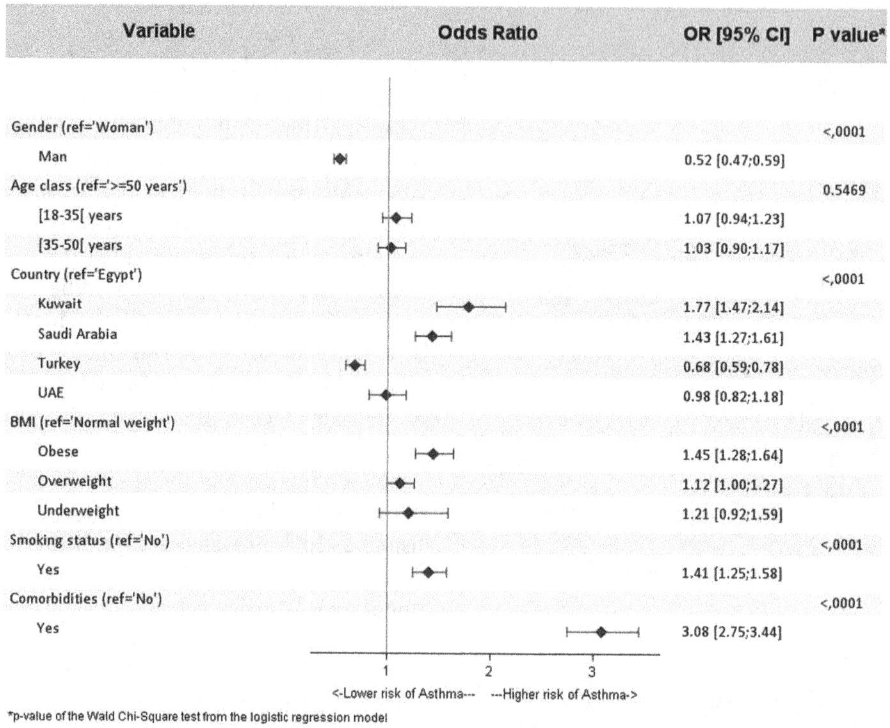

Fig. 3 Multivariate regression analysis investigating the risk factors for asthma: Asthma population (1931 subjects) versus non-asthma population (28,586 subjects); OR [95% CI] = odds ratio [95% Confidence Interval]. The results presented are adjusted for age (18–34,35–49, ≥50 years), gender and country (Egypt, Kuwait, Saudi Arabia, Turkey, UAE)

respective age groups [31]. This is in line with the findings presented here.

It has been documented that the prevalence of allergic disease is generally higher in urban compared to rural areas [32]. Consistent this with theory, the United Nations (UN) 2014 World Urbanisation report indicates that the Gulf countries that participated in this study have a higher urban population percentage than Turkey and Egypt, and this cluster reports the highest prevalence of asthma. However, The UN report estimates 43% of the Egyptian population are urban compared to 73% of the Turkish population, yet the reported prevalence of asthma in this study is higher in Egypt compared to Turkey [33]. Data from our study also describes regional variations in prevalence that cannot be explained solely by urbanisation. For example, whilst the regional asthma prevalence reported in Kuwait could correlate with the presence of increased urban extents as defined in the Global Rural-Urban Mapping Project (GRUMP) [34], this is not the case for Saudi Arabia, where the highest urban extents are reported in the western region [35], yet the highest asthma prevalence in this study was reported in central Saudi Arabia. The variations in prevalence between countries and regions reported in the SNAPSHOT study could be influenced by population density and urbanisation. However, these may not be the only factors involved; for example, elements such as air pollution, climate exposure and allergens could play a role.

Many studies have consistently shown a higher prevalence of asthma in women during adulthood [36, 37]. Consistent with this, the current prevalence of asthma reported in SNAPSHOT was higher among women compared to men, a trend observed across all the countries studied. Multiple hypotheses have been put forward to explain this difference. For example, it has been reported that the prevalence of asthma increases significantly after puberty for women and female sex hormones may play a role [38]. However, to date no single explanation can fully explain the differences observed.

Smoking is considered a major risk factor for several diseases, one of which is COPD [39], and COPD often presents with similar symptoms to asthma. This can make a differential diagnosis of asthma more challenging, particularly in general population surveys like SNAPSHOT with lay interviewers and no case ascertainment by a physician. There was no significant difference between the numbers of smokers in the asthma population compared to the non-asthma population, suggesting little or no contamination of this population with COPD patients who have been wrongly classified as subjects with asthma, and supporting the case definition of asthma used in the SNAPSHOT study. Interestingly, despite the fact that

Variable	No Asthma	Asthma	Odds Ratio	OR [95% CI]	P-value*
Cardiovascular disease (ref='No')					<0.0001
Yes	2457 (7.83%)	401 (18.88%)		2.11 [1.84;2.43]	
Nervous disease (ref='No')					0.0161
Yes	346 (1.1%)	47 (2.21%)		1.53 [1.08;2.17]	
Neurological disease (ref='No')					0.001
Yes	84 (0.27%)	20 (0.94%)		2.53 [1.46;4.40]	
Respiratory disease (ref='No')					<0.0001
Yes	105 (0.33%)	277 (13.04%)		44.6 [35.2;56.6]	
Gastrointestinal disease (ref='No')					<0.0001
Yes	472 (1.51%)	75 (3.53%)		1.78 [1.34;2.35]	
Diabetes (ref='No')					0.9901
Yes	192 (9.04%)	1740 (5.55%)		1.00 [0.84;1.20]	

*p-value of the Wald Chi-Square test from the logistic regression model

Fig. 4 Multivariate regression analysis investigating the impact of co-morbidities on the risk of asthma. Asthma population (2124 subjects) versus non-asthma population (31,362 subjects); OR [95% CI] = Odds Ratio [95% Confidence Interval]. The results presented are adjusted for age (18–34,35–49, ≥50 years), gender and country (Egypt, Kuwait, Saudi Arabia, Turkey, UAE)

there was no difference in the prevalence of asthma between smokers and non-smokers in this study, smoking was identified as a risk factor for asthma. One factor contributing to this could be that that the prevalence of smoking in the Middle East and North Africa is higher in men, as reported in the BREATHE study [40], whereas the prevalence of asthma is higher in women as reported here.

This study shows an association between certain co-morbidities and asthma, particularly allergic rhinitis (OR 6.4). The association between allergic rhinitis and asthma is supported in the literature [41]. The World Health organisation (WHO), through the Allergic Rhinitis and its Impact on Asthma (ARIA) program, has examined the impact of allergic rhinitis on asthma and

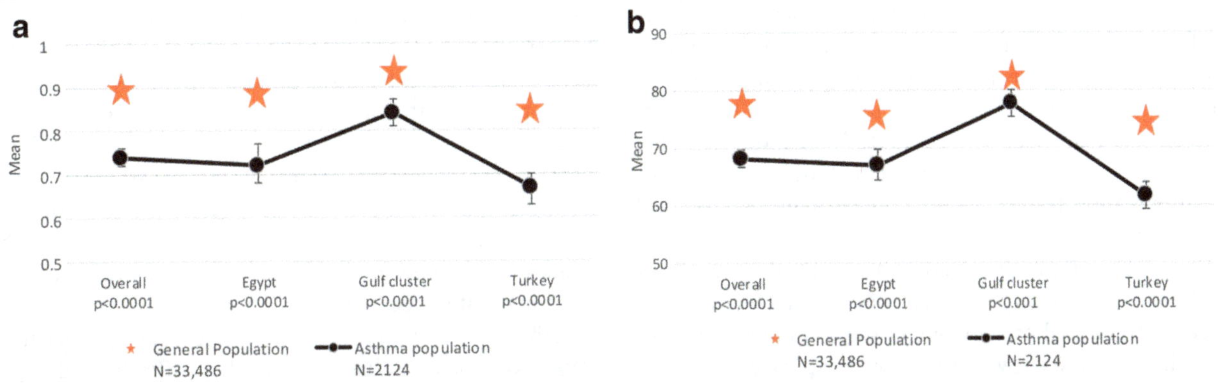

Fig. 5 Impact of asthma on quality of life. Quality of life was assessed using the three level EuroQol five-dimension questionnaire (EQ-5D-3L). Comparison of the EQ-5D-3L utility values (**a**) and EQ-VAS scores (**b**) between the asthma population and general population by country or cluster are shown. **a** For the asthma population ($n = 2124$) the data represent the mean EQ-5D-3L utility value with the 95% CI. For the general population ($N = 33,486$), the mean EQ-5D-3L utility value is presented. **b** For the asthma population (n = 2124) the data represent the mean EQ-VAS score with the 95% CI. For the general population ($n = 33,486$), the mean EQ-VAS score is presented

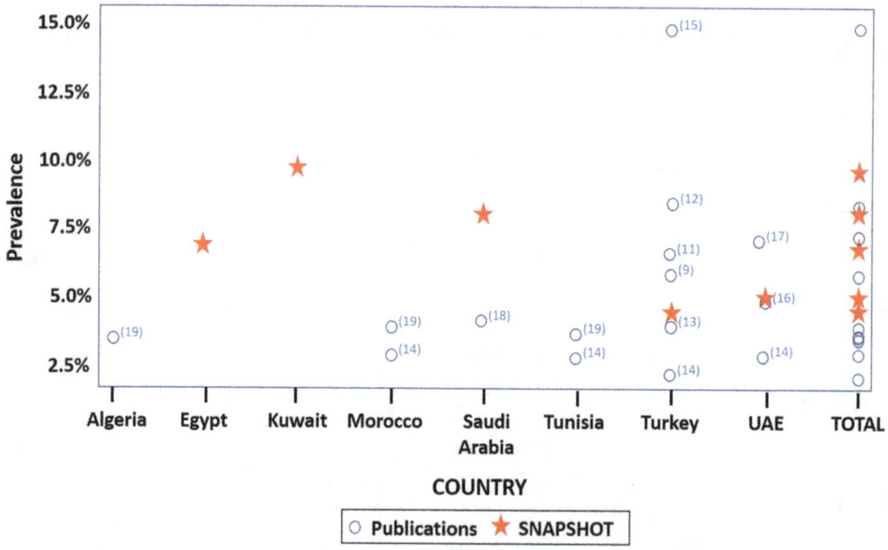

Fig. 6 Asthma prevalence in the Middle East. Prevalence of asthma as reported by SNAPSHOT and earlier studies in the Middle East and North Africa region. The inclusion criteria for the literature review were: article published between January 2000 and December 2015, population-based observational studies investigating the current prevalence of asthma in adults. The red star denotes the prevalence findings from the SNAPSHOT study. Note: two Turkish studies [9, 11] were carried out in urban centres only and were not national studies

concluded that both allergic and non-allergic rhinitis should be considered risk factors for asthma [42].

Overall, 54% of the screening population and 67.5% of the asthma population are overweight or obese. This is high compared to the global estimate from the WHO in 2014 which stated that 39% of adults aged 18 years and over were overweight and 13% of those were obese [43]. However, data from the 2013 Global Burden of Disease study demonstrates a higher prevalence of obesity in the MENA region compared to the global average [44]. An association between obesity and asthma has previously been reported; a meta-analysis of prospective epidemiological studies reported that those overweight were 38% more likely to develop asthma, rising to 92% of those who were obese [45]. Given the high incidence of obesity in the screening population the impact of cardiovascular disease is not unexpected since obesity predisposes subjects to cardiovascular disease. However, cardiovascular disease has also been linked to asthma independently. For example, a cohort study carried out in Northern California reported an association between asthma and increased risk of cardiovascular disease in women [46]; a large cross-sectional population-based study carried out in Adelaide, Australia also showed an association between asthma and cardiovascular disease independent of BMI, in a representative population sample aged 18 years and above [47]. An association between gastrointestinal disease and asthma was also reported in the SNAPSHOT study. Again, this could be linked to the high levels of obesity in the screening population and associated predisposition to gastro-oesophageal reflux disease (GERD). Indeed, there are numerous studies demonstrating an association between asthma and GERD. One such study has shown an independent association of GERD with poorly controlled asthma [48].

In addition to the co-morbidities mentioned above a significant correlation was also observed for nervous and neurological disease. Previously published studies have documented an association between asthma and diseases of the nervous system such as cerebrovascular disease. For example, the Atherosclerosis Risk in Communities (ARIC) study reported an association between asthma and stroke. Interestingly however, this study did not find an association between asthma and cardiovascular disease [49]. Neurological diseases such as dementia have also been previously linked to asthma. For example, a retrospective cohort study carried out in Taiwan reported an increased risk of developing dementia for those people with asthma compared to without asthma within a follow up period of 11 years [50]. The high levels of co-morbidities identified in the asthma population indicate that physicians need to check for co-morbidities as part of routine care and ensure they are managed correctly in all asthma patients as these conditions may influence asthma control.

Asthma is a condition that is known to have a negative impact on quality of life for those that suffer from the disease. Several disease specific questionnaires have been developed to assess the quality of life of patients with respiratory disease [51] and specifically asthma [52–56]. Both specific and generic quality of life measures [22, 57] have been used in a clinical setting to monitor the quality of life of asthma patients, and have demonstrated that asthma impairs quality of life with a more pronounced impact during exacerbations and in uncontrolled disease [58, 59]. However, general population studies investigating the effects of asthma on quality of life are scarce. The EQ-5D questionnaire is a widely used generic measure of health-related quality of life and is not specific to a particular disease, thus enabling comparisons between different disease areas. In addition, it is a brief, simple measure for patients to understand over the telephone in a general population setting. Previous studies with this questionnaire have demonstrated an impairment of quality of life in patients with respiratory disease [60]. The results of the SNAPSHOT study indicate that, across all countries studied, subjects with asthma suffer significant impairment in their quality of life. Whilst this observation is expected, it is the first time it has been shown in these countries on such a large scale in a general population setting.

The study has several strengths. It is a cross sectional, population-based study with a large sample size using consistent methodology across all countries, providing a standardised measure of prevalence in the Middle East. In addition, the case definition of asthma used is based on the global AIR surveys, and quality of life has been assessed using the EQ-5D questionnaire, which have been validated and used widely, enabling comparison with data collected elsewhere.

As with all studies, limitations do exist. These include the fact that the survey was telephone based, which could introduce a sampling bias if certain groups do not have access to a telephone, such as those in more remote, rural areas. However, the emergence of mobile telephones means that the majority of households in these countries have access to a telephone, and the SNAPSHOT program included both mobile and fixed landline telephone numbers. Another limitation was that the survey was conducted by trained lay interviewers; therefore, the diagnosis of asthma or other reported co-morbidities was not confirmed by a physician. In addition, reporting of a physician diagnosis of asthma was not one of the inclusion criteria for a positive screen. It is well-known that access to healthcare infrastructure and primary care is lower in the Middle East compared to Europe. Therefore, if the definition of asthma had been restricted to those subjects who had a confirmed asthma diagnosis by a physician, it would have excluded many subjects with undiagnosed asthma, as these subjects might experience issues around access to healthcare. The proportion of people with undiagnosed asthma is thought to be higher in this region compared to Europe. However, as part of the screening questionnaire, subjects were asked whether they had been told by a physician that they had asthma, and of the 2124 subjects with asthma included in the SNAPSHOT program, 70.2% ($n = 1490$) had a confirmed asthma diagnosis, validating the study findings based on the screening criteria used. As is the case for all studies that require participants to recall data, there is a risk of inaccuracy in the data collected. However, this is minimised by setting the inclusion criteria for the asthma population based on exacerbations and treatments over the last 12 months as opposed to simple symptom reporting.

Conclusion

This study provides an updated prevalence estimate for asthma within the adult general population of five countries in the Middle East region, using an identical methodology across all countries studied. The reported prevalence estimates suggest that the Middle East is a low/medium prevalence area compared to other regions in the world. Prevalence is higher among adult women than men and increases with age. A positive correlation was observed for co-morbidities such as allergic rhinitis. In addition, asthma was shown to have a negative impact on quality of life; the first time this has been shown in these countries through a large scale general population based study. The lack of reliable recent data on the prevalence and burden of disease is a major obstacle to the implementation of effective public health strategies for disease prevention and management. The results from this study can contribute to informed decision making when setting priorities public health policy and strategy to manage asthma in these countries.

Abbreviations

AIR: Asthma insights and reality; AIRMAG: Asthma insights and reality Maghreb; ARIA: Allergic rhinitis and its impact on asthma; ARIC: Atherosclerosis risk in communities; BMI: Body mass index; BPH: Benign prostatic hyperplasia; CAPI: Computer-assisted personal interviewing; CI: Confidence interval; COPD: Chronic obstructive pulmonary disease; CRO: Contract research organisation; ECRHS: European community respiratory health survey; EQ-5D: EuroQoL five dimension questionnaire; EQ-5D-3 L: 3 level EQ-5D questionnaire; EQ-VAS: EuroQol visual analogue scale; GA2LEN: Global allergy and asthma network of excellence; GEP: Good epidemiological practice; GERD: Gastro-oesophageal reflux disease; GRUMP: Global rural-urban mapping project; HTA: Health technology assessment; IQR: Inter quartile range; ISAAC: International study of asthma and allergies in childhood; OR: Odds ratio; SD: Standard deviation; SFAR: Score for allergic rhinitis; SFDA: Saudi food and drug authority; UAE: United Arab Emirates; UN: United Nations; WHO: World health organisation; WHS: World health survey

Acknowledgements

Editorial support in the form of manuscript development, collating of author comments, copy editing and referencing was provided by Sarah Osei-Ntem, an employee of Glaxo SmithKline (GSK). Data analysis input was provided by Leyla Depret-Bixio, a former employee of GSK.

The authors also wish to express their appreciation for the contributions of Ahmed Abu al Faraj*, Tamer Elfishawy, Hany Gamil*, Ridwaan Jhetam*, Saeed Noibi, Selda Özdemir*, Candice Pinto*, Nauman Rashid, Samer Talaat El Falaky, Indira Umareddy* (GSK), Sophie Abadie, Salaheddine El Khadiri, Maria José Lopez (MS Health), and the participating Contract Research Organisations (Infomine Research Middle East, Omega CRO) in different stages of the SNAPSHOT study.

Formerly employed at GSK.

Funding
Funding for this study was provided by GSK (GSK study number 201291, GSK study title: SNAPSHOT).

Authors' contributions
AEH, FA, and LT conceptualised the study. AEH, FA, LT, AD, HT*, OA, DM, MAB and BM contributed to the study design and interpretation of results, AL contributed to data collection and analysis. All authors contributed to and provided approval for the submitted manuscript.

Ethics approval and consent to participate
The study followed guidelines for good epidemiological practice (GEP) and pertinent local rules and regulations for each participating country. The protocol and amendments were submitted to the appropriate independent ethics committee in each country for approval. The following ethics committees approved the SNAPSHOT program: In Egypt, the Ministry of Health and Population, Central Directorate for Research and Health Development; In Kuwait, the Kuwait University Health Sciences Centre Ethical Committee; in Turkey, the Ankara University Medical Faculty Ethics Committee; and in the UAE, the Ethics and Research Committee of the University of Sharjah. In Saudi Arabia, no ethics approval was required, since SNAPSHOT was an epidemiological, cross sectional, population based study and as such is out of scope of the Saudi Food and Drug Authority (SFDA) approval and/or notification. The protocol specified that oral consent to participate in the study was required. At the start of the telephone call, subjects were asked to provide their consent to participate verbally, and this information was recorded in the CAPI system by the interviewee. Participants taking part in the study did not receive any financial compensation and participation in the study did not influence the medical management of the patient. It was not possible to link the telephone number dialled and the respondent's data in the study database. All data collected was kept confidential and anonymous.

Competing interests
AEH, FA, and LT are employees of and shareholders in GSK, which funded the SNAPSHOT study. HT is currently also employed by GSK but at the time the study was conducted he participated in his capacity as Professor of medicine and allergy at the University of Cairo. AL is a director of MS Health, the clinical and epidemiological research company that implemented this study on behalf of GSK. AD is a director of Foxymed, a medical communication and consultancy company which participated in the design of the study and the interpretation of the results on behalf of GSK. The authors declare to have no further conflict of interest.

Author details
[1]The Medical School, Cairo University, Cairo, Egypt. [2]Department of Chest Diseases, Division of Allergy and Immunology, Ankara University, School of Medicine, Ankara, Turkey. [3]Chest Medicine Department, Zain Hospital, Kuwait City, Kuwait. [4]College of Medicine, University of Sharjah, Sharjah, United Arab Emirates. [5]Department of Pulmonary Medicine, Rashid Hospital, Dubai, United Arab Emirates. [6]Foxymed, Paris, France. [7]MS Health, Rabat, Morocco. [8]GlaxoSmithKline, PO Box 50199, Dubai, United Arab Emirates.

References

1. The Global Asthma Report 2014. In.: Global asthma network; 2014.
2. Global surveillance, prevention and control of chronic respiratory diseases: a comprehensive approach. In.: World Health Organisation; 2007.
3. Worldwide variation in prevalence of symptoms of asthma, allergic rhinoconjunctivitis, and atopic eczema: ISAAC. The international study of asthma and allergies in childhood (ISAAC) steering committee. Lancet (London, England). 1998;351(9111):1225–32.
4. Lai CK, Beasley R, Crane J, Foliaki S, Shah J, Weiland S. Global variation in the prevalence and severity of asthma symptoms: phase three of the international study of asthma and allergies in childhood (ISAAC). Thorax. 2009;64(6):476–83.
5. Variations in the prevalence of respiratory symptoms, self-reported asthma attacks, and use of asthma medication in the European Community respiratory health survey (ECRHS). Eur Respir J. 1996;9(4): 687–95.
6. Witvliet M. World health survey: a useful yet underutilized Global Health data source. Austin J Public Health Epidemiology. 2014;1(3):1012.
7. Jarvis D, Newson R, Lotvall J, Hastan D, Tomassen P, Keil T, Gjomarkaj M, Forsberg B, Gunnbjornsdottir M, Minov J, et al. Asthma in adults and its association with chronic rhinosinusitis: the GA2LEN survey in Europe. Allergy. 2012;67(1):91–8.
8. Rabe KF, Adachi M, Lai CK, Soriano JB, Vermeire PA, Weiss KB, Weiss ST. Worldwide severity and control of asthma in children and adults: the global asthma insights and reality surveys. J Allergy Clin Immunol. 2004;114(1):40–7.
9. Sekerel BE, Gemicioglu B, Soriano JB. Asthma insights and reality in Turkey (AIRET) study. Respir Med. 2006;100(10):1850–4.
10. Khadadah M, Mahboub B, Al-Busaidi NH, Sliman N, Soriano JB, Bahous J. Asthma insights and reality in the Gulf and the near east. Int J Tuberc Lung Dis. 2009;13(8):1015–22.
11. Emri S, Turnagol H, Basoglu S, Bacanli S, Guven GS, Aslan D. Asthma-like symptoms prevalence in five Turkish urban centers. Allergol Immunopathol. 2005;33(5):270–6.
12. Kurt E, Metintas S, Basyigit I, Bulut I, Coskun E, Dabak S, Deveci F, Fidan F, Kaynar H, Kunt Uzaslan E, et al. Prevalence and risk factors of allergies in Turkey (PARFAIT): results of a multicentre cross-sectional study in adults. Eur Respir J. 2009;33(4):724–33.
13. OECD. Health at a Glance: Europe 2012. Paris: OECD Publishing; 2012. http://dx.doi.org/10.1787/9789264183896-en.
14. To T, Stanojevic S, Moores G, Gershon AS, Bateman ED, Cruz AA, Boulet LP. Global asthma prevalence in adults: findings from the cross-sectional world health survey. BMC Public Health. 2012;12:204.
15. Tug T, Acik Y. Prevalence of asthma, asthma-like and allergic symptoms in the urban and rural adult population in eastern Turkey. Asian Pac J Allergy Immunol/Allergy Immunol Soc Thailand. 2002;20(4):209–15.
16. Alsowaidi S, Abdulle A, Bernsen R, Zuberbier T. Allergic rhinitis and asthma: a large cross-sectional study in the United Arab Emirates. Int Arch Allergy Immunol. 2010;153(3):274–9.
17. Mahboub BH, Al-Hammadi S, Rafique M, Sulaiman N, Pawankar R, Al Redha AI, Mehta AC. Population prevalence of asthma and its determinants based on European Community respiratory health survey in the United Arab Emirates. BMC Pulm Med. 2012;12:4.
18. Moradi-Lakeh M, El Bcheraoui C, Daoud F, Tuffaha M, Kravitz H, Al Saeedi M, Basulaiman M, Memish ZA, AlMazroa MA, Al Rabeeah AA, et al. Prevalence of asthma in Saudi adults: findings from a national household survey, 2013. BMC Pulm Med. 2015;15:77.
19. Nafti S, Taright S, El Ftouh M, Yassine N, Benkheder A, Bouacha H, Fakhfakh H, Ali-Khoudja M, Texier N, El Hasnaoui A. Prevalence of asthma in North Africa: the asthma insights and reality in the Maghreb (AIRMAG) study. Respir Med. 2009;103(Suppl 2):S2–11.
20. Adeloye D, Chan KY, Rudan I, Campbell H. An estimate of asthma prevalence in Africa: a systematic analysis. Croat Med J. 2013;54(6):519–31.
21. Abdelkader El Hasnaoui FA, Tariq L, Lahlou A, Du Plessis D. An omnibus approach to assess the prevalence, burden and quality of life of multiple diseases in the general population: the snapshot program in the Middle East. Med Res Archives. 2018;6:2.
22. Rabin R, de Charro F. EQ-5D: a measure of health status from the EuroQol group. Ann Med. 2001;33(5):337–43.
23. Dolan P. Modeling valuations for EuroQol health states. Med Care. 1997; 35(11):1095–108.
24. Annesi-Maesano I, Didier A, Klossek M, Chanal I, Moreau D, Bousquet J. The score for allergic rhinitis (SFAR): a simple and valid assessment method in population studies. Allergy. 2002;57(2):107–14.
25. Duc AN, Wolbers M. Weighted analysis of composite endpoints with simultaneous inference for flexible weight constraints. Stat Med. 2017; 36(3):442–54.
26. Min SY, Park DW, Yun SC, Kim YH, Lee JY, Kang SJ, Lee SW, Lee CW, Kim JJ, Park SW, et al. Major predictors of long-term clinical outcomes after coronary revascularization in patients with unprotected left main coronary disease: analysis from the MAIN-COMPARE study. Circ Cardiovasc Interv. 2010;3(2):127–33.
27. Rabe KF, Vermeire PA, Soriano JB, Maier WC. Clinical management of asthma in 1999: the asthma insights and reality in Europe (AIRE) study. Eur Respir J. 2000;16(5):802–7.
28. Bourdin A, Doble A, Godard P. The asthma insights and reality in the Maghreb (AIRMAG) study: perspectives and lessons. Respir Med. 2009; 103(Suppl 2):S38–48.

29. Lai CK, De Guia TS, Kim YY, Kuo SH, Mukhopadhyay A, Soriano JB, Trung PL, Zhong NS, Zainudin N, Zainudin BM. Asthma control in the Asia-Pacific region: the asthma insights and reality in Asia-Pacific study. J Allergy Clin Immunol. 2003;111(2):263–8.
30. Abdul Salam A, Elsegaey I, Khraif R, Al-Mutairi A. Population distribution and household conditions in Saudi Arabia: reflections from the 2010 census. SpringerPlus. 2014;3:530.
31. Hamzacebi H, Unsal M, Kayhan S, Bilgin S, Ercan S. Prevalence of asthma and respiratory symptoms by age, gender and smoking behaviour in Samsun, north Anatolia Turkey. Tuberkuloz ve toraks. 2006;54(4):322–9.
32. Nicolaou N, Siddique N, Custovic A. Allergic disease in urban and rural populations: increasing prevalence with increasing urbanization. Allergy. 2005;60(11):1357–60.
33. United Nations DoEaSA, Population Division: World urbanization prospects: the 2014 revision, highlights (ST/ESA/SER.A/352). In.; 2014.
34. Center for International Earth Science Information Network - CIESIN - Columbia University, International Food Policy Research Institute - IFPRI, The World Bank, Centro Internacional de Agricultura Tropical - CIAT: Global rural-urban mapping project, version 1 (GRUMP), urban extents, Kuwait. In. Palisades, NY: CIESIN, Columbia University: NASA Socioeconomic Data and Applications Center (SEDAC); 2009.
35. Center for International Earth Science Information Network - CIESIN - Columbia University, International Food Policy Research Institute - IFPRI, The World Bank, Centro Internacional de Agricultura Tropical - CIAT: Global rural-urban mapping project, version 1 (GRUMP), urban extents, Saudi Arabia. In. Palisades, NY: CIESIN, Columbia University: NASA Socioeconomic Data and Applications Center (SEDAC); 2009.
36. Leynaert B, Sunyer J, Garcia-Esteban R, Svanes C, Jarvis D, Cerveri I, Dratva J, Gislason T, Heinrich J, Janson C, et al. Gender differences in prevalence, diagnosis and incidence of allergic and non-allergic asthma: a population-based cohort. Thorax. 2012;67(7):625–31.
37. de Marco R, Locatelli F, Sunyer J, Burney P. Differences in incidence of reported asthma related to age in men and women. A retrospective analysis of the data of the European respiratory health survey. Am J Respir Crit Care Med. 2000;162(1):68–74.
38. van den Berge M, Heijink HI, van Oosterhout AJ, Postma DS. The role of female sex hormones in the development and severity of allergic and non-allergic asthma. Clin Exp Allergy: J British Soc Allergy Clin Immunol. 2009; 39(10):1477–81.
39. Lundback B, Lindberg A, Lindstrom M, Ronmark E, Jonsson AC, Jonsson E, Larsson LG, Andersson S, Sandstrom T, Larsson K. Not 15 but 50% of smokers develop COPD?–report from the obstructive lung disease in northern Sweden studies. Respir Med. 2003;97(2):115–22.
40. Khattab A, Javaid A, Iraqi G, Alzaabi A, Ben Kheder A, Koniski ML, Shahrour N, Taright S, Idrees M, Polatli M, et al. Smoking habits in the Middle East and North Africa: results of the BREATHE study. Respir Med. 2012;106(Suppl 2):S16–24.
41. Scadding G, Walker S. Poor asthma control?–then look up the nose. The importance of co-morbid rhinitis in patients with asthma. Prim Care Respir J: J Gen Practice Airways Group. 2012;21(2):222–8.
42. Bousquet J, Van Cauwenberge P, Khaltaev N. Allergic rhinitis and its impact on asthma. J Allergy Clin Immunol. 2001;108(5 Suppl):S147–334.
43. Organisation WH: Global status report on noncommunicable diseases 2014. In.; 2014.
44. Ng M, Fleming T, Robinson M, Thomson B, Graetz N, Margono C, Mullany EC, Biryukov S, Abbafati C, Abera SF, et al. Global, regional, and national prevalence of overweight and obesity in children and adults during 1980-2013: a systematic analysis for the global burden of disease study 2013. *Lancet (London, England)*. 2014;384(9945):766–81.
45. Beuther DA, Sutherland ER. Overweight, obesity, and incident asthma: a meta-analysis of prospective epidemiologic studies. Am J Respir Crit Care Med. 2007;175(7):661–6.
46. Iribarren C, Tolstykh IV, Eisner MD. Are patients with asthma at increased risk of coronary heart disease? Int J Epidemiol. 2004;33(4):743–8.
47. Appleton SL, Ruffin RE, Wilson DH, Taylor AW, Adams RJ. Asthma is associated with cardiovascular disease in a representative population sample. Obes Res Clin Pract. 2008;2(2):71–142.
48. Liang B, Yi Q, Feng Y. Association of gastroesophageal reflux disease with asthma control. Dis Esophagus : official journal of the International Society for Diseases of the Esophagus / ISDE. 2013;26(8):794–8.
49. Iribarren C, Tolstykh IV, Miller MK, Sobel E, Eisner MD. Adult asthma and risk of coronary heart disease, cerebrovascular disease, and heart failure: a prospective study of 2 matched cohorts. Am J Epidemiol. 2012;176(11): 1014–24.
50. Chen MH, Li CT, Tsai CF, Lin WC, Chang WH, Chen TJ, Pan TL, Su TP, Bai YM. Risk of dementia among patients with asthma: a nationwide longitudinal study. J Am Med Dir Assoc. 2014;15(10):763–7.
51. Jones PW, Quirk FH, Baveystock CM, Littlejohns P. A self-complete measure of health status for chronic airflow limitation. The St. George's respiratory questionnaire. Am Rev Respir Dis. 1992;145(6):1321–7.
52. Juniper EF, Guyatt GH, Ferrie PJ, Griffith LE. Measuring quality of life in asthma. Am Rev Respir Dis. 1993;147(4):832–8.
53. Marks GB, Dunn SM, Woolcock AJ. A scale for the measurement of quality of life in adults with asthma. J Clin Epidemiol. 1992;45(5):461–72.
54. Hyland ME, Finnis S, Irvine SH. A scale for assessing quality of life in adult asthma sufferers. J Psychosom Res. 1991;35(1):99–110.
55. Maille AR, Kaptein AA, Koning CJ, Zwinderman AH. Developing a quality-of-life questionnaire for patients with respiratory illness. Monaldi archives for chest disease = Archivio Monaldi per le malattie del torace. 1994;49(1):76–8.
56. Creer TL, Wigal JK, Kotses H, McConnaughy K, Winder JA. A life activities questionnaire for adult asthma. J Asthma : official journal of the Association for the Care of Asthma. 1992;29(6):393–9.
57. Bousquet J, Knani J, Dhivert H, Richard A, Chicoye A, Ware JE Jr, Michel FB. Quality of life in asthma. I. Internal consistency and validity of the SF-36 questionnaire. Am J Respir Crit Care Med. 1994;149(2 Pt 1):371–5.
58. Lloyd A, Price D, Brown R. The impact of asthma exacerbations on health-related quality of life in moderate to severe asthma patients in the UK. Prim Care Respir J: journal of the General Practice Airways Group. 2007;16(1):22–7.
59. Chen H, Gould MK, Blanc PD, Miller DP, Kamath TV, Lee JH, Sullivan SD. Asthma control, severity, and quality of life: quantifying the effect of uncontrolled disease. J Allergy Clin Immunol. 2007;120(2):396–402.
60. Hazell M, Frank T, Frank P. Health related quality of life in individuals with asthma related symptoms. Respir Med. 2003;97(11):1211–8.

11

Evaluation of inhaler technique and achievement and maintenance of mastery of budesonide/ formoterol Spiromax® compared with budesonide/ formoterol Turbuhaler® in adult patients with asthma: the Easy Low Instruction Over Time (ELIOT) study

David B. Price[1,2*], Vicky Thomas[1], P. N. Richard Dekhuijzen[3], Sinthia Bosnic-Anticevich[4], Nicolas Roche[5], Federico Lavorini[6], Priyanka Raju[1], Daryl Freeman[1], Carole Nicholls[1], Iain R. Small[1], Erika Sims[1,7], Guilherme Safioti[8], Janice Canvin[8] and Henry Chrystyn[1,9]

Abstract

Background: Incorrect inhaler technique is a common cause of poor asthma control. This two-phase pragmatic study evaluated inhaler technique mastery and maintenance of mastery with DuoResp® (budesonide-formoterol [BF]) Spiromax® compared with Symbicort® (BF) Turbuhaler® in patients with asthma who were receiving inhaled corticosteroids/long-acting β2-agonists.

Methods: In the initial cross-sectional phase, patients were randomized to a 6-step training protocol with empty Spiromax and Turbuhaler devices. Patients initially demonstrating ≥1 error with their current device, and then achieving mastery with both Spiromax and Turbuhaler (absence of healthcare professional [HCP]-observed errors), were eligible for the longitudinal phase. In the longitudinal phase, patients were randomized to BF Spiromax or BF Turbuhaler. Co-primary endpoints were the proportions of patients achieving device mastery after three training steps and maintaining device mastery (defined as the absence of HCP-observed errors after 12 weeks of use). Secondary endpoints included device preference, handling error frequency, asthma control, and safety. Exploratory endpoints included assessment of device mastery by an independent external expert reviewing video recordings of a subset of patients.

(Continued on next page)

* Correspondence: dprice@opri.sg
[1]Observational and Pragmatic Research Institute Pte Ltd, Singapore, Singapore
[2]University of Aberdeen, Aberdeen, UK
Full list of author information is available at the end of the article

(Continued from previous page)

Results: Four hundred ninety-three patients participated in the cross-sectional phase, and 395 patients in the longitudinal phase. In the cross-sectional phase, more patients achieved device mastery after three training steps with Spiromax (94%) versus Turbuhaler (87%) (odds ratio [OR] 3.77 [95% confidence interval (CI) 2.05–6.95], $p < 0.001$). Longitudinal phase data indicated that the odds of maintaining inhaler mastery at 12 weeks were not statistically significantly different (OR 1.26 [95% CI 0.80–1.98], $p = 0.316$). Asthma control improved in both groups with no significant difference between groups (OR 0.11 [95% CI -0.09–0.30]). An exploratory analysis indicated that the odds of maintaining independent expert-verified device mastery were significantly higher for patients using Spiromax versus Turbuhaler (OR 2.11 [95% CI 1.25–3.54]).

Conclusions: In the cross-sectional phase, a significantly greater proportion of patients using Spiromax versus Turbuhaler achieved device mastery; in the longitudinal phase, the proportion of patients maintaining device mastery with Spiromax versus Turbuhaler was similar. An exploratory independent expert-verified analysis found Spiromax was associated with higher levels of device mastery after 12 weeks. Asthma control was improved by treatment with both BF Spiromax and BF Turbuhaler.

Keywords: Budesonide/formoterol, Dry-powder inhaler, Inhaler technique, Inhaler mastery, Intuitive, Pragmatic clinical trial, Asthma

Background

Asthma is a worldwide chronic inflammatory disorder of the airways with major adverse effects on affected individuals' quality of life [1]. Despite advances in therapy, suboptimal asthma control is commonplace and is associated with a substantial socioeconomic burden [2–6]. The causes of poor asthma control are multifactorial and include several patient-related factors. Smoking, poor treatment adherence, and device handling errors have all been shown to have a negative impact on asthma control [7–12].

Therapeutic efficacy of inhalation therapy is dependent on the drug(s) reaching the targeted areas of the lower lung [5]. There is a growing body of evidence suggesting that errors in inhaler technique can reduce drug delivery to the lungs and produce poor clinical outcomes [2, 10, 12–16]. Correct inhaler technique should therefore be considered an essential component in asthma management [5, 10, 14, 17] and has become an integral part of the management strategy set out by the Global Initiative for Asthma (GINA). However, despite the importance of patient training, many healthcare professionals (HCPs) themselves lack proficiency in correct inhaler use, are not confident in demonstrating proper inhaler technique and, consequently, patients are neither taught nor checked in follow-up visits [18–23]. As a result, poor inhaler technique continues to represent a barrier to achieving optimal asthma control among many patients with asthma, a situation that has not improved over the past 40 years [5, 14, 24–26].

Although the use of all inhalers involves techniques associated with the preparation of the device, inhalation and post-inhalation behaviors, some steps associated with the correct use of different inhalers are device-specific [2, 14, 27, 28]. The CRITIKAL study, which investigated the association between specific inhaler errors of different devices and asthma outcomes, enabled the identification of specific inhaler technique errors that were associated with lack of asthma control [16]. Other factors shown to be associated with poor asthma control when using the Turbuhaler® were not breathing out before an inhalation, not tilting the head or sealing the lips round the mouthpiece, not using a fast inhalation and no breath-holding after each inhalation [16].

Because inhaler technique errors have implications for disease control and HCPs do not always deliver inhaler technique education [29, 30], it is important that devices are as intuitive as possible. Additionally, many patients express preferences for inhaler devices that they are able to use easily and efficiently [5], but to date, only a few studies have investigated intuitiveness and the maintenance of device mastery with different inhalers by patients with asthma [31–33].

Combined use of an inhaled corticosteroid (ICS) and a long-acting β2–agonist (LABA) is considered to be recommended for patients with asthma at step 3 or higher of the GINA guidelines [1]. ICS/LABA fixed-dose combinations are available in a range of inhaler devices, including DuoResp® budesonide/formoterol (BF) Spiromax® and Symbicort® (BF) Turbuhaler. In Europe, these two products are approved for use in adult patients with asthma or chronic obstructive pulmonary disease where an inhaled ICS/LABA is indicated [34].

This Easy Low Instruction Over Time (ELIOT) study was a pragmatic trial designed to compare the intuitiveness of BF Spiromax and a real-life comparator, the BF Turbuhaler by assessing achievement and maintenance of correct inhaler technique (mastery), in adult patients with moderate-to-severe asthma.

Methods

The ELIOT study was a pragmatic 12-week, 2-stage, multicenter, open-label, randomized, parallel-group study designed to compare the achievement and maintenance of inhaler technique in adults with asthma. It was conducted between May 2014 and March 2015 at 68 centers in the UK. The study was divided into two parts: a cross-sectional phase at Visit 1, followed by a 12-week longitudinal phase with Visit 2 at the end.

Inclusion and exclusion criteria

Patients aged 18–75 years with a diagnosis of asthma in accordance with the GINA guidelines [1], as evidenced by the presence of an Asthma READ Code (UK diagnostic coding system), were eligible to participate in the study provided they were receiving step 3 or 4 therapy for asthma as defined by the British Thoracic Society (BTS) guidelines for persistent asthma [35]. Exclusion criteria included any previous use of BF Spiromax, use of the BF Turbuhaler device in the preceding 6 months, the presence of a significant chronic lower respiratory tract disease other than asthma, a significant asthma exacerbation, a prescription of oral corticosteroids or antibiotic treatment within the preceding 2 weeks.

Study design and procedures

As shown in Fig. 1, the study comprised an initial cross-sectional phase at Visit 1, followed by a 12-week longitudinal phase with Visit 2 at the end.

Cross-sectional phase

Prior to patient enrollment, HCPs conducting clinics involved in the study were trained to instruct patients on the correct use of the Spiromax and Turbuhaler devices. This included emphasizing the prescription dose (two inhalations, twice per day) and reminding patients to reload their device and take the second inhalation. This prior device training for HCPs was supported by a training manual and videos showing the proper use of each device as well as videos highlighting potential errors that patients could make when using them.

During Visit 1 (Fig. 1a) patients were evaluated on the handling of their current inhaler device and taught the proper use of empty Spiromax and Turbuhaler inhalers by the trained HCPs.

Assessments at this stage (Fig. 1b) included baseline demographic and clinical characteristics (including

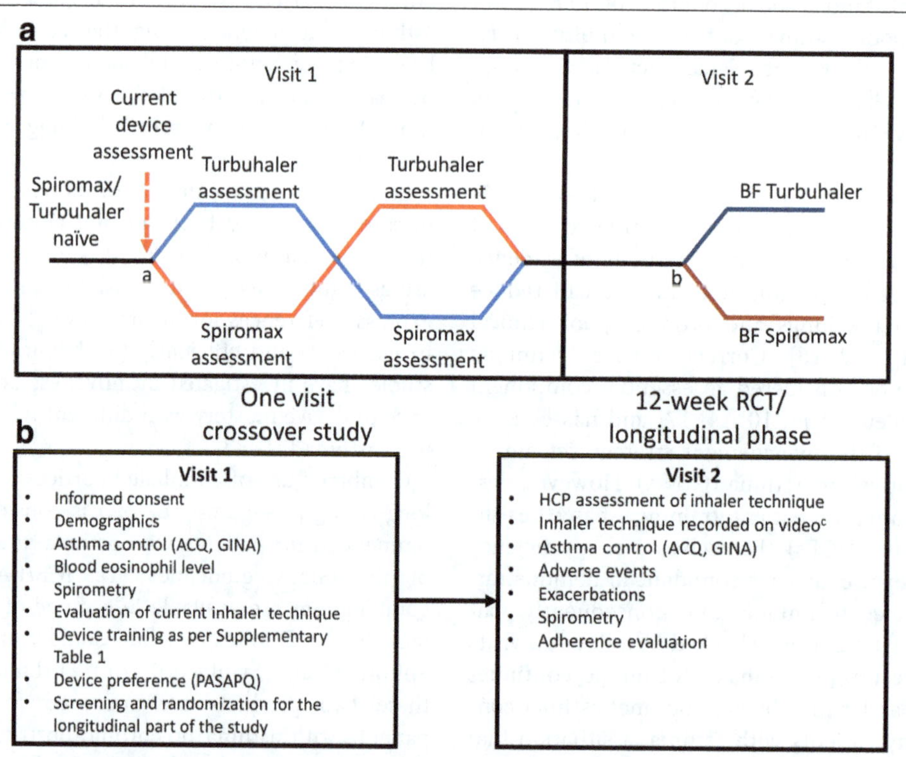

Fig. 1 Study design (**a**) and procedures (**b**). [a]Randomization into cross-over phase; [b]Randomization into longitudinal phase; patients meeting the inclusion criteria: step 3 or 4 asthma therapy as defined by BTS guidelines for persistent asthma, partially or poorly controlled asthma as defined by GINA, and ≥ 1 error on current device were included; [c]Video review was used only with patients who provided consent; patients not providing consent were able to continue in the study. ACQ: Asthma Control Questionnaire; BTS: British Thoracic Society; GINA: Global Initiative for Asthma; HCP: healthcare professional; PASAPQ: Patient Satisfaction and Preference Questionnaire; RCT: randomized control trial

medical history, prior and concomitant medications), recording of a patient's last peripheral blood eosinophil level (from medical records, if available), asthma review (completion of asthma review questionnaire and asthma control questionnaire [ACQ]), evaluation of current inhaler technique by HCP assessment and spirometry. Upon completion of these assessments, patients were randomized to receive device training with either empty Spiromax followed by empty Turbuhaler devices or vice versa. Randomization was accomplished using interactive response technology (IRT).

Details of how patients were trained in correct inhaler technique and how device mastery was determined and assessed are presented below.

Training on inhaler technique and device mastery After randomization, each patient was trained to use the empty Spiromax and Turbuhaler devices using a six-step approach (details provided in Additional file 1: Table S1), as follows: (1) intuitive use (prior to any training); (2) after reading patient information leaflet (as supplied to patients in standard clinical practice); (3) following instructional video; (4) following tuition by HCP; (5) following first repeat of tuition by HCP; (6) following second repeat of tuition by HCP.

After each training step, an assessment of device use was carried out by HCPs using a predefined list of inhaler errors (Additional file 1: Table S2) collated from the best available evidence (developed through steering committee discussion and consensus). The predefined list was split into sections relating to dose preparation and the inhalation maneuver, with separate assessments being made for inhalations 1 and 2.

Device mastery was defined as the absence of HCP-observed errors. Once this had been attained or all six steps had been completed for the first inhaler device, patients were trained on the second device according to the randomly assigned order.

Recording of patients' device preferences using the PASAPQ questionnaire After device training was completed, patients' preference for the Spiromax versus the Turbuhaler was assessed using the Patient Satisfaction and Preference Questionnaire (PASAPQ). The PASAPQ is a multi-item measure of respiratory inhalation device satisfaction and reference, designed and validated in patients with asthma and chronic obstructive pulmonary disease [36].

At the end of Visit 1, patients who met the required criteria for entry into the longitudinal phase of the study were then randomly assigned to receive treatment with a BF Spiromax or BF Turbuhaler at an equivalent dose to the patient's current ICS and retrained on that device [35] (Fig. 1).

Patients were eligible to proceed to the longitudinal phase if they made at least one inhaler technique error on their existing device (i.e. the one they were using when they entered the study) and had demonstrated mastery of both the Spiromax and Turbuhaler devices during the cross-sectional phase.

Longitudinal phase

In this second phase of the study, patients were randomly assigned to BF Spiromax or BF Turbuhaler for 12 weeks. Randomization to treatment was undertaken separately from randomization to device training order during the crossover phase of the study, but using the same IRT system. Patients were asked to return to the study center to have their technique checked again at Visit 2, which took place 12 weeks after Visit 1. In addition, patients' asthma control was followed-up by telephone at Weeks 4, 8 and 12 (no more than 3 days before Visit 2). During these calls, each patient self-reported the first 6 items of the ACQ, any adverse events (AEs) and use of concomitant medications to investigators who were blinded to the patient's randomized treatment assignment.

The maintenance of device mastery was assessed at Visit 2, 12 weeks after Visit 1. For those patients who had previously consented to video recording, a video recording of the patient's handling of the study device at Visit 2 was also made to enable additional review by an independent external device expert. Device mastery was defined as the absence of observed errors after 12 weeks of device use as assessed by trained HCPs, and by independent external experts viewing the video recordings.

Pulmonary function (forced expiratory volume in 1 s and forced vital capacity) was assessed by spirometry at Visit 2. Drug safety was monitored by AEs, recorded by the study investigator or a designee and coded according to the Medical Dictionary for Regulatory Activities (MedDRA version 17.0). Investigators were asked to rate the likelihood of an AE being related to the study medication as possibly, probably or definitely related. Treatment adherence was assessed by device dose counters which displayed the number of actuations remaining.

Endpoints

Co-primary

The cross-sectional phase co-primary endpoint was the proportion of patients in the full-analysis set (FAS; see below) achieving device mastery after training step 3 (instructional video) with Spiromax compared with Turbuhaler.

The longitudinal phase co-primary endpoint was the proportion of patients in the full-analysis set maintaining device mastery based on HCP observations with BF Spiromax compared with BF Turbuhaler after 12 weeks of device use.

Secondary

For the cross-sectional phase, secondary endpoints were: the proportion of patients achieving device mastery by steps 1 and 2, the number of steps required to achieve device mastery, the number of HCP-observed errors, and the patient device preference (PASAPQ score).

For the longitudinal phase, secondary endpoints were: the proportion of patients maintaining mastery after 12 weeks of device use when split into dose preparation and inhalation maneuver steps, total number of observed errors (assessed by HCP and technology), number of technology-observed inhalation errors, number of handling errors, adherence, efficacy (as assessed by ACQ scores, time to treatment failure [change of treatment or treatment for exacerbation or infection], exacerbations, impact of maintaining device mastery on time to treatment failure, use of concomitant medications), and AEs.

Exploratory (longitudinal phase only)

The first exploratory analysis was maintenance of device mastery at 12 weeks as defined by the absence of external expert- (video-)observed errors. Additional exploratory analyses included the number and type of HCP- and external expert-observed errors; aspects of asthma control (including symptoms and exacerbations) and current inhaler errors; aspects of asthma control and current inhaler errors.

Statistical analysis

The FAS comprised patients who completed the crossover stage of the study. Patient demographics and baseline characteristics were summarized using descriptive statistics. Outcomes for device mastery achievement and maintenance were compared using parametric or non-parametric tests, as appropriate. For variables measured on an interval or ratio scale, a t-test or Mann Whitney U-test (depending on the distribution of the variable) was used; for categorical variables a Pearson's Chi-square (or Fisher's exact test if sample sizes were too small) was used. The proportion of patients achieving device mastery was analyzed using a conditional logistic regression model to calculate an odds ratio (OR), 95% confidence interval (CI), and p-value to quantify any difference between devices. The proportion of patients achieving maintenance of device mastery was analyzed using logistic regression. Superiority was demonstrated if the logistic regression model showed that the proportion of patients maintaining device mastery was significantly greater (at the 5% level) with one device compared with the other. The number of steps taken to achieve mastery, counts of errors, and PASAPQ scoring were all analyzed using paired t-tests or Wilcoxon signed ranks tests, depending on the distributions of the count/score data. The number and type of HCP- and external expert-(video-)observed errors were tabulated and Cohen's Kappa Coefficient was used to quantify agreement of error counts between the assessors (HCP and external expert). HCP-observed errors were analyzed using a negative binomial regression model. The frequencies of errors after 12 weeks were tabulated by device. To assess the maintenance of device mastery according to external expert review of video recordings, the proportion of patients maintaining mastery of device across treatment groups was compared using a Chi-square test.

Sample size

For the assessment of device mastery, a sample size of 477 patients was needed to achieve 90% power to detect a difference in proportions of 0.08 when the proportion of discordant pairs is expected to be 0.282 and the method of analysis is a McNemar's test of equality of paired proportions with a 0.05 two-sided significance level [37, 38]. For the longitudinal phase, a two-group Chi-squared test would have 90% power to detect the difference between maintenance of device mastery of 61.2% for BF Turbuhaler [39] and maintenance of device mastery of 78.9% for BF Spiromax (OR 0.422) when the sample size in each group is 139.

Study populations

The FAS was the primary analysis set for all study assessments. For the cross-sectional phase, this included all randomized patients participating in the cross-sectional phase (cross-sectional phase intent-to-treat [ITT] population) who completed assessments on both study devices. The longitudinal phase FAS included all patients in the longitudinal phase ITT population who returned for assessment of maintenance of inhaler technique at Visit 2 (week 12), and who had at least 10 weeks of inhaler use to which they were randomly assigned. The safety population was specific to the longitudinal phase and included all patients randomly assigned to treatment and who received at least one dose of the study drug.

Results

Patients

A total of 540 patients with asthma receiving step 3 or 4 treatment as defined by BTS guidelines were screened, 493 were enrolled and randomized, and 481 were included in the cross-sectional phase FAS (Spiromax followed by Turbuhaler, $n = 240$; Turbuhaler followed by Spiromax, $n = 241$) (Fig. 2). Eleven patients did not have device assessment because empty Spiromax and Turbuhaler devices were not available at the site, and one

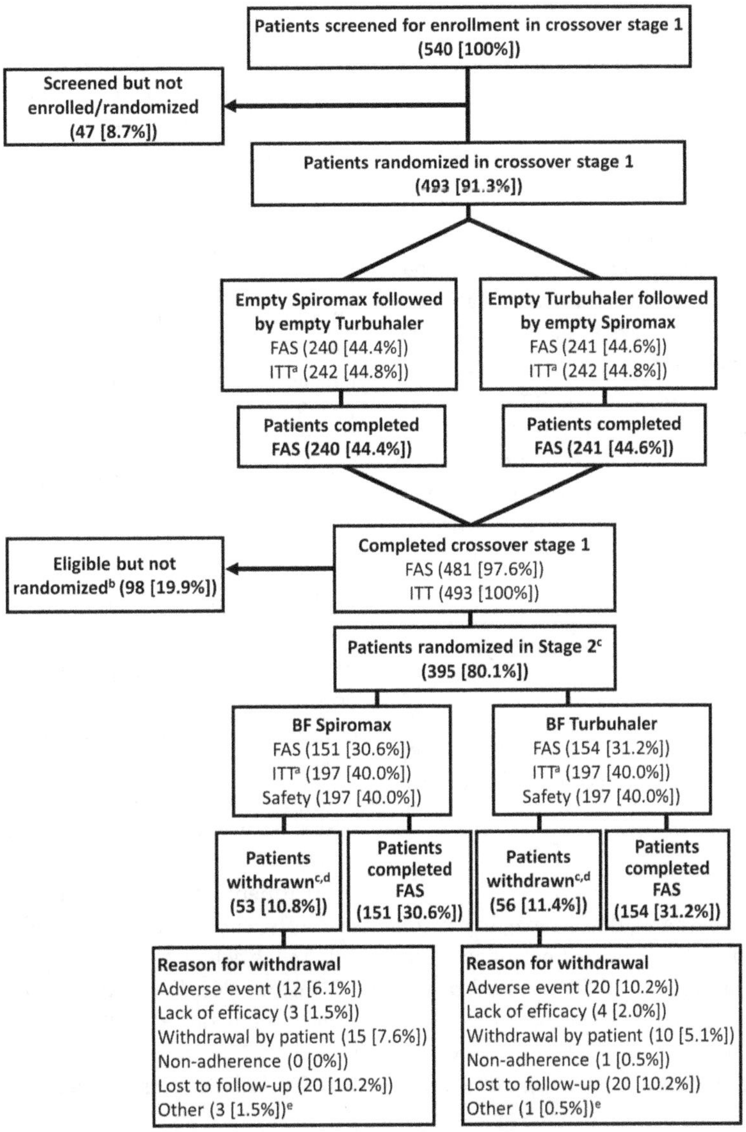

Fig. 2 Patient disposition in the cross-sectional phase and the longitudinal phase. [a]Eleven patients did not have device assessment because training devices were not available at the site. Withdrawals during the cross-sectional phase were not captured because of the study design. [b]One patient was eligible for the longitudinal phase and was included in the ITT analysis; however, no device was available at the visit and the patient withdrew consent before treatment was allocated. [c]Only patients who achieved device mastery on both devices could proceed to stage 2. [d]Data were captured retrospectively. [e]Other reasons for study withdrawal during the longitudinal phase included the following: Visit 2 was not scheduled and patient inclusion/exclusion criteria were not met. Note: Numbers in parentheses are numbers of patients. Percentages are based on the number of patients randomly assigned device order in the cross-sectional phase (n = 493). BF: budesonide formoterol; FAS: full analysis set; ITT: intent-to-treat

additional patient did not complete device assessment for reasons not recorded.

Prior to enrollment in this study, screened patients were using breath-actuated inhalers (Easi--breathe [$n = 2$], Autohaler [$n = 3$]), regular metered dose inhalers ($n = 436$), and dry powder inhalers (DPIs) (Diskus ($n = 56$), Novolizer ($n = 1$); prior inhaler use data were unavailable for 42 patients.

Of the 481 patients who completed the cross-sectional phase, 395 were randomized to the longitudinal phase and 305 were included in the longitudinal phase FAS (BF Spiromax, n = 151; BF Turbuhaler, n = 154) (Fig. 2). Of the latter group, 243 (80%) gave their consent to have their inhaler technique video-recorded; these patients were included in the FAS for the exploratory analysis, which entailed video review of their inhaler technique by an independent expert.

Patient demographics and baseline characteristics are summarized in Table 1. The most common comorbidity among participants in the cross-sectional phase was rhinitis (25% among patients randomized to use Spiromax followed by Turbuhaler; 24% in those randomized to Turbuhaler followed by Spiromax).

Device technique evaluations

Cross-sectional phase

The proportion of patients achieving device mastery (absence of errors) after step 3 (instructional video tuition) was significantly higher with Spiromax (94.4%) compared with Turbuhaler (86.9%; $p < 0.001$) (Table 2). Similarly, the proportion of patients achieving device mastery using the Spiromax versus the Turbuhaler in step 1 (intuitive use; 33.3% vs. 11.4%, respectively) and step 2 (after reading the patient information leaflet; 80.2% vs. 64.0%, respectively) was significantly higher with Spiromax compared with Turbuhaler. Furthermore, the number of steps taken to achieve device mastery and the number of HCP-observed errors were significantly lower with Spiromax compared with Turbuhaler (Table 2). Median PASAPQ scores (part 2 of the questionnaire) were statistically significantly higher for Spiromax versus Turbuhaler (89.8 vs. 85.7; $p < 0.001$). Higher levels of dose preparation mastery (97.3% vs. 92.1%; $p < 0.001$]) and inhalation maneuver mastery (96.3% vs. 92.5%, respectively; $p = 0.007$) at the end of step 3 were observed with Spiromax when compared with Turbuhaler (Table 2).

Longitudinal phase

Table 3 details the assessments of device mastery made during Visit 2 at the end of the longitudinal phase. The proportion of patients maintaining HCP-assessed device mastery over 12 weeks of device use was 58.9% with BF Spiromax and 53.2% with BF Turbuhaler; these values were not significantly different ($p = 0.316$). When the errors that impeded achievement of mastery were split into those relating to dose preparation and the inhalation maneuver, significantly fewer patients made dose preparation errors with Spiromax compared with Turbuhaler ($p = 0.007$) (Table 3).

In an exploratory investigation, independent external experts assessed device mastery using video review of HCP-observed errors for 243 of the 305 (79.7%) patients participating in the longitudinal phase. Maintenance of mastery according to this analysis was significantly higher with Spiromax than with Turbuhaler (66.4% vs. 48.4%, respectively; $p = 0.005$), with patients observed to make less than half as many errors on average with Spiromax compared with Turbuhaler (0.47 vs. 1.00 errors per patient; $p < 0.001$]) (Table 3). The total numbers of HCP- and video-assessed errors per patient were also significantly lower with BF Spiromax compared with BF Turbuhaler (Table 3).

The HCP assessments during Visit 2 of each error (described in Additional file 1: Table S1) are shown in Table 4. The most common errors made with both inhalers were not inhaling fast enough from the start (14–17% of patients) and incorrectly shaking the inhaler before or after dose preparation (12–13% of patients). Nineteen patients (12.3%) using Turbuhaler failed to twist and/or untwist the base correctly, an action that is not required for Spiromax dose preparation. Errors specific to preparation of the second dose were made by 9–10% of patients using both inhalers.

Treatment adherence, assessed using device dose counters, showed no statistically significant difference in adherence when using the BF Spiromax inhaler versus BF Turbuhaler. For both regimens, adherence was ≤50% in 40% of patients. Adherence to treatment was in the range 51–70% for 13 and 10% of patients with Spiromax and Turbuhaler, respectively, in the range 71–99% for

Table 1 Summary of baseline characteristics and demographics

	Cross-sectional phase			Longitudinal phase		
	Empty Spiromax followed by empty Turbuhaler ($N = 243^a$)	Empty Turbuhaler followed by empty Spiromax ($N = 242^a$)	P-value	BF Spiromax ($N = 197^a$)	BF Turbuhaler ($N = 197^a$)	P-value
Age, years, mean (SD)	54.4 (13.8)	53.1 (14.2)	0.309^b	53.3 (14.3)	53.1 (14.1)	0.758^b
Height, cm, mean (SD)	167.5 (9.1)	169.3 (9.4)	0.022^b	168.1 (8.9)	168.8 (9.5)	0.348^b
Sex, male, n (%)	91 (37.4)	108 (44.6)	0.108^c	81 (41.1)	82 (41.6)	0.919^c
FEV_1, mean (SD)	2.5 (0.8)	2.6 (0.8)	0.238^b	2.5 (0.8)	2.6 (0.9)	0.305^b
ACQ-7, mean (SD)	1.4 (0.9)	1.6 (0.9)	0.043^b	1.6 (1.0)	1.6 (0.9)	0.257^b
Eosinophil levels, mean cells/nL (SD)	0.3 (0.3)	0.3 (0.3)	0.279^b	0.3 (0.2)	0.3 (0.2)	0.595^b
Medications, n (%)						
Prior medication	199 (81.9)	195 (80.6)	0.711^c	179 (90.9)	184 (93.4)	0.350^c
Concomitant medication	240 (98.8)	240 (99.2)	0.656^c	194 (98.5)	196 (99.5)	0.315^c

ACQ-7 7-item asthma control questionnaire, *BF* budesonide formoterol, *FEV_1* forced expiratory volume in 1 second, *SD* standard deviation
[a]Intent-to-treat population
[b]Mann-Whitney U Test
[c]Chi-Squared Test

Table 2 Inhaler technique, device mastery and device preference in the cross-sectional phase

Device mastery	Empty Spiromax (*N* = 481)	Empty Turbuhaler (N = 481)	Odds ratio (95% CI)[a]	*P*-value
Step 1 (Intuitive use), n[b] (%) [No. of patients participating]	160 (33.3) [481]	55 (11.4) [481]	4.89 (3.23–7.40)	< 0.001
Step 2 (Patient information leaflet), n[b] (%) [No. of patients participating]	386 (80.2) [321]	308 (64.0) [426]	2.95 (2.06–4.22)	< 0.001
Step 3 (Instructional video), n[b] (%) [No. of patients participating]	454 (94.4) [95]	418 (86.9) [173]	3.77 (2.05–6.95)	< 0.001
Achievement of dose preparation device mastery (primary endpoint; all patients), n (%)	468 (97.3)	443 (92.1)	4.12 (1.91–8.93)	< 0.001
Achievement of inhalation maneuver device mastery (all patients), n (%)	463 (96.3)	445 (92.5)	2.50 (1.28–4.88)	0.007
Number of steps taken to achieve device mastery, median (range)	1 (1–6)	2 (1–5)	N/A	< 0.001
Number of HCP-observed errors, median (range)	1.91 (0–6)	2.36 (0–6)	N/A	< 0.001
Patient device preference: PASAPQ score [scale of 1–100], median (range)	89.8[c] (18.4–100)	85.7[c] (14.3–100)	N/A	< 0.001

[a]Odds ratios are derived from conditional logistic regression of data from paired patients
[b]Numbers of patients achieving mastery at each stage are cumulative (i.e. patients achieving mastery at previous step(s) are included). Patients demonstrating mastery did not proceed to the next step; they were either proceeded to the second inhaler or finished the study (if they were using the second inhaler)
[c]$n = 477$ for each. *CI* confidence interval, *HCP*, healthcare professional, *N/A* not applicable, *PASAPQ* Patient Satisfaction and Preference Questionnaire

46% of patients with both devices and reached 100% for just 1 and 4% of patients with these respective devices. Taking adherence into account, the average ICS daily dose in both groups was lower than the 800 μg/day inclusion criterion: 765 μg/day among BF Spiromax and 740 μg/day among BF Turbuhaler users who returned all of their devices ($n = 227$). All but nine patients returned at least one partially or completely full device.

Efficacy and safety

Asthma control improved after 12 weeks of treatment in both treatment groups: mean changes in the 7-item ACQ from baseline to week 12 showed no statistically significant differences between BF Spiromax (– 0.20) and BF Turbuhaler (– 0.31) (OR [95% CI]: 0.11 [– 0.09–0.30]; $p = 0.278$). Blood eosinophil levels were generally not correlated with baseline ACQ, asthma control, or inhaler errors (Spearman's correlation < 0.3).

Over 12 weeks of treatment, 57% of patients using BF Spiromax and 60% of patients using BF Turbuhaler experienced at least one AE (Table 5), most of which were mild or moderate in severity and deemed unrelated to treatment. The incidences of events considered by investigators to be possibly, probably or definitely related to study medication were 6.1% in the BF Spiromax group and 9.1% in the BF Turbuhaler group. Serious AEs were reported in 12 patients (4 on BF Spiromax and 8 on BF Turbuhaler) (Table 5; Additional file 1: Table S3), but these were generally deemed to be unrelated to study treatment. One serious AE (worsening of asthma, in a

Table 3 Maintenance of device mastery and inhalation errors after 12 weeks in the longitudinal phase

Outcome	BF Spiromax (*N* = 151)	BF Turbuhaler (*N* = 154)	Odds ratio (95% CI)	*P*-value[a]
HCP-observed errors				
Patients without errors (inhalations 1 & 2) (co-primary endpoint), n (%)	89 (58.9)	82 (53.2)	1.26 (0.80–1.98)[c]	0.316
Patients without errors related to dose preparation (inhalation 1), n (%)	128 (84.8)	111 (72.1)	2.16 (1.22–3.80)[c]	0.007
Patients without errors related to the inhalation maneuver (inhalation 1), n (%)	117 (77.5)	116 (75.3)	1.13 (0.66–1.92)[c]	0.657
Number of HCP-observed errors per patient, mean (SD)	0.50 (0.67)	0.81 (1.10)	0.61 (0.44–0.84)[d]	0.003
HCP-observed errors reassessed by video expert review (exploratory analysis)				
n[b]	119	124	–	–
Total number of errors observed by video expert	56	124	–	–
Patients without errors (inhalations 1 & 2), n (%)	79 (66.4)	60 (48.4)	2.11 (1.25–3.54)[c]	0.005
Number of video expert assessed errors per patient, mean (SD)	0.47 (0.78)	1.00 (1.26)	0.47 (0.34–0.64)[d]	< 0.001

BF budesonide formoterol, *CI* confidence interval, *HCP* healthcare professional, *SD* standard deviation
[a]Derived from Chi-squared test
[b]Note: Six patients for whom errors were reassessed by independent video review were not included in the full analysis set; data for these patients are not shown in the table
[c]Estimated from logistic regression models
[d]Estimated from negative binomial regression model

Table 4 Frequency of HCP-observed errors after 12 weeks of device use in the longitudinal phase

	BF Spiromax (*N* = 151)	BF Turbuhaler (*N* = 154)
Number of patients with at least one error, n (%)	62 (41.1%)	72 (46.8%)
Total errors, n	75[a]	125[a]
Does not hold the inhaler with the semi-transparent mouthpiece cover at the bottom	0	N/A
Spiromax: Does not open cap Turbuhaler: Does not remove cap	0	0
Dose preparation: A click is not heard when the cap is opened	0	N/A
Dose preparation: not twisting the base as far as possible, until it clicks and not turning it back to the original position	N/A	19 (12.3%)
Spiromax: Inhaler is not held upright when a dose is prepared (±90° is acceptable) Turbuhaler: Inhaler is not held upright (mouthpiece skywards ±45°) when a dose is prepared throughout dose preparation	4 (2.6%)	8 (5.2%)
Turbuhaler: Device not held upright (upright means mouthpiece pointed skywards ±45°) after the base is twisted until inhalation	N/A	8 (5.2%)
Vigorous shaking before or after dose preparation	19 (12.6%)	18 (11.7%)
Exhales into the inhaler before taking dose	8 (5.3%)	13 (8.4%)
Fails to put in mouth and seal lips around mouthpiece	1 (0.7%)	1 (0.6%)
Spiromax: Finger (or face) placed over the air inlet during an inhalation (at front above the mouthpiece) Turbuhaler: Fingers or mouth placed around air inlets (positioned around the base and above the mouthpiece)	2 (1.3%)	10 (6.5%)
Inhalation is not as fast as possible (from the start)	25 (16.6%)	22 (14.3%)
Errors involving a second dose error, n		
Spiromax: Does not close cap after the inhalation and load a new dose; a click is not heard when the cap is opened Turbuhaler: Does not load a new dose as described; dose preparation: not twisting the base as far as possible, until it clicks and not turning it back to the original position	14 (9.3%)	15 (9.7%)
Spiromax: Does not close the inhaler after taking the second dose Turbuhaler: Does not place the cap back on the inhaler after taking the second dose	1 (0.7%)	7 (4.5%)
Does not know how to read out the dose counter after asking the patient to check the number of doses left	0	4 (2.6%)

BF budesonide formoterol, *HCP* healthcare professional, *N/A* not applicable
[a]Cohen's Kappa Coefficient (measure the inter-rater (HCP and external) agreement of error) = – 0.606

Table 5 AEs occurring in ≥ 2% of patients

	BF Spiromax (*N* = 197)	BF Turbuhaler (*N* = 197)
Patients with at least 1 AE, n (%)	113 (57.4)	119 (60.4)
Infections and infestations		
Lower respiratory tract infection	17 (8.6)	31 (15.7)
Urinary tract infection	5 (2.5)	2 (1.0)
Nervous system disorders		
Headache	5 (2.5)	2 (1.0)
Respiratory, thoracic, and mediastinal disorders		
Asthma (worsening of asthma or asthma attack)	8 (4.1)	9 (4.6)
Cough	11 (5.6)	12 (6.1)
Dyspnea	5 (2.5)	5 (2.5)
Wheezing	4 (2.0)	3 (1.5)
Number of patients with at least 1 serious AE, n (%)	4 (2.0)	8 (4.1)

AE adverse event, *BF* budesonide formoterol

patient who received BF Spiromax) was considered by the investigator to be related to the study treatment. Withdrawals due to AEs were similar in the two study groups; the AEs most frequently causing withdrawal were cough, dyspnea, oral candidiasis, and worsening of asthma or asthma exacerbation.

Discussion

In this two-part pragmatic study, Spiromax was associated with higher levels of device mastery compared with Turbuhaler after training in the initial crossover phase. During this phase, patients were significantly less likely to make an HCP-observed error with the empty Spiromax device compared with the empty Turbuhaler device in intuitive use, after reading the patient information leaflet, and after viewing an instructional video. In addition, patients using the empty Spiromax achieved device mastery in fewer steps and made fewer errors overall.

In the longitudinal phase of the study, the proportion of patients maintaining device mastery (absence of HCP-observed errors upon assessment after 12 weeks of device use) was numerically higher with BF Spiromax than with BF Turbuhaler, but not statistically significantly so. However, in the exploratory analysis wherein an independent external expert viewed video recordings of participants' inhaler usage, higher levels of mastery than were reported by the HCPs were reported, suggesting that HCPs may have had a tendency to over-estimate the number of errors.

The findings of the cross-sectional phase support the hypothesis that patients may find it easier to attain mastery of Spiromax compared with Turbuhaler. Fewer errors were observed with both devices when patients received tuition by reading the patient information leaflet and watching the instructional video (step 3; verbal instruction and demonstration given) than after reading the leaflet alone (step 2; no verbal instructions given). Device mastery at step 2 was achieved in a significantly greater proportion of patients using Spiromax versus Turbuhaler, but rates of achievement of device mastery were markedly increased following viewing of the instructional video at step 3.

In a 'real-world' setting, many patients may not have access to video instructions, or they may be of variable quality. In contrast, all patients should receive the patient leaflet, so maximizing patient mastery of inhaler technique using this resource is an important objective. The outcomes of this study are in agreement with previously published findings that passive instructions alone (such as reading the patient information leaflet) are not as effective as verbal instructions or demonstration (such as watching an instructional video) in teaching patients correct inhaler technique, specifically in patients using inhalers for the first time [40–43]. Other instructional tools for the training of correct inhaler technique should be considered, including verbal instructions and multimedia educational materials (e.g. a link to a website-based instructional video could be included in the patient information leaflet). Demonstrations and practice sessions should also be considered in clinical practice to maximize the number of patients with correct inhaler technique [5, 31, 32, 41, 44–47]. Overall, in order to improve device mastery, HCPs should consider a range of factors including the inhaler type, the patient, the educator/teacher, and the method of teaching [48].

Possible reasons why the longitudinal phase mastery results (based on HCP-observed errors) did not demonstrate a significant difference between the two devices include the fact that many longitudinal phase participants had previous experience of using the Turbuhaler (albeit more than 6 months prior to the study), whereas none had used the Spiromax. Cross-sectional studies [16, 24, 25] have reported a much higher frequency of errors with Turbuhaler than that observed in this study. Another possible explanation is the frequent telephone follow-up of patients, a situation rather different from normal clinical practice, which could have had an impact on the proportion of patients maintaining correct technique. Maintenance of correct device technique may be influenced by patient motivation. Previous studies, in which patients received intensive inhaler technique education in a community pharmacy setting, and had their technique checked 1 month later back at the pharmacy, showed correct technique in about 45 to 60% of patients at this time [31, 45].

It could also be argued that HCP assessment is prone to human observational errors. The discrepancy between HCP-reported error rates and those obtained through independent expert assessment of video-recorded use that was observed in our exploratory analysis suggests that HCPs may be conservative with patient assessments or lack experience and require training in assessment themselves, potentially resulting in over-estimation of error rates. In real-life clinical settings, it could be beneficial for external experts to review each patient's inhaler technique with HCPs. The implementation of such assessment in busy clinics would be a challenge, and if this is not feasible, HCPs should ensure that they maintain their own inhaler technique mastery and periodically review each other's technique. In the future, smartphone apps (including video recording of inhalation technique at home or augmented reality facial mapping) could become an option, as well as new technologies incorporating electronic sensors to inhalers. This study therefore highlights the potential for technology-assisted methods to enhance teaching and assessment of inhaler technique. Our findings also suggest that HCPs should receive training on inhaler technique and its evaluation, to ensure that they monitor their patients in a standardized manner reflecting the approach of an inhalation device expert.

Another important aspect of this study was the analysis of specific aspects of device mastery such as dose preparation. Spiromax was associated with significantly higher levels of dose preparation mastery in the cross-sectional phase compared with Turbuhaler and significantly fewer HCP-observed errors after the longitudinal phase. Errors in dose preparation can significantly impair effective delivery of drug to the lungs, leading to a risk of inadequate treatment dosing (or even no drug dose) [5, 8, 14, 46]. Previous studies have reported that dose preparation errors are device-specific whereas errors in inhalation maneuvers are usually observed across different devices of a particular type (in this study, both devices were DPIs) [24, 25, 49]. Studies in which dose preparation errors have been specifically examined report error rates of between 24 and 49% with Turbuhaler in patients who use this device for their regular medication [16, 49] and in 16.7% of people who are using Turbuhaler for the first time and have read the patient leaflet [43]. The findings of the latter study are consistent with the outcomes from our research, in that both studies found that (1) Spiromax was associated with a lower rate of dose preparation errors compared with Turbuhaler, and (2) maximal device mastery is achieved after HCP education and demonstration [43]. Research shows that when patients learn correct inhaler technique and adhere to treatment for 7 days, they are more likely to maintain device mastery over time [50].

It has recently been shown that not using a fast inhalation when using dry powder inhalers is one of the principal errors related to a greater incidence of poor asthma control [16]. Dose emission from a DPI is affected by inhalation flow, but the extent of variability differs between devices, so that it may be beneficial to use an inhaler with low variability [51].

Participants were instructed to take two inhalations twice daily, and the preparation of the second dose formed an important part of the device mastery assessment. Many of the inhalation 2 errors were due to patients making two inhalations from the first dose that was prepared, instead of preparing a second dose. They made a second inhalation either without closing and opening the cap of the Spiromax inhaler or without rotating the base of the Turbuhaler. Patients were observed to make this type of error with both Spiromax and Turbuhaler with a similar frequency, suggesting that they may have misinterpreted the dosing instructions or had never properly been instructed. Further studies are therefore required to investigate if this is a problem that needs to be addressed. The role of HCPs in ensuring that patients are fully aware of all steps required, including those that apply when taking a second dose if applicable, and directing patients to suitable training material, must therefore be emphasized.

Patients are more likely to prefer a device that they consider easy to use and that they can use correctly, and patient satisfaction with an inhaler is correlated with clinical outcomes [5, 10, 17, 44, 48, 52]. Hence, selecting the correct inhaler device by matching the patient with the inhaler that they prefer and find more intuitive to use could potentially lead to improved adherence, better clinical outcomes and reduced costs for care [5, 13, 28, 48, 53].

Although the between-group difference was small, patient-reported PASAPQ scores for Spiromax and Turbuhaler were significantly in favor of the empty Spiromax (PASAPQ score 89.8 vs. 85.7 for Turbuhaler; $p < 0.001$), indicating higher device preference with Spiromax. Similar findings were reported in two recent studies [43, 54]. One of these was a clinical study comparing BF Spiromax with BF Turbuhaler in patients with asthma; PASAPQ scores showed that patients preferred the Spiromax device for its performance and that they were more willing to continue therapy with Spiromax beyond the 12-week study period [54]. In the other study, device preference questionnaire results from inhaler-naïve Finnish volunteers showed that the majority of participants found Spiromax easier to use than Easyhaler or Turbuhaler and, if they were prescribed an inhaler, they would prefer Spiromax [43]. In our study, device preference was only assessed in the cross-sectional phase. It would be relevant to know whether device preference or satisfaction was maintained after 12 weeks of using the active inhaler (i.e. by repeating the PASAPQ at the end of the study and comparing the outcomes with the cross-sectional phase).

One strength of the current study is the assessment of the maintenance of device mastery, which has been addressed in very few other pragmatic studies in asthma [31, 32, 45]. This begins to address a gap in the literature and provides a preliminary insight into the possible impact of inhaler technique and mastery on disease control. For a formal assessment, adjustment for confounding factors such as adherence will be required. Our study suggests that maintaining good inhaler technique could provide benefits to patients receiving high-dose ICS medication, as the daily dose of beclomethasone dipropionate-equivalent ICS in patients enrolled in this study was 800–2000 μg (fixed or free combinations with LABA). Dose modification and alternative choices for improving asthma control are generally limited in these patients. Another strength of this pragmatic study was the assessment of patients in real-life scenarios. In general, randomized clinical trials (RCTs) provide evidence from narrowly defined patient groups representing subsets of the real-life patient population; co-morbidities and lifestyle factors are not usually captured. Findings from pragmatic trials provide additional insight from a broader asthma population and can be combined with findings from conventional RCTs to provide a comprehensive picture of treatment efficacy and outcomes [55]. Among the limitations of this study are the open-label design, potential confounding associated with 4-weekly follow-up acting as a reminder to patients, and the subjective nature of some assessments such as HCP observations making it inherently prone to a degree of bias and personal judgment. The 4-weekly follow-up calls, in particular, may have had a positive influence on patients' device mastery, as previous research has shown that regular follow-up of patients affects device mastery over time [31, 50]. A regimen requiring two doses to be taken twice daily also represents a dosing frequency greater than that typically found in the clinic, where patients more usually administer one dose, twice daily. In addition, the findings are not necessarily applicable to mild asthma which was outside of the scope of this study.

Conclusions

In the cross-sectional phase of this study, Spiromax was associated with higher levels of device mastery compared with Turbuhaler in adult patients with moderate-to-severe asthma. No significant overall difference between the devices was observed by HCP assessment of inhaler technique in the longitudinal phase, though Spiromax users were observed to make fewer dose preparation errors than those using Turbuhaler. An exploratory investigation involving external expert assessment of inhalation technique by video reported higher levels of maintenance of device mastery during the longitudinal phase with Spiromax versus Turbuhaler. Improvements in asthma control, similar with both devices, were observed over 12 weeks of BF treatment, despite low adherence levels in both study groups. In accordance with previous studies, device preference was higher with Spiromax than with Turbuhaler. This study supports the use of active (e.g. verbal) training to minimize the likelihood of inhalation errors. Our findings also highlight the possible value of independent assessment using video to assist HCPs in evaluating patients' device mastery.

Abbreviations

ACQ: Asthma control questionnaire; AE: Adverse event; BF: Budesonide/formoterol; BTS: British Thoracic Society; CI: Confidence interval; DPI: Dry powder inhaler; ELIOT: Easy Low Instruction Over Time; FAS: Full-analysis set; GINA: Global Initiative for Asthma; HCP: Healthcare professional; ICS: Inhaled corticosteroid; IRT: Interactive response technology; ITT: Intent-to-treat; LABA: Long-acting β2–agonist; OR: Odds ratio; PASAPQ: Patient Satisfaction and Preference Questionnaire; RCT: Randomized clinical trial

Acknowledgments

The authors would like to thank Sandra Kreuzaler, Francis Appiagyei, Tanith Hjelmbjerg, Latife Hardaker, Miriam Cottle, Andrew McLoughlin, Christina Callan, Elwira Fidziukiewcz, Katy Savage, Jo Steele, Marjan Bojarnejad, and Tahreem Sarwar of the Observational and Pragmatic Research Institute Pte Ltd., Singapore for their contributions to the management, co-ordination and conduct of this study.
Medical writing support was provided by Nadia Korfali and Ian Grieve of Ashfield Healthcare Communications, part of UDG Healthcare plc, and was funded by Teva Branded Pharmaceutical Products R & D, Inc. (Frazer, PA). Teva provided a full review of the article.

Funding

Teva Branded Pharmaceutical Products R & D, Inc. (Frazer, PA).

Authors' contributions

Commissioning of study, DP, RD, ES. Study design, DP, VT, RD, SB-A, NR, ES, DF, HC. Acquisition of data, DP, ES, JC, HC. Analysis of the data: DP, VT, RD, IS, CN, PR, JC, GS, HC. Interpretation of data, DP, VT, RD, SB-A, NR, FL, IS, GS, JC, HC. Development of manuscript, critical review, and approval of final version: All authors.

Competing interests

David B. Price has board membership with Aerocrine, Amgen, AstraZeneca, Boehringer Ingelheim, Chiesi, Mylan, Mundipharma, Napp, Novartis, Regeneron Pharmaceuticals, Sanofi Genzyme and Teva Pharmaceuticals; consultancy agreements with Almirall, Amgen, AstraZeneca, Boehringer Ingelheim, Chiesi, GlaxoSmithKline, Mylan, Mundipharma, Napp, Novartis, Pfizer, Teva Pharmaceuticals, and Theravance; grants and unrestricted funding for investigator-initiated studies (conducted through Observational and Pragmatic Research Institute Pte Ltd) from Aerocrine, AKL Research and Development Ltd., AstraZeneca, Boehringer Ingelheim, British Lung Foundation, Chiesi, Mylan, Mundipharma, Napp, Novartis, Pfizer, Regeneron Pharmaceuticals, Respiratory Effectiveness Group, Sanofi Genzyme, Teva Pharmaceuticals, Theravance, UK National Health Service, and Zentiva (Sanofi Generics); payment for lectures/speaking engagements from Almirall, AstraZeneca, Boehringer Ingelheim, Chiesi, Cipla, GlaxoSmithKline, Kyorin, Mylan, Merck, Mundipharma, Novartis, Pfizer, Regeneron Pharmaceuticals, Sanofi Genzyme, Skyepharma, and Teva Pharmaceuticals; payment for manuscript preparation from Mundipharma and Teva Pharmaceuticals; payment for the development of educational materials from Mundipharma and Novartis; payment for travel/accommodation/meeting expenses from Aerocrine, AstraZeneca, Boehringer Ingelheim, Mundipharma, Napp, Novartis, and Teva Pharmaceuticals; funding for patient enrolment or completion of research from Chiesi, Novartis, Teva Pharmaceuticals, and Zentiva (Sanofi Generics); stock/stock options from AKL Research and Development Ltd. which produces phytopharmaceuticals; owns 74% of the social enterprise Optimum Patient Care Ltd. (Australia, and UK) and 74% of Observational and Pragmatic Research Institute Pte Ltd. (Singapore); and is peer reviewer for grant committees of the Efficacy and Mechanism Evaluation programme, and Health Technology Assessment.
Vicky Thomas has no competing interests to declare.
Richard Dekhuijzen has received grants and personal fees from Chiesi, AstraZeneca, Teva, Mundipharma, and Boehringer Ingelheim; grants from GlaxoSmithKline; and personal fees from Sandoz and Zambon. All are unrelated to the present work.
Sinthia Bosnic-Anticevich has received sponsorship to carry out studies, together with Board Membership, consultant agreements and honoraria for presentation, from several pharmaceutical companies that market inhaled products. These include AstraZeneca, GlaxoSmithKline, Meda, Mundipharma, and Teva. Research sponsorship has also been received from grant awarding bodies (Australian Research Council, The Commonwealth of Australia Department of Health and the National Health and Medical Research Council).
Nicolas Roche reports grants and personal fees from BoehringerIngelheim, Novartis, and personal fees from Teva, GSK, AstraZeneca, Chiesi, Mundipharma, Cipla, Sanofi, Sandoz, 3 M, Pfizer, Zambon, outside the presented work.
Federico Lavorini received fees for lectures and advisory board meetings from Astra Zeneca, Boehringer Ingelheim, Chiesi, Cipla, Menarini International, TEVA, Zentiva.

Priyanka Raju is an employee of OPRI, which has conducted paid research in respiratory disease on behalf of the following organizations in the past 5 years: Aerocrine, AKL Research and Development Ltd., Almirall, AstraZeneca, Boehringer Ingelheim, Chiesi, GlaxoSmithKline, Meda, Mundipharma, Napp, Novartis, Orion, Takeda, Teva, Zentiva (a Sanofi company).
Daryl Freeman has received speaking honoraria, support for conferences or consultant agreements with AstraZeneca, Chiesi, Mundipharma, and Pfizer.
Carole Nicholls is an employee of OPRI, which has conducted paid research in respiratory disease on behalf of the following organizations in the past 5 years: Aerocrine, AKL Research and Development Ltd., Almirall, AstraZeneca, Boehringer Ingelheim, Chiesi, GlaxoSmithKline, Meda, Mundipharma, Napp, Novartis, Orion, Takeda, Teva, Zentiva (a Sanofi company).
Iain Small has no competing interests to declare.
Erika Sims was an employee of Research In Real Life at the time the study was conducted.
Guilherme Safioti is an employee of Teva Pharmaceuticals.
Janice Canvin was an employee of Teva Pharmaceuticals at the time the study was conducted.
Henry Chrystyn has received sponsorship to carry out studies, together with Board Membership, consultant agreements and honoraria for presentation, from several pharmaceutical companies that market inhaled products. These include Almirall, AstraZeneca, Boehringer Ingelheim, Chiesi, GlaxoSmithKline, Innovata Biomed, Meda, Napp Pharmaceuticals, Mundipharma, NorPharma, Novartis, Orion, Sanofi, Teva, Truddell Medical International, UCB and Zentiva. Research sponsorship has also been received from grant awarding bodies (EPSRC and MRC). He is the owner of Inhalation Consultancy Ltd. and a consultant to the Observational and Pragmatic Research Institute Pte Ltd., Singapore.

Author details

[1]Observational and Pragmatic Research Institute Pte Ltd, Singapore, Singapore. [2]University of Aberdeen, Aberdeen, UK. [3]Radboud University Nijmegen Medical Center, Nijmegen, The Netherlands. [4]Woolcock Institute, University of Sydney and Sydney Local Health District, Sydney, NSW, Australia. [5]University Paris Descartes, Paris, France. [6]University of Florence, Florence, Italy. [7]Norwich Medical School, University of East Anglia, Norwich, UK. [8]Teva Pharmaceuticals Europe BV, Amsterdam, The Netherlands. [9]Inhalation Consultancy Ltd, Leeds, Yeadon, UK.

References

1. Global Initiative for Asthma. 2017 GINA report, global strategy for asthma management and prevention. 2017 update. https://ginasthma.org/wp-content/uploads/2016/01/wms-GINA-2017-main-report-tracked-changes-for-archive.pdf. Accessed 12 June 2018.
2. Haughney J, Price D, Barnes NC, Virchow JC, Roche N, Chrystyn H. Choosing inhaler devices for people with asthma: current knowledge and outstanding research needs. Respir Med. 2010;104:1237–45.
3. Mäkelä MJ, Backer V, Hedegaard M, Larsson K. Adherence to inhaled therapies, health outcomes and costs in patients with asthma and COPD. Respir Med. 2013;107:1481–90.
4. Price D, Fletcher F, van der Molen T. Asthma control and management in 8,000 European patients: the REcognise asthma and LInk to symptoms and experience (REALISE) survey. NPJ Prim Care Respir Med. 2014;24:14009.
5. Virchow JC, Akdis CA, Darba J, Dekhuijzen R, Hartl S, Kobelt G, et al. A review of the value of innovation in inhalers for COPD and asthma. J Mark Access Health Policy. 2015;3:28760.
6. Sastre J, Fabbri LM, Price D, Wahn HU, Bousquet J, Fish JE, et al. Insights, attitudes, and perceptions about asthma and its treatment: a multinational survey of patients from Europe and Canada. World Allergy Organ J. 2016;9:13.
7. Lavorini F, Magnan A, Dubus JC, Voshaar T, Corbetta L, Broeders M, et al. Effect of incorrect use of dry powder inhalers on management of patients with asthma and COPD. Respir Med. 2008;102:593–604.
8. Molimard M, Le Gros V. Impact of patient-related factors on asthma control. J Asthma. 2008;45:109–13.
9. Clatworthy J, Price D, Ryan D, Haughney J, Horne R. The value of self-report assessment of adherence, rhinitis and smoking in relation to asthma control. Prim Care Respir J. 2009;16:300–5.
10. Papi A, Haughney J, Virchow JC, Roche N, Palkonen S, Price D. Inhaler devices for asthma: a call for action in a neglected field. Eur Respir J. 2011; 37:982–5.
11. Papaioannou AI, Kostikas K, Zervas E, Kolilekas L, Papiris S, Gaga M. Control of asthma in real life: still a valuable goal? Eur Respir Rev. 2015;24:361–9.
12. Westerik J, Carter V, Chrystyn H, Burden A, Thompson SL, Ryan D, et al. Characteristics of patients making serious inhaler errors with a dry powder inhaler and association with asthma-related events in a primary care setting. J Asthma. 2016;53:321–9.
13. Price D, Roche N, Christian Virchow J, Burden A, Ali M, Chisholm A, et al. Device type and real-world effectiveness of asthma combination therapy: an observational study. J Asthma Allergy. 2011;4:37–47.
14. Al-Jahdali H, Ahmed A, Al-Harbi A, Khan M, Baharoon S, Bin Salih S, et al. Improper inhaler technique is associated with poor asthma control and frequent emergency department visits. Allergy Asthma Clin Immunol. 2013;9:8.
15. Giraud V, Roche N. Misuse of corticosteroid metered-dose inhaler is associated with decreased asthma stability. Eur Respir J. 2002;19:246–51.
16. Price DB, Román-Rodríguez M, McQueen RB, Bosnic-Anticevich S, Carter V, Gruffydd-Jones K, et al. Inhaler errors in the CRITIKAL study: type, frequency, and association with asthma outcomes. J Allergy Clin Immunol Pract. 2017; 5:1071–81.
17. Lavorini F, Fontana GA. Inhaler technique and patient's preference for dry powder inhaler devices. Expert Opin Drug Deliv. 2014;11:1–3.
18. Hanania NA, Wittman R, Kesten S, Chapman KR. Medical personnel's knowledge of and ability to use inhaling devices. Metered-dose inhalers, spacing chambers, and breath-actuated dry powder inhalers. Chest. 1994; 105:111–6.
19. Chopra N, Oprescu N, Fask A, Oppenheimer J. Does introduction of new "easy to use" inhalational devices improve medical personnel's knowledge of their proper use? Ann Allergy Asthma Immunol. 2002;88:395–400.
20. Basheti IA, Armour CL, Reddel HK, Bosnic-Anticevich SZ. Long-term maintenance of pharmacists' inhaler technique demonstration skills. Am J Pharm Educ. 2009;73:32.
21. Nguyen Y, Wainwright C, Basheti I, Willis M, Bosnic-Anticevich S. Do health professioanls on respiratory wards know how to use inhalers? J Pharm Pract Res. 2010;40:211–6.
22. Basheti IA, Bosnic-Anticevich SZ, Armour CL, Reddel HK. Checklists for powder inhaler technique: a review and recommendations. Respir Care. 2014;59:1140–54.
23. Alismail A, Song C, Terry M, Daher N, Almutairi W, Lo T. Diverse inhaler devices: a big challenge for health-care professionals. Respir Care. 2016;61:593–9.
24. Melani AS, Bonavia M, Cilenti V, Cinti C, Lodi M, Martucci P, et al. Gruppo Educazionale Associazione Italiana Pneumologi Ospedalieri. Inhaler mishandling remains common in real life and is associated with reduced disease control. Respir Med. 2011;105:930–8.
25. Molimard M, Raherison C, Lignot S, Depont F, Abouelfath A, Moore N. Assessment of handling of inhaler devices in real life: an observational study in 3811 patients in primary care. J Aerosol Med. 2003;16:249–54.
26. Sanchis J, Gich I, Pedersen S. Aerosol drug management improvement team (ADMIT). Systematic review of errors in inhaler use: has patient technique improved over time? Chest. 2016;150:394–406.
27. Price D, Thomas M. Breaking new ground; challenging existing asthma guidelines. BMC Pulm Med. 2006;6(1):S6.
28. Dekhuijzen PN, Vincken W, Virchow JC, Roche N, Agusti A, Lavorini F, et al. Prescription of inhalers in asthma and COPD: towards a rational, rapid and effective approach. Respir Med. 2013;107:1817–21.
29. Leung JM, Bhutani M, Leigh R, Pelletier D, Good C, Sin DD. Empowering family physicians to impart proper inhaler teaching to patients with chronic obstructive pulmonary disease and asthma. Can Respir J. 2015;22:266–70.
30. Lewis A, Torvinen S, Dekhuijzen PNR, Chrystyn H, Watson AT, Blackney M, Plich A. The economic burden of asthma and chronic obstructive pulmonary disease and the impact of poor inhalation technique with commonly prescribed dry powder inhalers in three European countries. BMC Health Serv Res. 2016;16:251.
31. Ovchinikova L, Smith L, Bosnic-Anticevich S. Inhaler technique maintenance: gaining an understanding from the patient's perspective. J Asthma. 2011;48:616–24.
32. Crane MA, Jenkins CR, Goeman DP, Douglass JA. Inhaler device technique can be improved in older adults through tailored education: findings from randomised controlled trial. NPJ Prim Care Respir Med. 2014;24:14034.
33. Bosnic-Anticevich S, Callan C, Chrystyn H, Lavorini F, Nikolaou V, Kritikos V, et al. Inhaler technique mastery and maintenance in healthcare professionals trained on different devices. J Asthma. 2017;23:1–10.
34. European Medicines Agency (EMA). DuoResp Spiromax Summary of Product Characteristics. 2014. http://www.ema.europa.eu/docs/en_GB/document_library/EPAR_-_Product_Information/human/002348/WC500167182.pdf. Accessed 12 June 2018.

35. BTS. British guideline on the management of asthma. 2014 Update https://www.brit-thoracic.org.uk/document-library/clinical-information/asthma/btssign-asthma-guideline-quick-reference-guide-2014/. Accessed 12 June 2018.
36. Kozma CM, Slaton TL, Monz BU, Hodder R, Reese PR. Development and validation of a patient satisfaction and preference questionnaire for inhalation devices. Treat Respir Med. 2005;4:41–52.
37. Schork M, Williams G. Number of observations required for the comparison of two correlated proportions. Communications in Statistics - Simulation and Computation. 1980;9:349–57.
38. Machin D, Campbell M, Fayers P, Pinol A. Sample size tables for clinical studies. 2nd ed. Malden, MA: Blackwell science; 1999.
39. Dupont WD. Power and sample size calculations: a review and computer program. Control Clin Trials. 1990;11:116–28.
40. Basheti IA, Reddel HK, Armour CL, Bosnic-Anticevich SZ. Counseling about Turbuhaler technique: needs assessment and effective strategies for community pharmacists. Respir Care. 2005;50:617–23.
41. Chrystyn H, Price DB, Molimard M, Haughney J, Bosnic-Anticevich S, Lavorini F, et al. Comparison of serious inhaler technique errors made by device-naïve patients using three different dry powder inhalers: a randomised, crossover, open-label study. BMC Pulm Med. 2016;16:12.
42. Van der Palen J, Klein JJ, Kerkhoff AH, van Herwaarden CL, Seydel ER. Evaluation of the long-term effectiveness of three instruction modes for inhaling medicines. Patient Educ Counsel. 1997;32(1):S87–95.
43. Sandler N, Holländer J, Långström D, Santtila P, Saukkonen A, Torvinen S. Evaluation of inhaler handling-errors, inhaler perception and preference with Spiromax, Easyhaler and Turbuhaler devices among healthy Finnish volunteers: a single site, single visit crossover study (Finhaler). BMJ Open Resp Res. 2016;3:e000119.
44. Crompton GK, Barnes PJ, Broeders M, Corrigan C, Corbetta L, Dekhuijzen R, et al. The need to improve inhalation technique in Europe: a report from the aerosol drug management improvement team. Respir Med. 2006;100:1479–94.
45. Bosnic-Anticevich SZ, Sinha H, So S, Reddel HK. Metered-dose inhaler technique: the effect of two educational interventions delivered in community pharmacy over time. J Asthma. 2010;47:251–6.
46. Giraud V, Allaert FA. Magnan a. A prospective observational study of patient training in use of the autohaler inhaler device: the sirocco study. Eur Rev Med Pharmacol Sci. 2011;15:563–70.
47. Aydemir Y. Assessment of the factors affecting the failure to use inhaler devices before and after training. Respir Med. 2015;109:451–8.
48. Price D, Harrow B, Small M, Pike J, Higgins V. Establishing the relationship of inhaler satisfaction, treatment adherence, and patient outcomes: a prospective, real-world, cross-sectional survey of US adult asthma patients and physicians. World Allergy Organ J. 2015;8:26.
49. Molimard M, Raherison C, Lignot S, Balestra A, Lamarque S, Chartier A, et al. Chronic obstructive pulmonary disease exacerbation and inhaler device handling: real-life assessment of 2935 patients. Eur Resp J. 2017;49:1601794.
50. Azzi E, Srour P, Armour C, Rand C, Bosnic-Anticevich S. Practice makes perfect: self-reported adherence a positive marker of inhaler technique maintenance. NPJ Prim Care Resp Med. 2017;27:29.
51. Chrystyn H, Safioti G, Keegstra JR, Gopalan G. Effect of inhalation profile and throat geometry on predicted lung deposition of budesonide and formoterol (BF) in COPD: an in-vitro comparison of Spiromax with Turbohaler. Int J Pharm. 2015;491:268–76.
52. Lenney J, Innes JA, Crompton GK. Inappropriate inhaler use assessment of use and patient preference of seven inhalation devices. EDICI Respir Med. 2000;94:496–500.
53. Small M, Anderson P, Vickers A, Kay S, Fermer S. Importance of inhaler-device satisfaction in asthma treatment: real-world observations of physician-observed compliance and clinical patient-reported outcomes. Adv Ther. 2011;28:202–12.
54. Virchow JC, Rodriguez-Roisin R, Papi P, Shah TP, Gopalan G. A randomized, double-blinded, double-dummy efficacy and safety study of budesonide–formoterol Spiromax® compared to budesonide–formoterol Turbuhaler® in adults and adolescents with persistent asthma. BMC Pulm Med. 2016;16:42.
55. Price D, Brusselle G, Roche N, Freeman D, Chisholm A. Real-world research and its importance in respiratory medicine. Breathe (Sheff). 2015b;11:26–38.

12

Early life vitamin D status and asthma and wheeze

Song-Ying Shen[1], Wan-Qing Xiao[1], Jin-Hua Lu[1], Ming-Yang Yuan[1], Jian-Rong He[1], Hui-Min Xia[2], Xiu Qiu[1*], Kar Keung Cheng[3] and Kin Bong Hubert Lam[4]

Abstract

Background: Vitamin D deficiency has been linked to an increased risk of asthma. This study aimed to quantify the effect of early life vitamin D status on asthma and wheeze later in life.

Methods: PubMed, Embase, CINAHL, and CNKI databases, the Cochrane Central Register of Controlled Trials, and Google Scholar were searched up to July 2017. We included randomized controlled trials (RCTs) and cohort studies with vitamin D level in blood (maternal or cord or infant) or intake (maternal intake during pregnancy or infant intake) and asthma and/or wheeze. Two reviewers independently extracted data. Fixed- and random-effects models were used to summarize the risk estimates of comparisons between highest vs. lowest vitamin D categories.

Results: Of the 1485 studies identified, three RCTs and 33 cohort studies were included. We did not include the RCTs (1619 participants) in the meta-analysis as the comparators and outcome definitions were heterogenous. Three RCTs reported a non-statistically significant effect of vitamin D supplementation during pregnancy on offspring wheeze/asthma at 3 years of age. Pooled estimates of cohort studies suggest no association between antenatal blood vitamin D levels or vitamin D intake and offspring asthma assessed either > 5 years or ≤ 5 years. The estimate for blood vitamin D remained unchanged when two studies assessing asthma in adulthood were excluded, but a significant inverse association emerged between vitamin D intake and childhood asthma. We found no association between antenatal vitamin D level and wheeze. On the other hand, vitamin D intake during pregnancy may have a protective effect against wheeze.

Conclusions: The pooled estimates from cohort studies show no association between antenatal blood vitamin D level and asthma/wheeze in later life. Whereas, the pooled estimates from cohort studies suggest that antenatal vitamin D intake may have an effect on childhood asthma > 5 years or childhood wheeze. The inconsistent results from studies assessing vitamin D either in blood or intake may be explained by previously reported non-linear association between blood vitamin D_3 and childhood asthma. Further trials with enough power and longer follow-up time should be conducted to confirm the results.

Keywords: Vitamin D, Asthma, Wheeze, Pregnancy, Fetal blood, Systematic review, Meta-analysis

* Correspondence: xiu.qiu@bigcs.org; qxiu0161@163.com
[1]Division of Birth Cohort Study, Guangzhou Women and Children's Medical Center, Guangzhou Medical University, 9 Junsui Road, Zhujiang Newtown, Tianhe District, Guangzhou 510623, China
Full list of author information is available at the end of the article

Background

Asthma is an important cause of disability and a major worldwide public health concern. The prevalence of asthma in developed countries rose rapidly in the 1960s and has remained high since [1]. More recently, the same rising trend has been observed in developing countries [2]. While asthma affects people of all ages, the surge among children has been most marked [3].

Among the environmental factors that contribute to asthma, vitamin D status has generated increasing interest for the vitamin's purported immunomodulatory properties.

Clinically, serum calcifediol [25(OH)D] is used as a marker of vitamin D level [4]. In various populations calcifediol levels in cord blood are strongly correlated with maternal levels during pregnancy [5], with maternal calcifediol as the source of the fetal vitamin D pool [6]. Vitamin D deficiency in pregnant women and infants is common worldwide, including both developed and developing countries, ranging from 45 to 90% in pregnant women and 61–94% in infants [5, 7–9]. Based on growing epidemiological evidence, vitamin D deficiency has been linked to an increased risk of respiratory infections and asthma [10]. However, it is still unclear if and to what extent antenatal or early postnatal vitamin D deficiency would affect the development of wheeze or asthma later in life. Previous reviews on vitamin D supplementation during pregnancy have given conflicting messages [11–13].

Given that there have been further published studies (including trials), we undertook a systematic review aiming to address whether antenatal or early postnatal vitamin D status (including intake and blood level, both maternal and in infant) has any impact on the risk of developing asthma and wheeze later in life.

Methods

We followed the Meta-analysis of Observational Studies in Epidemiology (MOOSE) [14] and the Preferred Reporting Items for Systematic Reviews and Meta-Analyses (PRISMA) guidelines [15] when conducting and presenting this systematic review and meta-analysis. PRISMA and MOOSE checklist can be found in Additional file 1: Supplement 1. The review protocol was registered previously with the International Prospective Register of Systematic Reviews (PROSPERO Registration No. CRD42013005559) [16]. The initial protocol considered asthma/wheeze, allergic rhinitis, atopic dermatitis (eczema), food allergy and atopic sensitization, but here we focus on asthma and wheeze.

Data sources and searches

We conducted a systematic literature search using PubMed, Embase, CINAHL, and CNKI (in Chinese) databases and Google Scholar for studies published up to 19th July 2017 and the Cochrane Central Register of Controlled Trials that reported data on antenatal or early postnatal vitamin D status or intervention and asthma and wheezing in children or adults. Details of the search strategy are provided in Additional file 1: Supplement 2.

Study selection

The present systematic review focused on the effect of vitamin D level in blood (maternal or cord or infant) and intake (maternal intake during pregnancy or infant intake) on asthma and wheeze. We included randomized controlled trials (RCTs), quasi-randomized controlled trials, non-randomized controlled trials, prospective and retrospective cohort studies that measured maternal vitamin D status during any trimester of pregnancy or cord blood or offspring vitamin D status during infancy, and having asthma or wheeze during childhood or adulthood as outcomes, which (i) were diagnosed by doctors (including parental or self-reports), or (ii) required the use of asthma medication, or (iii) as assessed by the International Study of Asthma and Allergies in Children (ISAAC) questionnaire (Additional file 1: Supplement 3). Two reviewers (SS and WX) independently screened the titles and abstracts and identified potentially relevant publications according to the selection criteria, of which full text was obtained and read (online Additional file 1: Supplement 4). The reference lists of all papers of interest were scrutinized to obtain other relevant articles. Disagreements over inclusion were resolved through consensus, and where necessary, a third reviewer (JL) was involved.

Data extraction and risk of Bias assessment

The same reviewers independently extracted data using a standard data extraction form. We collected data on the number of subjects with and without asthma or wheeze in the antenatal or early postnatal vitamin D exposed/intervention and non-exposed/control groups; risk estimates (crude and/or adjusted odds ratios [ORs], relative risks [RRs] and hazard ratios [HRs]) and the corresponding 95% confidence intervals (CIs) at any available age end point. Furthermore, we recorded information on the population, geographical location, inclusion and exclusion criteria, interval of follow up, exposure measurement, outcome definition, measurement and window of assessment, and confounders (more details in Additional file 1: Supplement 5). Study authors were contacted when missing data was an issue. Disagreements on data extraction were checked against the original articles and/or resolved by a third reviewer. The data extracted were entered into Review Manager software and were double checked by two reviewers. Risk of bias was assessed using the tool recommended by the Cochrane Collaboration [17, 18]. Two reviewers independently rated the risk of bias for each study as high, low, or unclear ('Definitely yes' in the tool was considered as 'low' risk, 'Definitely no' as 'high' risk, 'unclear' comprised 'probably yes' and 'probably no' as specified in the tools [18]). Disagreements were resolved by discussion or by involving a third reviewer. Each cohort study was classified into one of the following categories: high (more than two criteria not applied/met); moderate (one or two criteria not applied/met or unclear); and low risk of bias (all criteria applied/met).

Data synthesis and analysis

We pooled the original risk estimates as reported (most being ORs) and used adjusted risk estimates where available. When only frequency distributions were provided, we calculated unadjusted ORs and their 95% CIs from the outcome distribution of exposed and non-exposed groups. Where outcome assessment was done in multiple time points in a study, we chose the one with the longest follow-up period or the time point when the age of the participants was comparable to other studies.

We pooled the risk estimates from each study that compared the risk in the highest vitamin D concentration or intake category with the lowest (which is the referent category), and also the risk in vitamin D sufficiency (≥75 nmol/L [4]) with deficiency (< 50 nmol/L according to the Institute of Medicine (IOM) definition [19]). As it could be difficult to diagnose asthma in children below 5 years of age, we stratified the studies on asthma according to the age of outcome assessment (> 5 years and ≤ 5 years). For exploring the association between blood vitamin D status and childhood asthma, a sensitivity analysis was performed by excluding the studies assessing the outcome in adulthood. We contacted the authors of the studies ($n = 8$) that had different cut-off values, and asked them to re-analyze their data according to the above categorization scheme. Of the eight authors contacted, four responded and provided additional data [20–23].

Both fixed-effects and random-effects models were used to summarize the effect sizes. Heterogeneity was evaluated by using the Q ($P > 0.10$ in the Chi^2 test for low heterogeneity) and I^2 statistics (moderate heterogeneity for $I^2 > 30\%$ and considerable heterogeneity for ≥75%). We presented pooled ORs from random-effect models when considerable heterogeneity was observed. Stratified analyses by time window of vitamin D and outcome assessment (for wheeze only), latitude, geographical region, adjustment for family history of allergic disease, seasonality, and smoking status, methods of exposure and outcome ascertainment, and risk of bias were performed to explore the sources of heterogeneity. Funnel plots and Egger's test were used to explore the possibility of publication bias. Number needed to treat for preventing asthma by increasing from low to high levels of vitamin D or via supplementation was estimated by the baseline asthma prevalence estimates and pooled ORs [24]. Statistical analyses were performed with Review Manager software version 5.3 [25] and STATA version 13.

Results

Search results

We have identified 423 potentially relevant publications from PubMed, 855 from Embase, 36 from CNKI database, 105 from CINAHL and 66 from Google Scholar. After excluding duplicates and publication that did not meet the inclusion criteria, three RCTs [26–28] and 33 cohort studies [20–23, 29–57] were included (Fig. 1).

Study characteristics

The main characteristics of the eligible RCTs, cohort studies and those studies excluded during full text screening are shown in Tables 1 and 2 and Additional file 1: Table S1, respectively. Two of the three RCTs were single-center trials and recruited low-risk pregnant women. The other was a multicenter trial enrolling pregnant women who had history of allergic disease. The dose of vitamin D administration and outcome definition varied across the three trials (1619 participants) (Table 1). The median ages of outcome assessment in cohort studies that reported association between blood vitamin D level and asthma, vitamin D intake and asthma, blood vitamin D and wheeze, and vitamin D intake and wheeze were 6 years (range 1.5–25), 5 (1.5–31), 5 (1–10), and 3 (1–10), respectively. Only two studies assessed the outcome in adulthood [36, 57]. Of the cohort studies, 26 studies reported data on asthma and 17 on wheeze. Nineteen of these 26 asthma studies measured vitamin D levels (31,940 participants from 13 cohorts were included in the meta-analysis); the rest assessed dietary/supplement intake (41,952 participants). A variety of operational definitions of asthma were used, including parental reports of doctor-diagnosed asthma ($n = 7$), parental reports of asthma medication use ($n = 1$), a combination of both ($n = 2$), parental reports of doctor-diagnosed asthma with wheezing symptom ($n = 4$), parental reports of doctor-diagnosed asthma and wheezing and/or asthma medication use ($n = 5$) and doctor-diagnosed asthma or asthma medication use by medical record review ($n = 5$). Two studies did not report the definition of asthma. All 17 studies on wheeze assessed maternal vitamin D status during pregnancy, with 12 measuring blood vitamin D levels (8123 participants from 8 cohorts were meta-analyzed) and 6 recorded intake (5678 participants). Most wheeze studies defined outcome using parental reports of wheezing symptoms in the past 12 months (Table 2).

Early life vitamin D status and asthma

Two RCTs [27, 28] reported non-significant trends of vitamin D supplementation during pregnancy on preventing

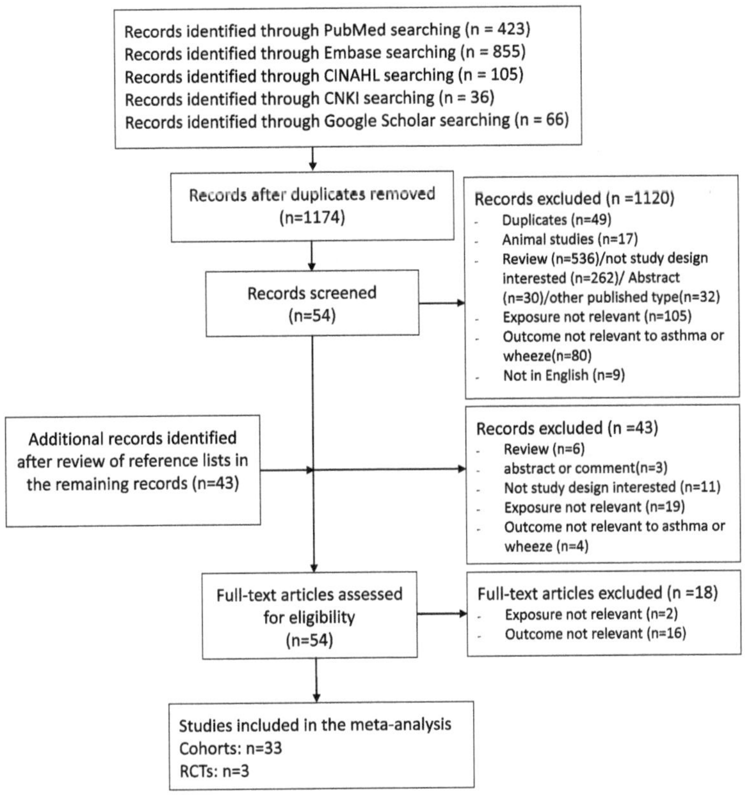

Fig. 1 Summary of literature search and study selection

Table 1 Characteristics of the randomized controlled trials

Reference	Design	Patients characteristics	Intervention (Number of participants)	Comparator (Number of participants)	Outcomes assessment and definition (Age of outcome assessment)
Goldring, 2013 [26]	Single-center non-blinded non-placebo RCT	Pregnant women in London (51°N) (27 weeks gestation, Asian, Middle Eastern, Black and White) without sarcoidosis, osteomalacia, renal dysfunction or tuberculosis	1. Daily vitamin D (800 IU ergocalciferol until delivery) ($n = 60$) 2. Bolus vitamin D (a single oral dose of 200,000 IU cholecalciferol ($n = 60$)	No treatment ($n = 60$)	1.Wheeze ever (ISAAC, at age 3) 2. Recurrent wheezing (≥2 episodes of reported wheezing since birth, at age 3) 3. Wheeze in the year prior to assessment (ISAAC, at age 3) 4. Wheeze with a positive asthma predictive index (loose criteria, at age 3)
Chawes, 2016 [27]	Single-center double-blinded RCT	Pregnant women in Denmark (55°43′N) (≤26 gestational week) without any endocrine, cardiovascular, or nephrological disorders; or vitamin D3 (cholecalciferol) intake more than 600 IU/d	Daily dose of 2400 IU vitamin D3 supplementation (24 gestational week to 1 week postpartum) ($n = 315$)	Matching placebo tablets (Camette A/S) (24 gestational week to 1 week postpartum) ($n = 308$)	1.Persistent wheeze (diagnosed according to a previously validated quantitative algorithm, from birth to age 3 years) 2.Asthma (doctor diagnosed in children fulfilling the persistent wheeze criteria at age 3)
Litonjua, 2016 [28]	Multicenter double-blinded placebo RCT	Pregnant women in Boston (52°58′N), Washington (38°53′N), San Diego (32°43′ N) (age 18–39,10–18 gestational week, nonsmoker, English or Spanish speaking, who or whose partner had a history of allergic disease, with intent to participate for 4 years)	Daily 4000 IU of vitamin D plus a multivitamin with 400 IU of vitamin D ($n = 440$)	Placebo (daily placebo pill plus a multivitamin with 400 IU of vitamin D) ($n = 436$)	Asthma or recurrent wheeze in first 3 y of life (parental report, every 3 months)

Table 2 Characteristics of cohort studies investigating the relationship between antenatal and early postnatal vitamin D exposure and asthma/wheeze

Reference	Location (latitude)	Exposure	Exposure assessment (vitamin D form)	Period of exposure assessment	Median (IQR) of vitamin D status	Outcome assessment and definition (Age outcome assessment), sample size
Pike, 2012 * [22]	Southampton, UK (50°54′N)	Maternal blood	Radioimmunoassay (Total 25(OH)D)	34 wk. gestation	59.0 (IQR, 40.5–84.9) nmol/L	Asthma (6y): Maternal report of doctor diagnosed asthma, $n = 860$ Wheeze (6, 12, 24, 36mo, 6y): Maternal report of wheezing symptom in the last 12 months (ISAAC questionnaire), n = 860
De Jongh, 2014* [29]	Southampton, UK, (50°54′N)	Maternal blood	Radioimmunoassay (Total 25(OH)D)	34 wk. gestation	59.0 (IQR, 40.6–84.3) nmol/L	Wheeze (0–6, 6–12, 12-24mo): Parental report of one or more episodes of chest wheezing/whistling, $n = 856$
Morales, 2012 [30]	4 study areas in Spain (39°N, 39°N, 41°N, 44°N)	Maternal blood	HPLC (25(OH)D3)	77%:12–23 wk.22%:< 12 wk.1%: 24–36 wk	73.8 (IQR,56.3–92.8) nmol/L	Asthma (4-6y): Mother report of medication for asthma or wheezing, $n = 1233$ Wheeze (1, 4y): parental report of wheezing symptom in the last 12 months (questionnaire), n = 1233
Gale, 2008 [20]	Southampton, UK (50°54′N)	Maternal blood	Radioimmunoassay (Total 25(OH)D)	Late pregnancy	50 (IQR,30 to 75.3) nmol/L	Asthma(9y): Unclear, $n = 178$
Zosky, 2014 [31]	Perth, Australia (31°57′S)	Maternal blood	ELISA (Total 25(OH)D)	16–20 wk. gestation; mean 18 wk	NA	Current asthma (6, 14y): maternal report of doctor diagnosis of asthma at any time, with wheeze and use of any asthma medication in the past 12 months. $n = 291$ Current wheeze (6, 14y): questionnaire, n = 291
Maslova, 2014 [32]	Nationwide, Denmark (55.4°N)	Maternal blood (prediction score)	LC-MS/MS (Total 25(OH)D) (use of prediction model)	25 wk. gestation in 1497 pregnant women	58.7(IQR,49.2–69.0) nmol/L	Asthma (18 months): parental report of doctor-diagnosed asthma, $n = 24{,}662$ Current asthma (7y): doctor diagnosis of asthma and parental report of wheeze in the past 12 months, $n = 21{,}194$
Wills, 2013 [33]	South West of England (50–51.5°N)	Maternal blood	HPLC-MS/MS (Total 25(OH)D: sum of 25(OH)D2 and 25(OH)D3)	34 wk. gestation (Translation by model)	NA	Asthma (7.5y): Maternal report of doctor-diagnosis of asthma plus report of wheeze or asthma (questionnaire), $n = 4648$ Wheeze (7.5y): Maternal report of wheezing symptom in the last 12 months, $n = 4696$
Magnus, 2013 [34]	Nationwide, Norway (57°54′ -70°55′ N)	Maternal blood	LC-MS/MS (Total 25(OH)D: sum of 25(OH)D2 and 25(OH)D3)	Approximately 18 wk. gestation	73.7 (SD 23.7) nmol/L	Asthma (3y): Maternal report of asthma plus name of medication for asthma (questionnaire), $n = 1246$
Chiu, 2015 [35]	Taiwan (25°N)	maternal blood, cord blood	electrochemiluminescence-based assay	before delivery, cord blood	Maternal blood: 58.3 (SD 19.3) nmol/L Cord blood: 59.5 (SD 23.8) nmol/L	Asthma (at 4y): ever having asthma, with the occurrence of recurrent wheeze in the last 12 months, or current use of asthma medication (only the results of maternal blood and children blood at 4y were reported), $n = 119$
Hansen, 2015 [36]	Aarhus, Denmark (56°9′ N)	maternal blood	LC-MS/MS	third trimester of pregnancy	76 (IQR 57) nmol/L	Asthma: medication use (at 25y), medical record hospitalizations (at 25y), medical record self-reported lifetime doctor's diagnosis of asthma(at 20y) Current asthma medication use (at 20y), $n = 850$
			LC-MS/MS	mid-gestation delivery		Asthma (6 y): parent reported physician-diagnosed, $n = 158$

Table 2 Characteristics of cohort studies investigating the relationship between antenatal and early postnatal vitamin D exposure and asthma/wheeze *(Continued)*

Reference	Location (latitude)	Exposure	Exposure assessment (vitamin D form)	Period of exposure assessment	Median (IQR) of vitamin D status	Outcome assessment and definition (Age outcome assessment), sample size
Gazibara, 2016 [37]	Rotterdam, the Netherlands (51°55′ N)	maternal blood cord blood			Maternal blood: 62.8 (range 2.3–193.2) nmol/L Cord blood: 40.2 (range 0.1–144.9) nmol/L	Persistent wheezing(1, 2, 3, 4 and 6 y): at least 1 wheezing episode in the first 3 years of life and 1 episode of wheezing at 4 or 6 years of age (ISAAC), $n = 255$
Baiz, 2014# [38]	Poitiers (46°35′N), Nancy (48°41′N), France	Cord blood	Immunochemiluminescent immunoassay (Total 25(OH)D)	Delivery	44.5 (IQR 37.8) nmol/L	Asthma (5y): parental report of a doctor's diagnosis of asthma plus either 1 or more attacks of wheeze or use of asthma medication in the last 12 month, $n = 239$ Wheeze (1, 2, 3, 5 y): parental report of wheezing in the past 12 months (ISAAC phase I questionnaire), n = 239
Rothers, 2011 [23]	Tucson, Arizona, USA (32°N)	Cord blood	LC-MS/MS (Total 25(OH)D: sum of 25(OH)D2 and 25(OH)D3)	Delivery	64 (IQR 49–81) nmol/L	Asthma (1, 2, 3, 5y): Parental report of doctor diagnosed asthma, $n = 194$
Camargo, 2011 # [39]	Wellington (41°S), Christchurch (43°S), New Zealand	Cord blood	Automated chemiluminescent immunoassay (Total 25(OH)D)	Delivery	44 (IQR, 29–78) nmol/L	Asthma (3,15 mo, 2, 3, 4, 5y): Any previous report of doctor-diagnosed asthma by 5y plus either a history of inhaler use or wheeze since 4y, $n = 181$ Wheeze (15mo, 2, 3, 4, 5y): Parental report of wheeze at any time before, $n = 533$
Stelmach, 2015 [40]	8 different regions of Poland (54°22 N)	Cord blood	HPLC (Total 25(OH)D)	Delivery	15.8 (IQR, 10.4, 21.3) nmol/L	Viral-induced wheezing (2 y): wheeze ever appearing during infection. Multi-triggered wheezing (2 y): wheezing triggered by two or more factors (e.g., viral infection, weather, activity) (ISAAC based questionnaire with information from medical chart), $n = 190$
Chawes, 2014 [41]	Copenhagen, Denmark (55°43′N)	Cord blood	LC-MS/MS (Total 25(OH)D: sum of 25(OH)D2 and 25(OH)D3)	Delivery	47.6 (range, 10–145) nmol/L	Asthma (7y): Doctor diagnosed, $n = 257$
Jones, 2012 [21]	Perth, Australia (31° 57′S)	1. Cord blood 2. Maternal intake (total/diet/ supplement)	1. LC-MS/MS (25(OH)D3) 2. FFQ	Last trimester of pregnancy	Blood: 58.4 (SD, 24.1) nmol/L Intake: 200 (SD, 248) IU/d	Wheeze (12mo): Unclear, $n = 231$
Junge, 2015 [42]	Leipzig, Germany (51.4 N)	Cord blood Infant blood-one year, two year	HPLC-MS/MS (25(OH)D 3)	Delivery Infant-one year Infant -two year	Cord blood: 27.4 (IRQ, 17.5, 43.5) nmol/L One year: 83.0 (IRQ, 70.5, 97.7) nmol/L two year: 55.6 (IRQ, 42.2, 70.7) nmol/L	Wheezing ever, Wheezing recurrent (0–36 months;12–36 months;24–36 month) Unclear, $n = 367$
Palmer, 2015 # [43]	Adelaide, Australia (34°51′ S)	Cord blood	LC-MS/MS (25(OH)D3)	Delivery	55.9 (SD, 28.4) nmol/L	Asthma (1, 3 y): as a history of 3 or more episodes of wheeze with the episodes less than 6 weeks apart and/or daily use of asthma medication (medical review), $n = 8123$

Table 2 Characteristics of cohort studies investigating the relationship between antenatal and early postnatal vitamin D exposure and asthma/wheeze *(Continued)*

Reference	Location (latitude)	Exposure	Exposure assessment (vitamin D form)	Period of exposure assessment	Median (IQR) of vitamin D status	Outcome assessment and definition (Age outcome assessment), sample size
Visness, 2015 # [44]	URECA: (Baltimore 39°17′N, Boston 52°58′N, New York40°44′N, and St Louis 38°4′N) COAST (Madison, Wisconsin 43°05′N)	Cord blood	Unclear	Delivery	URECA cohort:20.1 (rang, 4.2–54.6) nmol/L COAST cohort: 21.1 (range, 4.0–77.7) nmol/L	Recurrent wheeze (URECA cohort, every 3 months): at least two episodes of wheezing during the first three years of life with at least one episode during the third year (parent reported), $n = 435$. Any wheeze (COAST cohort, annual): unclear definition (phone contacts & questionnaire), n = 258 Current asthma (COAST cohort, 6y): doctor diagnosed, $n = 258$.
Wolsk, 2017 [45]	Boston (52°58′N), Washington (38°53′N), San Diego (32°43′ N)	Maternal blood	chemiluminescence immunoassay	weeks 10–18 of gestation	56.3 (SD 25.3) nmol/L	Asthma or recurrent wheeze in first 3 y of life (parental report, every 3 months), $n = 712$
Hollams, 2016# [46]	Western Australia(31°57′S)	Vitamin D over the first decade of life	LC-MS/MS (25(OH)D3)	Birth, 6 months, 1 year, 2 years, 3 years, 4 years, 10 years	Birth:26.2 (IQR 20.3, 36.9) nmol/L 6 months: 68.7 (IQR 55.4, 80.5) nmol/L 1 year: 62.1 (IQR 50.1 to 74.6) nmol/L 2 years: 58.6 (IQR 49.6, 68.0) nmol/L 3 years: 58.6 (IQR 46.5, 67.5) nmol/L 4 years: 57.5 (IQR 47.4 to 67.6) nmol/L 5 years: 89.0 (IQR 71.5, 97.4) nmol/L 10 years:76.2 (IQR 64.1, 87.6) nmol/L	Current asthma (from age 3 to 10 years): parent reported wheeze in the last 12 months in children who had ever been given a diagnosis of asthma by a doctor. $n = 216$ Wheeze (from age 1 to 10 years): parent reported wheezing symptom in the last 12 months, $n = 235$
Wegienka, 2015# [47]	Detroit, Michigan (42°19′N)	maternal blood cord blood infant blood at 2 age	HPLC (Total 25(OH)D: sum of 25(OH)D2 and 25(OH)D3)	pregnancy, delivery (cord blood) and at age 2 years	Prenatal; 58 (SD 29.3) nmol/L Cord: 27 (18.5) nmol/L 2 years: 59.5 (20.3) nmol/L	Asthma (3–6 years): parent-reported diagnosed, $n = 635$
Miyake, 2010 [48]	Neyagawa, Japan (34°45′58″N)	Maternal intake (diet)	FFQ	During pregnancy (5~ 39 wk)	6.2 (SD 3.7) μg/d	Wheeze (16-24mo): Maternal report wheezing symptom in the last 12 months (ISAAC phase-I questionnaire), $n = 763$
Devereux, 2007** [49]	Grampian region, Aberdeen, UK (57°N)	Maternal intake (total)	FFQ	32 wk. gestation	128 (IQR, 99–170) IU/d	Asthma (5y): Maternal report of doctor-diagnosed asthma Wheeze (2, 5y):

Table 2 Characteristics of cohort studies investigating the relationship between antenatal and early postnatal vitamin D exposure and asthma/wheeze *(Continued)*

Reference	Location (latitude)	Exposure	Exposure assessment (vitamin D form)	Period of exposure assessment	Median (IQR) of vitamin D status	Outcome assessment and definition (Age outcome assessment), sample size
						Maternal report of wheezing symptom in the last 12 months (ISAAC questionnaire), $n = 1212$
Allan, 2015** [50]	Grampian region, Aberdeen, UK (57°N)	Maternal intake (total)	FFQ	32 wk. gestation	3.60 (95% CI 3.50–3.71) µg/d	Asthma (10y): 1. Parental report of doctor-diagnosed asthma 2. Current asthma: asthma and wheeze in the previous year, $n = 919$ Wheeze (10y): Parental report of wheeze in the past 12 months (ISAAC based questionnaire), $n = 924$
Camargo, 2007 [51]	Eastern Massachusetts, USA (41°10′N to 42°53′N)	Maternal intake (total/diet/supplement)	FFQ	During the first and second trimesters	548 (SD 167) IU/d	Wheeze (1, 2, 3y): Parental report of recurrent wheeze as ≥2 wheezing attacks (summed from the 1-, 2-, and 3-y annual questionnaires) in children with a personal diagnosis of eczema or parental history of asthma, $n = 1194$
Maslova, 2013 [52]	Nationwide, Denmark (55.4°N)	Maternal intake (total/diet/supplement)	FFQ	25wk (mid-pregnancy)	11.7 (5th -95th percentile, 3.0–19.4) µg/d	Asthma (18mo): Maternal report of doctor diagnosed asthma (questionnaire), $n = 28{,}421$ Asthma (7y): Combination of lifetime doctor diagnosis of asthma and wheezing symptoms in the past 12 months (ISAAC questionnaire), $n = 24{,}382$
Erkkola, 2009 [53]	Turku (60°27′N), Oulu (65° 0′46″N), Tampere (61° 5′ N), Finland	Maternal intake (total/diet/supplement)	FFQ	8th month of pregnancy	6.5 (SD 3.8) µg/d	Asthma (5y): Maternal report of doctor diagnosed asthma plus medication for wheezing or asthma (questionnaire), $n = 1669$
Miyake, 2014 [54]	Kyushu Island, Okinawa Prefecture, Japan (33°N, 26°33′N)	Maternal intake (diet)	FFQ	During pregnancy (during the preceding month among women at the 5 and 39 wk. gestation)	5.8 (SD 3.0) µg/d	Asthma (23–29 mo): physician-diagnosed asthma, $n = 1354$ Wheeze (at 23–29 mo): Maternal report wheezing symptom in the last 12 months (ISAAC questionnaire), n = 1354
Anderson, 2015 [55]	Toronto, Ontario, Canada (43°40′N)	Maternal vitamin D supplementation	questionnaire	(1) During pregnancy (retrospective review at 0–5 ages) (2) 0–5 ages	Yes/no	Asthma (2.3 years after baseline): parent-reported diagnosed, $n = 2478$ Wheezing(2.3 years after baseline): parent-reported (ISAAC questionnaire), $n = 484$
Back, 2009 [56]	Umeå, Sweden (63°49′N)	Infantile intake (total)	FFQ	5, 7 and 10 months during infancy	Low (≤13.0 µg/d)/ high (> 13.0 µg/d) dose	Asthma (6y): Unclear definition (ISAAC questionnaire), $n = 123$
Hypponen, 2004 [57]	Oulu (65° 0′46″N), Lapland (61°2′45″N), Finland	Infantile intake (supplement)	Maternal report	Infancy	None or irregularly/ regularly	Asthma (31y): Self-report of asthma with wheezing or by current use of asthma medication, $n = 6722$

BMI: body mass index; ELISA: enzyme-linked immunosorbent assay; FFQ: food frequency questionnaire; HPLC: high performance liquid chromatography; ISAAC: The International Study of Asthma and Allergies in Children; LC-MS/MS: liquid chromatography-tandem mass spectrometry, IQR: interquartile range, SD: standard deviation

***Results from the same study: pooled estimates of asthma and wheeze at >3y using results from Pike et al.; wheeze at <3y from De Jongh et al.**

****Results from the same study: pooled estimates of asthma using results from Allan et al.; wheeze from Devereux et al.**

 # Not included in the meta-analysis of blood vitamin D levels as the continuous variables did not provide sufficient data to calculate estimates

the development of offspring asthma (OR, 0.82; 95% CI 0.50–1.36 and HR, 0.8; 95% CI, 0.6–1.0, respectively). As the intervention and the outcome definition were different, we did not pool the effect size. Apart from having insufficient information to assess allocation concealment, risk of bias was low in both RCTs (Additional file 1: Figure S1).

Figure 2 and Table 3 show the results from cohort studies as well as overall and subgroup summary ORs for the relationship between blood vitamin D and the risk of asthma assessed at > 5 years of age. Fix-effects ORs were not significant for the highest vs. the lowest categories of blood vitamin D concentrations (8 cohort studies, 28,436 participants, Fig. 2a) and for the sufficient vs. deficient groups (5 cohort studies, 23,339 participants, Fig. 2b), with moderate heterogeneity. The pooled estimate did not change materially (OR 0.91, 95% CI 0.73, 1.12, I^2 = 32%, for highest vs. lowest; OR 1.02, 95% CI 0.84, 1.24, I^2 = 47% for sufficient vs. deficient groups) after excluding one study assessing asthma in adulthood. Little heterogeneity was observed across subgroups, in studies measuring cord blood vitamin D level, adjusted for family history of allergic disease, or seasonality, those with exposure measured by liquid chromatography-tandem mass spectrometry (LC-MS/MS), and studies with moderate risk of bias (Table 3).

Figure 3 and Table 3 show the results from cohort studies and the overall and subgroup summary ORs for the relationship between blood vitamin D and the risk of asthma assessed at ≤5 years of age. The fixed-effects ORs were 0.81 (95% CI 0.65, 1.01, I^2 = 0%, 6 cohort studies, 27,776 participants, Fig. 3a) for the highest vs. lowest categories of blood vitamin D concentrations and 0.93 for the sufficient vs. deficient groups (95% CI 0.85, 1.03, I^2 = 36%, 6 cohort studies, 27,776 participants, Fig. 3b). Although higher maternal blood vitamin D level during pregnancy was significantly associated with lower risk of asthma assessed at ≤5 years, we did not observe any

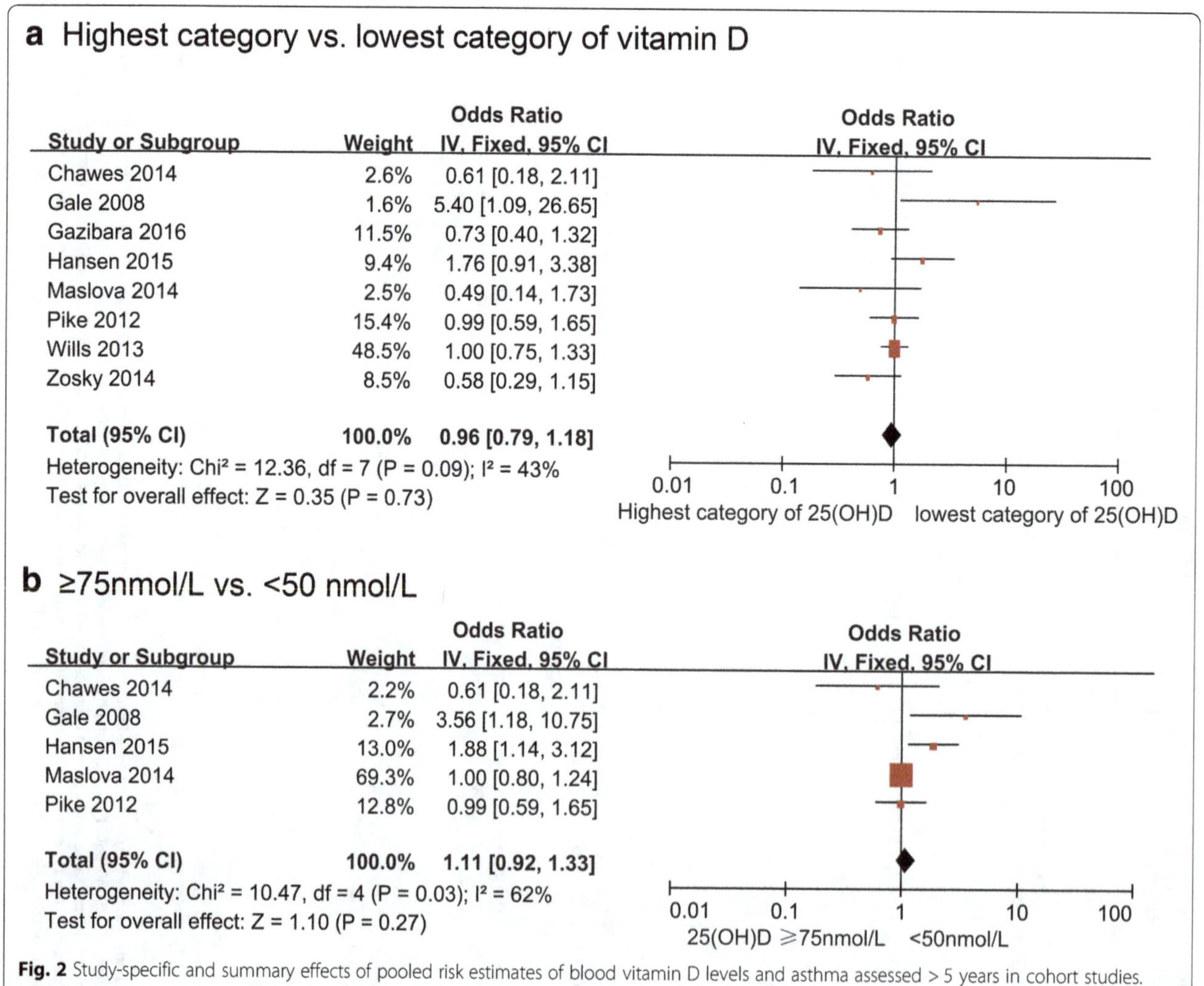

Fig. 2 Study-specific and summary effects of pooled risk estimates of blood vitamin D levels and asthma assessed > 5 years in cohort studies. **a** Highest category vs. lowest category of vitamin D; **b** ≥75 nmol/L vs. < 50 nmol/L

Table 3 Summary ORs of asthma and early life blood vitamin D levels (highest versus lowest category) in cohort studies, according to selected subgroups

Age at outcome assessment >5y					Age at outcome assessment ≤5y			
Subgroup	Studies (Ref. no.)	No. of studies	OR (95% CI)	I^2	Studies (Ref. no.)	No. of studies	OR (95% CI)	I^2
Window of exposure assessment								
During pregnancy (mother)	[20, 22, 31–33, 36, 37]	7	0.98 [0.80, 1.20]	19%	[30, 32, 34, 35, 45]	5	0.79 [0.63, 0.99]	0%
Cord blood	[37, 41]	2	1.03 [0.60, 1.79]	0%	[23]	1	2.00 [0.48, 8.31]	–
Period of outcome assessment								
At an end point (e.g. at age 1y)	[20, 22, 31–33, 41]	6	0.94 [0.75, 1.17]	39%	[30, 32, 34]	3	0.81 [0.64, 1.02]	20%
Up to an end point (e.g. by age 1y)	[32, 36, 37]	3	1.12 [0.77, 1.64]	49%	[23, 35, 45]	3	0.83 [0.40, 1.75]	17%
Latitude								
Tropics or subtropics (more intense UVR) (≤40°N/S)	[31]	1	0.58 [0.29, 1.15]	–	[23, 30, 35, 45]	4	0.87 [0.61, 1.24]	0%
Temperate (40–66.5°N/S)	[20, 22, 32, 33, 36, 37, 41]	7	1.01 [0.82, 1.25]	40%	[32, 34]	2	0.77 [0.57, 1.03]	54%
Region								
Europe	[20, 22, 32, 33, 36, 37, 41]	7	1.01 [0.82, 1.25]	40%	[30, 32, 34]	3	0.81 [0.64, 1.02]	20%
USA/Canada					[23]	1	2.00 [0.48, 8.31]	–
Australia	[31]	1	0.58 [0.29, 1.15]	–	[45]	1	0.74 [0.26, 2.14]	–
Asia					[35]	1	0.40 [0.09, 1.80]	–
Adjusted for family history of atopy								
No	[20, 33, 36]	3	1.14 [0.88, 1.48]	67%	[23, 34, 35]	3	0.70 [0.50, 0.96]	25%
Yes	[22, 31, 32, 37, 41]	5	0.75 [0.55, 1.03]	0%	[30, 32, 45]	3	0.93 [0.68, 1.28]	0%
Adjusted for seasonality								
No	[20, 22, 31]	3	0.92 [0.62, 1.37]	69%	[30, 45]	2	0.87 [0.60, 1.26]	0%
Yes	[32, 33, 36, 37, 41]	5	0.98 [0.78, 1.24]	30%	[23, 32, 34, 35]	4	0.78 [0.59, 1.03]	35%
Adjusted for smoking statues								
No	[20, 22, 33]	3	1.04 [0.81, 1.33]	52%	[35, 45]	2	0.60 [0.25, 1.44]	0%
Yes	[31, 32, 36, 37, 41]	5	0.84 [0.60, 1.18]	44%	[23, 30, 32, 34]	4	0.83 [0.66, 1.04]	26%
Outcome assessment								
Maternal report of doctor diagnosed or medication only	[22, 36, 37]	3	1.04 [0.75, 1.45]	49%	[23, 30, 45]	3	0.92 [0.64, 1.32]	0%
Maternal report of doctor diagnosed plus medication and/or wheeze symptom	[31–33]	3	0.90 [0.69, 1.16]	33%	[32, 34, 35]	3	0.75 [0.57, 1.00]	31%
Doctor diagnosed or medical review	[41]	1	0.61 [0.18, 2.13]	–				
Other definition	[20]	1	5.40 [1.09, 26.65]	–				
Blood 25(OH)D measurement								

Table 3 Summary ORs of asthma and early life blood vitamin D levels (highest versus lowest category) in cohort studies, according to selected subgroups *(Continued)*

	Age at outcome assessment >5y				Age at outcome assessment ≤5y			
Subgroup	Studies (Ref. no.)	No. of studies	OR (95% CI)	I^2	Studies (Ref. no.)	No. of studies	OR (95% CI)	I^2
LC-MS/MS (gold standard)	[32, 33, 36, 37, 41]	5	0.98 [0.78, 1.24]	30%	[23, 30, 32, 34, 45]	5	0.82 [0.66, 1.03]	2%
Other method	[20, 22, 31]	3	0.92 [0.62, 1.37]	69%	[35]	1	0.40 [0.09, 1.80]	–
Risk of bias								
Moderate	[22, 30, 32, 33, 36, 37, 41]	6	0.98 [0.80, 1.21]	13%	[23, 30, 32, 34, 45]	5	0.82 [0.66, 1.03]	2%
High	[20, 31]	2	1.57 [0.18, 13.80]	84%	[35]	1	0.40 [0.09, 1.80]	–
Overall	[20, 22, 31–33, 36, 37, 41]	8	0.96 [0.79, 1.18]	43%	[23, 30, 32, 34, 35, 45]	6	0.81 [0.65, 1.01]	0%

ISAAC: The International Study of Asthma and Allergies in Children; LC-MS/MS: liquid chromatography-tandem mass spectrometry; UVR: ultraviolet radiation

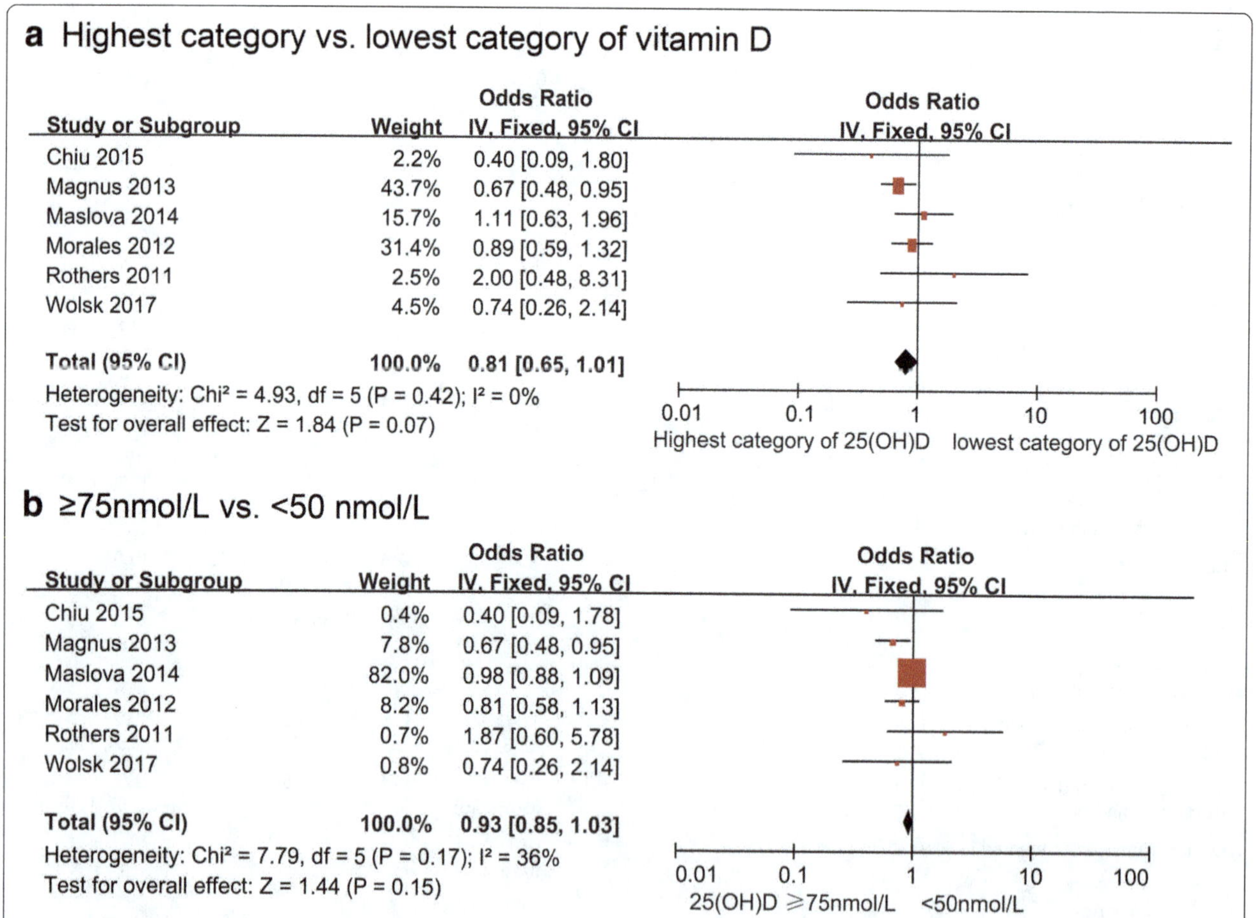

Fig. 3 Study-specific and summary effects of pooled risk estimates of blood vitamin D levels and asthma assessed ≤5 years in cohort studies. **a** Highest category vs. lowest category of vitamin D; **b** ≥75 nmol/L vs. < 50 nmol/L

Table 4 Summary ORs of asthma and early life vitamin D intake (highest versus lowest category) in cohort studies, according to selected subgroups

Age at outcome assessment >5y					Age at outcome assessment ≤5y			
Subgroup	Studies (Ref. no.)	No. of studies	OR (95% CI)	I^2	Studies (Ref. no.)	No. of studies	OR (95% CI)	I^2
Window of exposure assessment								
During pregnancy (mother)	[50, 57]	2	1.21 [0.90, 1.62]	64%	[49, 53, 55, 56]	4	0.89 [0.77, 1.04]	68%
During infancy	[52]	1	0.74 [0.56, 0.96]	–	[52, 54]	2	0.95 [0.85, 1.06]	27%
Period of outcome assessment								
At an end point (e.g. at age 1y)	[50, 52, 57]	3	0.90 [0.56, 1.45]	77%	[54]	1	0.60 [0.27, 1.31]	–
Up to an end point (e.g. by age 1y)	[50]	1	0.60 [0.32, 1.11]	–	[49, 52, 53, 55, 56]	5	0.94 [0.86, 1.02]	60%
Latitude								
Tropics or subtropics (more intense UVR) (≤40°N/S)	–	–	–	–	[54]	1	0.60 [0.27, 1.31]	–
Temperate (40–66.5°N/S)	[50, 52, 57]	3	0.90 [0.56, 1.45]	77%	[49, 52, 53, 55, 56]	5	0.94 [0.86, 1.02]	60%
Region								
Europe	[50, 52, 57]	3	0.90 [0.56, 1.45]	77%	[49, 52, 53, 56]	4	0.96 [0.88, 1.05]	47%
USA/Canada					[55]	1	0.65 [0.46, 0.93]	–
Asia					[54]	1	0.60 [0.27, 1.31]	–
Adjusted for family history of atopy								
No	[57]	1	1.33 [0.97, 1.82]	–	[55]	1	0.65 [0.46, 0.93]	–
Yes	[50, 52]	2	0.73 [0.56, 0.94]	0%	[49, 52–54, 56]	5	0.95 [0.87, 1.04]	43%
Adjusted for seasonality								
No	[57]	1	1.33 [0.97, 1.82]	–	[53–56]	4	0.64 [0.48, 0.86]	29%
Yes	[50, 52]	2	0.73 [0.56, 0.94]	0%	[49, 52]	2	0.97 [0.88, 1.06]	0%
Adjusted for smoking statues								
No	[57]	1	1.33 [0.97, 1.82]	–	[56]	1	3.16 [0.61, 16.32]	–
Yes	[50, 52]	2	0.73 [0.56, 0.94]	0%	[49, 52–55]	5	0.93 [0.85, 1.01]	56%
Outcome assessment								
Maternal report of doctor diagnosed or medication only	[50]	1	0.60 [0.32, 1.11]	–	[52, 53]	2	0.94 [0.85, 1.05]	71%
Maternal report of doctor diagnosed plus medication and/or wheeze symptom	[50, 52, 57]	3	0.90 [0.56, 1.45]	77%	[49, 55]	2	0.82 [0.55, 1.24]	77%
Doctor diagnosed or medical review	–	–	–	–	[54]	1	0.60 [0.27, 1.31]	–
Based on ISAAC questionnaire	–	–	–	–	[56]	1	3.16 [0.61, 16.32]	–
Risk of bias								
Moderate	[52, 57]	2	0.98 [0.55, 1.75]	87%	[49, 52, 54, 56]	4	0.96 [0.88, 1.06]	14%
High	[50]	1	0.63 [0.28, 1.44]	–	[53, 55]	2	0.61 [0.45, 0.84]	0%
Overall	[50, 52, 57]	3	0.90 [0.56, 1.45]	77%	[49, 52–56]	6	0.93 [0.85, 1.02]	56%

ISAAC: The International Study of Asthma and Allergies in Children; LC-MS/MS: liquid chromatography-tandem mass spectrometry; UVR: ultraviolet radiation significant associations in the stratified analyses for studies that had more robust methodology (adjusting for further confounders, e.g. family history of atopy, seasonality, smoking status; blood calcifediol measured by the gold standard LC-MS/MS; studies with lower risk of bias) (Table 3). Six eligible cohort studies [38, 39, 43, 44, 46, 47] analyzed blood vitamin D as a continuous variable and we found no association with childhood asthma.

There was no association between vitamin D intake and asthma at ≤5 years (6 cohorts, 35,257 participants) or > 5 years (3 cohorts, 32,023 participants) (Table 4). A significant inverse association between vitamin D intake and asthma at ≤5 years of age emerged when we restricted our analysis to studies that did not adjust for seasonality or had high risk of bias, with low heterogeneity within these subgroups; and between vitamin D intake and asthma at > 5 years of age when we restricted to studies that adjusted for family history of atopy, seasonality or smoking status, or those that assessed outcome in childhood (OR 0.73, 95% CI 0.56, 0.94, $I^2 = 0\%$, 25,301 participants from 2 studies, for highest vs. lowest) (Table 4). The number needed to treat to prevent one case of asthma was 39 (range 25–93) via maternal vitamin D supplementation (Additional file 1: Table S2).

Studies that measured blood vitamin D concentrations generally had a low risk of bias except for attrition bias due to incomplete outcome data, confounding bias, and detection bias in the assessment of prognostic factors (Additional file 1: Figures S2 and S3). Several studies that assessed vitamin D intake had a high risk of detection bias due to recall of vitamin D intake, confounding bias, and attrition bias due to incomplete outcome data. (Additional file 1: Figures S4 and S5). No evidence of publication bias was found from the funnel plots or Egger's tests for blood ($P = 0.963$ for asthma > 5 years and $P = 0.655$ for asthma ≤5 years) and intake ($P = 0.913$ for asthma > 5 years and $P = 0.410$ for asthma ≤5 years) (Additional file 1: Table S3).

Early life vitamin D status and wheeze

All three RCTs [26–28] used wheeze as primary outcome (one combined with asthma [28]). Two RCTs found no definitive effect of vitamin D supplementation during pregnancy on wheeze among offspring by 3 years of age

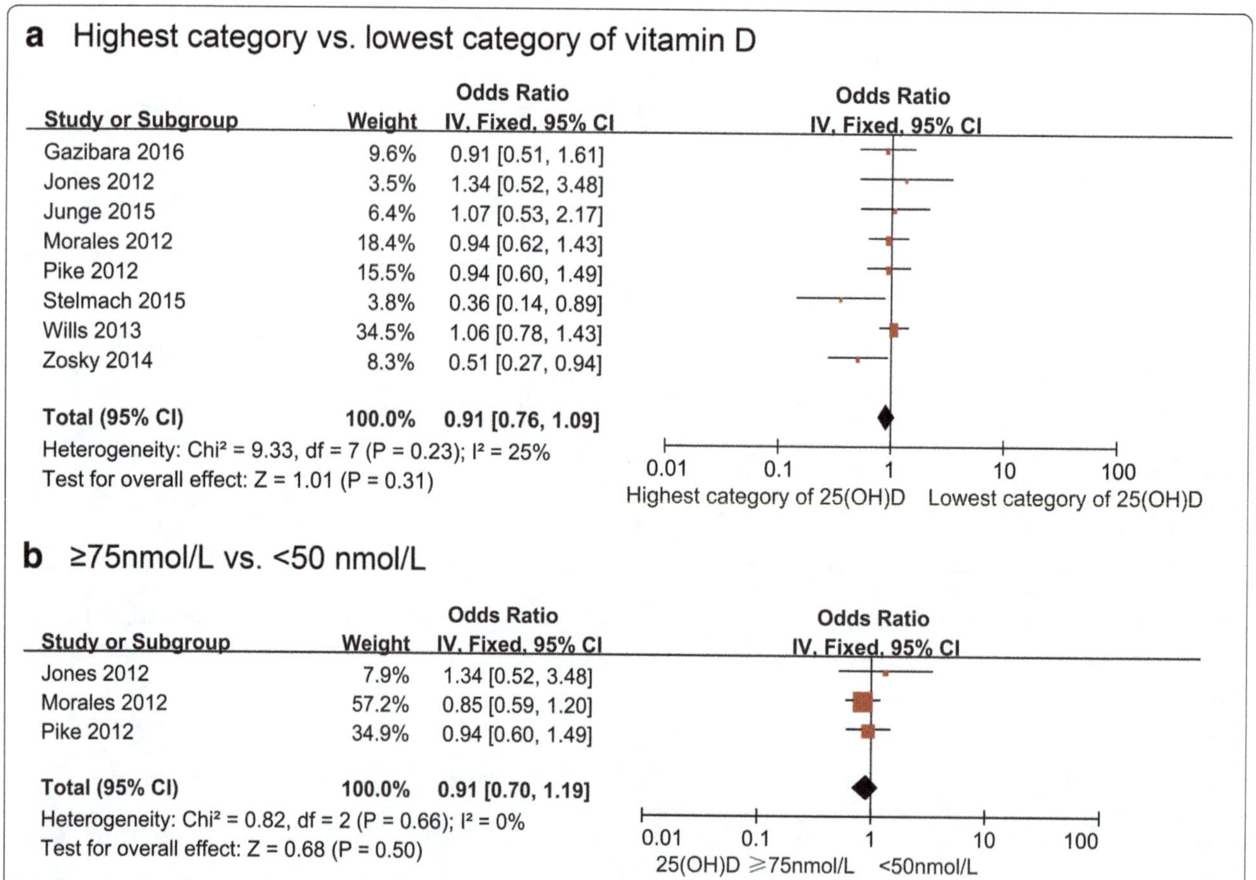

Fig. 4 Study-specific and summary effects of pooled risk estimates of blood vitamin D levels and wheeze in cohort studies. **a** Highest category vs. lowest category of vitamin D; **b** ≥75 nmol/L vs. < 50 nmol/L

(OR 0.86; 95% CI 0.49, 1.50; HR 0.76; 95% CI 0.52, 1.12) and one found a borderline statistical significance association (HR 0.8; 95% CI 0.6, 1.0). We did not perform pooled analysis for wheeze because of the major differences in intervention. Risks of performance and attrition bias were considered to be high due to missing outcome data and the lack of blinding in the trial conducted by Goldring et al. [26] (Additional file 1: Figure S1).

We did not observe significant association between maternal vitamin D concentrations during pregnancy and offspring wheeze in cohort studies (8123 participants from 8 studies, OR 0.91, 95% CI 0.76, 1.09 for highest vs. lowest levels, $I^2 = 25\%$; 2324 participants from 3 studies, OR 0.91, 95% CI 0.70, 1.19 for ≥75 nmol/L vs. < 50 nmol/L, $I^2 = 0\%$) (Fig. 4). Similar results were observed in stratified analyses (Table 5). Within-group inconsistency disappeared or was attenuated in studies that measured vitamin D intake during pregnancy or adjusted for family history of atopy or seasonality or blood calcifediol measured by LC-MS/MS or studies with moderate risk of bias. The overall fixed-effects OR of wheeze relating to maternal vitamin D intake was 0.66 (95% CI 0.53, 0.82; 5238 participants from 6 studies, $I^2 = 52\%$, Table 5). The association remained statistically significant when restricting to studies that: assessed outcome at or before 3 years of age and after 3 years of age, were conducted in a temperate area, adjusted for family history of atopy or seasonality, and those that had lower risk of bias. The Baiz paper [38] did not find an association in early transient, late onset or persistent wheeze, while Camargo et al. [39] reported a significant protective effect by 5 years of age (OR 0.95, 95% CI 0.91,

Table 5 Summary ORs of wheeze and vitamin D status (highest versus lowest category) in cohort studies, according to selected subgroups

	Early life blood vitamin D levels				Early life vitamin D intake			
Subgroup	Studies (Ref. no.)	No. of studies	OR (95% CI)	I^2	Studies (Ref. no.)	No. of studies	OR (95% CI)	I^2
Window of exposure assessment								
During pregnancy (mother)	[22, 30, 31, 33, 37]	5	0.93 [0.76, 1.12]	9%	[21, 48, 49, 51, 54, 55]	6	0.66 [0.53, 0.82]	52%
Cord blood	[21, 40, 42]	3	0.83 [0.51, 1.35]	58%	–	–	–	–
During infancy (infant)	[42]	1	1.88 [0.89, 3.98]					
Age at outcome assessment								
≤3y	[21, 29, 30, 37, 40, 42]	6	0.93 [0.77, 1.12]	26%	[21, 48, 51, 54]	4	0.68 [0.53, 0.88]	63%
> 3y	[22, 30, 31, 33, 37]	5	1.09 [0.89, 1.33]	11%	[49, 55]	2	0.57 [0.35, 0.93]	48%
Latitude								
Tropics or subtropics (more intense UVR) (≤40°N/S)	[21, 30, 31]	3	0.83 [0.60, 1.14]	47%	[21, 48, 54]	3	0.81 [0.61, 1.07]	7%
Temperate (40–66.5°N/S)	[22, 33, 37, 40, 42]	5	0.95 [0.77, 1.18]	21%	[49, 51, 55]	3	0.47 [0.33, 0.68]	35%
Adjusted for family history of atopy								
No	[40]	1	0.36 [0.14, 0.89]	–	[21, 55]	2	0.84 [0.47, 1.49]	46%
Yes	[21, 22, 30, 31, 33, 37, 42]	7	0.95 [0.79, 1.14]	0%	[48, 49, 51, 54]	4	0.63 [0.49, 0.80]	61%
Adjusted for seasonality								
No	[22, 30, 31, 40]	4	0.78 [0.60, 1.01]	51%	[21, 48, 54, 55]	4	0.79 [0.61, 1.03]	0%
Yes	[21, 33, 37, 42]	4	1.05 [0.82, 1.33]	0%	[49, 51]	2	0.37 [0.24, 0.58]	0%
Blood 25(OH)D measurement								
LC-MS/MS (gold standard)	[21, 30, 33, 37, 40, 42]	6	0.97 [0.79, 1.19]	10%	–	–	–	–
Other methods	[22, 31]	2	0.76 [0.53, 1.10]	60%	–	–	–	–
Risk of bias								
Moderate	[22, 30, 33, 37]	4	0.99 [0.81, 1.21]	0%	[48, 49, 51, 54]	4	0.63 [0.49, 0.80]	61%
High	[21, 31, 40, 42]	4	0.69 [0.47, 1.01]	52%	[21, 55]	2	0.84 [0.47, 1.49]	46%
Overall	[21, 22, 30, 31, 33, 37, 40, 42]	8	0.91 [0.76, 1.09]	25%	[21, 48, 49, 51, 54, 55]	6	0.66 [0.53, 0.82]	52%

LC-MS/MS: liquid chromatography-tandem mass spectrometry

0.99), but this has not been consistent in earlier time windows reported in the studies by Camargo et al. [39] and Visness et al. [44]

The 12 cohort studies that investigated blood vitamin D levels and wheeze were evaluated to have low risk of bias, in terms of participant selection, exposure assessment, and window of outcome assessment and co-intervention. Some studies had high or unclear risk of confounding bias, detection bias and attrition bias (Additional file 1: Figure S6, a and b). Overall, the studies on vitamin D intake had higher risk of bias, due to their inadequacy in exposure assessment, assessment and adjustment for prognostic factors, and outcome follow-up (Additional file 1: Figure S7, a and b). There was no evidence of publication bias from the funnel plots or Egger's tests for blood ($P = 0.772$) and intake ($P = 0.954$) (Additional file 1: Table S3).

Discussion

This meta-analysis of cohort studies found no statistically significant association between vitamin D levels in maternal or cord blood or intake in early life and asthma either at > 5 or ≤ 5 years of age, with no evidence of publication bias. Of the cohort studies included, only two studies assessed asthma in adulthood [36, 57]. The exclusion of these two studies did not change the pooled estimate for blood vitamin D levels, while a significant inverse association between early life vitamin intake and childhood asthma at > 5 years emerged. We found no association between early life vitamin D level and risk of wheeze in later life. On the other hand, findings from cohort studies seemed to suggest a lower risk of wheeze associated with maternal vitamin D intake during pregnancy.

Variations in the intervention and outcome definition in three identified RCTs made it difficult to pool the effect size for wheeze or asthma associated with vitamin D supplementation during pregnancy. Two more recent trials [27, 28] with lower risk of bias also found non-statistically significant benefit for persistent/recurrent wheeze or asthma in the first 3 years of life. The results of RCTs were in line with the results of our meta-analysis of cohort studies, where we found non-significant trends of vitamin D supplementation for preventing offspring asthma at ≤5 years. However, our findings from cohort studies also suggest that early-life vitamin D intake may have an effect on childhood asthma at age > 5 years and childhood wheeze. Longer follow-up time for assessing the effect of vitamin D intake against asthma is required in future RCTs to confirm these results [58].

There are two opposing views regarding the relationship between vitamin D exposure and asthma. One school of thought, based on growing epidemiological evidence, hypothesized a link between vitamin D deficiency in early life and development of asthma and other allergic diseases [59], thought to have begun as sunlight exposure decreased with industrialization and urbanization. Others argued, however, that the current asthma and allergic disease pandemic might have been the consequence of widespread vitamin D supplementation in food, backed by some historical evidence [60]. Coincidentally, both low and high levels of vitamin D were reported to be related to asthma, in a U-shaped manner [32]. Another study by Rothers et al. also found that both low (< 50 nmol/L) and high (≥100 nmol/L) levels of cord blood calcifediol were associated with increased IgE, which was related to subsequent risk of wheeze/asthma [23]. In the present meta-analysis, the inconsistent results from studies assessing vitamin D either in blood or intake for childhood asthma/wheeze risk may be explained by the previously reported non-linear association between blood vitamin D_3 and childhood asthma, which tends to be non-statistically significant by comparing the highest with lowest vitamin D levels [32]. However, the dichotomized exposure in the present study limited the exploration of non-linear association.

The sources of heterogeneity, as indicated by the results from stratified analyses were: window of exposure assessment, whether family history of atopy or seasonality have been adjusted for, definition of outcome, risk of bias, and the method of assessing blood calcifediol. As suggested by Autier et al. [61], vitamin D level could be a biomarker and proxy for overall health and wellbeing of mothers and infants. However, as most of the cohort studies included did not adjust for health status of the participants, we were unable to exclude such potential confounding. In most of the studies included, tobacco smoking was adjusted for in the analysis, but other important confounders including family history of atopic diseases, seasonal variations in blood vitamin D levels, sedentary lifestyle and obesity [62–64] were less commonly considered. Nevertheless, results from our sensitivity analysis on studies reporting blood vitamin D level, which included only studies that adjusted for family history and seasonal variations, showed no material difference in the summary estimates compared with our main findings. Three of the cohort studies [35, 42, 47] measured serum calcifediol in both prenatal and postnatal periods, but these studies analyzed the associations between vitamin D measured at different time points with outcome separately and failed to explore the effect of persistent vitamin D deficiency on asthma. While the half-life of serum calcifediol is only about two weeks [65], it is possible that such misclassification in vitamin D status measured at only one time point could have biased the findings towards the null. A recent study conducted by Hollams et al. used mixed-effects logistic regression and found no longitudinal association between calcifediol concentrations as a continuous variable and asthma from 3 to 10 years of age [46].

On the issue of case definition, ascertaining childhood asthma in epidemiological studies has been challenging given the lack of definitive diagnostic criteria [66, 67]. Most studies defined asthma by either maternal report of doctor-diagnosed asthma, asthma medications use, or a combination of doctor-diagnosed asthma and either asthma medication or wheezing symptoms within the past year. Although not without caveats, such as under-reporting both diagnosed and undiagnosed conditions [68] and variable agreement with clinical records [67], these definitions have been widely used in research [69]. In two studies asthma definition was not specified, adding further variability to outcome assessment and increased heterogeneity in our pooled analyses.

In general, studies investigating blood vitamin D levels had relatively low risk of bias in most domains except for confounding, detection, and attrition biases, whereas studies that used food frequency questionnaire to quantify vitamin D intake were at risk of misclassification bias as pregnant women often had to recall their dietary history from a few months previous.. Apart from detection bias, most vitamin D intake studies were also at risk of attrition bias for their inadequate follow-up duration or unknown difference between missing and available outcome data, as well as confounding bias in some studies which did not include major confounders. In addition to variation over time, different methods of blood vitamin D level quantification employed in different studies might also introduce inter-study variability. In the stratified analysis, we compared the risk estimates derived from studies that used the gold standard LC-MS/MS with those using other methods and found no material difference between the pooled estimates. Studies that investigated antenatal vitamin D intake and asthma at > 5 years of age tended to be small and their inclusion in the meta-analysis may explain the weak evidence observed.

Compared to previous related systematic reviews [11–13, 70], we have identified more cohort studies and included two recently published RCTs in the analysis. Only six cohort studies [20, 22, 23, 30, 33, 39] measuring maternal serum calcifediol during pregnancy or from cord blood and asthma risk were identified by Cassim et al. [70], but we have included 13 more studies [31, 32, 34–38, 41, 43–47], plus an additional 13 cohort studies [21, 22, 29–31, 33, 37–40, 42, 44, 46] to explore the association between calcifediol level in maternal blood or cord blood and wheeze risk. As a consequence of our more comprehensive approach in including various exposure metrics (intake and blood level, both maternal and in infant) in the search strategy and a critical risk of bias assessment using the risk of bias tool recommended by the Cochrane Collaboration [17, 18], we were able to demonstrate the existence of heterogeneity between studies in the findings, which lead us to a more conservative conclusion. In addition, we further studied the association between antenatal or early postnatal vitamin D level and asthma and wheeze using commonly accepted clinical cut-off values. We found no difference of risk of asthma or wheeze between sufficient and deficient vitamin D level groups, implying the optimal threshold for bone health may not necessarily be applicable for the respiratory and immune systems.

One of the limitations of this work is that we were unable to retrieve sufficient information for calculating pooled estimates from six eligible studies that analyzed vitamin D level as a continuous variable. We were able to identify one study that has examined infant blood vitamin D levels and their relationship to wheeze but none for asthma. Studies investigating the association between infant vitamin D levels and risk of childhood asthma should be encouraged, with designs that minimize detection, confounding, and follow-up biases.

Conclusions

The pooled estimates from cohort studies show no association between antenatal blood vitamin D level and asthma/wheeze in later life. On the other hand, although the interventional studies found a non-statistically significant benefit for asthma/wheeze in first 3 years of life, the pooled estimates from cohort studies suggest that early life vitamin D intake may have an effect on childhood asthma > 5 years or childhood wheeze. Should that be the case, this may point to a cost-effective intervention for childhood asthma. Further trials with enough power and longer follow-up time should be conducted to confirm the results.

Abbreviations

BMI: body mass index; CIs: confidence intervals; ELISA: enzyme-linked immunosorbent assay; FFQ: food frequency questionnaire; HPLC: high performance liquid chromatography; HR: hazard ratio; IOM: Institute of Medicine; ISAAC: The International Study of Asthma and Allergies in Children; LC-MS/MS: liquid chromatography-tandem mass spectrometry; MOOSE: Meta-analysis of Observational Studies in Epidemiology; OR: odds ratio; PRISMA: Preferred Reporting Items for Systematic Reviews and Meta-Analyses; RCT: randomized controlled trial; RR: relative risk; UVR: ultraviolet radiation

Acknowledgements

The authors would like to thank Professor Susan L. Prescott (Centre for Child Health Research, University of Western Australia, Perth, Australia), Dr. Anderson P. Jones (Centre for Child Health Research, University of Western Australia, Perth, Australia), Professor Anne L. Wright (Arizona Respiratory Center, at the University of Arizona, Tucson, AZ), Dr. Debra A. Stern (Arizona Respiratory Center, at the University of Arizona, Tucson, AZ), Dr. Jane SA Lucas (Clinical and Experimental Sciences Academic Unit, University of Southampton Faculty of Medicine, Southampton, UK), Dr. Katharine C Pike (Clinical and Experimental Sciences Academic Unit, University of Southampton Faculty of Medicine, Southampton, UK), Dr. Catharine R Gale (MRC Epidemiology Resource Centre (University of Southampton),

Southampton General Hospital, Southampton) for re-analyzing and sending the data requested from their manuscripts. We also thank Professor Carlos A. Camargo, Jr., Dr. Andrew Wills and Dr. Bo L. Chawes for clarifying our queries relating to their manuscripts and Mr. Ian Henderson for helping the language editing of the manuscript.

Funding
This work was supported by the Guangzhou Science and Technology Bureau, Guangzhou, China (2012 J5100038, 201807010086). The funders had no role in study design, data collection and analysis, decision to publish, interpretation of data and preparation of the manuscript.

Authors' contributions
XQ, HX, KC and SS acquired funding. XQ, SS, KC and KL conceived the study. SS and KL developed the protocol of the systematic review and conducted the electronic database searches. SS and WX screened titles and abstracts, extracted relevant data, performed the quality grading and drafted the manuscript. SS, JL, JH, and YM performed statistical analysis. SS wrote the manuscript and KL revised the manuscript. KC, XQ and HX contributed to the interpretation of the findings. All authors reviewed and approved the final manuscript.

Consent for publication
Not applicable.

Competing interests
The authors declare that they have no competing interests.

Author details
[1]Division of Birth Cohort Study, Guangzhou Women and Children's Medical Center, Guangzhou Medical University, 9 Junsui Road, Zhujiang Newtown, Tianhe District, Guangzhou 510623, China. [2]Department of Pediatric Surgery, Guangzhou Women and Children's Medical Center, Guangzhou Medical University, Guangzhou, China. [3]Institute of Applied Health Research, University of Birmingham, Birmingham, UK. [4]Clinical Trial Service Unit and Epidemiological Studies Unit, Nuffield Department of Population Health, University of Oxford, Oxford, UK.

References
1. Eder W, Ege MJ, von Mutius E. The asthma epidemic. N Engl J Med. 2006; 355(21):2226–35.
2. Song WJ, Kang MG, Chang YS, Cho SH. Epidemiology of adult asthma in Asia: toward a better understanding. Asia Pac Allergy. 2014;4(2):75–85.
3. Akinbami LJ, Moorman JE, Bailey C, Zahran HS, King M, Johnson CA, Liu X. Trends in asthma prevalence, health care use, and mortality in the United States, 2001–2010. NCHS data brief, no 94. Hyattsville, MD: National Center for Health Statistics. 2012(94):1–8.
4. Holick MF. Vitamin D deficiency. N Engl J Med. 2007;357(3):266–81.
5. Halicioglu O, Aksit S, Koc F, Akman SA, Albudak E, Yaprak I, Coker I, Colak A, Ozturk C, Gulec ES. Vitamin D deficiency in pregnant women and their neonates in spring time in western Turkey. Paediatr Perinat Epidemiol. 2012; 26(1):53–60.
6. Salle BL, Delvin EE, Lapillonne A, Bishop NJ, Glorieux FH. Perinatal metabolism of vitamin D. Am J Clin Nutr. 2000;71(5 Suppl):1317S–24S.
7. Vandevijvere S, Amsalkhir S, Van Oyen H, Moreno-Reyes R. High prevalence of vitamin D deficiency in pregnant women: a national cross-sectional survey. PLoS One. 2012;7(8):e43868.
8. Khuri-Bulos N, Lang RD, Blevins M, Kudyba K, Lawrence L, Davidson M, Faouri S, Halasa NB. Vitamin D deficiency among newborns in Amman, Jordan. Glob J Health Sci. 2014;6(1):162–71.
9. Vieth Streym S, Kristine Moller U, Rejnmark L, Heickendorff L, Mosekilde L, Vestergaard P. Maternal and infant vitamin D status during the first 9 months of infant life-a cohort study. Eur J Clin Nutr. 2013;67(10):1022–8.
10. Bozzetto S, Carraro S, Giordano G, Boner A, Baraldi E. Asthma, allergy and respiratory infections: the vitamin D hypothesis. Allergy. 2012;67(1):10–7.
11. Nurmatov U, Devereux G, Sheikh A. Nutrients and foods for the primary prevention of asthma and allergy: systematic review and meta-analysis. J Allergy Clin Immunol. 2011;127(3):724–733 e721–730.
12. Harvey NC, Holroyd C, Ntani G, Javaid K, Cooper P, Moon R, Cole Z, Tinati T, Godfrey K, Dennison E, et al. Vitamin D supplementation in pregnancy: a systematic review. Health Technol Assess. 2014;18(45):1–190.
13. Beckhaus AA, Garcia-Marcos L, Forno E, Pacheco-Gonzalez RM, Celedon JC, Castro-Rodriguez JA. Maternal nutrition during pregnancy and risk of asthma, wheeze, and atopic diseases during childhood: a systematic review and meta-analysis. Allergy. 2015;70(12):1588–604.
14. Stroup DF, Berlin JA, Morton SC, Olkin I, Williamson GD, Rennie D, Moher D, Becker BJ, Sipe TA, Thacker SB. Meta-analysis of observational studies in epidemiology: a proposal for reporting. Meta-analysis of observational studies in epidemiology (MOOSE) group. JAMA. 2000;283(15):2008–12.
15. Moher D, Liberati A, Tetzlaff J, Altman DG. Preferred reporting items for systematic reviews and meta-analyses: the PRISMA statement. J Clin Epidemiol. 2009;62(10):1006–12.
16. Shen SY, Xiao WQ, Lu JH, Lam KB, Qiu X, Cheng KK. Maternal and infant vitamin D status in relation to asthma and allergic diseases: a systematic review and meta-analysis. 2013, http://www.crd.york.ac.uk/prospero/display_record.asp?ID=CRD42013005559#.U458kySS1dg. Accessed August, 2017.
17. Higgins JPT, Altman DG, JAC S. Chapter 8 Assessing risk of bias in included studies. In: JPT H, Green S, editors. Cochrane Handbookfor systematic reviews of interventions. London: Cochrane Collaboration; 2011.
18. Cochrane. Tool to Assess Risk of Bias in Cohort Studies. 2013; http://methods.cochrane.org/bias/sites/methods.cochrane.org.bias/files/public/uploads/Tool%20to%20Assess%20Risk%20of%20Bias%20in%20Cohort%20Studies.pdf. Accessed August, 2017.
19. Ross AC, Manson JE, Abrams SA, Aloia JF, Brannon PM, Clinton SK, Durazo-Arvizu RA, Gallagher JC, Gallo RL, Jones G, et al. The 2011 report on dietary reference intakes for calcium and vitamin D from the Institute of Medicine: what clinicians need to know. J Clin Endocrinol Metab. 2011;96(1):53–8.
20. Gale CR, Robinson SM, Harvey NC, Javaid MK, Jiang B, Martyn CN, Godfrey KM, Cooper C. Maternal vitamin D status during pregnancy and child outcomes. Eur J Clin Nutr. 2008;62(1):68–77.
21. Jones AP, Palmer D, Zhang G, Prescott SL. Cord blood 25-hydroxyvitamin D3 and allergic disease during infancy. Pediatrics. 2012;130(5):e1128–35.
22. Pike KC, Inskip HM, Robinson S, Lucas JS, Cooper C, Harvey NC, Godfrey KM, Roberts G. Maternal late-pregnancy serum 25-hydroxyvitamin D in relation to childhood wheeze and atopic outcomes. Thorax. 2012;67(11):950–6.
23. Rothers J, Wright AL, Stern DA, Halonen M, Camargo Jr CA: Cord blood 25-hydroxyvitamin D levels are associated with aeroallergen sensitization in children from Tucson, Arizona. J Allergy Clin Immunol 2011, 128(5):1093–1099.e1095.
24. Cates CJ. Simpson's paradox and calculation of number needed to treat from meta-analysis. BMC Med Res Methodol. 2002;2:3.
25. Cochrane. Revman 5. 2014; http://community.cochrane.org/tools/review-production-tools/revman-5. Accessed August, 2017.
26. Goldring ST, Griffiths CJ, Martineau AR, Robinson S, Yu C, Poulton S, Kirkby JC, Stocks J, Hooper R, Shaheen SO, et al. Prenatal vitamin d supplementation and child respiratory health: a randomised controlled trial. PLoS One. 2013;8(6):e66627.
27. Chawes BL, Bonnelykke K, Stokholm J, Vissing NH, Bjarnadottir E, Schoos AM, Wolsk HM, Pedersen TM, Vinding RK, Thorsteinsdottir S, et al. Effect of vitamin D3 supplementation during pregnancy on risk of persistent wheeze in the offspring: a randomized clinical trial. JAMA. 2016;315(4):353–61.
28. Litonjua AA, Carey VJ, Laranjo N, Harshfield BJ, McElrath TF, O'Connor GT, Sandel M, Iverson RE Jr, Lee-Paritz A, Strunk RC, et al. Effect of prenatal supplementation with vitamin D on asthma or recurrent wheezing in offspring by age 3 years: the VDAART randomized clinical trial. JAMA. 2016;315(4):362–70.
29. de Jongh RT, Crozier SR, D'Angelo S, Pike KC, Roberts G, Lucas JS, Inskip H, Godfrey KM, Cooper C, Harvey NC. Maternal 25-hydroxyvitamin D levels in relation to offspring respiratory symptoms and infections. Eur Respir J. 2014; 43(4):1181–3.
30. Morales E, Romieu I, Guerra S, Ballester F, Rebagliato M, Vioque J, Tardon A, Rodriguez Delhi C, Arranz L, Torrent M, et al. Maternal vitamin D status in pregnancy and risk of lower respiratory tract infections, wheezing, and asthma in offspring. Epidemiology. 2012;23(1):64–71.
31. Zosky GR, Hart PH, Whitehouse AJ, Kusel MM, Ang W, Foong RE, Chen L, Holt PG, Sly PD, Hall GL. Vitamin D deficiency at 16 to 20 weeks' gestation is

associated with impaired lung function and asthma at 6 years of age. Ann Am Thorac Soc. 2014;11(4):571–7.
32. Maslova E, Hansen S, Thorne-Lyman AL, Jensen CB, Strom M, Cohen A, Nielsen NO, Olsen SF. Predicted vitamin D status in mid-pregnancy and child allergic disease. Pediatr Allergy Immunol. 2014;25(7):706–13.
33. Wills AK, Shaheen SO, Granell R, Henderson AJ, Fraser WD, Lawlor DA. Maternal 25-hydroxyvitamin D and its association with childhood atopic outcomes and lung function. Clin Exp Allergy. 2013;43(10):1180–8.
34. Magnus MC, Stene LC, Nafstad P, Stigum H, London SJ, Nystad W. Prospective study of maternal mid-pregnancy 25-hydroxyvitamin D level and early childhood respiratory disorders. Paediatr Perinat Epidemiol. 2013; 27(6):532–41.
35. Chiu CY, Huang SY, Peng YC, Tsai MH, Hua MC, Yao TC, Yeh KW, Huang JL. Maternal vitamin D levels are inversely related to allergic sensitization and atopic diseases in early childhood. Pediatr Allergy Immunol. 2015;26(4):337–43.
36. Hansen S, Maslova E, Strom M, Linneberg A, Halldorsson TI, Granstrom C, Dahl R, Hoffmann HJ, Olsen SF. The long-term programming effect of maternal 25-hydroxyvitamin D in pregnancy on allergic airway disease and lung function in offspring after 20 to 25 years of follow-up. J Allergy Clin Immunol. 2015;136(1):169–76. e162
37. Gazibara T, den Dekker HT, de Jongste JC, McGrath JJ, Eyles DW, Burne TH, Reiss IK, Franco OH, Tiemeier H, Jaddoe VW, et al. Associations of maternal and fetal 25-hydroxyvitamin D levels with childhood lung function and asthma: the generation R study. Clin Exp Allergy. 2016;46(2):337–46.
38. Baiz N, Dargent-Molina P, Wark JD, Souberbielle JC, Annesi-Maesano I. Cord serum 25-hydroxyvitamin D and risk of early childhood transient wheezing and atopic dermatitis. J Allergy Clin Immunol. 2014;133(1):147–53.
39. Camargo CA Jr, Thadhani R, Silvers KM, Pattemore PK, Espinola JA, Crane J, Dench C, Duignan M, Epton MJ, Fishwick D, et al. Cord-blood 25-hydroxyvitamin D levels and risk of respiratory infection, wheezing, and asthma. Pediatrics. 2011;127(1):e180–7.
40. Stelmach I, Majak P, Jerzynska J, Podlecka D, Stelmach W, Polanska K, Gromadzinska J, Wasowicz W, Hanke W. Cord serum 25-hydroxyvitamin D correlates with early childhood viral-induced wheezing. Respir Med. 2015; 109(1):38–43.
41. Chawes BL, Bonnelykke K, Jensen PF, Schoos AM, Heickendorff L, Bisgaard H. Cord blood 25(OH)-vitamin D deficiency and childhood asthma, allergy and eczema: the COPSAC2000 birth cohort study. PLoS One. 2014;9(6):e99856.
42. Junge KM, Bauer T, Geissler S, Hirche F, Thurmann L, Bauer M, Trump S, Bieg M, Weichenhan D, Gu L, et al. Increased vitamin D levels at birth and in early infancy increase offspring allergy risk-evidence for involvement of epigenetic mechanisms. J Allergy Clin Immunol. 2016;137(2):610–3.
43. Palmer DJ, Sullivan TR, Skeaff CM, Smithers LG, Makrides M. Higher cord blood 25-hydroxyvitamin D concentrations reduce the risk of early childhood eczema: in children with a family history of allergic disease. World Allergy Organ J. 2015;8(1):28.
44. Visness CM, Sandel MT, O'Connor G, Gern JE, Jaffee KF, Wood RA, Kattan M, Bloomberg GR, Dresen A, Gergen PJ, et al. Cord blood vitamin D concentrations are unrelated to atopy and wheeze in 2 diverse birth cohort studies. J Allergy Clin Immunol. 2015;136(4):1108–10. e1102
45. Wolsk HM, Harshfield BJ, Laranjo N, Carey VJ, O'Connor G, Sandel M, Strunk RC, Bacharier LB, Zeiger RS, Schatz M, et al. Vitamin D supplementation in pregnancy, prenatal 25(OH)D levels, race, and subsequent asthma or recurrent wheeze in offspring: secondary analyses from the vitamin D antenatal asthma reduction trial. J Allergy Clin Immunol. 2017;140(5):1423–29.e5.
46. Hollams EM, Teo SM, Kusel M, Holt BJ, Holt KE, Inouye M, De Klerk NH, Zhang G, Sly PD, Hart PH, et al. Vitamin D over the first decade and susceptibility to childhood allergy and asthma. J Allergy Clin Immunol. 2017; 139(2):472–81. e479
47. Wegienka G, Havstad S, Zoratti EM, Kim H, Ownby DR, Johnson CC. Association between vitamin D levels and allergy-related outcomes vary by race and other factors. J Allergy Clin Immunol. 2015;136(5):1309–1314 e1301-1304.
48. Miyake Y, Sasaki S, Tanaka K, Hirota Y. Dairy food, calcium and vitamin D intake in pregnancy, and wheeze and eczema in infants. Eur Respir J. 2010; 35(6):1228–34.
49. Devereux G, Litonjua AA, Turner SW, Craig LCA, McNeill G, Martindale S, Helms PJ, Seaton A, Weiss ST. Maternal vitamin D intake during pregnancy and early childhood wheezing. Am J Clin Nutr. 2007;85(3):853–9.
50. Allan KM, Prabhu N, Craig LC, McNeill G, Kirby B, McLay J, Helms PJ, Ayres JG, Seaton A, Turner SW, et al. Maternal vitamin D and E intakes during pregnancy are associated with asthma in children. Eur Respir J. 2015;45(4):1027–36.
51. Camargo CA Jr, Rifas-Shiman SL, Litonjua AA, Rich-Edwards JW, Weiss ST, Gold DR, Kleinman K, Gillman MW. Maternal intake of vitamin D during pregnancy and risk of recurrent wheeze in children at 3 y of age. Am J Clin Nutr. 2007;85(3):788–95.
52. Maslova E, Hansen S, Jensen CB, Thorne-Lyman AL, Strom M, Olsen SF. Vitamin D intake in mid-pregnancy and child allergic disease – a prospective study in 44,825 Danish mother-child pairs. BMC Pregnancy Childbirth. 2013;13(1):199.
53. Erkkola M, Kaila M, Nwaru BI, Kronberg-Kippila C, Ahonen S, Nevalainen J, Veijola R, Pekkanen J, Ilonen J, Simell O, et al. Maternal vitamin D intake during pregnancy is inversely associated with asthma and allergic rhinitis in 5-year-old children. Clin Exp Allergy. 2009;39(6):875–82.
54. Miyake Y, Tanaka K, Okubo H, Sasaki S, Arakawa M. Maternal consumption of dairy products, calcium, and vitamin D during pregnancy and infantile allergic disorders. Ann Allergy Asthma Immunol. 2014;113(1):82–7.
55. Anderson LN, Chen Y, Omand JA, Birken CS, Parkin PC, To T, Maguire JL. Vitamin D exposure during pregnancy, but not early childhood, is associated with risk of childhood wheezing. J Dev Orig Health Dis. 2015;6(4):308–16.
56. Back O, Blomquist HK, Hernell O, Stenberg B. Does vitamin D intake during infancy promote the development of atopic allergy? Acta Derm Venereol. 2009;89(1):28–32.
57. Hypponen E, Sovio U, Wjst M, Patel S, Pekkanen J, Hartikainen AL, Jarvelinb MR. Infant vitamin d supplementation and allergic conditions in adulthood: northern Finland birth cohort 1966. Ann N Y Acad Sci. 2004;1037:84–95.
58. von Mutius E, Martinez FD. Inconclusive results of randomized trials of prenatal vitamin D for asthma prevention in offspring: curbing the enthusiasm. JAMA. 2016;315(4):347–8.
59. Litonjua AA, Weiss ST. Is vitamin D deficiency to blame for the asthma epidemic? J Allergy Clin Immunol. 2007;120(5):1031–5.
60. Wjst M. Is vitamin D supplementation responsible for the allergy pandemic? Curr Opin Allergy Clin Immunol. 2012;12(3):257–62.
61. Autier P, Boniol M, Pizot C, Mullie P. Vitamin D status and ill health: a systematic review. Lancet Diabetes Endocrinol. 2014;2(1):76–89.
62. Burke H, Leonardi-Bee J, Hashim A, Pine-Abata H, Chen Y, Cook DG, Britton JR, McKeever TM. Prenatal and passive smoke exposure and incidence of asthma and wheeze: systematic review and meta-analysis. Pediatrics. 2012; 129(4):735–44.
63. King ME, Mannino DM, Holguin F. Risk factors for asthma incidence. A review of recent prospective evidence. Panminerva Med. 2004;46(2):97–110.
64. Kasahara AK, Singh RJ, Noymer A. Vitamin D (25OHD) serum seasonality in the United States. PLoS One. 2013;8(6):e65785.
65. Jones KS, Assar S, Vanderschueren D, Bouillon R, Prentice A, Schoenmakers I. Predictors of 25(OH)D half-life and plasma 25(OH)D concentration in the Gambia and the UK. Osteoporos Int. 2015;26(3):1137–46.
66. Pekkanen J, Pearce N. Defining asthma in epidemiological studies. Eur Respir J. 1999;14(4):951–7.
67. Canova C, Harris JM, Mills P, White C, Moffat S, Shread L, Cullinan P. Epidemiological measures of childhood asthma: cross-sectional and longitudinal consistency. Respir Med. 2012;106(9):1226–35.
68. Depner M, Fuchs O, Genuneit J, Karvonen AM, Hyvarinen A, Kaulek V, Roduit C, Weber J, Schaub B, Lauener R, et al. Clinical and epidemiologic phenotypes of childhood asthma. Am J Respir Crit Care Med. 2014;189(2):129–38.
69. Cornish RP, Henderson J, Boyd AW, Granell R, Van Staa T, Macleod J. Validating childhood asthma in an epidemiological study using linked electronic patient records. BMJ Open. 2014;4(4):e005345.
70. Cassim R, Russell MA, Lodge CJ, Lowe AJ, Koplin JJ, Dharmage SC. The role of circulating 25 hydroxyvitamin D in asthma: a systematic review. Allergy. 2015;70(4):339–54.

13

Cell distribution and cytokine levels in induced sputum from healthy subjects and patients with asthma after using different nebulizer techniques

Sinem Koc-Günel[1,2*], Ralf Schubert[1], Stefan Zielen[1] and Martin Rosewich[1]

Abstract

Background: Sputum induction is an important noninvasive method for analyzing bronchial inflammation in patients with asthma and other respiratory diseases. Most frequently, ultrasonic nebulizers are used for sputum induction, but breath-controlled nebulizers may target the small airways more efficiently. This treatment may produce a cell distribution similar to bronchoalveolar lavage (less neutrophils and more macrophages) and provide deeper insights into the underlying lung pathology. The goal of the study was to compare both types of nebulizer devices and their efficacy in inducing sputum to measure bronchial inflammation, i.e., cell composition and cytokines, in patients with mild allergic asthma and healthy controls.

Methods: The population of this study consisted of 20 healthy control subjects with a median age of 17 years, range: 8–25 years, and 20 patients with a median age of 12 years, range: 8–24 years, presenting with mild, controlled allergic asthma who were not administered an inhaled steroid treatment. We induced sputum in every individual using both devices on two separate days. The sputum weight, the cell composition and cytokine levels were analyzed using a cytometric bead assay (CBA) and by real-time quantitative PCR (qRT-PCR).

Results: We did not observe significant differences in the weight, cell distribution or cytokine levels in the sputum samples induced by both devices. In addition, the Bland-Altman correlation revealed good concordance of the cell distribution. As expected, eosinophils and IL-5 levels were significantly elevated in patients with asthma.

Conclusions: The hypothesis that sputum induction with a breath-controlled "smart" nebulizer is more efficient and different from an ultrasonic nebulizer was not confirmed. The Bland-Altman correlations showed good concordance when comparing the two devices.

Keywords: Induced sputum, Bronchial inflammation, Cell distribution, Smart nebulizer, Ultrasonic nebulizer, Allergic asthma, Cytokines

* Correspondence: sinem.koc-guenel@kgu.de
[1]Department for Children and Adolescents, Division for Allergology, Pneumology and Cystic Fibrosis, University Hospital Goethe University, Theodor-Stern-Kai 7, 60590 Frankfurt am Main, Germany
[2]Department of Internal Medicine, Division of Pneumology, University Hospital Goethe University, Theodor-Stern-Kai 7, Frankfurt am Main 60590, Germany

Background

Sputum induction is a well-known, noninvasive method for analyzing bronchial inflammation in patients with asthma and other respiratory diseases [1, 2]. Standardized induction protocols, including specifications for saline concentrations, the duration and time of induction, and laboratory requirements for sputum processing have been previously described for measuring cell composition, gene expression levels and cytokine patterns [1, 3–6].

Although sputum protocols have been developed to optimize the duration of inhalation and saline concentrations used, few protocols have compared different nebulizers [7, 8]. Davidson et al. compared a vibrating mesh nebulizer with an ultrasonic nebulizer in a previous study but did not detect any differences in sputum cell composition [9].

Several nebulizers are available, and the size of produced respirable particles is important for lung deposition. Conventional nebulizers deliver aerosol particles of approximately 5–10 μg in size, and most droplets are shed in the upper and larger airways. Ultrasonic nebulizers provide smaller droplets of 2–5 μg, and these droplets may be inhaled more easily in the lower airway. For ultrasonic nebulizers, such as the Omron nebulizer, a number of published studies have shown superior efficiency [10]. In addition to particle size, the timing and depth of inhalation are important factors for particle deposition in the lower airways. Recently, so-called smart nebulizers have been developed to more precisely define the breathing maneuvers of patients and target aerosol delivery to specific lung regions [11]. In addition, the use of a smart nebulizer to deliver dornase alpha was recently reported to significantly improve FEF 75% in children with stable cystic fibrosis [12].

Therefore, the technical standardization of sputum induction seems to become more important for more efficiently targeting the small airways and providing deeper insights into lung pathology, comparable to BAL. Based on this information, we investigated whether sputum induction with a smart nebulizer and its technical settings produce a sputum cell distribution similar to BAL. In the present study, we compared sputum weight, cell composition and cytokine levels following treatment with an optimized smart nebulizer and an ultrasonic nebulizer.

Methods

Patients

The study included 20 healthy control subjects with a median age of 17 years, range: 8–25 years, and 20 patients with a median age of 12 years, range: 8–24 years, who presented with mild, controlled allergic asthma but were not receiving an inhaled steroid treatment [Table 1]. The patients were recruited from the pediatric outpatient clinic of Goethe University, Frankfurt am Main, Germany, and control subjects were recruited by a public posting. The diagnosis of asthma was based on the Global Initiative for Asthma (GINA).

Table 1 Characteristics of patients with allergic asthma and controls

	Controls	Asthmatics
Number	(n = 20)	(n = 20)
Gender [f/m]	9/11	7/13
Age [age]*	17 (8–25)	13 (8–24)
eNO [ppb]*	15.0 (2.2–35.5)	64.4 (30.4–192.1)
Total IgE [IU/ml]*	72.5 (2–230)	292 (17–1927)
FEV1 [%]*	104.8 (90.1–136.6)	101.5 (51.5–130.5)
VCin [%]*	100.4 (70.7–115.6)	100.5 (69.9–136.2)
FEV1/VCmax [%]*	89.0 (76.25–99.26)	81.9 (51.74–98.15)
RV/TLC [%]*	106.3 (59.58–181.4)	121.2 (54.69–206.3)
MEF 25 [%]*	101.0 (62.7–203.3)	67.5 (20.8–151)

*Data are presented as medians and ranges

The inclusion criteria were: age between 6 and 25 years, informed consent, ability to perform lung function tests, well-controlled allergic asthma, and an exhaled NO (eNO) of eNO > 30 ppb. The exclusion criteria included an acute respiratory illness within four weeks prior to the investigation, other chronic infectious diseases, pregnancy, alcohol/drug/medication abuse and the inability to realize consequences or participation in another study. One patient was excluded due to an asthma exacerbation that was treated with systemic corticosteroids between visits 1 and 2, and another patient did not fulfill the inclusion criteria for allergic asthma. Additionally, one healthy subject did not complete the study because of an infection identified during visit 2.

After providing informed consent, each patient underwent two nonrandomized visits, each of which included a detailed physical examination to evaluate the present status and medical history. Lung function tests, airway reversibility testing and the eNO test were performed. Then, induced sputum was generated as described [13]. Sputum was induced with an ultrasonic nebulizer at visit 1. One week (7 + 5 days) later, at visit 2, lung function and eNO tests were repeated, and sputum was induced with a smart nebulizer.

Study design

This study was an open, nonblinded explorative study.

Lung function tests

The lung function tests and reversibility testing were performed using a body plethysmograph (VIASYS Healthcare GmbH, Hoechberg, Germany). The VCmax, FVC, FEV1, FEV1/VC, 25% of the maximum expiratory flow (MEF

25%), RV, and RV/TLC were registered. Lung function tests adhered to the standards of the American Thoracic Society und der European Respiratory Society.

Exhaled nitric oxide test

Measurements of exhaled NO were conducted using NIOX1 (Aerocrine, Solna, Sweden). NIOX1 measures the eNO in exhaled air, according to the American Thoracic Society guidelines [14]. This chemiluminescence gas analyzer is sensitive to eNO concentrations ranging from 1.5 to 200 ppb and exhibits a deviation from the mean value of + 2.5 ppb at NO 50 ppb or + 5% of the measured value at 150 ppb.

Description of nebulizers

The ultrasonic device (NE-U17, OMRON® Healthcare Europe, Hoofddorp, Netherlands) uses an ultrasonic frequency of approximately 1.7 MHz to nebulize a volume of up to 4 ml/minute and a particle size of 4.7 μm mass median aerodynamic diameter (MMAD). The airflow and nebulization volumes are adjustable. We used the maximum output of the device for our study, with an airflow velocity of 10 l/s and a nebulization volume of 10 ml/minutes.

The smart nebulizer (AKITA® Jet, Activaero, Gemünden/Wohra, Germany) controls the flow rate and inhalation volume and guides the patient through inhalation [11]. A smart card can be programmed to define the optimal dose of the inhaled particles. In addition, the smart nebulizer provides feedback when the patient, for example, inhales too quickly. The nebulizer creates an individual breathing pattern to optimize the drug delivery with a particle size of 3.8 μm, as measured by the manufacturer.

Nebulization with the ultrasonic nebulizer was tested in a mechanical lung by Activaero GmbH in Gemünden/Wohra, Germany to compare the ultrasonic nebulizer with the smart nebulizer. Measurements showed a delivery of 4 ml NaCl in the lung during an inhalation period of 7 min. The smart nebulizer outputs for our study were adjusted by programming a smart card based on the results, and a peripheral deposition of the aerosol was coded.

Sputum collection, processing and cell analysis

The patients and controls inhaled saline solutions of 3, 4 and 5% every 7 min, as recently described [13, 15]. During visit 1, subjects inhaled through the ultrasonic nebulizer, and at visit 2, they inhaled through the optimized smart nebulizer.

Shortly after inhalation, the sputum was quantified, and sputum plugs were selected from the samples. Then, 4 × 0.1% (weight/volume) dithiothreitol (DTT) was added, and the samples were processed for 15 min on ice before the subsequent addition of 2 x weight/volume of phosphate-buffered saline (PBS). After centrifuging each sample for 10 min at 790 x *g*, the supernatants were removed by pipette and stored at − 80 °C until further protein analyses. The slides used to analyze cellular differentiation were generated from these samples. Four hundred cells per slide were identified using the Leucodiff 800plus instrument (Instrumentation Laboratory, Bedford, MA, USA), and the percentages of neutrophils, lymphocytes, eosinophils, and macrophages were quantified [13].

Cytometric bead array (CBA)

The concentrations of four cytokines, IL-5, IL-8, TNF-α and IFN-γ, in sputum samples were determined using the BD™ CBA Flex Set System (BD Biosciences-PharMingen, San Diego, CA, USA). Each BD™ CBA Flex Set contained a one-bead population with distinct fluorescence intensity and both the appropriate phycoerythrin (PE) detection reagent and the standard. The tests were performed according to the manufacturer's instructions, and samples were tested in duplicate. We added the same concentration of DTT (0.025%) as in the sputum supernatant to the standard curve and the enzyme immunoassay buffer as previously described to analyze the cytokine levels ([13, 15]). The lower detection limits of the cytokines were as follows: IL-8, 1.2 pg/ml; IL-5, 1.1 pg/ml; TNF-α, 0.7 pg/ml and IFN-γ, 1.8 pg/ml.

RNA extraction

Total RNA was extracted from induced sputum samples using the Qiagen RNeasy Mini Kits (Qiagen, Hamburg, Deutschland), according to the manufacturer's instructions. All sputum plugs were processed with RNAprotect cell reagent and PBS, according to the manufacturer's instructions. Before reverse transcription, a DNase treatment was performed using DNase I (Qiagen, Hilden, Germany), as described recently ([15]). The processed RNA samples were supplemented with 9 μL of a master mix of 1 μL of iScript Reverse Transcriptase (Bio-Rad, Hercules, CA, USA), a random hexamer and oligo-dT mix, 4 μL of 10 × iScript RT buffer and 4 μL of nuclease-free water. Then, samples were incubated in a thermocycler at 25 °C for 5 min for an initial incubation step, at 42 °C for 30 min and finally at 85 °C for 5 min.

Real-time qRT-PCR

Transcripts were quantified using two-step real-time RT-PCR with an Eppendorf Mastercycler RealPlex S detection system (Eppendorf, Hamburg-Eppendorf, Germany) in Greiner 25 μL 96-well reaction plates (Greiner, Germany). The expression of the IL-5, IL-8, TNF-α and IFN-γ mRNAs was normalized to the endogenous control glyceraldehyde-3-phosphate-dehydrogenase (GAPDH), and the relative quantification and calculation of range of confidence was performed using the comparative threshold cycle (2 – ΔΔCt) method (relative gene expression). All amplifications were performed in at least duplicate reactions. The expression data and statistical analysis of the genes involved in immune cells and inflammatory markers were analyzed as previously described [13, 15].

Data analysis

The data were analyzed with Microsoft Excel (Microsoft Corporation, Redmond, USA), GraphPad Prism 5.0 (GraphPad Software Inc., La Jolla, CA, USA) and BIAS for Windows 11.0 software (Epsilon-Verlag GbR, Hochheim Darmstadt, Germany). The results are presented as medians ± ranges. The differences between the nebulizers were calculated using the Wilcoxon matched-pairs test and the Bland-Altman method. The differences between the patients with asthma and the controls were calculated using the Mann-Whitney test.

Results

Sample characteristics

The demographic and clinical characteristics are shown in Table 1. The study population comprised 20 healthy control subjects and 20 patients with mild, controlled allergic asthma who were not receiving steroid treatment. Eighteen patients and 19 healthy subjects completed the study, according to the protocol.

Sputum

Sputum weight

The analysis of the sputum weight [g] did not reveal statistically significant differences between the two devices. The median preprocessing sputum weight of the controls was 5.64 [g] (2.77–22.09) at V1 and 6.60 [g] (2.72–14.10) at V2. For patients with asthma, the median preprocessing sputum weight was 5.14 [g] (2.55–8.09) at V1 and 4.97 [g] (2.64–10.52) at V2. The median weight of the induced sputum in the group of controls was 3.19 [g] (1.22–6.6) at V1 and 3.85 [g] (1.89–7.82) at V2. In patients with asthma, the median weight was 2.90 [g] (1.71–5.03) at V1 and 3.18 [g] (1.82–7.19) at V2 [Fig. 1a and b].

Sputum cell count

Total cell counts [106 cells/ml] were compared between the controls and patients with asthma and between the nebulizers. A difference in the total cell counts in induced sputum was not observed between the devices in either group (controls: $p = 0.41$; patients with asthma: $p = 0.33$) [Fig. 2].

Sputum cell composition

Each cell subtype was compared between the sputum collected with the ultrasonic and smart nebulizers. A comparison of the percentage of macrophages after induction with the ultrasonic or the smart nebulizer did not show significant differences in either group (controls: $p = 0.605$; patients with asthma: $p = 0.737$). Additionally, a significant difference in the percentage of neutrophils after the use of the different devices was not observed in either group (controls: $p = 0.670$; patients with asthma: $p = 0.816$). The percentages of eosinophils did not differ between sputum collected with the different devices (controls: $p = 0.344$; patients with asthma: $p = 0.224$), but the percentage of eosinophils differed significantly between patients with asthma and controls based on the inclusion criteria ($p < 0.0001$ at V1; $p = 0.0003$ at V2). The results are shown in Fig. 3.

Estimation of cytokine levels

The cytokine levels measured by qRT-PCR and CBA were compared between the devices. No significant differences were observed for levels of the cytokine proteins and mRNAs between the sputum collected with the two devices. As expected, qRT-PCR revealed that patients with asthma had significantly higher levels of IL-5 than controls ($p = 0.0360$ at V1 and $p = 0.0115$ at V2) [Fig. 4]. IL-8 and IFN-γ expression (IL-8 in controls $p = 0.420$ vs. IL-8 in patients with asthma $p = 0.7439$ and IFN-γ in controls $p = 0.695$ vs. IFN-γ in patients with asthma $p = 0.327$) were not different between the patient groups. In addition, no differences in cytokine levels measured using CBA were identified between the two nebulizers.

Bland-Altman correlation

The correlation between both devices was analyzed using the Bland-Altman method, which compares differences in two methods using their means. We compared the cell counts obtained after the use of both devices. A small bias of – 0.2441 and a SD of 9.614 were found for the macrophage population, and a bias of – 0.5075 and a SD of 8.016 were identified for the neutrophils. The results are shown in Table 2.

Discussion

Because sputum induction is a noninvasive method for evaluating bronchial inflammation, particularly for diagnostic research purposes, the induction methods, including devices and their technical settings, must be standardized [16]. For this purpose, the sputum weight, cell composition and cytokine levels were compared in patients using the ultrasonic and smart nebulizers. Interestingly, we did not observe differences between the different sputum induction devices.

The total deposition of aerosols in the lungs depends on the particle size, breathing pattern, and lung volume [17]. In addition, factors such as saline concentrations and the duration of inhalation influence both the cell distribution and the quality of sputum [18–20]. Several studies have reported an increasing percentage of macrophages for longer time intervals of sputum induction, reflecting a cell distribution consistent with the peripheral airways [18].

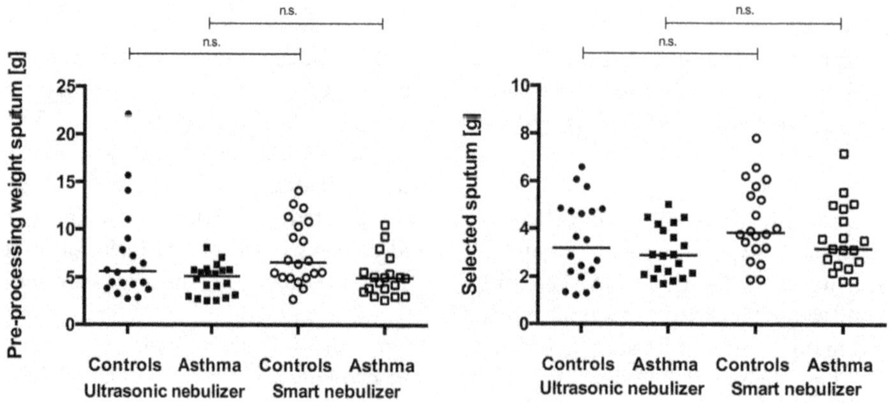

Fig. 1 Sputum weight produced using different nebulizers. Data are presented as medians. No differences were observed in preprocessed sputum from the controls ($p = 0.522$) and patients with ($p = 0.298$) [Fig. 1a] or for selected sputum from controls ($p = 0.143$) and patients with asthma ($p = 0.113$) [Fig. 1b] between the ultrasonic and smart nebulizers

According to the study by Gershman et al., shorter induction periods produce a higher percentage of neutrophils, which represent the large airways, but longer induction periods result in an increasing percentage of macrophages, which are most likely derived from the small airways [5]. More recently, smart nebulizers have been able to guide patients to inhale slowly and deeply to more effectively deposit inhaled particles in the small airways [12, 21, 22].

However, the hypothesis that sputum induction with a smart nebulizer, here, the Akita Jet, and its technical settings produce a sputum cell distribution similar to BAL was not confirmed in our study. In addition, significant differences in any of the investigated parameters, including gene expression levels and cytokine patterns, were not observed between the two devices. One criticism is that the nonrandomized design of our study may induce a small learning effect in favor for the Akita Jet results. However, when we considered the difference in handling of both nebulizers, the learning effect was neglected. The Bland-Altman correlations showed good concordance when comparing the two devices. This finding is contradictory to previous studies showing that smart nebulizers are more efficient drug delivery devices that deposit larger amounts of the inhaled dose in the small airways [12, 21, 23, 24].

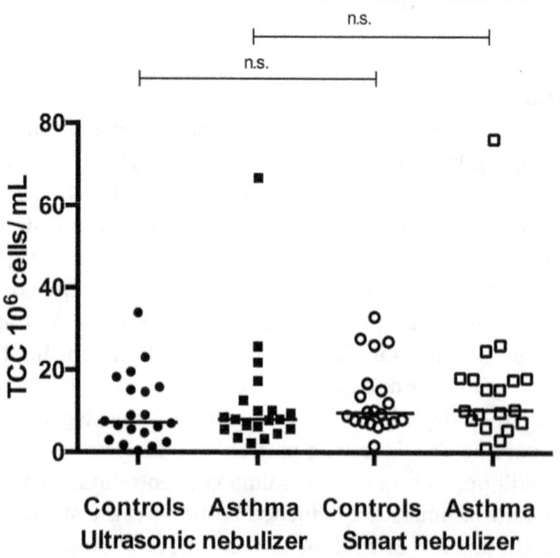

Fig. 2 Total cell counts obtained using different nebulizers. Data are presented as medians. In the controls, $p = 0.325$ when comparing ultrasonic and smart nebulizers. In patients with asthma, $p = 0.275$

One possible explanation for this discrepancy is related to the saline particles. Hygroscopic particles such as NaCl tend to increase in size when passing through the lung due to humidity, thus limiting the diameter for the minimum deposition in the peripheral lung [25]. Additionally, the initial diameter of the particle sizes creates a difference in deposition [25]. Although the use of small particle sizes (0.1 μm) shows a similar distribution, regardless of the presence of nonhygroscopic or hygroscopic particles, because their primary deposition mechanism is diffusion, the use of larger sizes (1 μm) alters the deposition due to particle growth, thereby altering the deposition pattern [25]. Further investigations are necessary to evaluate the effect of NaCl particle sizes on sputum induction.

Conversely, the inhalation of an aerosol, regardless of whether it is deposited in central or peripheral airways, must not lead to a higher expectoration of sputum and inflammatory cells. Because the underlying pathological mechanism of asthma involves hyperplasia of the smooth muscle, the expectoration of peripheral sputum is likely limited due to decreases in the diameter of the lumen, which might retain secretions. Indeed, Pavia et al. have identified a positive correlation between patients' FEV1 and the depth of deposition [26–28]. In addition, cough is

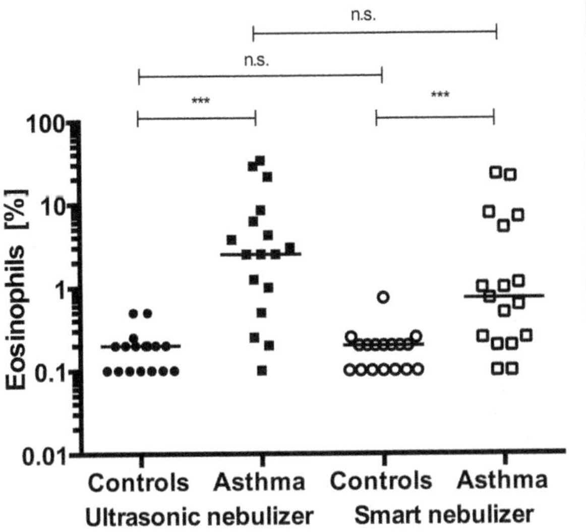

Fig. 3 Percentage of eosinophils obtained after the use of different nebulizers. Data are presented as medians. Zero values were increased to 0, 1/0, or 2 for visualization. In the controls, $p = 0.670$ when comparing ultrasonic and smart nebulizers. In the patients with asthma, $p = 0.816$. The percentage of eosinophils was significantly elevated in patients with asthma compared to that in controls

less effective in the small airways of the lung, as shown in the study by Alexis et al. [29]. The authors showed that induced sputum samples are predominantly derived from the central airways, and little or no clearance is associated with sputum induction when a radio aerosol was targeted to the alveolar region.

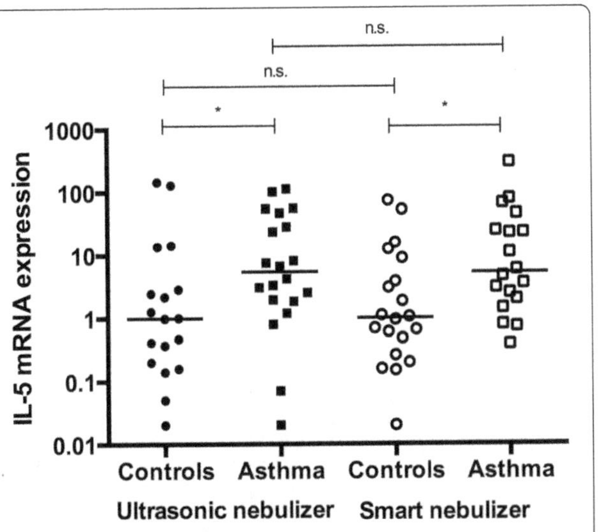

Fig. 4 IL-5 mRNA expression measured after the use of different nebulizers. Data are presented as medians. In the controls, $p = 0.3927$ when comparing the Omron and Akita nebulizers. In the patients with asthma, $p = 0.4307$. qRT-PCR revealed a significant elevation in IL-5 levels in patients with asthma compared with levels in controls

Table 2 Bland-Altman analysis of both nebulizers

	Macrophages	Neutrophils	All cell types
Bias	−0.2441	−0.5075	− 0.001625
SD of bias	9.614	8.016	6.153
95% limits of agreement			
From	−19.09	−16.22	−12.06
To	18.60	15.20	12.06

Finally, breathing patterns have been shown to influence lung deposition in several studies [25, 27, 30]. Although the subjects were instructed to avoid shallow breathing and to take deep breaths in each session, the breathing patterns were not identical for both nebulizers. During inhalation with the smart nebulizer, the subjects made small pauses due to the previously programmed breathing pattern, but the subjects inhaled continuously when using the ultrasonic nebulizer. A tidal breathing pattern that precludes any deep breaths during inhalation may enhance the degree of induced bronchoconstriction [31]. In contrast, the smart nebulizer guided subjects to pause and take the mouth piece out to open up the lungs using a deeper inhalation strategy. Surprisingly, although breathing patterns were optimized by the smart nebulizer, the expectorated sputum did not differ sonic nebulizer.
from that samples produced after the use of the ultra-

Conclusions

In conclusion, we did not detect differences in sputum induction between the ultrasonic nebulizer and smart nebulizer. The sputum weight, the cell composition and cytokine levels showed good concordance when comparing the two devices. In particular, for academic purposes, additional investigations aiming to standardize the technical settings of sputum induction should be performed in the future.

Abbreviations

BAL : Bronchoalveolar lavage; BIAS: Bias function; CBA: Cytometric bead array; DNA : Deoxyribonucleic acid; DTT: Dithiothreitol; ECP: Eosinophil cationic protein; EnO: Exhaled nitric oxide; FEV1: Forced expiratory volume in 1 s; FEV1/VC: Tiffeneau index; FVC: Forced vital capacity (FVC); IFN- γ: Interferon gamma; IL-5: Interleukin-5; IL-8: Interleukin-8; MEF25 : 25% of the maximal expiratory flow; MMAD: Mass median aerodynamic diameter; mRNA: Messenger ribonucleic acid; NaCl: Sodium chloride; PBS: Phosphate-buffered saline; PCR: Polymerase chain reaction; RV: Residual volume; RV/TLC: Functional residual volume; SD: Standard deviation; V1: Visit 1; V2: Visit 2; VC: Vital capacity

Acknowledgements

All equipment for the Akita Jet smart nebulizer was supplied free of charge by Activaero GmbH, Gemünden/Wohra, Germany.

Authors' contributions

SKG recruited patients, performed the experiments, generated data from the research database, analyzed the data and wrote the manuscript. RS analyzed the data, reviewed the manuscript and provided a scientific critique of the data. SZ and MR conceived and designed the study, analyzed the data and wrote and critically reviewed the manuscript. All authors read and approved the final manuscript.

Consent for publication
Not applicable.

Competing interests
The authors declare that they have no competing interests. No author has a financial relationship with a commercial entity with an interest in the subject of this manuscript.

References

1. Eickmeier O, Huebner M, Herrmann E, Zissler U, Rosewich M, Baer PC, et al. Sputum biomarker profiles in cystic fibrosis (CF) and chronic obstructive pulmonary disease (COPD) and association between pulmonary function. Cytokine. 2010;50(2):152–7.
2. Araujo L, Moreira A, Palmares C, Beltrao M, Fonseca J, Delgado L. Induced sputum in children: success determinants, safety, and cell profiles. J Investig Allergol Clin Immunol. 2011;21(3):216–21.
3. Pizzichini E, Pizzichini MM, Efthimiadis A, Evans S, Morris MM, Squillace D, et al. Indices of airway inflammation in induced sputum: reproducibility and validity of cell and fluid-phase measurements. Am J Respir Crit Care Med. 1996;154(2 Pt 1):308–17.
4. Fahy JV, Wong H, Liu J, Boushey HA. Comparison of samples collected by sputum induction and bronchoscopy from asthmatic and healthy subjects. Am J Respir Crit Care Med. 1995;152(1):53–8.
5. Gershman NH, Liu H, Wong HH, Liu JT, Fahy JV. Fractional analysis of sequential induced sputum samples during sputum induction: evidence that different lung compartments are sampled at different time points. J Allergy Clin Immunol. 1999;104(2 Pt 1):322–8.
6. Reinhardt N, Chen CI, Loppow D, Schink T, Kleinau I, Jorres RA, et al. Cellular profiles of induced sputum in children with stable cystic fibrosis: comparison with BAL. Eur Respir J. 2003;22(3):497–502.
7. Holz O, Richter K, Jorres RA, Speckin P, Mucke M, Magnussen H. Changes in sputum composition between two inductions performed on consecutive days. Thorax. 1998;53(2):83-6.
8. Gershman NH, Wong HH, Liu JT, Mahlmeister MJ, Fahy JV. Comparison of two methods of collecting induced sputum in asthmatic subjects. Eur Respir J. 1996;9(12):2448–53.
9. Davidson WJ, Dennis J, The S, Litoski B, Pieron C, Leigh R. Identification and validation of nebulized aerosol devices for sputum induction. Can Respir J. 2014;21(2):101–6.
10. Harvey CJ, O'Doherty MJ, Page CJ, Thomas SH, Nunan TO, Treacher DF. Comparison of jet and ultrasonic nebulizer pulmonary aerosol deposition during mechanical ventilation. Eur Respir J. 1997;10(4):905–9.
11. Scheuch G, Siekmeier R. Novel approaches to enhance pulmonary delivery of proteins and peptides. J Physiol Pharmacol. 2007;58(Suppl 5 (Pt 2)):615–25.
12. Bakker EM, Volpi S, Salonini E, van der Wiel-Kooij EC, Sintnicolaas CJ, Hop WC, et al. Improved treatment response to dornase alfa in cystic fibrosis patients using controlled inhalation. Eur Respir J. 2011;38(6):1328–35.
13. Rosewich M, Zissler UM, Kheiri T, Voss S, Eickmeier O, Schulze J, et al. Airway inflammation in children and adolescents with bronchiolitis obliterans. Cytokine. 2015;73(1):156–62.
14. ATS/ERS recommendations for standardized procedures for the online and offline measurement of exhaled lower respiratory nitric oxide and nasal nitric oxide, 2005. American journal of respiratory and critical care medicine. 2005;171(8):912–30.
15. Schulze J, Voss S, Zissler U, Rose MA, Zielen S, Schubert R. Airway responses and inflammation in subjects with asthma after four days of repeated high-single-dose allergen challenge. Respir Res. 2012;13:78.
16. Kips JC, Inman MD, Jayaram L, Bel EH, Parameswaran K, Pizzichini MM, et al. The use of induced sputum in clinical trials. Eur Respir J Suppl. 2002;37:47s–50s.
17. Heyder J. Deposition of inhaled particles in the human respiratory tract and consequences for regional targeting in respiratory drug delivery. Proc Am Thorac Soc. 2004;1(4):315-20.
18. Holz O, Jorres RA, Koschyk S, Speckin P, Welker L, Magnussen H. Changes in sputum composition during sputum induction in healthy and asthmatic subjects. Clin Exp Allergy. 1998;28(3):284–92.
19. Belda J, Hussack P, Dolovich M, Efthimiadis A, Hargreave FE. Sputum induction: effect of nebulizer output and inhalation time on cell counts and fluid-phase measures. Clin Exp Allergy. 2001;31(11):1740–4.
20. Bacci E, Cianchetti S, Paggiaro PL, Carnevali S, Bancalari L, Dente FL, et al. Comparison between hypertonic and isotonic saline-induced sputum in the evaluation of airway inflammation in subjects with moderate asthma. Clin Exp Allergy. 1996;26(12):1395–400.
21. Brand P, Beckmann H, Maas Enriquez M, Meyer T, Mullinger B, Sommerer K, et al. Peripheral deposition of alpha1-protease inhibitor using commercial inhalation devices. Eur Respir J. 2003;22(2):263–7.
22. Brand P, Schulte M, Wencker M, Herpich CH, Klein G, Hanna K, et al. Lung deposition of inhaled alpha1-proteinase inhibitor in cystic fibrosis and alpha1-antitrypsin deficiency. Eur Respir J. 2009;34(2):354–60.
23. Brand P, Meyer T, Haussermann S, Schulte M, Scheuch G, Bernhard T, et al. Optimum peripheral drug deposition in patients with cystic fibrosis. J Aerosol Med. 2005;18(1):45–54.
24. Griese M, Ramakers J, Krasselt A, Starosta V, Van Koningsbruggen S, Fischer R, et al. Improvement of alveolar glutathione and lung function but not oxidative state in cystic fibrosis. Am J Respir Crit Care Med. 2004;169(7):822–8.
25. Xu GB, Yu CP. Theoretical lung deposition of hygroscopic NaCl aerosols. Aerosol Sci Technol. 1985;4(4):455–61.
26. Pavia D, Thomson ML, Clarke SW, Shannon HS. Effect of lung function and mode of inhalation on penetration of aerosol into the human lung. Thorax. 1977;32(2):194–7.
27. Labiris NR, Dolovich MB. Pulmonary drug delivery. Part I: physiological factors affecting therapeutic effectiveness of aerosolized medications. Br J Clin Pharmacol. 2003;56(6):588–99.
28. Smaldone GC, Perry RJ, Bennett WD, Messina MS, Zwang J, Ilowite J. Interpretation of '24 hour lung retention' in studies of mucociliary clearance. J Aerosol Med Pulm Drug Deliv. 2009;1(1):11–20.
29. Alexis NE, Hu SC, Zeman K, Alter T, Bennett WD. Induced sputum derives from the central airways: confirmation using a radiolabeled aerosol bolus delivery technique. Am J Respir Crit Care Med. 2001;164(10 Pt 1):1964–70.
30. Zanen P, Go LT, Lammers JW. The optimal particle size for beta-adrenergic aerosols in mild asthmatics. Int J Pharm. 1994;107:211–7.
31. Fish JE, Ankin MG, Kelly JF, Peterman VI. Regulation of bronchomotor tone by lung inflation in asthmatic and nonasthmatic subjects. J Appl Physiol Respir Environ Exerc Physiol. 1981;50(5):1079–86.

14

Agreement in reporting of asthma by parents or offspring – the RHINESSA generation study

Ingrid N. Kuiper[1*], Cecilie Svanes[2,1], Bryndis Benediktsdottir[3], Randi J. Bertelsen[1,11], Lennart Bråbäck[4], Shyamali C. Dharmage[5], Mathias Holm[6], Christer Janson[7], Rain Jõgi[8], Andrei Malinovschi[9], Melanie Matheson[5], Jesús Martínez Moratalla[10], Francisco Gómez Real[11,12], José Luis Sánchez-Ramos[13], Vivi Schlünssen[14,15], Signe Timm[14] and Ane Johannessen[2,1]

Abstract

Background: Self-report questionnaires are commonly used in epidemiology, but may be susceptible to misclassification, especially if answers are given on behalf of others, e.g. children or parents. The aim was to determine agreement and analyse predictors of disagreement in parents' reports of offspring asthma, and in offspring reports of parents' asthma.

Methods: In the Respiratory Health in Northern Europe, Spain and Australia (RHINESSA) generation study, 6752 offspring (age range 18–51 years) and their parents (age range 39–66 years) reported their own and each other's asthma status. Agreement between asthma reports from offspring and parents was determined by calculating sensitivity, specificity, positive and negative predictive value and Cohen's kappa. The participants' own answers regarding themselves were defined as the gold standard. To investigate predictors for disagreement logistic regression analyses were performed to obtain odds ratios (OR) with 95% confidence intervals (CI) for sex, smoking status, education, comorbidity and severity of asthma.

Results: Agreement was good for parental report of offspring early onset asthma (< 10 years, Cohen's kappa 0.72) and moderate for offspring later onset asthma (Cohen's kappa 0.46). Specificity was 0.99 for both, and sensitivity was 0.68 and 0.36, respectively. For offspring report of maternal and paternal asthma the agreement was good (Cohen's kappa 0.69 and 0.68), specificity was 0.96 and 0.97, and sensitivity was 0.72 and 0.68, respectively. The positive predictive value (PPV) was lowest for offspring report of maternal asthma (0.75), and highest for parents' report of early onset asthma in the offspring (0.83). The negative predictive value (NPV) was high for all four groups (0.94–0.97). In multivariate analyses current smokers (OR = 1.46 [95% CI 1.05, 2.02]) and fathers (OR = 1.31 [95% CI 1.08, 1.59]) were more likely to report offspring asthma incorrectly. Offspring wheeze was associated with reporting parental asthma incorrectly (OR = 1.60 [95% CI 1.21, 2.11]), both under- and over reporting.

Conclusions: Asthma reports across generations show moderate to good agreement, making information from other generations a useful tool in the absence of direct reports.

Keywords: Agreement, Validation, Asthma, Questionnaire, Self-report, Transgenerational

* Correspondence: ingrid.kuiper@gmail.com; ingrid.nordeide.kuiper@helse-bergen.no
[1]Department of Occupational Medicine, Haukeland University Hospital, N-5021 Bergen, Norway
Full list of author information is available at the end of the article

Background

Asthma is the most common non-communicable disease among children and one of the most prevalent chronic diseases worldwide [1, 2]. The World Health Organization [3] estimated in 2011 that 235 million people suffer from asthma, but later studies have indicated numbers as high as 300 million and projected that the worldwide prevalence will increase to 400 million by 2025 [4].

The investigation of asthma is complex. Questionnaires are often preferred in epidemiological studies to determine disease occurrence because they are cost-efficient and simple to perform compared to clinical examination. Questionnaire data on the prevalence of asthma have been used for epidemiological research since the mid 1960s. In 1995 the International Study of Asthma and Allergies in Childhood [5] developed a standardized questionnaire to improve the investigation of asthma in an epidemiological setting [5–7]. Even though clinical examination has been regarded as the gold standard for assessing asthma, recent studies show that questionnaires are a useful epidemiological tool, being reasonably valid [8–10].

Nevertheless, self-reported information is susceptible to misclassification such as recall bias, and it may be particularly susceptible to misclassification if participants are asked to provide information on behalf of others, for example their children or their parents [11, 12]. At the same time, in absence of direct reports, asthma reports on behalf of family members can be highly valuable in a clinical setting if the patient cannot report on behalf of himself/herself or in absence of prior patient history. However, validity of such intergenerational reports with regard to asthma has been poorly investigated, mostly focusing on current asthma status asked at the same time, and only including young children and adolescents [13, 14]. With an increasing interest in intergenerational risk factors [15–19] more attention should be given to validate this kind of information across generations.

The Respiratory Health in Northern Europe, Spain and Australia generation study (RHINESSA) uses questionnaires, interviews, and clinical examinations to study asthma and lung health throughout the lifespan and across generations. Participants are asked to provide information about themselves as well as their children and parents. To underpin the research of RHINESSA and to shed light on this important part of epidemiological methodology, the aim of the present paper was to assess agreement between parental report of offspring asthma as compared to offspring's own report, to assess agreement between offspring's report of parent's asthma as compared to parents' own report, and to investigate predictors for discrepant answers.

Methods

Study design and population

This agreement study compares questionnaires about asthma from two generations. The primary sources of data are parents from the Respiratory Health in Northern Europe study (RHINE, www.rhine.nu) and the European Community Respiratory Health Survey (ECRHS, www.ecrhs.org) and their offspring included in the RHINESSA study (www.rhinessa.net). The parent and offspring pairs provided information on asthma status regarding both themselves and each other.

Parent population

RHINE is a prospective questionnaire-based cohort study comprising subjects from seven Northern European centres: Reykjavik (Iceland), Bergen (Norway), Umea, Uppsala and Gothenburg (Sweden), Aarhus (Denmark) and Tartu (Estonia). All subjects participated in stage 1 of the ECRHS I in 1990, together with many other centres, among others Melbourne (Australia) and Huelva and Albacete (Spain) [20, 21]. Both ECRHS and RHINE had follow-ups after 10 and 20 years, and have investigated incidence, prevalence and risk factors for respiratory diseases, allergies and symptoms related to asthma and chronic obstructive pulmonary disease (COPD) throughout this time period. Response rate in RHINE III was 61%. The ECRHS subjects from the Spanish and Australian study centres filled in the ECRHS stage 3 screening questionnaire; which includes identical questions as in RHINE III for all characteristics needed in the present study.

Offspring population

In the period 2013–2015 questionnaires were sent to all adult offspring (> 18 years) of parents from the RHINE centres and the Spanish and Australian ECRHS centres, and a sub-sample was invited for clinical examination. The questionnaires were web-based in all centres except Sweden where they used postal questionnaires. Overall response rate was 33.5%, varying across centres from 18.6% in Tartu to 73.7% in Melbourne (See Additional file 1: Table S1).

Predictors and outcomes

The main outcome in this agreement study was physician diagnosed asthma self-reported by the participants. Reports of one's own asthma were "doctors-diagnosed asthma" while reports of asthma in others were "ever asthma". In more detail, the asthma outcomes were built on the following wordings:

> Parents reported doctor-diagnosed asthma about themselves by answering yes to the questions "Do you

have or have you ever had asthma?" and "Has it been confirmed by a medical doctor?"

Parents reported asthma about their offspring by answering yes to the questions "For each child, please tick yes if they had asthma before 10 years" and/or "For each child, please tick yes if they had asthma after 10 years". The former was classified as early onset asthma in the offspring, while the latter was classified as late onset asthma.

Offspring reported doctor-diagnosed asthma about themselves by answering yes to the questions "Do you have or have you ever had asthma?" and "Has it been confirmed by a medical doctor?"

Offspring were also asked how old they were when they first experienced asthma symptoms.

Offspring reported asthma about their parents defined by answering yes to the questions "Did your mother ever suffer from asthma?" and "Did your father ever suffer from asthma?". Questionnaires are available from www.rhinessa.net.

A discrepant asthma report by parents was defined as parents reporting absence of asthma in their offspring when the offspring report presence of asthma, or parents reporting presence of asthma in their offspring when the offspring state they do not have asthma. In the same manner, a discrepant asthma report by offspring was defined as offspring reporting absence of asthma in their parents when the parents report presence of asthma, or offspring reporting presence of asthma in their parents when the parents themselves state they do not have asthma.

Predictors for discrepant reports between parent and offspring pairs were investigated for the following covariates in each generation: smoking status (never-, ex- or current smoker), education (primary school, secondary school or college/university), respiratory symptoms (wheeze, wheeze with shortness of breath, awoken with tightness in chest, awoken with attack of cough in the past 12 months and currently taking medication) and comorbidities (hypertension, stroke, ischemic heart disease, diabetes mellitus, COPD and serious respiratory infections before the age of 5 years).

Statistical analyses

All analyses were performed using Stata version 14.0.

The overall agreement between asthma reports from offspring and parents was calculated by Cohen's kappa. The following interpretation categories were used: poor agreement, < 0.2; fair, 0.21–0.40; moderate, 0.41–0.60; good, 0.61–0.80; and very good, 0.81–1.00 [22]. Sensitivity, specificity and predictive values were calculated using the participants' own answers regarding themselves as the golden standard. Descriptive analyses and estimations of Cohen's kappa, sensitivity, specificity and predictive values were performed stratified by sex to investigate any specific differences between mothers and fathers, and between daughters and sons.

We performed univariate logistic regressions with each covariate as predictor and discrepant report (yes/no) in parent-offspring pairs as outcome. The participants' own answers regarding themselves were considered the gold standard also in these analyses. Significant predictors ($p < 0.05$) from the univariate analyses were carried forward to multivariate logistic regression. Separate models were constructed for discrepant reports by parents and discrepant reports by offspring. In addition, the multivariate analyses were adjusted for study centre and sibling status (siblings in RHINESSA/no siblings in RHINESSA).

Ethical approval

In all study centres written informed consent was obtained from each participant, and the study was approved by regional committees of medical research ethics in each study centre according to national legislations.

Results

Reports of 6752 offspring and their parents who had answered questions regarding their own and each other's asthma status were included from the ten study centres. Table 1 shows the characteristics of the study population by parents and offspring. A slight majority of the population was female. The mean age for the mothers and fathers were 54.0 (±6.5) and 54.7 (±6.1) respectively. More mothers than fathers and more daughters than sons reported having asthma. For the offspring, mean age was 30 years and did not differ significantly between males and females. More mothers than fathers and more daughters than sons had obtained university education. Slightly more mothers than fathers were current smokers, whereas in offspring more sons than daughters smoked. The reports of respiratory symptoms were comparable across gender for the parents, but in the offspring, all respiratory symptoms, except the symptoms awoken with attack of breathlessness and wheeze with shortness of breath, were significantly higher for the daughters (Table 1).

Figure 1 summarizes offspring early/late onset asthma and the corresponding parent report (Fig. 1a and b), as well as paternal and maternal asthma and the corresponding offspring report (Fig. 1c and d). The vast majority of parents answered correctly concerning their offspring's asthma status: in 4798 (90%) of the reports on early onset asthma, both parents and offspring

Table 1 Study population characteristics, 5907 parents and 6752 offspring included in the RHINESSA generation study

Characteristics	Parents (RHINE/ECRHS)			Children (RHINESSA)		
	Mother N (%)	Father N (%)	P[a]	Daughter N (%)	Son N (%)	P[a]
N (%)	3377 (57)	2530 (43)		3910 (58)	2842 (42)	
Albacete	39 (57)	30 (43)		39 (53)	34 (47)	
Bergen	593 (53)	518 (47)		706 (60)	480 (40)	
Gothenburg	413 (56)	322 (44)		491 (53)	439 (47)	
Huelva	42 (69)	19 (31)		44 (64)	25 (36)	
Melbourne	96 (55)	80 (45)		42 (62)	26 (38)	
Reykjavik	409 (55)	328 (45)		543 (61)	342 (39)	
Tartu	205 (68)	97 (32)		177 (60)	119 (40)	
Umea	629 (60)	423 (40)		735 (57)	545 (43)	
Uppsala	602 (59)	420 (41)		713 (56)	556 (44)	
Aarhus	349 (54)	293 (46)		420 (60)	276 (40)	
Mean age (SD)	54.0 (6.5)	54.7 (6.1)	**< 0.001**	30.3 (7.7)	30.4 (7.8)	0.930
Asthma (%)	478 (14)	292 (12)	**0.004**	671 (17)	420 (15)	**0.008**
Smoking			**0.009**			**< 0.001**
Never-smokers	1496 (46)	1155 (47)		2602 (67)	1942 (69)	
Ex-smokers	1400 (43)	1100 (45)		850 (22)	503 (18)	
Current smokers	337 (10)	197 (8)		445 (11)	382 (14)	
Education			**< 0.001**			**< 0.001**
Primary school	385 (12)	296 (12)		97 (3)	91 (3)	
Secondary school	1224 (38)	1029 (44)		1282 (33)	1259 (44)	
College/university	1576 (50)	1068 (45)		2521 (65)	1487 (52)	
Parental asthma			0.058			**< 0.001**
Mother	295 (10)	206 (9)		476 (12)	272 (10)	
Father	218 (7)	124 (6)		309 (8)	179 (6)	
No one	2518 (83)	1922 (85)		3038 (79)	2333 (83)	
Both	12 (0.4)	12 (0.5)		39 (2)	23 (1)	
Other diseases[b]						
Comorbidity	892 (26)	778 (31)	**< 0.001**	165 (4)	124 (4)	0.770
Hypertension	778 (23)	659 (26)	**0.005**	120 (3)	96 (4)	0.390
Stroke	54 (2)	46 (2)	0.510	–	–	–
Ischemic heart disease	64 (2)	116 (5)	**< 0.001**	5 (0.1)	8 (0.3)	0.150
Diabetes mellitus	106 (3)	107 (5)	**0.027**	53 (1)	30 (1)	0.270
COPD	73 (2)	60 (2)	0.600	10 (0.3)	5 (0.2)	0.490
Serious childhood infection < 5 years	254 (8)	126 (5)	**< 0.001**	331 (9)	185 (7)	**< 0.001**
Respiratory symptoms			0.246			**0.001**
Wheeze[c]	669 (20)	530 (21)	0.330	697 (18)	468 (17)	0.150
Wheeze with shortness of breath[c]	421 (13)	297 (12)	0.380	457 (62)	256 (49)	**< 0.001**
Awoken with tightness in chest[c]	364 (11)	245 (10)	0.170	497 (13)	286 (10)	**< 0.001**
Awoken with attack of breathlessness[c]	220 (7)	126 (5)	**0.013**	173 (4)	136 (5)	0.48
Awoken with attack of cough[c]	1093 (33)	533 (21)	**< 0.001**	1343 (34	562 (20)	**< 0.001**
Currently taking asthma medication	327 (10)	216 (9)	0.130	383 (10)	212 (8)	**< 0.001**

[a]All *p*-values < 0.05 = significant and are marked bold. *P*-values are estimated from two-group mean comparison test (unpaired t-test) for continuous values and chi-squared test for categorical values

[b]Comorbidity includes the variables: hypertension, stroke, ischemic heart disease, diabetes mellitus, COPD, serious childhood infection < 5 years. Questions about stroke and COPD were not included in the offspring-questionnaires

[c]In the past 12 months

answered "no" and 323 (6%) "yes" to the presence of asthma in the offspring. The reports about late onset asthma followed the same pattern: in 4816 (90%) reports both parents and offspring answered "no asthma" in the offspring, and both parts reported late onset asthma in the offspring among 185 (3%). Parents' discrepant answers were most often that they reported no asthma for asthmatic offspring rather than reporting asthma for non-asthmatic offspring (Fig. 1a and b).

In 86% of the cases, both offspring and fathers reported absence of paternal asthma, compared to 83% for maternal asthma status. In 8% of the reports, offspring and fathers both reported a present asthma diagnosis; the corresponding frequency for maternal asthma was 10%. It was also more common for offspring to report no asthma in asthmatic parents than to report asthma in non-asthmatic parents.

The specificity was high for all four groups (Table 2), while sensitivity was lower. The sensitivity was lowest for the late onset asthma in the offspring (0.36), and highest for the maternal asthma (0.72). The positive predictive value (PPV) was lowest for the maternal asthma (0.75), and highest for the early onset asthma in the offspring (0.83). The negative predictive value (NPV) was high for all four groups (0.94–0.97).

Agreement between the parental reports and early onset asthma in offspring was good (Cohen's kappa 0.72), and moderate for late onset asthma in offspring (Cohen's kappa 0.46). The agreement between offspring reports and maternal and paternal asthma were both good (Cohen's kappa 0.69 and 0.68, respectively). Additional analyses stratified by study centres are given in the additional file (See Additional file 1: Table S2) and show some variability between the centres. To investigate if offspring reports of parental asthma differed in agreement with the parental reports according to age of asthma onset in parents, we performed an additional analysis (See Additional file 1: Table S3) stratifying by the timing of parental asthma onset. This analysis showed that offspring reported asthma in their parents more correctly if the parents had their asthma before the children were 20 years old, than if the parents got their asthma diagnosis after their offspring were 20 years old.

Table 3 shows univariate and multivariate logistic regression analyses of the association between covariates and offspring/parent discrepant asthma reports. In the univariate analyses regarding parent-reported offspring asthma, several parental factors were associated with reporting incorrect: male gender, current smoker, ex-smoker, ischemic heart disease, diabetes, COPD, wheeze and wheeze with shortness of breath. In the univariate analyses regarding the offspring-reported parental asthma, the following factors on the offspring level were associated with

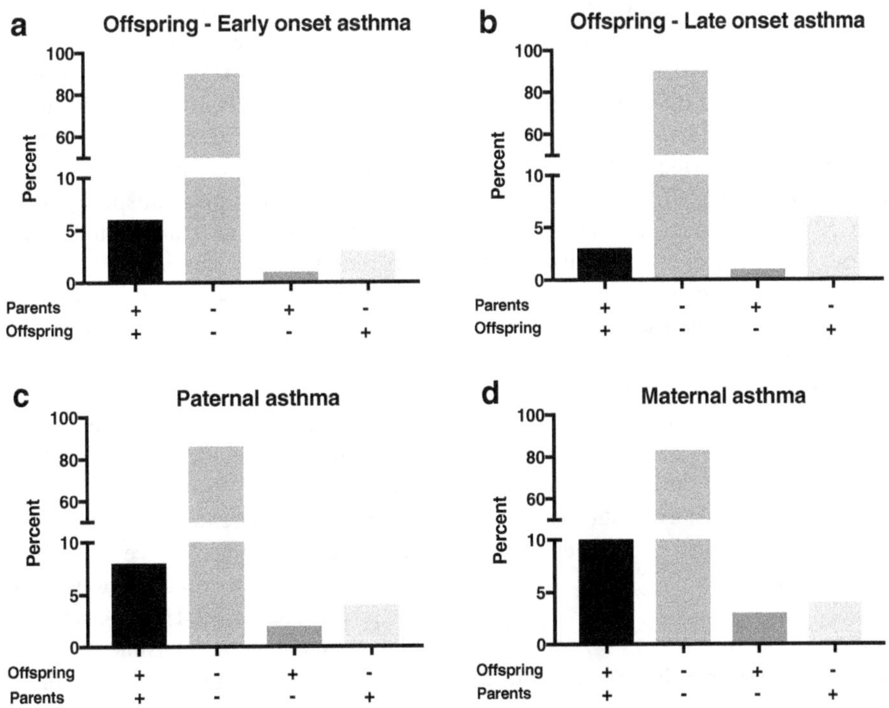

Fig. 1 Parent-reported offspring asthma as compared to offspring's own report (**a**, **b**); and offspring-reported paternal (**c**) and maternal (**d**) asthma as compared to parents' own report

Table 2 Parameter estimates (95% CI) for Cohen's kappa, sensitivity, specificity, PPV and NPV for offspring-reported parental asthma and parent-reported offspring asthma

Offspring asthma	Agreement[a] N (%)	Disagreement[b] N (%)	Cohens kappa	Sensitivity	95% CI	Specificity	95% CI	PPV	95% CI	NPV	95% CI
Early onset asthma	5121 (96)	219 (4)	0.72	0.68	0.64, 0.72	0.99	0.98, 0.99	0.83	0.79, 0.86	0.97	0.96, 0.97
Mother	2935 (96)	110 (4)	0.75	0.72	0.66, 0.77	0.99	0.98, 0.99	0.83	0.77, 0.88	0.98	0.97, 0.98
Father	2186 (95)	109 (5)	0.69	0.64	0.57, 0.70	0.99	0.98, 0.99	0.83	0.76, 0.88	0.96	0.95, 0.97
Late onset asthma	5001 (93)	376 (7)	0.46	0.36	0.32, 0.41	0.99	0.98, 0.99	0.79	0.73, 0.84	0.94	0.93, 0.94
Mother	2891 (94)	199 (6)	0.53	0.43	0.37, 0.49	0.99	0.98, 0.99	0.82	0.75, 0.88	0.94	0.93, 0.95
Father	2110 (92)	177 (8)	0.36	0.26	0.21, 0.33	0.99	0.98, 0.99	0.73	0.61, 0.82	0.93	0.92, 0.94
Parental asthma											
Maternal	3477 (93)	276 (7)	0.69	0.72	0.68, 0.75	0.96	0.95, 0.97	0.75	0.71, 0.79	0.95	0.95, 0–96
Daughter	2009 (92)	163 (8)	0.69	0.75	0.69, 0.79	0.95	0.94, 0.96	0.71	0.66, 0.76	0.96	0.95, 0.97
Son	1468 (93)	113 (7)	0.70	0.68	0.61, 0.74	0.97	0.96, 0.98	0.81	0.75, 0.86	0.95	0.93, 0.96
Paternal	2817 (94)	182 (6)	0.68	0.68	0.63, 0.73	0.97	0.96, 0.98	0.76	0.71, 0.80	0.96	0.95, 0.97
Daughter	1637 (94)	101 (6)	0.71	0.72	0.65, 0.78	0.97	0.96, 0.98	0.77	0.70, 0.83	0.96	0.95, 0.97
Son	1180 (94)	81 (6)	0.64	0.63	0.54, 0.71	0.97	0.96, 0.98	0.74	0.65, 0.82	0.96	0.94, 0.97

[a]Agreement: when both parents and offspring answered the same (yes/yes or no/no)
[b]Disagreement: when parents and offspring answered differently (yes/no or no/yes)

reporting incorrectly: ex-smoker, wheeze, currently taking asthma medication and late onset of own asthma.

The statistically significant predictors from the univariate analyses were included in the multivariate logistic regression. After adjustment, the only predictors associated with reporting incorrectly for the parent-reported offspring asthma were gender (OR 1.31 for fathers versus mothers, 95% CI 1.08–1.59) and current smoker (OR 1.46, 1.05–2.02). For the offspring-reported parental asthma, only wheeze was associated with reporting incorrectly in the multivariate model (OR 1.60, 1.21–2.11). No factors were associated with reporting correctly for either the parent-reported offspring asthma or the offspring-reported parental asthma.

Further inspection of the discrepant answers given by offspring with wheeze, showed that they reported both asthma in non-asthmatic parents as well as *no* asthma in asthmatic parents slightly more often than offspring with no wheeze (Table 4). Fathers and smoking parents, on the other hand, (See Additional file 1: Table S4) showed that fathers and current smokers were more likely to report *no* asthma in asthmatic offspring than the mothers and never-smokers were. With regard to reporting asthma in non-asthmatic offspring, however, the fathers and current smokers were as correct as the mothers and never-smokers.

Discussion

In this study, agreement between self-reported asthma and asthma reported by family-members were moderate to good. The specificity was high in both offspring reports of parental asthma and parent reports of offspring asthma, suggesting a high fraction of non-asthmatics correctly identified as such by their relatives. Conversely, the sensitivity was lower for all groups, especially for the late onset asthma in the offspring i.e. a lower fraction of those with asthma after 10 years of age are correctly identified as asthmatics by their parents. The same trend was observed for the offspring; a lower fraction of asthmatic parents are correctly identified as asthmatics, while a higher fraction of the non-asthmatic parents are correctly identified. Overall, however, the vast majority of parents and offspring were in accordance with each other when reporting each other's asthma status. In multivariate analyses, never smokers and mothers were more likely to report offspring asthma correctly. In offspring, wheeze was associated with incorrect reports of parental asthma status.

Our results showed that parents seem to have more knowledge about the asthma status of their offspring than the offspring have about their parents' asthma condition. This may be reasonable if we assume that parents are in general more concerned with their children's health than the children are with their parents' health. In addition, the offspring's awareness of the respiratory health of their parents likely depends on the severity of the parents' asthma. Where asthma in the past was a disease with severe exacerbations, it is today a disease mostly without hospital admissions, indicating that parental asthma may be "invisible" for the offspring.

To our knowledge this is the first agreement study comparing generational reports on each other's adult asthma status in general. Previous studies have only addressed parent-reports of current offspring asthma

Table 3 Odds ratios for discrepant answers in offspring/parent asthma reports, univariate and multivariate logistic regression analysis

Predictor	Univariate analyses Parents		Multivariate analyses[a] Parents		Univariate analyses Offspring		Multivariate analyses[a] Offspring	
	OR (95% CI)	p	OR (95% CI)	p	OR (95% CI)	p	OR (95% CI)	p
Male gender	1.33 (1.11, 1.60)	**0.002**	1.31 (1.08, 1.59)	**0.007**	1.01 (0.84, 1.23)	0.905		
Age	1.00 (0.99, 1.02)	0.630			1.01 (1.00, 1.02)	0.058		
Smoking								
Never smoker	1.00		1.00		1.00			
Current smoker	1.51 (1.11, 2.05)	**0.009**	1.46 (1.05, 2.02)	**0.023**	1.14 (0.85, 1.52)	0.392		
Ex-smoker	1.28 (1.05, 1.56)	**0.013**	1.22 (0.99, 1.50)	0.062	1.31 (1.04, 1.64)	**0.021**	1.22 (0.95, 1.55)	0.114
Education								
College/university	1.00				1.00			
Primary school	1.25 (0.94, 1.66)	0.127			1.59 (0.97, 2.59)	0.065		
Secondary school	1.04 (0.86, 1.28)	0.641			1.03 (0.85, 1.26)	0.756		
Comorbidity								
Hypertension	0.93 (0.75, 1.15)	0.505			1.42 (0.89, 2.28)	0.140		
Stroke	1.03 (0.52, 2.06)	0.930			–	–		
Ischemic heart	1.88 (1.23, 2.86)	**0.003**	1.54 (0.96, 2.46)	0.071	–	–		
Diabetes	1.64 (1.09, 2.46)	**0.018**	1.46 (0.96, 2.24)	0.077	1.07 (0.47, 2.48)	0.868		
COPD	1.75 (1.07, 2.87)	**0.026**	1.49 (0.89, 2.50)	0.129	–	–		
Serious childhood infection < 5 years	1.12 (0.99, 1.27)	0.080			1.11 (0.98, 1.25)	0.106		
Respiratory symptoms								
Wheeze	1.32 (1.07, 1.63)	**0.010**	1.02 (0.72, 1.46)	0.902	1.58 (1.26, 1.97)	**< 0.001**	1.60 (1.21, 2.11)	**0.001**
Wheeze with shortness of breath	1.47 (1.15, 1.89)	**0.002**	1.22 (0.81, 1.84)	0.343	1.37 (0.92, 2.04)	0.127		
Awoken with tightness in chest	1.01 (0.76, 1.36)	0.924			1.16 (0.87, 1.53)	0.313		
Awoken with attack of breathlessness	1.26 (0.89, 1.80)	0.193			1.11 (0.72, 1.72)	0.634		
Awoken with attack of cough	1.28 (1.05, 1.55)	**0.013**	1.25 (1.00, 1.57)	**0.046**	0.94 (0.76, 1.16)	0.557		
Currently taking asthma medication	1.32 (1.00, 1.76)	0.058			1.42 (1.06, 1.91)	**0.020**	0.95 (0.60, 1.49)	0.823
Age of onset								
Early onset	–	–			1.12 (0.78, 1.62)	0.528		
Late onset	–	–			1.76 (1.32, 2.34)	**< 0.001**	1.45 (1.01, 2.07)	**0.042**

[a]Adjusted for all predictors that were significant in the univariate analyses as well as for study centre and sibling status

and not vice versa, and the children have been young [1, 23–25]. The observed high validity in parent-reported offspring asthma is in accordance with for instance a study by Cornish et al. [26] comparing parent-reported asthma to electronic patient records. That parent-reports of children's asthma has high specificity although not so high sensitivity has also been observed in a relatively recent Canadian study [24]. High validity in parent reports of offspring atopic disease status has also been reported [27].

Cohen's kappa and sensitivity were both lower for late onset asthma compared to early onset asthma, which may be explained by the fact that parents are more aware of their offspring's health while they are young and still living at home. The impact on the parents and their ability to recall may be less when an offspring is diagnosed with asthma as a grownup. This is rendered particularly likely with a disease such as asthma, which is not continuously visible, but comes in attacks of various intervals – sometimes with a substantial amount of time between each attack.

In the same manner, it is likely to suspect offspring reporting their parents' asthma more correctly if they witnessed asthma in the parents during childhood when they saw their parents on a daily basis, then if the parents developed asthma after the offspring had grown up and left home. This suspicion was confirmed in the additional analysis (See Additional file 1: Table S3), where we analysed separately offspring-reported parental asthma with onset *after* the offspring was 20 years old, and with onset *before* the offspring was 20 years old. Offspring reported asthma in their parents more correctly if the parents had their asthma during the offspring's childhood.

Table 4 Frequency (absolute and relative) of discrepant asthma reports according to wheezing/non-wheezing

Discrepant asthma reports	N (%)
Offspring with wheeze reporting asthma in their non-asthmatic mothers	31/655 (4.7)
Offspring without wheeze reporting asthma in their non-asthmatic mothers	94/3091 (3.0)
Offspring with wheeze reporting no asthma in their asthmatic mothers	33/655 (5.0)
Offspring without wheeze reporting no asthma in their asthmatic mothers	117/3091 (3.8)
Offspring with wheeze reporting asthma in their non-asthmatic fathers	22/510 (4.3)
Offspring without wheeze reporting asthma in their non-asthmatic fathers	52/2483 (2.1)
Offspring with wheeze reporting no asthma in their asthmatic fathers	24/510 (4.7)
Offspring without wheeze reporting no asthma in their asthmatic fathers	83/2483 (3.3)

We found that never-smokers and mothers were more likely to report offspring asthma correctly. Non-smokers have higher health-risk awareness than smokers [28], thus it is plausible that this group also have more knowledge regarding their offspring health. That mothers report more correctly than fathers may be explained by them generally being the primary care givers of children and consequently spending more time with them in the daily life. Today this is probably not as rigid a pattern as before, but the present agreement study is based on a parent population born between 1945 and 1973, and their offspring born between 1963 and 1997.

Wheeze in the offspring is a significant predictor for incorrect reports of parental asthma. One could speculate that offspring with wheeze over-report asthma in their parents because of a hyper alertness concerning asthma and its symptoms. This would be in accordance with what has been observed for instance in atopic diseases, where fathers were more likely to recall their own atopic disease history if their children currently had severe atopic diseases [29]. In addition, Danell et al. [30] showed that children reported more asthma-related issues than their parents regarding their own symptoms. However, in our study, the discrepant answers given by offspring with wheeze were associated with both under-reporting and over-reporting (See Additional file 1: Table S4), and further studies are needed to appropriately investigate the mechanisms behind these discrepancies. Although seemingly random, the observed misclassification may lead to a bias towards the null and yield weaker associations than what actually exist in real life.

Regarding the parents, we observed an increased risk for differential misclassification of offspring asthma among men and smokers, with a tendency for under-estimating asthma in their offspring. As suspected, we also observed that this type of misclassification was more widespread regarding late onset asthma in the offspring than early onset asthma. The same pattern was also observed for offspring reporting parental asthma with onset after the offspring had grown up and left home.

Apart from male gender and current smoking in parents, and wheeze in offspring, we did not observe any other significant predictors for discrepant asthma reports across generations. This leads us to believe that discrepant reports concerning offspring health status are mostly due to minor and random misclassification with little consequences for the validity of asthma reports.

Nevertheless, the observed predictors for discrepant answers should be taken into consideration in any future studies relying on asthma reports on behalf of family members.

The main strengths of this study are population size and study design; to our knowledge RHINESSA is the largest population-based generational study so far, and this is the first study to compare self-report questionnaires across generations. In addition to the agreement analyses, we also identified predictors for disagreement, which was possible through the large dataset collected in the RHINE, ECRHS and RHINESSA.

However, some limitations to our study should also be acknowledged. First, the response rate in the offspring population was low: Only a third of the offspring of ECRHS/RHINE participants agreed to participate in the RHINESSA generation study. However, the offspring population was not severely skewed in any direction – distribution of demographic characteristics such as sex, smoking habits and educational level did not seem to differ substantially from that of a general population in the same age range. We also examined distribution of sex, smoking habits, educational level and asthma status of parents with participating offspring and parents with non-participating offspring to further examine any potential response bias. Our data showed that the groups were very similar. There was a miniscule overrepresentation in RHINESSA of offspring who had parents with asthma (13.6% versus 11.5% in non-participating offspring), parents who were non-smokers (84.3% versus 80.6%), and female parents (mothers, 55.3% versus 50.6%). In addition, slightly less parents with higher education had offspring who participated in RHINESSA (46.1% versus 47.9% of the parents with non-participating offspring). These very small differences are reassuring, and do not provide any evidence of differential misclassification due to response bias. In addition, we were not aiming to assess disease prevalence in the present study, but to assess associations between two variables (parent reports and offspring reports). Although a low response rate may have impact on prevalence rates, internal exposure-outcome associations are less affected [20, 31]. However, we cannot be entirely certain that the observed differences in agreement between centres (Additional file 1: Table S2a and b), are valid for the general populations in these centres or if they apply only to the select group of participants.

Secondly, self-report questionnaires are susceptible to misclassification in the form of recall bias, especially if the outcomes date far back in time. Through comparing offspring-reports on parental asthma and parent-reports on offspring asthma, we set as a prerequisite that the reports they have given regarding themselves are correct. A comparison with primary care records for the study participants would have helped us assess presence or absence of recall bias in our study. Other possibilities would be to use prescription registry data. Data on dispensed antiasthmatics from the Norwegian Prescription Database (NorPD) has previously been validated in the Norwegian mother and child cohort study (MoBa), and they found that the use of prescription data for 7-year old children had high validity [32]. Unfortunately, such data was not available in our study. However, while clinical assessment is often considered the best method for validating self-reported asthma, recent studies presented self-report questionnaires to be a reliable tool in an epidemiological setting [8, 26].

Thirdly, we used "doctor-diagnosed asthma" when subjects reported about themselves, but "ever asthma" when subjects reported about each other. A recent Danish study showed how asthma prevalence in children is highly dependent on the method of measuring asthma, being lowest when measured with hospitalization data and highest when measured with prescription data, and with self-reports by parents in between the two other methods [4].

Since the asthma report on behalf of the other generation in our study was ever asthma and not doctor-diagnosed, one could suspect an over-report of asthma on behalf of the other generation. However, the results of our study did not show any such tendency. This is in line with previous research by de Marco et al., who found that the question "Do you have or have you ever had asthma?" gave prevalence estimates comparable to clinical diagnosis [33].

Furthermore, in RHINESSA only one of the parents is included, while ideally both parents should have been included. However, mothers and fathers were approximately equally distributed in RHINESSA and consequently we have no reason to believe that there is a gender bias present.

Conclusion

In conclusion, this agreement study shows a moderate to good agreement between the self-reported asthma and asthma reported by family-members, although we observed some risk of under-report. In the absence of direct reports, offspring asthma status reported by parents and parental asthma status reported by offspring may be used as a proxy, both in epidemiological studies and in a clinical setting before undergoing further clinical examination.

Additional file

Additional file 1: Table S1. Response rates of the offspring population, RHINESSA. **Table S2a and 2b.** Parameter estimates and 95% confidence intervals for Cohen's kappa, sensitivity, specificity, positive predictive value (PPV), and negative predictive value (NPV) for offspring-reported parental asthma and parent- reported offspring asthma, stratified by study centers. **Table S3.** Parameter estimates and 95% confidence intervals for sensitivity, specificity, positive predictive value (PPV), and negative predictive value (NPV) for offspring-reported parental asthma and parent-reported offspring asthma, according to timing of parental asthma onset. **Table S4.** Frequency (absolute and relative) of discrepant asthma reports according to fathers/mothers, and current smoking parents/never-smoking parents.

Abbreviations

CI: Confidence interval; COPD: Chronic obstructive lung disease; ECRHS: European Community Respiratory Health Survey; MoBa: Norwegian mother and child cohort study; NorPD: The Norwegian Prescription Database; NPV: Negative predictive value; OR: Odds ratio; PPV: Positive predictive value; RHINE: Respiratory Health in Northern Europe; RHINESSA: Respiratory Health in Northern Europe, Spain and Australia

Acknowledgements

Open access was funded by the University of Bergen.

Funding

This work was supported by the following funding: The first author received a recruitment grant from Western Norway Regional Health Authorities (grant No 912011). The RHINESSA generation study has received funding from Norwegian Research Council, Bergen Medical Research Foundation, Western Norway Regional Health Authorities, Norwegian Labor Inspection, Wood Foundation, Danish Working Environment Authority, Swedish Lung Foundation, Swedish Asthma and Allergy Foundation, Estonian Research Council PUT No 562, Australian National Health Medical Research Council, Sociedad Espanola de Neumologia y Cirurgia Toracica. For more information, please see www.rhinessa.net.

Authors' contributions

INK: Principal author, conception and design of the work, statistical analysis, interpretation of data, drafting the work. CS, BB, RJB, LB, SCD, MH, CJ, RJ, AM, MM, JMM, FGR, JLSR, VS, ST, AJ: Conception and design of the work, acquisition and interpretation of data and revising for important intellectual content. All authors read and approved the final manuscript.

Consent for publication

Not applicable.

Competing interests

The last author, Ane Johannessen is a member of the Editorial Board of BMC Pulmonary Medicine. All of the other authors declare that they have no competing interests.

Author details

[1]Department of Occupational Medicine, Haukeland University Hospital, N-5021 Bergen, Norway. [2]Centre for International Health, Department of Global Public Health and Primary Care, University of Bergen, Bergen, Norway. [3]Faculty of medicine, University of Iceland, Reykjavik, Iceland. [4]Occupational and Environmental Medicine, Umeå University, Umeå, Sweden. [5]Allergy and Lung Health Unit, Melbourne School of Population and Global Health, University of Melbourne, Melbourne, Australia. [6]Department of Occupational and Environmental Medicine, University of Gothenburg, Gothenburg, Sweden. [7]Department of Medical Sciences: Respiratory Allergy and Sleep Research, Uppsala University, Uppsala, Sweden. [8]Lung Clinic, Tartu University Hospital, Tartu, Estonia. [9]Department of Medical Sciences: Clinical Physiology, Uppsala University, Uppsala, Sweden. [10]Servicio de Salud de Castilla, Servicio de Neumología del Complejo Hospitalario Univerisitario de Albacete, La Mancha, Albacete, Spain. [11]Department of Clinical Science, University of Bergen, Bergen, Norway. [12]Department of Gynecology and Obstetrics, Haukeland University Hospital, Bergen, Norway. [13]Facultad de Enfermeria, University of Huelva, Huelva, Spain. [14]Department of Public Health, Danish Ramazzini Center, Aarhus University, Aarhus, Denmark. [15]National Research Center for the Working Environment, Copenhagen, Denmark.

References

1. Strippoli MP, Silverman M, Michel G, Kuehni CE. A parent-completed respiratory questionnaire for 1-year-old children: repeatability. Arch Dis Child. 2007;92(10):861–5.
2. Beasley R, Semprini A, Mitchell EA. Risk factors for asthma: is prevention possible? Lancet. 2015;386(9998):1075–85.
3. Soubry A, Hoyo C, Jirtle RL, Murphy SK. A paternal environmental legacy: evidence for epigenetic inheritance through the male germ line. BioEssays. 2014;36(4):359–71.
4. Hansen S, Strom M, Maslova E, Mortensen EL, Granstrom C, Olsen SF. A comparison of three methods to measure asthma in epidemiologic studies: results from the Danish national birth cohort. PLoS One. 2012;7(5):e36328.
5. Asher MI, Keil U, Anderson HR, Beasley R, Crane J, Martinez F, et al. International study of asthma and allergies in childhood (ISAAC): rationale and methods. Eur Respir J. 1995;8(3):483–91.
6. Minasyan A, Babajanyan A, Campbell DE, Nanan R. Validation of a comprehensive early childhood allergy questionnaire. Pediatr Allergy Immunol. 2015;26(6):522–9.
7. Kim MH, Kwon JW, Kim HB, Song Y, Yu J, Kim WK, et al. Parent-reported ISAAC written questionnaire may underestimate the prevalence of asthma in children aged 10-12 years. Pediatr Pulmonol. 2012;47(1):36–43.
8. Hansen TE, Evjenth B, Holt J. Validation of a questionnaire against clinical assessment in the diagnosis of asthma in school children. J Asthma. 2015; 52(3):262–7.
9. Pekkanen J, Pearce N. Defining asthma in epidemiological studies. Eur Respir J. 1999;14(4):951–7.
10. Brozek G, Zejda J, Farnik M, Wypych-Slusarska A, Skoczynski S. Validation of simple and composed screening test of childhood asthma. Eur Respir J. 2016;48(suppl 60). https://doi.org/10.1183/13993003.congress-2016.PA4231.
11. Sundblad GM, Saartok T, Engstrom LM. Child-parent agreement on reports of disease, injury and pain. BMC Public Health. 2006;6:276.
12. Miller JE. Predictors of asthma in young children: does reporting source affect our conclusions? Am J Epidemiol. 2001;154(3):245–50.
13. Sole D, Vanna AT, Yamada E, Rizzo MC, Naspitz CK. International study of asthma and allergies in childhood (ISAAC) written questionnaire: validation of the asthma component among Brazilian children. J Investig Allergol Clin Immunol. 1998;8(6):376–82.
14. Braun-Fahrlander C, Gassner M, Grize L, Minder CE, Varonier HS, Vuille JC, et al. Comparison of responses to an asthma symptom questionnaire (ISAAC core questions) completed by adolescents and their parents. SCARPOL-Team. Swiss Study on Childhood Allergy and Respiratory Symptoms with respect to Air Pollution. Pediatr Pulmonol. 1998;25(3):159–66.
15. Li YF, Langholz B, Salam MT, Gilliland FD. Maternal and grandmaternal smoking patterns are associated with early childhood asthma. Chest. 2005; 127(4):1232–41.
of the asthma component among Brazilian children. J Investig Allergol Clin Immunol. 1998;8(6):376–82.
14. Braun-Fahrlander C, Gassner M, Grize L, Minder CE, Varonier HS, Vuille JC, et al. Comparison of responses to an asthma symptom questionnaire (ISAAC core questions) completed by adolescents and their parents. SCARPOL-Team. Swiss Study on Childhood Allergy and Respiratory Symptoms with respect to Air Pollution. Pediatr Pulmonol. 1998;25(3):159–66.
15. Li YF, Langholz B, Salam MT, Gilliland FD. Maternal and grandmaternal smoking patterns are associated with early childhood asthma. Chest. 2005; 127(4):1232–41.
16. Miller LL, Henderson J, Northstone K, Pembrey M, Golding J. Do grandmaternal smoking patterns influence the etiology of childhood asthma? Chest. 2014;145(6):1213–8.
17. Svanes C, Koplin J, Skulstad SM, Johannessen A, Bertelsen RJ, Benediktsdottir B, et al. Father's environment before conception and asthma risk in his children: a multi-generation analysis of the respiratory health in northern Europe study. Int J Epidemiol. 2017;46(1):235–45.
18. Arshad SH, Karmaus W, Zhang H, Holloway JW. Multigenerational cohorts in patients with asthma and allergy. J Allergy Clin Immunol. 2017;139(2):415–21.
19. Lodge CJ, Braback L, Lowe AJ, Dharmage SC, Olsson D, Forsberg B. Grandmaternal smoking increases asthma risk in grandchildren: a nationwide Swedish cohort. Clin Exp Allergy. 2018;48(2):167-74.
20. Johannessen A, Verlato G, Benediktsdottir B, Forsberg B, Franklin K, Gislason T, et al. Longterm follow-up in European respiratory health studies - patterns and implications. BMC Pulm Med. 2014;14:63.
21. Toren K, Gislason T, Omenaas E, Jogi R, Forsberg B, Nystrom L, et al. A prospective study of asthma incidence and its predictors: the RHINE study. Eur Respir J. 2004;24(6):942–6.
22. D A. Practical statistics for medical research. London: Chapman and Hall; 1991.
23. Brunekreef B, Groot B, Rijcken B, Hoek G, Steenbekkers A, de Boer A. Reproducibility of childhood respiratory symptom questions. Eur Respir J. 1992;5(8):930–5.
24. Yang CL, To T, Foty RG, Stieb DM, Dell SD. Verifying a questionnaire diagnosis of asthma in children using health claims data. BMC Pulm Med. 2011;11:52.
25. Hederos CA, Hasselgren M, Hedlin G, Bornehag CG. Comparison of clinically diagnosed asthma with parental assessment of children's asthma in a questionnaire. Pediatr Allergy Immunol. 2007;18(2):135–41.
26. Cornish RP, Henderson J, Boyd AW, Granell R, Van Staa T, Macleod J. Validating childhood asthma in an epidemiological study using linked electronic patient records. BMJ Open. 2014;4(4):e005345.
27. Vissing NH, Jensen SM, Bisgaard H. Validity of information on atopic disease and other illness in young children reported by parents in a prospective birth cohort study. BMC Med Res Methodol. 2012;12:160.
28. Lund KE, Helgason AR. Environmental tobacco smoke in Norwegian homes, 1995 and 2001: changes in children's exposure and parents attitudes and health risk awareness. Eur J Pub Health. 2005;15(2):123–7.
29. Kulig M, Bergmann R, Edenharter G, Wahn U, Multicenter Allergy Study Group. Does allergy in parents depend on allergy in their children? Recall bias in parental questioning of atopic diseases. J Allergy Clin Immunol. 2000;105(2 Pt 1):274–8.
30. Danell CS, Bergstrom A, Wahlgren CF, Hallner E, Bohme M, Kull I. Parents and school children reported symptoms and treatment of allergic disease differently. J Clin Epidemiol. 2013;66(7):783–9.
31. Nilsen RM, Suren P, Gunnes N, Alsaker ER, Bresnahan M, Hirtz D, et al. Analysis of self-selection bias in a population-based cohort study of autism spectrum disorders. Paediatr Perinat Epidemiol. 2013;27(6):553–63.
32. Furu K, Karlstad O, Skurtveit S, Haberg SE, Nafstad P, London SJ, et al. High validity of mother-reported use of antiasthmatics among children: a comparison with a population-based prescription database. J Clin Epidemiol. 2011;64(8):878–84.
33. de Marco R, Cerveri I, Bugiani M, Ferrari M, Verlato G. An undetected burden of asthma in Italy: the relationship between clinical and epidemiological diagnosis of asthma. Eur Respir J. 1998;11(3):599–605.

15

Bronchial thermoplasty reduces gas trapping in severe asthma

David Langton[1,2*], Alvin Ing[3,4], Kim Bennetts[1], Wei Wang[2], Claude Farah[3,5], Matthew Peters[3,4], Virginia Plummer[1,2] and Francis Thien[2,6]

Abstract

Background: In randomized controlled trials, bronchial thermoplasty (BT) has been proven to reduce symptoms in severe asthma, but the mechanisms by which this is achieved are uncertain as most studies have shown no improvement in spirometry. We postulated that BT might improve lung mechanics by altering airway resistance in the small airways of the lung in ways not measured by FEV_1. This study aimed to evaluate changes in measures of gas trapping by body plethysmography.

Methods: A prospective cohort of 32 consecutive patients with severe asthma who were listed for BT at two Australian university hospitals were evaluated at three time points, namely baseline, and then 6 weeks and 6 months post completion of all procedures. At each evaluation, medication usage, symptom scores (Asthma Control Questionnaire, ACQ-5) and exacerbation history were obtained, and lung function was evaluated by (i) spirometry (ii) gas diffusion (KCO) and (iii) static lung volumes by body plethysmography.

Results: ACQ-5 improved from 3.0 ± 0.8 at baseline to 1.5 ± 0.9 at 6 months (mean ± SD, $p < 0.001$, paired t-test). Daily salbutamol usage improved from 8.3 ± 5.6 to 3.5 ± 4.3 puffs per day ($p < 0.001$). Oral corticosteroid requiring exacerbations reduced from 2.5 ± 2.0 in the 6 months prior to BT, to 0.6 ± 1.3 in the 6 months after BT ($p < 0.001$). The mean baseline FEV_1 was 57.8 ± 18.9%predicted, but no changes in any spirometric parameter were observed after BT. KCO was also unaltered by BT. A significant reduction in gas trapping was observed with Residual Volume (RV) falling from 146 ± 37% predicted at baseline to 136 ± 29%predicted 6 months after BT ($p < 0.005$). Significant improvements in TLC and FRC were also observed. These changes were evident at the 6 week time period and maintained at 6 months. The change in RV was inversely correlated with the baseline FEV_1 ($r = 0.572$, $p = 0.001$), and in patients with a baseline FEV_1 of < 60%predicted, the RV/TLC ratio fell by 6.5 ± 8.9%.

Conclusion: Bronchial thermoplasty improves gas trapping and this effect is greatest in the most severely obstructed patients. The improvement may relate to changes in the mechanical properties of small airways that are not measured with spirometry.

Keywords: Bronchial thermoplasty, Severe asthma, Residual volume, Small airways dysfunction

* Correspondence: davidlangton@phcn.vic.gov.au
[1]Department of Thoracic Medicine, Frankston Hospital, Peninsula Health, 2 Hastings Road, Frankston, VIC 3199, Australia
[2]Faculty of Medicine, Nursing and Health Sciences, Monash University, Clayton, Vic, Australia
Full list of author information is available at the end of the article

Background

Bronchial thermoplasty (BT) offers an alternative therapeutic option for patients with severe asthma, defined by the Global Initiative for Asthma (GINA) as those with persistent symptoms requiring step 5 of controller treatment [1].

Performed during bronchoscopy, radiofrequency thermal impulses are delivered to airways ranging in size from 2 to 10 mm, with the intention of inducing atrophy in hypertrophied airway smooth muscle. Histological studies in both canine and humans have demonstrated that this occurs [2–5]. Three randomized controlled trials have established that patients feel better after this treatment, with fewer asthma symptoms, reduced exacerbations and improved quality of life [6–8]. However, two of these three clinical trials showed no effect of BT on the one-second forced expiratory volume (FEV_1) [6, 7].

How is it then, that large numbers of asthmatic patients in a controlled clinical trial can experience an improvement in their symptoms and quality life, without improvement in physiological parameters such as FEV_1? One explanation might lie in the placebo effect, known to be a powerful force in surgical treatment [9]. However, this would not explain the significantly better results observed in the active arm of a double blind, sham controlled study, namely the AIR2 trial [6]. An alternative hypothesis might be that BT leads to physiological changes which are not measured by spirometry - such as might occur in the peripheral airways.

Smaller airways, less than 2 mm in diameter, have been histologically shown to be involved in asthma [10]. These smaller airways make up a large portion of the cross-sectional area of the lung, and as a result resistance in these airways is not easily detected by changes in FEV_1 [11, 12].

A number of methods exist to evaluate physiological changes in the small airways [13]. These include (i) plethysmography (ii) impulse oscillometry (iii) inert gas washout and (iv) sophisticated imaging techniques such as hyperpolarized magnetic resonance imaging. In this study, we report changes in plethysmographic lung volumes as measures of response to BT.

Methods

Participants

This was a prospective evaluation of consecutive patients selected for BT at two Australian university teaching hospitals, between June 2014 and January 2017. Participants were referred for BT by their treating respiratory physician if they had frequent symptoms despite optimized asthma therapy including high dose inhaled corticosteroids and two long acting bronchodilators. All patients were required to meet at least one of the 4 European Respiratory Society/American Thoracic Society (ERS/ATS) criteria for the definition of severe asthma, before the procedure would be considered [14].

The baseline characteristics of the patients were collated, including age, gender, body mass index (BMI), medication usage, exacerbation history, and the disease specific quality of life tool, the Asthma Control Questionnaire score (ACQ-5). The ACQ-5 was chosen as it has an established place as an evaluative tool in asthma and is known to be sensitive to change [15].

Measurements

Lung function testing was conducted in accredited respiratory laboratories by experienced scientific staff and according to ERS/ATS standards [16], with instrument calibration immediately prior to testing. All tests were performed in the morning, and prior to the administration of any bronchodilators that day. Tests were conducted in the seated position using the Jaeger Masterscreen Body (Carefusion, Hoechberg, Germany). For spirometry, at least three acceptable maneuvers were obtained, with the FEV_1 and the forced vital capacity (FVC) measurement values within 0.15 L of each other during repeated testing. For body plethysmography, at least three acceptable measurements were performed with functional residual capacity (FRC) values within 5% of each other. After the administration of 400mcg salbutamol, the single breath diffusing capacity (DLCO) was tested, and at least two acceptable maneuvers within 3 ml/min/mmHg of each other were required. Post bronchodilator spirometry was then performed. The predicted equations used were Quanjer [17] for spirometry, and ECCS 1993 [18] for all other tests. Testing was conducted at baseline, in the 4 weeks prior to BT being undertaken, then at 6 weeks and 6 months after the final BT procedure. Exacerbations of asthma were recorded if the patient reported a deterioration in their asthma requiring an increase in, or the commencement of, oral corticosteroids.

Procedure

BT was performed by experienced bronchoscopists, trained in using the Alair Bronchial Thermoplasty System (Boston Scientific, NSW, Australia), using the Olympus BF-Q190 bronchoscope (Olympus Medical Systems, Tokyo, Japan) and conducted according to the previously published technique [19]. All bronchoscopies were performed under general anesthesia. Consistent with the standard protocol, each patient was treated in three sessions, three to 4 weeks apart. The right lower lobe was treated first, followed by the left lower lobe, and then both upper lobes during the final bronchoscopy. The right middle lobe was not treated. The number of radiofrequency actuations delivered was recorded for each patient. Prednisolone was prescribed for 3 days prior, and continued for 3 days after each BT procedure. All patients were electively admitted to hospital for the night immediately following treatment.

Outcomes

The primary outcomes in this study were the changes in lung function parameters measured 6 months post procedure when compared to baseline. Secondary outcomes related to changes in ACQ-5 score, reliever and preventer medication use, and exacerbation history at 6 months. Re-evaluation at the 6 month time point was chosen so as to allow for any structural effects from BT to have been completed, yet to have avoided patients being lost to follow up or started on new medication.

Analysis

SPSS version 24 (IBM corporation, New York, USA) was used for all statistical analyses. Grouped data refers to all 32 patients and is reported throughout as mean ± standard deviation. A paired t-test was used for paired sets of data, whilst an unpaired t-test was used to compare groups. Analysis of variance was used to compare baseline data with repeated tests over time. Pearson's Correlation Coefficient was calculated to evaluate bivariate continuous normally distributed data. For multivariate linear regression a stepwise backward model was created. Statistical significance was taken throughout as $p < 0.05$ for a two-tailed test.

Ethical considerations

Approval to collate and audit data as part of quality assurance was provided by the Human Research Ethics Committee at both participating institutions. All participants provided informed consent for treatment and data collection. Specific permission to use the ACQ-5 in this project was granted by its author, Elizabeth Juniper.

Results

Baseline characteristics

Thirty-two consecutive patients undergoing this study protocol were available for inclusion, 15 males, 17 females. No patients were lost to follow up, nor excluded. The mean age was 60.1 ± 11.7 yrs. The mean BMI was 30.4 ± 7.1 kg/m^2. Every patient selected for treatment met the ERS/ATS definition for severe asthma, by fulfilling at least one of the four criteria. Specifically, all cases (100%) had baseline ACQ-5 scores > 1.5; 22 cases (69%) had ≥2 prednisolone courses in the previous year; and 29 cases (91%) demonstrated a baseline prebronchodilator $FEV_1 < 80\%$ predicted. All patients had been prescribed high doses of inhaled corticosteroids, mean beclomethasone equivalent dose of 1947 ± 728 mcg daily. Sixteen patients (50%) were taking maintenance oral prednisolone, mean dose 11.0 ± 5.5 mg. All patients (100%) were taking long-acting beta$_2$ agonists and long-acting muscarinic antagonists. Despite this treatment, patients used a mean of 8.3 ± 6.0 salbutamol puffs daily for rescue reliever therapy. Seven patients had been receiving stable therapy with omalizumab, for the preceding 12 months, and no patient commenced a monoclonal antibody during study period from immediately prior to BT to the 6 month re-evaluation.

The baseline prebronchodilator FEV_1 was 57.8 ± 18.9% predicted, and the mean improvement in FEV_1 after 400μg inhaled salbutamol was 10.9 ± 13.8%. The mean forced expiratory ratio was 53.3 ± 12.3%. The mean baseline DLCO was 85.5 ± 14.1%predicted, and the gas transfer per lung unit (KCO) was 99.5 ± 17.7%predicted. In this group of patients, twenty-four patients (75%) were never smokers, 5 patients had a pack year history of less than 10, and 3 patients had a pack year history of greater than 10. There were no current cigarette smokers.

Procedure

The average total number of radiofrequency activations delivered per patient was 209 ± 59. No patient required treatment in the Intensive Care after the procedure, and there were no instances of prolonged hospital stay post procedure. One patient was readmitted to hospital with radiologically proven right upper lobe pneumonia 6 days after upper lobe treatment. Intravenous antibiotics were prescribed and the patient was discharged on the fourth hospital day, without further incident. One patient developed lobar collapse after BT, twice, and each time required an additional bronchoscopic procedure for suction and airway clearance.

Outcomes

At the six-month reevaluation, the ACQ-5 had improved from 3.0 ± 0.8 to 1.5 ± 0.9 (mean difference 1.5, CI 1.1–1.9, $p < 0.001$). Only 5 patients (15.6%) did not show an improvement in ACQ-5 of greater than 0.5 units (the minimal clinically significant difference). The requirement for salbutamol rescue therapy had reduced from a mean of 8.3 ± 5.6 puffs per day to 3.5 ± 4.3 puffs per day ($p < 0.001$, paired t-test). Of 16 patients who required maintenance prednisolone pre-procedure, 12 were completely weaned from prednisolone at the 6 month follow up. A further two patients had reduced their daily prednisolone dose from 15 to 20 mg/day to 5 mg/day. The frequency of oral steroid requiring exacerbations improved from 2.5 ± 2.0 exacerbations in the 6 months prior to commencement of BT, to 0.6 ± 1.3 exacerbations in the 6 months after BT completion ($p < 0.001$, paired t- test).

Dynamic lung function: Spirometry

Table 1 shows the effect of BT at 6 months across a range of spirometric parameters. There was no detectable effect on any variable.

Diffusion capacity

BT did not alter pulmonary diffusion capacity. The baseline KCO was 99.5 ± 17.7% predicted, and at the 6 month reassessment was 100 ± 15.8% predicted.

Static lung function

Consistent with the obstructed spirometry, the static lung function tests demonstrated marked gas trapping with a mean Residual Volume (RV) of 146 ± 37% predicted. The mean RV contributed 50% of the Total Lung Capacity (TLC) (Table 2). Following BT significant improvements were observed in TLC, RV and Functional Residual Capacity (FRC). The effect size was greatest in RV where a 7% reduction was observed. The RV at 6 weeks post BT was 139 ± 38%predicted, and at 6 months post BT was 136 ± 29% predicted. Using ANOVA for repeated measures, Wilks' Lambda was $p = 0.002$, and the multivariate partial eta squared was 0.355, indicating a strong effect. Pairwise comparisons showed the significant change occurred between baseline and 6 weeks ($p = 0.02$) after which there was no further significant change.

Subgroup analysis by airflow obstruction

To assess whether the reduction in RV was distributed evenly across the spectrum of airflow obstruction, a scatterplot was constructed showing the percentage change in RV plotted against the baseline FEV_1% predicted, and this is shown in Fig. 1. The graph demonstrates that the greatest improvements in RV were evident at the lower end of the baseline FEV_1 range, with flattening of effect at the higher range of FEV_1. The best model which described this relationship is given by the equation $y = 13–930/x$ where y = percentage change in RV and x = FEV_1 percent predicted, $r^2 = 0.33$, $p = 0.001$.

To assess whether the reduction in RV was accompanied by a reduction in RV/TLC ratio, a scatterplot was constructed showing the percentage change in the RV/TLC ratio after BT plotted against the baseline FEV_1%-predicted, and this is shown in Fig. 2. The best model to describe this relationship was given by $y = 20.5–1148/x$, where y = percentage change in RV/TLC ratio and x = FEV_1 percent predicted, $r^2 = 0.37$, p = 0.001.

Table 1 Dynamic Lung Function Pre and Post BT

Parameter	Baseline	6 months post	p
Prebronchodilator FEV_1 (litres)	1.50 ± 0.54	1.50 ± 0.56	NS
Prebronchodilator FEV_1 (%pred)	57.8 ± 18.9	58.7 ± 18.2	NS
Prebronchodilator VC (litres)	2.80 ± 0.90	2.80 ± 0.90	NS
Prebronchodilator VC (%pred)	88.2 ± 17.8	87.5 ± 18.2	NS
Prebronchodilator FEV_1/VC (%)	53.3 ± 12.3	53.9 ± 12.4	NS
Bronchodilator response FEV_1 (%)	10.9 ± 13.8	10.6 ± 16.0	NS
Postbronchodilator FEV_1 (litres)	1.65 ± 0.63	1.62 ± 0.69	NS

FEV_1 forced expiratory volume in 1 s, *VC* vital capacity, *%pred* percent predicted value

Table 2 Static Lung Function Pre bronchodilator

Parameter	Baseline	6 months	p
TLC (litres)	5.92 ± 1.42	5.73 ± 1.41	0.008
TLC (%pred)	107 ± 16	103 ± 14	0.002
RV (litres)	3.00 ± 0.99	2.80 ± 0.83	0.003
RV (%pred)	146 ± 37	136 ± 29	0.002
RV/TLC (%)	50 ± 10	49 ± 9	NS
FRC (litres)	3.72 ± 1.08	3.57 ± 1.01	0.005

TLC total lung capacity, *RV* residual volume, *FRC* functional residual capacity *%pred* percent predicted value

To better understand the effect of baseline FEV_1 on response to BT, patients were divided into two groups, around the inflection point demonstrated in Figs. 1 and 2, of baseline FEV_1 equal to 60% predicted. These two groups are compared in Table 3. A stepwise backward multivariate linear regression model was created to examine factors predictive of percentage change in RV at 6 months post BT. The following variables had no significant effect: age, gender, baseline ACQ-5, BMI and activations. Only the baseline FEV_1%predicted was significantly related to the change in RV (beta coefficient + 0.257, $p = 0.002$).

Discussion

This study recruited a group of subjects with severe asthma, persistent lung function impairment, high current symptom burden and frequent exacerbations. All were at GINA Step 5 treatment, with 50% requiring maintenance oral corticosteroids. Following BT, there was a marked improvement in current asthma control, as reflected in ACQ. Whereas no subject had an ACQ5 < 1.5 at baseline, 18/32 (56%) had achieved this at 6 months ($p < 0.001$, Chi-square). This improvement was accompanied by a 76% reduction in oral steroid requiring asthma exacerbations. Further, amongst 16 patients requiring maintenance oral corticosteroids pretreatment, 75% had been able to discontinue oral steroids by the 6-month re-evaluation.

Despite the substantive clinical improvement observed in this study, no change was seen in any spirometric parameter. This has been a consistent finding in the published literature in relation to BT [5, 6, 20, 21]. It highlights our lack of understanding of the pathophysiology of the response to BT, and underscores our desire to evaluate the effect of BT on the peripheral airways. Reassuringly, Table 1 demonstrates that BT does not attenuate the response to short

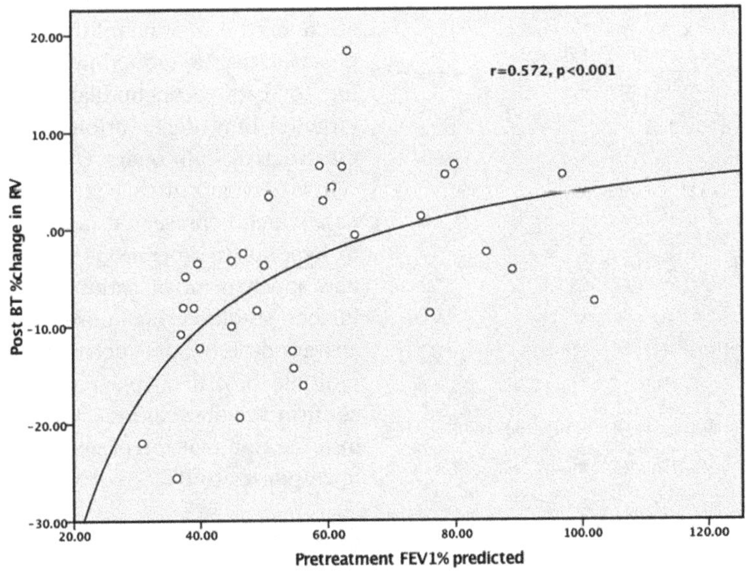

Fig. 1 Percentage change in RV versus baseline FEV_1% predicted

acting bronchodilator- something which might otherwise have been anticipated from treatment causing atrophy of airway smooth muscle. This demonstrates that the reason that patients use less reliever medication after BT is not because the reliever medication is in any way less effective.

The absence of change in pulmonary gas diffusion following BT is also reassuring from a safety perspective. It is consistent with the normality of the lung parenchyma observed by CT scans at 5 year follow up in the AIR2 study [22], and also with reports by Thomson of diffusion capacity in the AIR trial [23].

The novel findings in this study relate to the changes in gas trapping as measured by body plethysmography. Surprisingly this aspect of lung function has not been previously reported in detail following BT, but there has been a suggestion from one CT study [24] that a reduction in total lung volume might be occurring. In the current study it is clear that BT reduces RV, and that this effect is greatest in the most obstructed patients at baseline. Accompanying the reduction in RV, a reduction in TLC and FRC are observed. The magnitude of the reduction in RV in the overall group is 7%, and this is modest but comparable to the effect of bronchodilators in this patient group. In the more severely obstructed patients, the reduction in RV is accompanied by a reduction in RV/TLC ratio. Multivariate analysis suggests that

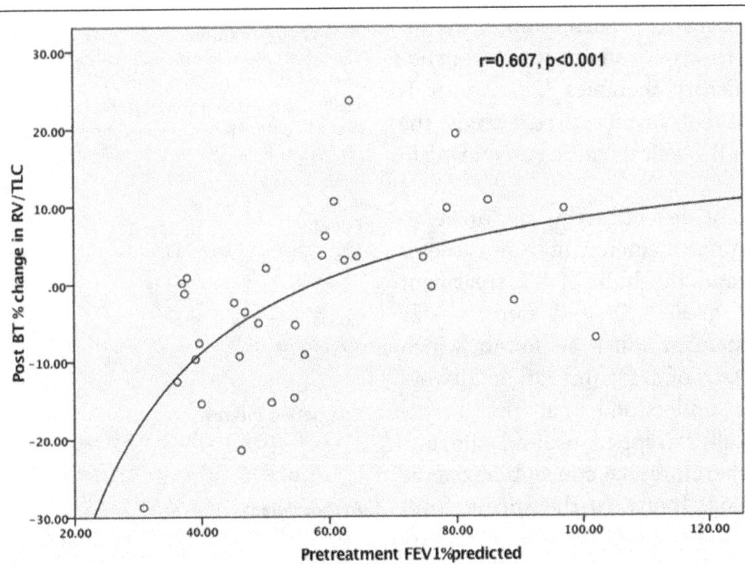

Fig. 2 Percentage change in RV/TLC ratio versus FEV_1% predicted

Table 3 Subgroup comparison by baseline FEV_1

Parameter	Group A $FEV_1 < 60$	Group B $FEV_1 \geq 60$	p
n	20	12	
age	61.5 ± 11.3	57.9 ± 12.5	NS
BMI kg/m^2	30.6 ± 7.6	30.2 ± 6.5	NS
RF activations	207 ± 62	210 ± 57	NS
Baseline ACQ-5	3.0 ± 0.8	3.0 ± 0.9	NS
Baseline FEV_1 (%predicted)	45.8 ± 8.3	77.7 ± 13.7	–
Baseline RV (litres)	3.5 ± 0.9	2.1 ± 0.4	< 0.001
Baseline RV (%predicted)	164 ± 34	114 ± 18.7	< 0.001
Baseline RV/TLC (%)	55.4 ± 8.6	42.3 ± 6.5	< 0.001
Post BT delta RV (mls)	– 326 ± 338	+ 40 ± 144	< 0.001
Post BT change RV (%)	–8.6 ± 8.4	+ 2.0 ± 7.4	< 0.001
Post BT change RV/TLC (%)	–6.5 ± 8.9	+ 7.1 ± 8.8	< 0.001

p unpaired t-test

it was only the baseline FEV_1 which was predictive of the fall in RV, with age, gender, BMI, activations and baseline ACQ-5 all having no effect. Figures 1 and 2, and Table 3 suggest that a ceiling in this effect is observed beyond a baseline FEV_1 of 60% predicted.

Reduction in RV, without any change in spirometry, is a signal that BT may be exerting an effect in the small peripheral airways of the lung. These airways constitute a very large part of the total cross sectional area of the lung yet contribute only 10% of the total airway resistance [25]. For this reason, airways obstruction in these airways is not detected by spirometry [13]. These small airways lack the cartilaginous support of the larger airways and their premature closure leads to elevation of the RV [13]. It is well established the small airways are pathologically involved in asthma [26] and that the RV rises as the severity increases [27]. Furthermore, the increased RV is amenable to improvement with bronchodilator and anti-inflammatory therapies [28, 29]. It is entirely feasible therefore that, in this current study, the improvement in RV after BT reflects an improvement in small airways function.

Exactly how this might be occurring is open to speculation. The minimum diameter of the catheter used in BT is 1.5 mm and the bulk of BT treatment is delivered to airways greater than 2 mm in size [30]. Therefore, a mechanism must be found which would propagate the effect of BT from larger airways to small airways. It is understood that the airway smooth muscle is helically wrapped around the airways [31], and could therefore be conceptualized as acting like a coiled spring. Injury to the spring from BT would therefore weaken the apparatus along its whole length, and thus influence distal airway diameter. Alternatively, Pretolani [5] has demonstrated a marked reduction in the autonomic neural innervation of the airway following BT, and therefore it is possible that a reduction in cholinergic tone is leading to distal bronchodilatation, in the same way that targeted lung denervation is being applied in Chronic Obstructive Pulmonary Disease [32].

It is recognized that it is uncontrolled, observational data which is presented in this study. As such, its role is in hypothesis generation- in this case, about a potential new mechanism of action of BT. It is anticipated that further studies using more sensitive measures of small airways dysfunction, such as impedance oscillometry and multiple breath nitrogen washout, will be necessary to confirm the observations made and yield further insights into the role that the peripheral airways might be playing in responses to BT.

Conclusion

The substantive clinical response to BT without any accompanying change in spirometry suggests that BT affects small peripheral airway function. Support for this concept is seen by the reduction in Residual Volume after treatment, accompanied by a reduction in RV/TLC ratio in more obstructed patients.

Abbreviations

ACQ-5: Asthma control questionnaire-5 item version; BMI: Body Mass Index; BT: Bronchial thermoplasty; DLCO: Diffusion Capacity for carbon monoxide; ERS/ATS: European Respiratory Society/American Thoracic Society; FEV_1: Forced expiratory volume in 1 s; FRC: Functional Residual Capacity; KCO: Gas transfer per lung unit; RV: Residual Volume; TLC: Total Lung Capacity; VC: Vital Capacity

Acknowledgements

The authors wish to acknowledge the assistance of Ms. Ceri Banks in patient assessments and care co-ordination.

Author contributions

DL had access to all study data and takes responsibility for data integrity and analysis. DL and AI performed all BT procedures. KB supervised lung function testing. WW assisted with statistical review. All authors, including CF, MP, VP and FT contributed to manuscript preparation and intellectual input. All authors read and approved the final manuscript.

Funding

D.L. is the recipient of a Monash University post-graduate scholarship.

Consent for publication

Not applicable.

Competing interests

The authors declare that they have no competing interests.

Author details

[1]Department of Thoracic Medicine, Frankston Hospital, Peninsula Health, 2 Hastings Road, Frankston, VIC 3199, Australia. [2]Faculty of Medicine, Nursing and Health Sciences, Monash University, Clayton, Vic, Australia. [3]Faculty of Medicine and Health Sciences, Macquarie University, Sydney, NSW, Australia.

[4]Department of Thoracic Medicine, Concord Hospital, Concord, NSW, Australia. [5]Sydney Medical School, University of Sydney, Sydney, NSW, Australia. [6]Department of Respiratory Medicine, Eastern Health, Vic, Boxhill, Australia.

References

1. Global initiative for asthma. Global strategy for asthma management and prevention, 2017. Available from: www.ginasthma.org.
2. Danek CJ, Lombard CM, Dungworth DL, Cox PG, Miller JD, Biggs MJ, Keast TM, Loomas BE, Wizeman WJ, Hogg JC. Reduction in airway hyperresponsiveness to methacholine by the application of RF energy in dogs. J Appl Physiol (1985). 2004;97(5):1946–53.
3. Pretolani M, Dombret MC, Thabut G, Knap D, Hamidi F, Debray MP, Taille C, Chanez P, Aubier M. Reduction of airway smooth muscle mass by bronchial thermoplasty in patients with severe asthma. Am J Respir Crit Care Med. 2014;190(12):1452–4.
4. Chakir J, Haj-Salem I, Gras D, Joubert P, Beaudoin E-L, Biardel S, Lampron N, Martel S, Chanez P, Boulet L-P, Laviolette M. Effects of bronchial Thermoplasty on airway smooth muscle and collagen deposition in asthma. Annals ATS. 2015;12(11):1612–8.
5. Pretolani M, Bergqvist A, Thabut G, Dombret M-C, Knapp D, Hamidi F, Alavoine L, Taille C, Chanez P, Erjefait J, Aubier M. Effectiveness of bronchial thermoplasty in patients with severe refractory asthma: clinical and histopathological correlations. JACI. 2017;139:1176–85.
6. Castro M, Rubin AS, Laviolette M, Fiterman J, De Andrade Lima M, Shah P, Fiss E, Olivenstein R, Thomson N, Niven R. Effectiveness and safety of bronchial thermoplasty in the treatment of severe asthma: a multicenter, randomized, double-blind, sham-controlled clinical trial. Am J Respir Crit Care Med. 2010;181(2):116–24.
7. Cox G, Thomson NC, Rubin AS, Niven RM, Corris PA, Olivenstein R, Pavord ID, McCormack D, Chaudhuri R. Asthma control during the year after bronchial thermoplasty. N Engl J Med. 2007;356(13):1327–37.
8. Pavord ID, Cox G, Thomson NC, Rubin AS, Corris PA, Niven RM, Chung KF, Laviolette M. Safety and efficacy of bronchial thermoplasty in symptomatic, severe asthma. Am J Respir Crit Care Med. 2007;176(12):1185–91.
9. Harris Ian. Surgery, the ultimate placebo: a surgeon cuts through the evidence. Coogee NSW, New South Publishing. 2016.
10. Hamid Q. Pathogenisis of small airways in asthma. Respiration. 2012;84:4–11.
11. Thien F. Measuring and imaging small airways dysfunction in asthma. Asia Pac Allergy. 2013;3:224–30.
12. Perez T, Chanez P, Dusser D, Devillier P. Small airway impairment in moderate to severe asthmatics without significant proximal airway obstruction. Respir Med. 2013;107:1667–74.
13. McNulty W, Usmani O. Techniques of assessing small airways dysfunction. Euro Clin Resp J. 2014;1:25898.
14. Chung KF, Wenzel SE, Brozek JL, Bush A, Castro M, Sterk PJ, Adcock IM, Bateman ED, Bel EH, Bleeker ER, Boulet LP, Brightling C, Chanez P, Dahlen SE, Djukanovic R, Frey U, Gaga M, Gibson P, Hamid Q, Jajour NN, Mauad T, Sorkness RL, Teague WG. International ERS/ATS guidelines on definition, evaluation and treatment of severe asthma. ERJ. 2014;43:343–73.
15. Juniper EF, Svensson K, Mörk AC, Ståhl E. Measurement properties and interpretation of three shortened versions of the asthma control questionnaire. Respir Med. 2005;99(5):553–8.
16. Miller MR, Hankinson J, Brusasco V, Burgos F, Casaburi R, Coates A, Crapo R, Enright P, van der Grinten CP, Gustafsson P, et al. ATS/ERS task force. Standardisation of spirometry. Eur Respir J. 2005;26(1):319–38.
17. Quanjer PH, Stanojevic S, Cole TJ, Bauer X, Hall GL, Culver BH, Enright PL, Hankinson JL, MSM I, Zheng J, Stocks J. Multi-ethnic reference values for spirometry for 3-95 year age range: the global lung function 2012 equations. ERJ. 2012;40(6):1324–43.
18. Quanjer PH, Tammeling GJ, Cotes JE, Pedersen OF, Peslin R, Yernault JC. Lung volumes and forced ventilatory flows. Report working party standardization of lung function tests, European Community for steel and coal. Official statement of the European Respiratory Society. Eur Respir J Suppl. 1993;16:5–40.
19. Mayse ML, Laviolette M, Rubin AS, Lampron N, Simoff M, Duhamel D, Musani A, Yung R, Mehta A. Clinical pearls for bronchial thermoplasty. J Bronchol. 2007;14(2):115–23.
20. Chupp G, Laviolette M, Cohn L, McEvoy C, Bansal S, Shifren A, Khatri S, Grubb M, McMullen E, Strauven R, Kline J. Long-term outcomes of bronchial thermoplasty in subjects with severe asthma: a comparison of 3-year follow-up results from twp prospective multicentre studies. Eur Respir L. 2017;50: 1700017.
21. Thomson NC, Chanez P. How effective is bronchial thermoplasty for severe asthma in clinical practice? Eur Respir J. 2017;50:1701140.
22. Wechsler ME, Laviolette M, Rubin AS, Fiterman J, Lapa e Silva JR, Shah PL, Fiss E, Olivenstein R, Thomson NC, Niven RM. Bronchial thermoplasty:long-term safety and effectiveness in patients with severe persistent asthma. J Allergy Clin Immunol. 2013;132:1295–302.
23. Thomson N, Rubin A, Niven R, Corris P, Siersted H, Olivenstein R, Pavord I, McCormack D, laviolette M, Shargill N, Cox G. Long-term (5 year) safety of bronchial thermoplasty: asthma intervention Resaerch (AIR) trial. BMC Pulmonary Medicine. 2011;11:8.
24. Zanon M, Strieder D, Rubin A, Watte G, Marchiori E, cardoso PF, Hochhegger B. Use of MDCT to assess the results of bronchial thermoplasty. Am J Roentgenology. 2017;209:752–6.
25. Macklem P. The physiology of small airways. Am J Respir Crit Care Med. 1998;157:S181–3.
26. Tulic MK, Christodoulopoulos P, Hamid Q. Small airway inflammation in asthma. Respir Res. 2001;2:333–9.
27. Irvin C, Bates JH. Physiologic dysfunction of the asthmatic lung. Proc Am Thorac Soc. 2009;6(3):306–11.
28. Newton MF, O'Donnell DE, Forkert L. Response of lung volumes to inhaled salbutamol in a large population of patients with severe hyperinflation. Chest. 2002;121:1042–50.
29. Kraft M, Cairns CB, Ellison MC, Pak J, Irvin C, Wenzel S. Improvement in distal lung function correlate with asthma symptoms after treatment with oral montelukast. Chest. 2006;130:1726–32.
30. Cox G. Bronchial thermoplasty. Clin Chest Med. 2010;31:135–40.
31. Gunst SJ, Tang D. The contractile apparatus and mechanical properties of airway smooth muscle. Eur Respir J. 2000;15:600–16.
32. Slebos D-J, Klooster K, Koegelenberg CF, Theron J, Styen D, Valipour A, Mayse M, Bolliger C. Targeted lung denervation for moderate to severe COPD: a pilot study. Thorax. 2015;0:1–9.

Detailed analysis of sputum and systemic inflammation in asthma phenotypes: are paucigranulocytic asthmatics really non-inflammatory?

Sophie Demarche[1,2,3*], Florence Schleich[1,2], Monique Henket[1,2], Virginie Paulus[1,2], Thierry Van Hees[3] and Renaud Louis[1,2]

Abstract

Background: The technique of induced sputum has allowed to subdivide asthma patients into inflammatory phenotypes according to their level of granulocyte airway infiltration. There are very few studies which looked at detailed sputum and blood cell counts in a large cohort of asthmatics divided into inflammatory phenotypes. The purpose of this study was to analyze sputum cell counts, blood leukocytes and systemic inflammatory markers in these phenotypes, and investigate how those groups compared with healthy subjects.

Methods: We conducted a retrospective cross-sectional study on 833 asthmatics recruited from the University Asthma Clinic of Liege and compared them with 194 healthy subjects. Asthmatics were classified into inflammatory phenotypes.

Results: The total non-squamous cell count per gram of sputum was greater in mixed granulocytic and neutrophilic phenotypes as compared to eosinophilic, paucigranulocytic asthma and healthy subjects ($p < 0.005$). Sputum eosinophils (in absolute values and percentages) were increased in all asthma phenotypes including paucigranulocytic asthma, compared to healthy subjects ($p < 0.005$). Eosinophilic asthma showed higher absolute sputum neutrophil and lymphocyte counts than healthy subjects ($p < 0.005$), while neutrophilic asthmatics had a particularly low number of sputum macrophages and epithelial cells. All asthma phenotypes showed an increased blood leukocyte count compared to healthy subjects ($p < 0.005$), with paucigranulocytic asthmatics having also increased absolute blood eosinophils compared to healthy subjects ($p < 0.005$). Neutrophilic asthma had raised CRP and fibrinogen while eosinophilic asthma only showed raised fibrinogen compared to healthy subjects ($p < 0.005$).

Conclusions: This study demonstrates that a significant eosinophilic inflammation is present across all categories of asthma, and that paucigranulocytic asthma may be seen as a low grade inflammatory disease.

Keywords: Asthma, Phenotypes, Healthy subjects, Sputum cytology, Blood leukocyte count, CRP, Fibrinogen

* Correspondence: sophie.demarche@ulg.ac.be
[1]Department of Respiratory Medicine, CHU Liege, Sart-Tilman B35, 4000 Liege, Belgium
[2]GIGA I[3] Research Group, University of Liege, Liege, Belgium
Full list of author information is available at the end of the article

Background

The technique of induced sputum has been pivotal in the emergence of the concept of inflammatory asthma phenotypes. Although it is technically demanding and time-consuming, several centers have applied the technique of induced sputum to characterize asthma inflammatory phenotypes in routine [1–7]. It has been suggested that airway inflammation may be subdivided into four phenotypes according to the level of granulocyte airway infiltration: eosinophilic, neutrophilic, mixed granulocytic and paucigranulocytic [2, 3]. This latter has been considered as a non-inflammatory type of asthma as the sputum analysis of these patients was suggested not to differ from healthy subjects [8].

These inflammatory phenotypes have been analyzed with respect to their demographic, functional and clinical characteristics in several studies [2, 3, 9, 10]. However, there has been fewer studies looking in detail at sputum cells [2], blood leukocytes [11], systemic inflammatory markers or at these variables in combination in a large cohort of asthmatics classified according to the extent of airway granulocytic inflammation, and investigating how those groups compared with healthy subjects.

Here, in a retrospective analysis, we report on sputum cell counts, blood leukocytes, C-reactive protein (CRP) and fibrinogen in a large series of asthmatics seen in daily practice of a University Clinic and compare the results with those in healthy subjects.

Our results show that paucigranulocytic asthmatics may display a low grade airway and systemic inflammation.

Methods

Study design, setting and participants

We conducted a retrospective cross-sectional study on asthmatic patients and healthy subjects recruited from the University Asthma Clinic of Liege. Asthmatic patients were eligible for the study if they had a first visit with a successful sputum analysis between 1 October 2003 and 5 February 2015. The diagnosis of asthma was based on the presence of typical symptoms (wheezing, breathlessness, chest tightness, cough) and at least one of the following: forced expiratory volume in one second (FEV_1) increase of ≥12 % and 200 ml after inhalation of 400 μg salbutamol or a provocative concentration of methacholine causing a 20 % fall in FEV_1 (PC20M) less than 16 mg/ml. Atopy was defined by the presence of at least one positive specific IgE (>0.35 kU/L; Phadia; Groot-Bijgaarden, Belgium) to one or more common aeroallergen (cat, dog, grass pollen, tree pollen, house dust mite and a mixture of moulds). Fractional exhaled nitric oxide (FENO) measurements were performed at 50 ml/s of flow rate (NIOX, Aerocrine, Sweden). Healthy subjects were recruited by advertisement and in the hospital staff, during this 12-year period of study. They had no diagnosis of respiratory disease, a $FEV_1 \geq 80$ % and a Tiffeneau index ≥0.7. Only healthy subjects with a successful sputum analysis were selected. This retrospective study was conducted with the approval from the ethics committee of the University Hospital of Liege (Reference 2015/193). Informed consents were obtained from healthy subjects. As for asthmatic patients, all procedures were performed in the context of clinical practice and the retrospective data collection was conducted with the approval from the above-mentioned ethics committee.

Sputum induction and analysis

Sputum was induced and processed as previously described [12]. Briefly, sputum was induced by hypertonic (5 %) or isotonic saline with salbutamol when post-bronchodilator FEV_1 was >65 % or ≤65 % predicted, respectively. Sputum was then processed using the whole expectorate technique. Dithiothreitol (DTT) was used as the mucolytic agent. Sputum sample was considered as adequate for cell count when squamous cell count was <80 % [13]. Differential cell count was performed on cytospins after a Diff-Quick staining.

Asthma phenotypes

Threshold values used to define the eosinophilic and neutrophilic phenotypes were a sputum eosinophil count ≥3 % and a sputum neutrophil count ≥76 %, respectively [14]. The mixed granulocytic phenotype was defined as both raised sputum eosinophil and neutrophil counts and the paucigranulocytic one as sputum eosinophil and neutrophil counts lower than the thresholds.

Statistical analysis

Results were expressed as frequencies and percentages for categorical variables and as median (interquartile range) or mean ± standard deviation for continuous variables. Comparisons were performed using a Pearson's chi-squared test for categorical variables, an ANOVA or a Student's t-test for parametric variables, and a Kruskal-Wallis test for non-parametric variables. The Pearson correlation coefficient was used to measure the association between the percentage of sputum neutrophils and eosinophils, and the number of pack-years in asthmatics. For this parametric test, sputum eosinophils were logtransformed and the 0 values replaced by 0.1. A p value <0.05 was considered statistically significant. When multiple tests were performed, the statistically significant level was corrected according to the Bonferroni principle. Statistical analysis was done using STATA version 13.0 (Statistical Software, College Station, TX: StataCorp LP).

Results

Subject characteristics

The demographic, functional and treatment characteristics of asthmatics and healthy subjects are given in Table 1. In our cohort of asthmatics with a successful sputum analysis ($n = 833$), inflammatory phenotypes were distributed as follows: 42 % of patients were eosinophilic, 16 % neutrophilic, 4 % mixed granulocytic and 38 % paucigranulocytic. The group of neutrophilic asthma presented a higher proportion of women while eosinophilic asthma had a lower proportion of women. Paucigranulocytic asthmatics were the youngest and had the best FEV_1 (% predicted) and FEV_1/forced vital capacity (FVC) ratio. All asthma subgroups had a higher prevalence of atopy as compared to healthy subjects ($p < 0.005$: level of statistical significance after Bonferroni correction).

Sputum cell counts and viability

The sputum cell counts and viability of asthma phenotypes and healthy subjects are shown in Table 2. The total non-squamous cell count per gram of sputum and the cell viability were greater in mixed granulocytic and neutrophilic phenotypes compared to eosinophilic, paucigranulocytic asthma and healthy subjects. Eosinophilic asthmatics also had significantly greater total sputum cell counts than paucigranulocytic asthmatics and healthy subjects. The fraction of squamous cells was less than 20 % in a majority of the patients, and was particularly low in eosinophilic, neutrophilic and mixed granulocytic asthma. While levels were obviously the highest in eosinophilic and mixed granulocytic phenotypes compared to other asthmatics, sputum eosinophils (in absolute values and percentages) were increased in all asthma phenotypes, compared to healthy subjects (Table 2 and Fig. 1a). Absolute neutrophil counts were increased not only in neutrophilic and mixed granulocytic asthma, but also in eosinophilic asthma subjects, compared with healthy subjects. The group of neutrophilic asthma was the only one to have a lower absolute sputum macrophage count than eosinophilic, paucigranulocytic asthmatics and healthy subjects. Absolute sputum lymphocyte count was greater in eosinophilic asthma ($p < 0.005$, versus paucigranulocytic asthma and healthy subjects), while absolute epithelial cell count was remarkably lower in case of intense neutrophilic inflammation ($p < 0.005$, versus paucigranulocytic and eosinophilic asthma, Table 2 and Fig. 1b).

Table 1 Demographic, functional and treatment characteristics of asthmatics classified by phenotypes and healthy subjects

	Eosinophilic asthma	Neutrophilic asthma	Mixed granulocytic asthma	Paucigranulocytic asthma	Healthy subjects	p value
N (% of asthmatics)	350 (42)	134 (16)	31 (4)	318 (38)	194	-
Women, N (%)	184 (53)	95 (71)‡†	19 (61)	197 (62)	105 (54)	0.002
Age, years	49 (34–60)*	52 (41–61)‡*	61 (43–71)‡*	43 (30–54)	45 (27–56)	0.0001
BMI	25.9 ± 4.9‡	25.3 ± 5.4	25.5 ± 4.6	26.1 ± 4.8‡	24.3 ± 4.1	0.0004
Atopy, N (%)	213 (63)‡	69 (52)‡	17 (57)‡	165 (53)‡	46 (28)	<0.001
Smoking status, N (%)						
Non-smokers	190 (54)	73 (55)	19 (61)	162 (52)	109 (57)	>0.05
Current smokers	64 (18)	26 (20)	5 (16)	76 (24)	35 (18)	
Ex-smokers	96 (27)	33 (25)	7 (23)	75 (24)	47 (25)	
FEV_1, % predicted	81.2 ± 20.9‡*	81.6 ± 22.0‡*	81.6 ± 20.6‡	89.2 ± 18.2‡	108.0 ± 13.3	0.0001
FEV_1/FVC, %	70.7 ± 11.1‡*	71.7 ± 11.5‡*	70.1 ± 10.5‡*	76.2 ± 9.0‡	82.1 ± 6.5	0.0001
FENO, ppb	43 (23–82)*	20 (13–33)†§	36 (21–75)*	16 (12–29)	/	0.0001
ICS therapy, N (%)	227 (65)	87 (65)	18 (58)	195 (61)	/	>0.05
ICS dose[a]	500 (0–1000)	800 (0–2000)	800 (0–1600)	400 (0–1000)	/	>0.05
OCS therapy, N (%)	21 (6)	9 (7)	2 (6)	14 (4)	/	>0.05
LABA, N (%)	209 (60)	80 (60)	20 (65)	181 (57)	/	>0.05
LTRA, N (%)	75 (21)	37 (28)	9 (29)	73 (23)	/	>0.05
Theophylline, N (%)	11 (3)	7 (5)	0 (0)	11 (3)	/	>0.05

$^{‡}p < 0.005$, comparison with healthy subjects
$^{*}p < 0.005$, comparison with paucigranulocytic asthma
$^{†}p < 0.005$, comparison with eosinophilic asthma
$^{§}p < 0.005$, comparison with mixed granulocytic asthma
[a]ICS dose in beclomethasone dipropionate - chlorofluorocarbon equivalents

Abbreviations: *BMI* body mass index; *FENO* fractional exhaled nitric oxide; *FEV_1* forced expiratory volume in 1 s; *FVC* forced vital capacity; *ICS* inhaled corticosteroid; *LABA* long-acting β2-agonist; *LTRA* leukotriene receptor antagonist; *OCS* oral corticosteroid

Table 2 Sputum cell counts and viability of asthmatics classified by phenotypes and healthy subjects

	Eosinophilic asthma Sp. eosinophils ≥3 % Sp. neutrophils <76 %	Neutrophilic asthma Sp. eosinophils <3 % Sp. neutrophils ≥76 %	Mixed granulocytic asthma Sp. eosinophils ≥3 % Sp. neutrophils ≥76 %	Paucigranulocytic asthma Sp. eosinophils <3 % Sp. neutrophils <76 %	Healthy subjects	*p* value (Kruskal-Wallis test)
Total non-squamous cell count ($\times 10^6$/g)	1.18 (0.56–2.85)$^{\ddagger *}$	1.84 (0.82–5.52)$^{\ddagger * \dagger}$	4.10 (1.07–12.00)$^{\ddagger * \dagger}$	0.81 (0.40–2.07)	0.64 (0.37–1.30)	0.0001
Viability (%)	64 (50–75)	79 (68–88)$^{\ddagger * \dagger}$	81 (67–86)$^{\ddagger * \dagger}$	64 (48–75)	67 (53–78)	0.0001
Squamous cells (%)	13 (5–25)$^{\ddagger *}$	12 (3–28)$^{\ddagger *}$	6 (2–23)$^{\ddagger *}$	18 (8–35)	18 (10–31)	0.0001
Eosinophils						
x 10^3/g	201 (64–636)$^{\ddagger *}$	3 (0–27)$^{\ddagger \dagger \S}$	271 (46–685)$^{\ddagger *}$	3 (0–10)‡	0 (0–2)	0.0001
% of non-squamous cells	17.1 (7.4–38.0)$^{\ddagger *}$	0.2 (0.0–1.0)$^{\ddagger \dagger \S}$	5.2 (3.4–8.8)$^{\ddagger * \dagger}$	0.4 (0.0–1.0)‡	0.0 (0.0–0.4)	-
Neutrophils						
x 10^3/g	335 (135–823)‡	1504 (707–4728)$^{\ddagger * \dagger}$	3272 (881–10992)$^{\ddagger * \dagger}$	270 (90–795)	210 (63–563)	0.0001
% of non-squamous cells	33 (16–50)*	87 (82–93)$^{\ddagger * \dagger}$	83 (79–88)$^{\ddagger * \dagger}$	42 (21–58)	36 (13–63)	-
Macrophages						
x 10^3/g	288 (144–648)	169 (52–425)$^{\ddagger * \dagger}$	218 (77–607)	337 (167–853)	285 (120–568)	0.0001
% of non-squamous cells	27 (16–43)$^{\ddagger *}$	9 (4–13)$^{\ddagger * \dagger}$	6 (3–9)$^{\ddagger * \dagger}$	46 (29–61)	46 (30–67)	0.0001
Lymphocytes						
x 10^3/g	19 (5–52)$^{\ddagger *}$	12 (2–41)	19 (0–88)	10 (3–31)	10 (4–26)	0.0012
% of non-squamous cells	1.7 (0.6–3.2)	1.0 (0.3–1.6)$^{\ddagger * \dagger}$	0.6 (0.0–1.8)$^{\ddagger \dagger}$	1.4 (0.5–2.8)	1.8 (0.8–3.4)	0.0001
Epithelial cells						
x 10^3/g	56 (20–140)‡	18 (3–67)$^{\ddagger * \dagger}$	15 (0–106)$^{* \dagger}$	50 (23–115)‡	35 (12–86)	0.0001
% of non-squamous cells	5.0 (2.0–8.6)*	1.0 (0.4–2.0)$^{\ddagger * \dagger}$	0.6 (0.2–1.8)$^{\ddagger * \dagger}$	6.0 (2.8–13.0)	4.8 (2.2–11.8)	0.0001

$^{\ddagger}p < 0.005$, comparison with healthy subjects
$^{*}p < 0.005$, comparison with paucigranulocytic asthma
$^{\dagger}p < 0.005$, comparison with eosinophilic asthma
$^{\S}p < 0.005$, comparison with mixed granulocytic asthma
Abbreviation: *Sp.* sputum

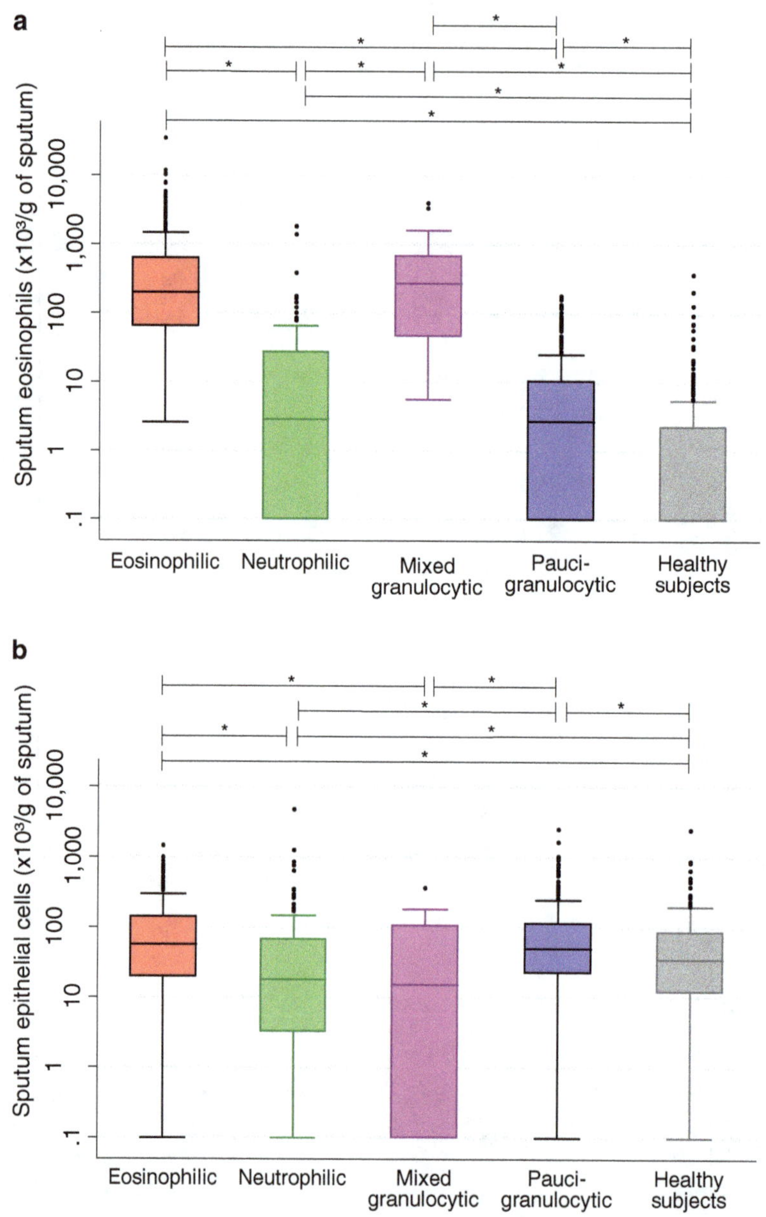

Fig. 1 Absolute sputum eosinophils (**a**) and absolute sputum epithelial cells (**b**) in asthma phenotypes and healthy subjects. * $p < 0.005$. Values of 0 were assigned to 0.1 because of the use of a logarithmic scale

Blood leukocyte counts and systemic inflammatory markers

The blood leukocyte counts and systemic inflammatory markers of asthma phenotypes and healthy subjects are shown in Table 3. All subgroups of asthmatics showed an increased level of blood leukocytes compared with healthy subjects (Table 3 and Fig. 2a). As expected, eosinophilic and mixed granulocytic asthmatics had higher blood eosinophils (in absolute values and percentages) than neutrophilic, paucigranulocytic asthma and healthy subjects, but paucigranulocytic asthmatics also showed higher levels of absolute blood eosinophils than healthy subjects. Neutrophilic asthmatics had the highest level of blood neutrophils, compared to eosinophilic, paucigranulocytic asthma and healthy subjects, but both eosinophilic and paucigranulocytic asthmatics also had greater absolute blood neutrophils than healthy subjects. Absolute lymphocyte counts were mainly increased in eosinophilic and paucigranulocytic asthma. Only the group of eosinophilic asthma had increased absolute blood basophil counts compared to healthy subjects. Neutrophilic asthma was characterized by raised CRP and fibrinogen levels, while eosinophilic asthma had raised fibrinogen only, compared with healthy subjects (Table 3 and Fig. 2b).

Table 3 Blood leukocyte counts and systemic inflammatory markers of asthmatics classified by phenotypes and healthy subjects

	Eosinophilic asthma Sp. eosinophils ≥3 % Sp. neutrophils <76 %	Neutrophilic asthma Sp. eosinophils <3 % Sp. neutrophils ≥76 %	Mixed granulocytic asthma Sp. eosinophils ≥3 % Sp. neutrophils ≥76 %	Paucigranulocytic asthma Sp. eosinophils <3 % Sp. neutrophils <76 %	Healthy subjects[a]	*p* value (Kruskal-Wallis test)
Blood leukocytes (x 10^3/μL)	7.76 (6.52–8.87)‡	7.75 (6.43–10.00)‡	8.02 (6.16–10.83)‡	7.25 (6.02–8.75)‡	6.12 (5.03–7.37)	0.0001
Blood eosinophils						
/μL	315 (202–513)$^{\ddagger *}$	129 (79–228)$^{\dagger \S}$	289 (216–449)$^{\ddagger *}$	140 (85–227)‡	106 (68–172)	0.0001
%	4.2 (2.8–6.2)$^{\ddagger *}$	1.7 (1.0–3.0)$^{\dagger \S}$	3.9 (2.7–5.8)$^{\ddagger *}$	2.0 (1.1–3.0)	1.8 (1.0–3.0)	0.0001
Blood neutrophils						
/μL	4045 (3204–5140)‡	4847 (3260–6323)$^{\ddagger * \dagger}$	4207 (2834–6610)	3971 (3156–5280)‡	3416 (2610–4188)	0.0001
%	54.0 (47.6–60.1)*	59.5 (52.5–69.3)$^{* \dagger}$	57.6 (44.4–62.4)	56.5 (50.3–62.2)	54.4 (49.6–62.1)	0.0001
Blood monocytes						
/μL	515 (396–667)$^{\ddagger *}$	492 (408–656)‡	564 (448–775)‡	461 (362–608)	399 (330–550)	0.0001
%	6.7 (5.1–8.3)	6.5 (5.4–8.2)	7.2 (5.6–9.0)	6.4 (5.1–8.2)	7.1 (5.7–8.2)	>0.05
Blood lymphocytes						
/μL	2358 (1918–2809)‡	2249 (1765–2807)	2180 (1887–2869)	2337 (1894–2904)‡	2009 (1611–2386)	0.0001
%	31.8 (26.0–38.3)	29.4 (22.5–37.1)$^{\ddagger *}$	29.1 (21.0–38.2)	32.7 (27.3–38.2)	33.9 (26.5–37.7)	0.006
Blood basophils						
/μL	42 (29–63)$^{\ddagger *}$	35 (23–51)†	39 (27–55)	34 (24–52)	34 (24–46)	0.0001
%	0.6 (0.4–0.8)*	0.5 (0.3–0.6)$^{\ddagger \dagger}$	0.5 (0.4–0.7)	0.5 (0.3–0.7)	0.5 (0.4–0.8)	0.0001
CRP (mg/L)[b]	1.4 (0.6–3.6)	1.9 (0.8–5.3)‡	2.9 (0.6–8.9)	1.6 (0.6–4.5)	1.1 (0.4–2.4)	0.034
Fibrinogen (g/L)[c]	3.2 (2.8–3.8)‡	3.2 (2.8–3.7)‡	3.3 (2.7–3.9)	3.1 (2.7–3.6)	2.9 (2.6–3.2)	0.0008

[a]Data available for 96 healthy subjects
[b]Data available for 208 eosinophilic, 92 neutrophilic, 23 mixed granulocytic, 186 paucigranulocytic and 63 healthy subjects
[c]Data available for 194 eosinophilic, 85 neutrophilic, 21 mixed granulocytic, 174 paucigranulocytic and 59 healthy subjects
$^{\ddagger}p < 0.005$, comparison with healthy subjects
$^{*}p < 0.005$, comparison with paucigranulocytic asthma
$^{\dagger}p < 0.005$, comparison with eosinophilic asthma
$^{\S}p < 0.005$, comparison with mixed granulocytic asthma
Abbreviations: *CRP* C-reactive protein; *Sp.* sputum

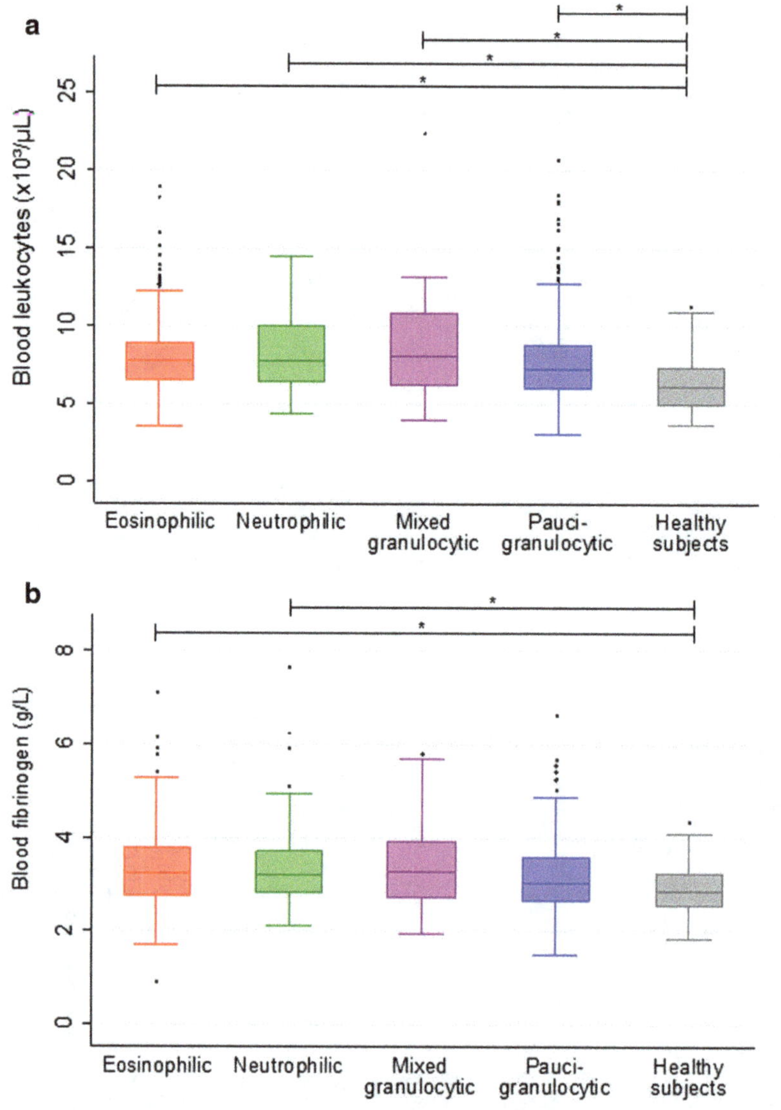

Fig. 2 Blood leukocytes (**a**) and blood fibrinogen (**b**) in asthma phenotypes and healthy subjects. * $p < 0.005$

Analysis of asthma phenotypes according to treatment with inhaled corticosteroids (ICS) and comparison with healthy subjects

For each phenotype, we compared sputum and blood cell counts between patients treated and not treated with ICS and we also compared these subgroups with healthy subjects (Table 4 and Additional file 1: Table S1). In steroid-naïve paucigranulocytic patients, as in the whole group of paucigranulocytic asthma, there was an increase in sputum eosinophil counts, compared to healthy subjects. With respect to systemic inflammation, blood leukocyte, eosinophil and lymphocyte counts were increased in steroid-naïve paucigranulocytic asthmatics, compared to healthy subjects ($p < 0.0042$: level of statistical significance after Bonferroni correction, Table 4). Paucigranulocytic asthmatics receiving inhaled corticosteroids showed an increase in sputum eosinophils and epithelial cells, and an increase in blood leukocyte, neutrophil and lymphocyte numbers ($p < 0.0042$, Table 4). We did not find any statistically significant difference between patients treated and not treated with ICS in the subgroups of paucigranulocytic, neutrophilic and mixed granulocytic asthma ($p > 0.0042$, Table 4 and Additional file 1: Table S1). In eosinophilic asthmatics, patients treated with ICS presented higher levels of sputum epithelial cells, blood leukocytes and blood neutrophils, as compared with eosinophilic patients not treated with ICS ($p < 0.0042$, Additional file 1: Table S1).

Analysis of asthma phenotypes classified with a threshold of sputum eosinophils of 1.01 %

We also used 1.01 % as the threshold of sputum eosinophils to define asthma phenotypes. When using this cutoff value,

Table 4 Sputum and blood cell counts of non-eosinophilic phenotypes classified by ICS treatment and healthy subjects

	Paucigranulocytic asthma, not treated with ICS	Paucigranulocytic asthma, treated with ICS	ICS- vs ICS+	Neutrophilic asthma, not treated with ICS	Neutrophilic asthma, treated with ICS	ICS- vs ICS+	Healthy subjects
N	123	195	-	47	87	-	194
Sputum total non-squamous cell count (x 10^6/g)	0.93 (0.43–2.12)	0.69 (0.36–1.61)	NS	1.45 (0.82–4.65)[‡]	2.10 (0.75–8.02)[‡]	NS	0.64 (0.37–1.30)
Sputum viability (%)	65 (48–78)	64 (48–75)	NS	78 (68–87)[‡]	80 (68–88)[‡]	NS	67 (53–78)
Sputum squamous cells (%)	16 (7–30)	19 (10–37)	NS	18 (5–30)	7 (2–27)[‡]	NS	18 (10–31)
Sputum eosinophils (x 10^3/g)	4 (0–15)[‡]	2 (0–10)[‡]	NS	2 (0–28)[‡]	4 (0–27)[‡]	NS	0 (0–2)
Sputum neutrophils (x 10^3/g)	315 (97–994)	245 (86–710)	NS	1197 (707–3776)[‡]	1879 (593–7060)[‡]	NS	210 (63–563)
Sputum macrophages (x 10^3/g)	451 (188–864)[‡]	280 (154–853)	NS	127 (33–396)[‡]	182 (52–436)	NS	285 (120–568)
Sputum lymphocytes (x 10^3/g)	12 (3–45)	10 (2–24)	NS	15 (4–41)	11 (1–39)	NS	10 (4–26)
Sputum epithelial cells (x 10^3/g)	48 (19–113)	52 (25–120)[‡]	NS	19 (4–44)	18 (3–73)	NS	35 (12–86)
Blood leukocytes (x10^3/μL)[a]	6.87 (5.85–8.51)[‡]	7.47 (6.32–9.06)[‡]	NS	7.87 (6.41–9.93)[‡]	7.71 (6.44–10.06)[‡]	NS	6.12 (5.03–7.37)
Blood eosinophils (/μL)[a]	145 (101–217)[‡]	139 (74–229)	NS	172 (63–293)	123 (80–215)	NS	106 (68–172)
Blood neutrophils (/μL)[a]	3598 (2924–5119)	4211 (3392–5392)[‡]	NS	4804 (3158–6021)[‡]	4885 (3403–6969)[‡]	NS	3416 (2610–4188)
Blood monocytes (/μL)[a]	461 (353–592)	463 (370–615)[‡]	NS	476 (387–648)	519 (419–669)[‡]	NS	399 (330–550)
Blood lymphocytes (/μL)[a]	2352 (1891–2967)[‡]	2321 (1900–2855)[‡]	NS	2518 (1989–3035)[‡]	2167 (1675–2726)	NS	2009 (1611–2386)
Blood basophils (/μL)[a]	35 (25–52)	33 (24–51)	NS	40 (29–53)	33 (22–50)	NS	34 (24–46)

[a] Data available for 96 healthy subjects
[‡] $p < 0.0042$, comparison with healthy subjects
Abbreviation: *ICS* inhaled corticosteroid

there was no statistically significant difference in sputum and blood eosinophils (in absolute values and percentages) between neutrophilic or paucigranulocytic asthma, and healthy subjects (the level of statistical significance after Bonferroni correction being a p value <0.005, Table 5). However, there was a strong trend for greater absolute sputum eosinophil count in paucigranulocytic asthmatics versus healthy subjects ($p = 0.005$). In the paucigranulocytic asthma subgroup defined with this cutoff value, absolute sputum epithelial cells (50 (24-115) $\times 10^3$/g), blood leukocytes (7.21 (5.82–8.66) $\times 10^3/\mu L$), absolute blood neutrophils (3900 (3083–5299)/μL) and absolute blood lymphocytes (2334 (1891–2904)/μL) were still greater than in healthy subjects ($p < 0.005$).

Analysis according to atopy

The blood and sputum eosinophil counts of asthmatics and healthy subjects according to their atopic status are presented in Table 6. We did not observe any statistically significant difference in these cells between atopic and non-atopic healthy subjects or asthmatics (the level of statistical significance after Bonferroni correction being a p value <0.0083).

Analysis according to smoking habits

The proportion of asthma inflammatory phenotypes was analyzed according to the smoking status of patients (Fig. 3), and was not different between non-smokers, ex-smokers and current smokers ($p = 0.6$). There was however a correlation between the number of pack-years and the percentage of sputum neutrophils but this correlation was absent with sputum eosinophils (Fig. 4).

Discussion

Our study shows that the four inflammatory asthma phenotypes display raised sputum eosinophilia compared to healthy subjects. Eosinophilic asthma showed higher levels of absolute sputum neutrophils and lymphocytes than healthy subjects, while neutrophilic asthmatics had a reduced number of sputum macrophages and epithelial cells. In addition, all phenotypes had increased systemic inflammation reflected by raised total circulating leukocyte counts, mainly accounted for by raised granulocytic blood cell counts compared to healthy subjects.

As previously shown [2], our data indicate that neutrophilic and mixed granulocytic inflammation is more intense than pure eosinophilic and paucigranulocytic ones as the total number of cells per gram of sputum was clearly increased in these two first forms of groups. This might be related to the larger pool of circulating neutrophils and the variety of stimuli able to recruit neutrophils into the airways [15]. Our results showing greater viability in neutrophilic and mixed granulocytic asthma are also in keeping with those reported by Simpson et al. [2]. It may seem paradoxical as neutrophils are recognized to be more fragile than eosinophils in cell culture [16], but this may suggest greater cell turnover and short time of residency of neutrophils in the airways [17].

It has been suggested that non-eosinophilic asthmatics are poorly responsive to inhaled corticosteroids [8, 18]. One interesting finding of our study is the fact that the so called "non-eosinophilic phenotypes" (neutrophilic and paucigranulocytic phenotypes) actually had more sputum eosinophils than healthy subjects, pointing to a low grade

Table 5 Eosinophilic inflammation of asthmatics classified by phenotypes (with a sputum eosinophil cutoff of 1.01 %) and healthy subjects

	Eosinophilic asthma	Neutrophilic asthma	Mixed granulocytic asthma	Paucigranulocytic asthma	Healthy subjects	p value (Kruskal-Wallis test)
	Sp. eosinophils ≥1.01 %	Sp. eosinophils <1.01 %	Sp. eosinophils ≥1.01 %	Sp. eosinophils <1.01 %		
	Sp. neutrophils <76 %	Sp. neutrophils ≥76 %	Sp. neutrophils ≥76 %	Sp. neutrophils <76 %		
N (% of asthmatics)	429 (51)	106 (13)	59 (7)	239 (29)	194	-
Sputum eosinophils						
x 10^3/g	127 (38–471)[‡*]	0 (0–9)[†§]	77 (31–380)[‡*]	0 (0–5)[‡‡]	0 (0–2)	0.0001
% of non-squamous cells	11.8 (4.0–30.8)[‡*]	0.0 (0.0–0.5)[†§]	3.0 (1.8–6.0)[‡*†]	0.2 (0.0–0.5)	0.0 (0.0–0.4)	0.0001
Blood eosinophils[a]						
/μL	289 (181–444)[‡*]	123 (62–220)[†§]	266 (126–430)[‡*]	133 (78–200)	106 (68–172)	0.0001
%	3.8 (2.4–5.6)[‡*]	1.7 (0.9–3.0)[†§]	2.9 (1.8–5.6)[‡*]	1.9 (1.0–2.7)	1.8 (1.0–3.0)	0.0001

[a]Data available for 96 healthy subjects
[‡]$p < 0.005$, comparison with healthy subjects
[‡‡]$p = 0.005$, comparison with healthy subjects
[*]$p < 0.005$, comparison with paucigranulocytic asthma
[†]$p < 0.005$, comparison with eosinophilic asthma
[§]$p < 0.005$, comparison with mixed granulocytic asthma
Abbreviation: *Sp.* sputum

Table 6 Eosinophilic inflammation of asthmatics and healthy subjects according to atopy

	Non-atopic asthmatics	Atopic asthmatics	Non-atopic healthy subjects	Atopic healthy subjects	p value (Kruskal-Wallis test)
N	344	464	118	46	-
Sputum eosinophils					
x 10^3/g	19 (1–173)[‡*]	34 (3–181)[‡*]	0 (0–3)	0 (0–4)	0.0001
% of non-squamous cells	1.6 (0.2–9.6)[‡*]	2.8 (0.2–13.8)[‡*]	0.0 (0.0–0.4)	0.0 (0.0–0.5)	0.0001
Blood eosinophils[a]					
/μL	188 (109–327)[‡]	217 (124–375)[‡*]	93 (62–135)	134 (80–202)	0.0001
%	2.6 (1.4–4.0)[‡]	3.0 (1.7–4.7)[‡]	1.5 (0.9–2.9)	2.1 (1.6–3.0)	0.0001

[a]Data available for 54 non-atopic healthy subjects and 31 atopic healthy subjects
[‡]$p < 0.0083$, comparison with non-atopic healthy subjects
[*]$p < 0.0083$, comparison with atopic healthy subjects

eosinophilic inflammation in these phenotypes. This could explain the fact that some patients with non-eosinophilic asthma responded to inhaled corticosteroids in the study of Cowan et al. [19], even though a limitation of this study was the absence of placebo-controlled design. Also of interest is the fact that eosinophilic asthmatics had more absolute sputum neutrophils compared to healthy subjects. It is likely to reflect that pathways leading to the recruitment of eosinophils and neutrophils in the airways may co-exist or act through a same effector in asthma [20].

It is noteworthy that absolute sputum lymphocyte counts were increased when there was significant eosinophilic infiltration. Although little attention has been paid to lymphocytes in sputum so far because of their small number (representing approximately 1–2 %), our finding is in keeping with the role of lymphocytes in organizing eosinophilic inflammation, a concept which has been established by bronchial biopsy and bronchoalveolar lavage analyses [21, 22].

A particularly low absolute number of macrophages was observed in neutrophilic asthma. Further to this decreased amount of macrophages in the airways, Simpson et al. [23] described an impaired capacity of sputum macrophages to phagocytose apoptotic material in non-eosinophilic asthma, which may explain chronic inflammation and accumulation of airway neutrophils.

In keeping with epithelial alteration in asthma [24], we found an increased epithelial cell number in sputum from eosinophilic and paucigranulocytic asthma. By contrast, epithelial cell count was particularly low in the groups displaying intense neutrophilic inflammation. The presence of epithelial cells in sputum samples may reflect epithelial desquamation. Therefore, it is somewhat surprising to find lower epithelial cell counts in neutrophilic asthma. Our clinical feeling is that the cough effort during sputum induction may favor epithelial shedding and our experience is that effort to produce sputum is less when patients have intense neutrophilic inflammation, which may prevent epithelial cell desquamation.

In contrast to COPD [25], little attention has been paid to systemic inflammation in asthma, so far. Our data show striking elevation of total blood leukocyte counts in all asthmatic phenotypes compared to healthy subjects. There was however no difference between asthma phenotypes in this respect, which is in keeping with the recent study of Zhang et al. [11]. Although raised circulating leukocytes might have been expected in patients with eosinophilic, neutrophilic and mixed granulocytic asthma, this finding was somewhat more surprising in paucigranulocytic asthma.

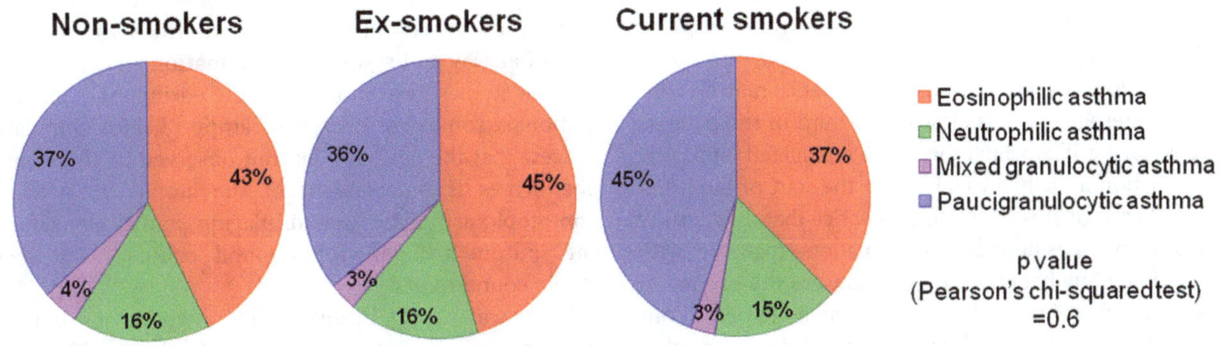

Fig. 3 Proportion of asthma inflammatory phenotypes according to the smoking status of asthmatics

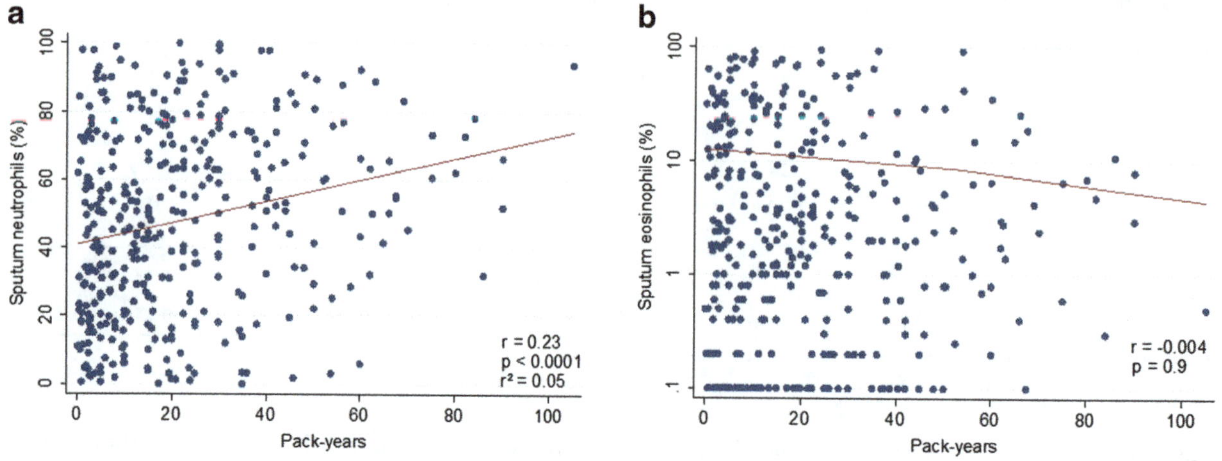

Fig. 4 Relationship between sputum neutrophils (**a**) and eosinophils (**b**) and the number of pack-years in ex- and current smoker asthmatics. For sputum eosinophils, values of 0 were assigned to 0.1 because of the use of a logarithmic scale

As previously shown [3, 11], patients with a raised sputum eosinophilic inflammation also had the highest levels of blood eosinophils (absolute values or percentages). Moreover, we found that the highest levels of absolute blood neutrophils were observed in neutrophilic and mixed granulocytic asthma, although the results did not reach statistical significance in this last phenotype, probably due to the small number of patients. Interestingly, paucigranulocytic asthmatics also had raised absolute circulating eosinophils and neutrophils compared to healthy subjects. Overall it points to a granulocytic inflammation in all asthma phenotypes.

Like in sputum, absolute lymphocyte counts were increased in blood of patients with eosinophilic asthma. Interestingly, levels of absolute blood basophils were also higher in these patients, which is consistent with a previous report showing a concomitant increase in circulating eosinophils and basophils after allergen inhalation in atopic asthmatics [26].

Supporting the concept of low grade systemic inflammation in asthma, we found a mild but significant increase in fibrinogen levels in eosinophilic and neutrophilic asthma, while increase in CRP was essentially observed in asthmatics with intense airway neutrophilic infiltration, as previously shown [27].

The group of paucigranulocytic asthmatics may be considered heterogeneous as almost two third of the patients were receiving ICS, which may have attenuated an airway inflammation initially present before the start of the treatment. Therefore, it is interesting to notice that mild airway and systemic eosinophilic inflammation, together with raised circulating lymphocyte number, were still present in those patients not treated with ICS. One limitation of our study is the retrospective design that precludes any further phenotypic characterization of circulating lymphocytes.

Several interventional studies have shown that ICS therapy decreases sputum eosinophils [28, 29] and increases sputum neutrophils [19]. In our study, we did not find any statistically significant difference in these sputum cells between patients treated and not treated with ICS. However, because of its cross-sectional design, our study does not question the impact of ICS on eosinophil and neutrophil counts. We believe that the persistence of significant sputum eosinophilia in ICS treated asthmatics reflects the severity of the inflammatory process in these patients.

Paucigranulocytic asthma is defined as a sputum eosinophil count <3 % in our study. Others have proposed a cutoff at 1.01 % [2]. When choosing this cutoff in our patients, we increase the proportion of eosinophilic asthma from 42 to 51 % and we correspondingly decrease the proportion of paucigranulocytic asthma from 38 to 29 %. With this cutoff at 1.01 %, the group of paucigranulocytic asthmatics still displayed signs of airway and systemic inflammation, although they did not show increased circulating blood eosinophils anymore. It is interesting to postulate that the paucigranulocytic phenotype may be composed of some asthmatics presenting low grade inflammation and others without any sign of airway and systemic inflammation.

Some studies have shown that the eosinophilic inflammation is somewhat related to atopy [3, 30]. Our data suggest that the eosinophilic trait observed in all asthma phenotypes is independent of the atopic status with non-atopic asthmatics not displaying statistically different sputum and blood eosinophil counts from their atopic counterparts.

There was no significant change in the proportion of inflammatory phenotypes according to the smoking status. However, in contrast to sputum eosinophils, sputum neutrophil count appears to be partly associated with the cumulative smoking history expressed as pack-years. Previous studies failed to find this relationship [31, 32] but they were performed on a limited number of patients. This association remains however rather limited based on our results, where pack-years can only account for 5 % of the neutrophil variability.

It is known that asthma inflammatory phenotypes may somewhat vary over time [2, 33]. One limitation of our study is its cross-sectional design with sputum analyzed at only one time point.

Conclusions

Overall, this study demonstrates that a significant eosinophilic inflammation is present across all categories of asthma, and that paucigranulocytic asthma may be seen as a low grade inflammatory disease. Whether steroid-naïve or a part of steroid-treated paucigranulocytic asthmatics may do without ICS should be investigated in long term trials, but our data incite to be cautious in clinical practice for now.

Ethics approval and consent to participate

This retrospective study was conducted with the approval from the ethics committee of the University Hospital of Liege (Reference 2015/193). Informed consents were obtained from healthy subjects. As for asthmatic patients, all procedures were performed in the context of clinical practice and the retrospective data collection was conducted with the approval from the above-mentioned ethics committee.

Consent for publication

Not applicable.

Abbreviations

BMI: body mass index; CRP: C-reactive protein; FENO: fractional exhaled nitric oxide; FEV_1: forced expiratory volume in 1 second; FVC: forced vital capacity; ICS: inhaled corticosteroid; LABA: long-acting β2-agonist; LTRA: leukotriene receptor antagonist; OCS: oral corticosteroid; PC20M: provocative concentration of methacholine causing a 20 % fall in FEV_1.

Competing interests

The authors declare that they have no competing interests.

Authors' contributions

SD designed the study, helped to collect the data, analyzed and interpreted the data and drafted the manuscript. FS collected the data, helped to draft the manuscript and revised it critically for important intellectual content. MH and VP collected the data and revised the manuscript critically for important intellectual content. TVH helped to analyze the data and revised the manuscript critically for important intellectual content. RL designed the study, collected the data, interpreted the data and drafted the manuscript. All authors read and approved the final manuscript.

Acknowledgements

We acknowledge the Fonds Léon Fredericq for funding training in statistics.

Funding

This work was supported by a federal grant IAP P7/30.

Author details

[1]Department of Respiratory Medicine, CHU Liege, Sart-Tilman B35, 4000 Liege, Belgium. [2]GIGA I[3] Research Group, University of Liege, Liege, Belgium. [3]Department of Clinical and Hospital Pharmacy, University of Liege, Liege, Belgium.

References

1. Pavord ID, Pizzichini MM, Pizzichini E, Hargreave FE. The use of induced sputum to investigate airway inflammation. Thorax. 1997;52:498–501.
2. Simpson JL, Scott R, Boyle MJ, Gibson PG. Inflammatory subtypes in asthma: assessment and identification using induced sputum. Respirol Carlton Vic. 2006;11:54–61.
3. Schleich FN, Manise M, Sele J, Henket M, Seidel L, Louis R. Distribution of sputum cellular phenotype in a large asthma cohort: predicting factors for eosinophilic vs neutrophilic inflammation. BMC Pulm Med. 2013;13:11.
4. in't Veen JC, de Gouw HW, Smits HH, Sont JK, Hiemstra PS, Sterk PJ, et al. Repeatability of cellular and soluble markers of inflammation in induced sputum from patients with asthma. Eur Respir J. 1996;9:2441–7.
5. Bacci E, Cianchetti S, Carnevali S, Bartoli ML, Dente FL, Di Franco A, et al. Induced sputum is a reproducible method to assess airway inflammation in asthma. Mediators Inflamm. 2002;11:293–8.
6. Vlachos-Mayer H, Leigh R, Sharon RF, Hussack P, Hargreave FE. Success and safety of sputum induction in the clinical setting. Eur Respir J. 2000;16:997–1000.
7. Green RH, Brightling CE, Woltmann G, Parker D, Wardlaw AJ, Pavord ID. Analysis of induced sputum in adults with asthma: identification of subgroup with isolated sputum neutrophilia and poor response to inhaled corticosteroids. Thorax. 2002;57:875–9.
8. Haldar P, Pavord ID. Noneosinophilic asthma: a distinct clinical and pathologic phenotype. J Allergy Clin Immunol. 2007;119:1043–52. quiz 1053-4.
9. Hastie AT, Moore WC, Meyers DA, Vestal PL, Li H, Peters SP, et al. Analyses of asthma severity phenotypes and inflammatory proteins in subjects stratified by sputum granulocytes. J Allergy Clin Immunol. 2010;125:1028–36. e13.
10. Porsbjerg C, Lund TK, Pedersen L, Backer V. Inflammatory subtypes in asthma are related to airway hyperresponsiveness to mannitol and exhaled NO. J Asthma Off J Assoc Care Asthma. 2009;46:606–12.
11. Zhang X-Y, Simpson JL, Powell H, Yang IA, Upham JW, Reynolds PN, et al. Full blood count parameters for the detection of asthma inflammatory phenotypes. Clin Exp Allergy J Br Soc Allergy Clin Immunol. 2014;44:1137–45.
12. Delvaux M, Henket M, Lau L, Kange P, Bartsch P, Djukanovic R, et al. Nebulised salbutamol administered during sputum induction improves bronchoprotection in patients with asthma. Thorax. 2004;59:111–5.
13. Gershman NH, Wong HH, Liu JT, Mahlmeister MJ, Fahy JV. Comparison of two methods of collecting induced sputum in asthmatic subjects. Eur Respir J. 1996;9:2448–53.
14. Louis R, Godinas L, Schleich F. Induced Sputum - Towards Normal Values. Non Invasive Assessment of airways inflammation in asthma and COPD. Athens: Paschalidis Medical Publications; 2011. p. 113–23.
15. Douwes J, Gibson P, Pekkanen J, Pearce N. Non-eosinophilic asthma: importance and possible mechanisms. Thorax. 2002;57:643–8.
16. Meagher LC, Cousin JM, Seckl JR, Haslett C. Opposing effects of glucocorticoids on the rate of apoptosis in neutrophilic and eosinophilic granulocytes. J Immunol Baltim Md 1950. 1996;156:4422–8.
17. Kamath AV, Pavord ID, Ruparelia PR, Chilvers ER. Is the neutrophil the key effector cell in severe asthma? Thorax. 2005;60:529–30.
18. Louis R, Schleich F, Barnes PJ. Corticosteroids: still at the frontline in asthma treatment? Clin Chest Med. 2012;33:531–41.
19. Cowan DC, Cowan JO, Palmay R, Williamson A, Taylor DR. Effects of steroid therapy on inflammatory cell subtypes in asthma. Thorax. 2010;65:384–90.
20. Cosmi L, Liotta F, Maggi E, Romagnani S, Annunziato F. Th17 cells: new players in asthma pathogenesis. Allergy. 2011;66:989–98.

21. Bradley BL, Azzawi M, Jacobson M, Assoufi B, Collins JV, Irani AM, et al. Eosinophils, T-lymphocytes, mast cells, neutrophils, and macrophages in bronchial biopsy specimens from atopic subjects with asthma: comparison with biopsy specimens from atopic subjects without asthma and normal control subjects and relationship to bronchial hyperresponsiveness. J Allergy Clin Immunol. 1991;88:661–74.
22. Walker C, Kaegi MK, Braun P, Blaser K. Activated T cells and eosinophilia in bronchoalveolar lavages from subjects with asthma correlated with disease severity. J Allergy Clin Immunol. 1991;88:935–42.
23. Simpson JL, Gibson PG, Yang IA, Upham J, James A, Reynolds PN, et al. Impaired macrophage phagocytosis in non-eosinophilic asthma. Clin Exp Allergy J Br Soc Allergy Clin Immunol. 2013;43:29–35.
24. Al-Muhsen S, Johnson JR, Hamid Q. Remodeling in asthma. J Allergy Clin Immunol. 2011;128:451–62. quiz 463-4.
25. Dickens JA, Miller BE, Edwards LD, Silverman EK, Lomas DA, Tal-Singer R, et al. COPD association and repeatability of blood biomarkers in the ECLIPSE cohort. Respir Res. 2011;12:146.
26. Gibson PG, Manning PJ, O'Byrne PM, Girgis-Gabardo A, Dolovich J, Denburg JA, et al. Allergen-induced asthmatic responses. Relationship between increases in airway responsiveness and increases in circulating eosinophils, basophils, and their progenitors. Am Rev Respir Dis. 1991;143:331–5.
27. Wood LG, Baines KJ, Fu J, Scott HA, Gibson PG. The neutrophilic inflammatory phenotype is associated with systemic inflammation in asthma. Chest. 2012;142:86–93.
28. Berry M, Morgan A, Shaw DE, Parker D, Green R, Brightling C, et al. Pathological features and inhaled corticosteroid response of eosinophilic and non-eosinophilic asthma. Thorax. 2007;62:1043–9.
29. Jatakanon A, Kharitonov S, Lim S, Barnes PJ. Effect of differing doses of inhaled budesonide on markers of airway inflammation in patients with mild asthma. Thorax. 1999;54:108–14.
30. Lewis SA, Pavord ID, Stringer JR, Knox AJ, Weiss ST, Britton JR. The relation between peripheral blood leukocyte counts and respiratory symptoms, atopy, lung function, and airway responsiveness in adults. Chest. 2001;119:105–14.
31. Boulet L-P, Lemière C, Archambault F, Carrier G, Descary MC, Deschesnes F. Smoking and asthma: clinical and radiologic features, lung function, and airway inflammation. Chest. 2006;129:661–8.
32. Telenga ED, Kerstjens HAM, Ten Hacken NHT, Postma DS, van den Berge M. Inflammation and corticosteroid responsiveness in ex-, current- and never-smoking asthmatics. BMC Pulm Med. 2013;13:58.
33. McGrath KW, Icitovic N, Boushey HA, Lazarus SC, Sutherland ER, Chinchilli VM, et al. A large subgroup of mild-to-moderate asthma is persistently noneosinophilic. Am J Respir Crit Care Med. 2012;185:612–9.

17

Childhood asthma prevalence and risk factors in three Eastern European countries - the Belarus, Ukraine, Poland Asthma Study (BUPAS)

Grzegorz Brozek[1], Joshua Lawson[2*], Andrei Shpakou[3], Olga Fedortsiv[4], Leonid Hryshchuk[5], Donna Rennie[6] and Jan Zejda[1]

Abstract

Background: The prevalence of asthma and other allergic diseases among children living in Eastern is not well described. Our objective was to estimate and compare the prevalence of asthma, respiratory symptoms and allergic diseases in children in Belarus, Ukraine, and Poland as well as to identify risk factors for these conditions. We also sought to profile and compare children with asthma between locations.

Methods: Data were collected as a part of an international, multicenter, cross-sectional study of childhood asthma: The Belarus Ukraine Poland Asthma Study (BUPAS). Subjects were children aged 7–13 years attending primary and secondary schools in the urban and surrounding rural area of Grodno (Belarus), Ternopil (Ukraine) and Silesia Region (Poland). Physician-diagnosed respiratory diseases and symptoms as well as allergic diseases were ascertained using the ISAAC questionnaire completed by the parents.

Results: In total there were 4019 children from Belarus (rural: 2018, urban: 2001), 4493 from Ukraine (1972; 2521), and 4036 from Poland (2002, 2034). The overall response rate was 76.7 %. Groups were similar in case of gender and age ($p > 0.05$). Almost all analyzed respiratory and allergic conditions differed significantly between countries including asthma [Poland (rural, urban): 3.5 %, 4.1 %; Ukraine: 1.4 %, 2.1 %; Belarus: 1.4 %, 1.5 %], spastic bronchitis (Poland: 2.7 %, 3.2 %; Ukraine: 7.5 %, 6.5 %; Belarus: 6.4 %, 7.9 %), and chest wheeze in the last year (Poland: 4.8 %, 5.2 %; Ukraine: 11.5 %, 13.0 %; Belarus: 10.7 %, 10.0 %). These differences remained after adjustment for potential confounders. Risk factor associations were generally similar between outcomes. Symptom characteristics of children with asthma between countries were not consistent. The ratio of current wheeze:diagnosis of asthma differed by country: (Rural areas: Belarus: 10.9:1, Ukraine: 17.3:1, Poland: 2.4:1; Urban areas: Belarus: 8.1:1, Ukraine: 7.3:1 Poland: 1.9:1).

Conclusions: The findings show large between-country differences and relatively low prevalence of asthma and allergic diseases in children of Western Belarus and Ukraine. There is evidence for underdiagnosis of asthma in these regions.

* Correspondence: josh.lawson@usask.ca
[2]Department of Medicine and Canadian Center for Health and Safety in Agriculture, University of Saskatchewan, Saskatoon, Canada
Full list of author information is available at the end of the article

Background

Geographic variation in childhood asthma prevalence has been reported [1, 2] with the global prevalence of asthma and related symptoms has ranged between approximately 2 and 37 % [1]. One difficulty in assessing asthma prevalence is potential differential use of labels for asthma. As such, it is important to symptoms, which do not require a diagnostic label and alternate labels for asthma and the potential of differences in asthma prevalence due to labeling differences.

While some investigation of asthma prevalence has been completed in Eastern Europe, including a regional investigation of countries from Eastern and Central Europe [3] which showed between-country variation in prevalence was more dominant than within-country variation along with some indication of diagnostic labeling explaining differences by region, there has been very little work completed in countries outside the EU including Ukraine and Belarus. Previously, we have described investigations of asthma prevalence separately in Ukraine [4] and Belarus [5] as part of the Belarus, Ukraine, and Poland Asthma Study (BUPAS). In each of these locations, there was some evidence of asthma underdiagnosis [4, 5] Qualitatively, the prevalence of asthma was lower in these countries compared to Western European nations, with possible underdiagnosis occurring. These observations, along with societal changes towards a Westernized lifestyle, which has been associated with higher asthma prevalence, make it likely that the prevalence of asthma will increase in the future. Indeed, we have some evidence suggesting increases of asthma prevalence in Eastern Europe [6]. Thus, asthma may be poised to increase as a public health problem in this region. Identification of reasons for geographic differences and risk factors for asthma, including consistency between regions, in these locations will help develop our etiologic understanding of asthma and may help our future management strategies for children with lung disease.

We further our previous work of BUPAS countries by combining the data from each country, which were based on data collection using the same questionnaires and study design. Specifically, we sought to: 1) compare prevalence of diagnosed asthma, diagnosed spastic bronchitis, respiratory symptoms, and allergic disorders between the three BUPAS countries; 2) To compare the prevalence and strength of association of risk factors for diagnosed asthma, wheeze, and spastic bronchitis between the three BUPAS countries; 3) To analyze the magnitude of urban–rural differences in the occurrence of diagnosed asthma in the three BUPAS countries; and 4) To compare symptoms profiles of children with diagnosed asthma between the three BUPAS countries. While we have previously described asthma prevalence and its determinants in Belarus and Ukraine as part of the BUPAS program, [4, 5] we have expanded on our previous investigations. First, the focus of the current paper is on between country differences, which allow us to make quantitative comparisons between regions. Second, this will be the first time where results from the Polish data are presented. Third, while minor, we focus on a slightly narrower age range than the previous studies in order to be able to include comparative data from all countries.

Methods

Study design and study population

Data were collected as a part of an international, multicenter, cross-sectional study of childhood asthma: The Belarus Ukraine Poland Asthma Study (BUPAS). Subjects were children aged 7–13 years attending primary and secondary schools in the urban and surrounding rural area of Ternopil (Ukraine), Grodno (Belarus) and Katowice (Poland). This age group was chosen given that this is generally when asthma prevalence is highest, it allows reasonable responses based on proxy report (i.e., parents), and for comparison, is comparable to ages consistently considered in other studies evaluating asthma prevalence in childhood. Schools were randomly selected from the urban center and the rural region, which included villages where agricultural activity was the primary industry, surrounding each urban area from which 3000 urban children and 3000 rural children were approached. This included 36 schools from urban areas in Belarus (10), Ukraine (11), and Poland (15) and 79 schools from rural areas in Belarus (20), Ukraine (23), and Poland (36). The number of schools included in each region differ due to differences in the number of students attending each school as participation rates were similar. Children from selected schools and their parents or legal guardians were invited to participate in the project. Questionnaires, accompanied by a letter explaining the study objectives and an informed written consent, were distributed to parents/guardians through the schools. Upon completion of the questionnaire, they were returned to the school where they were picked up by the research team. The study protocol was approved by the adequate local ethics committees at the State Medical University of Ternopil (Ukraine), Yanka Kupala University in Grodno (Belarus) and Medical University of Silesia in Katowice (Poland). None of the authors have any competing interests related to this manuscript.

Study instrument and operational definitions

The questionnaire included standard questions from the International Study of Asthma and Allergy in Children (ISAAC) respiratory questionnaire [2, 7] All questions were translated from English to Ukrainian, Russian and Polish respectively and their syntax was verified by back-translation. The ISAAC questionnaire has been used internationally and validated in many languages [8]. ISAAC questions have been used in Polish and Russian speaking populations previously [8]. The questionnaire included questions about established respiratory and allergic diagnoses, respiratory and allergic symptoms, family history of respiratory and allergic disorders, and socio-economic status. Location of dwelling was classified as urban or rural based on whether the child lived in the city (Grodno, Ternopil, Katowice) or the surrounding agricultural area. This was accounted for by targeting schools in these regions.

The list of analyzed allergic and respiratory diseases included diagnoses established during the child's lifetime by a physician and reported by subjects' parents for asthma and spastic bronchitis. Spastic bronchitis is a traditional diagnosis of the region and is used to describe chronic or recurrent asthmatic symptoms such as "wheezy bronchitis". Respiratory symptoms in the past 12 months were also assessed by report on the questionnaire.

Several variables were considered as potential correlates of respiratory outcomes. Parental asthma, allergic rhinitis, eczema were separately defined by a report of a positive history of physician diagnosed disease by either the mother or father. Current smoking and highest level of education were obtained for each of the mother and the father. Exposure to tobacco smoke was present when at least one family member smoked at home. Additional exposures were assessed by responses on the questionnaire based on the presence or absence of these exposures and included using coal or wood for cooking or heating, smoking during pregnancy, passive smoking during pregnancy, the presence of dog and cat in the home, and dampness at home. Evaluation of health care utilization and morbidity was based on answers to questions regarding medication use for breathing, specialist or general practitioner visits for breathing conditions, completion of spirometry testing, and completion of skin prick testing, all in the past 12 months.

Height (cm) and weight (kg) were reported on the questionnaire. From these measures, body mass index (BMI) was calculated based on the equation: [BMI = weight (kg)/ height (m)^2] [9]. Weight status was classified based on categorization of body mass index (BMI) using values described by Cole et al. [10] which base the cutoff value as the predicted adult (at 18 years of age) equivalent of a BMI of 25 for overweight and of 30 for obese.

Statistical analysis

All analyses were completed using SPSS 20. Statistical significance was defined by an alpha level of 0.05. Continuous variables were described by arithmetic mean values and standard deviations. Categorical variables were described by frequencies and proportions. Descriptive and comparative analyses were completed after stratification by urban/ rural status because of the method of sampling. Statistical significance of between-group differences in mean values was assessed by *t*-test and ANOVA, or nonparametric tests when distribution was not normal. When using categorical variables statistical significance was assessed by means of the independent samples chi-squared test. Initially, comparisons of personal and environmental factors were made between locations and between urban and rural status for each location. Following this analysis, comparisons of condition and symptom prevalence were made between locations and between urban and rural status for each location.

Multiple logistic regression was then completed to investigate the association between report of diagnosed asthma, diagnosed spastic bronchitis, and wheeze in the past 12 months with location and urban/rural status after adjusting for potential confounders. A multiple logistic model was fitted for each health outcome independently. Potential confounders were included based on their previously reported associations with asthma and availability on the questionnaire. For each model, the same fixed set of independent variables was tested to examine their association with the dependent variable and to control for potential confounding: age, sex, parental education, parental history of allergic disease, exposure to tobacco smoke at home, mother smoking during pregnancy, location of dwelling (urban or rural), use of coal or wood for cooking or heating, dampness, and dog or cat at home. The strength of the associations between the independent and dependent variables were quantified by odds ratios and their 95 % confidence intervals (CI). Statistical inference was based on the criterion $p < 0.05$. Interaction between location and each of the personal and environmental factors was tested using the Likelihood ratio test to assess if associations were consistent between locations. These results were also presented by stratified analyses.

Finally, among children with a previous diagnosis of asthma, we compared indicators of asthma severity and morbidity including hospitalization for asthma, visiting a physician for asthma, assessment by spirometry, assessment by skin prick testing and the presence of asthma-related symptoms between locations. This was completed using independent samples chi-squared tests.

Results

In total there were 4019 children from Belarus (rural: 2018, urban: 2001), 4493 children from Ukraine (rural: 1972, urban: 2521), and 4036 children from Poland (rural: 2002, urban: 2034). The response rate was 79.2 % in Ukraine, 77.8 % in Belarus and 75.4 % in Poland and was similar (>0.05) between urban and rural areas from each region. When comparing differences in the frequency of personal and environmental characteristics between countries (Table 1), there were many statistically significant differences. Among urban and rural dwellers, there were differences between countries for mother's and father's education levels, parental history of allergic disease, parental smoking, maternal smoking during pregnancy, use of coal or wood for cooking or heating, presence of mold or

Table 1 Personal characteristics of the study population by country and location of residence

	Urban			Rural		
	Belarus ($n = 2001$)	Ukraine ($n = 2521$)	Poland ($n = 2034$)	Belarus ($n = 2018$)	Ukraine ($n = 1972$)	Poland ($n = 2002$)
% Female	47.4	50.9	50.9**	49.8	51.5	51.8
% Mother with > high school	46.9*	54.1*	19.2*, **	19.7	41.9	13.0***
% Father with > high school	38.8*	45.7*	13.4*, **	16.3	32.0	6.8***
Obesity status						
% Not overweight or obese	87.1	87.8	86.8	88.3	85.9	88.2
% Overweight	11.5	10.7	11.8	10.0	11.2	10.4
% Obese	1.4	1.5*	1.5	1.7	3.0	1.5***
% Any parental history of allergic disease	14.7*	11.7*	30.7*, **	8.8	8.0	20.0***
% Either parent currently smoking	50.1*	50.9	46.5*, **	57.8	53.4	43.0***
% Maternal smoking during pregnancy	2.5	0.9	7.0*, **	2.4	1.1	4.4***
% Using coal or wood for cooking or heating	4.8*	1.4*	10.6*, **	28.3	6.8	28.2***
% Any mold or dampness in the home	30.5	47.9*	34.2*, **	29.9	55.8	27.5***
% With a cat	34.6*	27.9*	34.4*, **	61.4	64.2	43.9***
% With a dog	23.7*	17.2*	50.2*, **	45.6	54.2	55.1***
Mean age, years (SD)	10.2 (1.9)	10.4 (1.9)*	10.2 (1.9)**	10.2 (1.9)	10.2 (1.9)	10.3 (1.9)

* $p < 0.05$ comparing urban to rural within country
** $p < 0.05$ comparing across countries among urban children
*** $p < 0.05$ comparing across countries among rural children

dampness, and presence of a cat or dog. However, the differences were not always consistent in direction or magnitude. In addition to this, a lower proportion of urban dwelling children from Belarus were female compared to urban children from Ukraine or Poland and urban dwelling children from Ukraine were older than urban children from Belarus or Poland (Table 1).

The prevalence of asthma differed significantly by country for both urban and rural dwellers with the highest prevalence consistently in Poland (Rural: 3.5 %, Urban: 4.1 %) followed by Ukraine (Rural: 1.4 %, Urban: 2.1 %) and Belarus (Rural: 1.4 %, Urban: 1.5 %). The difference was not statistically significant between urban and rural dwellers in any country. Almost all other respiratory and allergic conditions considered differed significantly between countries for both urban and rural dwellers (Table 2). Similar to asthma, a higher prevalence of allergic conditions and symptoms, with the exception of eczema or skin allergy, was found in Poland compared to Ukraine and Belarus. While differences between countries were statistically significant, the direction of the differences was not entirely consistent when comparing respiratory symptoms. However, diagnosis of spastic bronchitis was consistently lower in Poland compared to Belarus and Ukraine.

Table 3 presents the findings from adjusted analyses for report of diagnosed asthma (primary interest), wheeze in the past 12 months (symptom reflective of asthma), and diagnosed spastic bronchitis (a diagnostic label thought to be used in place of asthma in the region). Compared to Belarus, children in Poland were at a higher risk of diagnosed asthma but a lower risk of wheeze in the past 12 months and spastic bronchitis while children from Ukraine were at increased risk of wheeze in the past 12 months. Females were at lower risk of any of the three outcomes with similar strengths of associations. There was a consistent increased risk of any of the three outcomes with the presence of parental history of allergic disease and mold or dampness in the home. Maternal smoking during pregnancy increased the risk of asthma and spastic bronchitis but this was only statistically significant for asthma. While having a dog was inversely associated with all three outcomes, it was only statistically significant for spastic bronchitis. Finally, increasing age was associated with an increased risk of diagnosed asthma but a reduced risk of wheeze in the past 12 months and spastic bronchitis.

We assessed the presence of interaction between country and the personal and environmental variables. When considering asthma as the outcome, there was statistically significant interaction between country and sex ($p = 0.03$) as well as home mold or dampness ($p = 0.04$). When considering wheeze in the past 12 months as the outcome, there was statistically significant interaction between country and home mold or dampness as well as age ($p < 0.001$). When considering spastic bronchitis there was statistically significant interaction between parental history of allergic disease ($p = 0.004$) as well as home mold or dampness ($p = 0.002$). Because of these results, we reran the adjusted analysis after stratification by country and presented the results for the

Table 2 Distribution of asthma, asthma-like conditions, and allergic conditions by country and location of residence

	Urban			Rural		
	Belarus (*n* = 2001)	Ukraine (*n* = 2521)	Poland (*n* = 2034)	Belarus (*n* = 2018)	Ukraine (*n* = 1972)	Poland (*n* = 2002)
Ever diagnosed with asthma	1.5	2.1	4.1†	1.4	1.4	3.5***
Asthma attacks in the past 12 months	0.7	0.9	1.8**	0.7	0.7	1.2
Woken by asthma attacks in the past 3 months	0.5	0.4	1.4*, **	0.3	0.7	0.7
Spastic bronchitis	7.9	6.5	3.2**	6.4	7.5	2.7***
Ever had chest wheeze	10.2	32.9*	14.7*, **	10.7	30.0	11.9***
Chest wheeze in the past 12 months	10.0	13.0	5.2**	10.7	11.5	4.8***
SOB with exercise in the past 12 months	4.0	6.6	4.7*, **	3.6	5.8	3.1***
Nocturnal SOB in the past 12 months	1.7*	1.8	3.5*, **	1.0	1.7	2.2***
Cough in the past 12 months	58.4*	73.4*	68.8**	65.1	70.5	67.8***
Productive cough in the past 12 months	34.0*	46.0	52.5*, **	39.4	44.3	42.8***
Ever diagnosed with rhinitis	5.3*	3.6	22.8*, **	2.1	4.4	14.7***
Ever diagnosed with eczema	12.6*	7.0	12.7*, **	8.6	6.8	7.4
Ever diagnosed with any allergy	17.7*	12.0	24.3*, **	10.7	13.1	16.1***
Ever had symptoms of allergic rhinitis or hayfever	3.7*	7.9*	20.6*, **	1.1	4.7	14.2***
Ever had sneezing with congestion or intense runny nose apart from a cold	10.0*	14.3*	21.1*, **	7.0	9.7	13.6***
Ever had skin allergy or itching	15.3*	14.1*	11.2*, **	12.7	11.7*	7.1***

*$p < 0.05$ comparing urban to rural within country
**$p < 0.05$ comparing across countries among urban children
***$p < 0.05$ comparing across countries among rural children

interaction variables in Fig. 1. In general, we found similar associations in Belarus and Poland and weaker, non-statistically significant associations within Ukraine.

Finally, we profiled the clinical characteristics of children with asthma and compared these by rural–urban status and by country (Table 4). When comparing characteristics of children with asthma by country, among rural dwellers, there were differences by country for diagnosis of rhinitis, rhinitis symptoms, taking breathing medication in the past 12 months, using asthma medication in the past 12 months, and being hospitalized for breathing troubles in the past 12 months (Table 4). Among urban children with asthma, differences by country existed for diagnosis of spastic bronchitis, diagnosis of rhinitis, diagnosis of any allergy, ever had a skin allergy or itching, using asthma medication in the past 12 months, being hospitalized for breathing troubles in the past 12 months, and having spirometry testing in the past 12 months (Table 4). Finally, to further consider some issues that may be related to diagnosis, we calculated the proportion of children with wheeze in the past 12 months who had a diagnosis of asthma. Belarus and Ukraine had lower proportions of those with wheeze in the past 12 months having an asthma diagnosis than in Poland for both rural (Belarus: 8.4 %, Ukraine: 5.5 %, Poland: 29.0 %) and urban regions (Belarus: 10.9 %, Ukraine: 12.1 %, Poland: 34.7 %). Related to these results, we considered the ratio of (current wheeze):(previous diagnosis of asthma). In rural areas this ratio was 10.9:1 in Belarus, 17.3:1 in Ukraine, and 2.4:1 in Poland. Similar patterns were observed in the urban areas (Belarus: 8.1:1, Ukraine: 7.3:1 Poland: 1.9:1).

In general, urban children with a report of doctor diagnosed asthma had a higher prevalence of conditions present than rural children. In Belarus we found urban children with a report of doctor diagnosed asthma to have a higher proportion of spastic bronchitis and allergic conditions or symptoms. In Ukraine, urban children with a report of doctor diagnosed asthma had a higher prevalence of wheeze in the past 12 months and cough in the past 12 months. In Poland, urban children with a report of doctor diagnosed asthma had a higher prevalence of asthma attacks in the past 12 months, had been woken by asthma attacks in the past 3 months, and had nocturnal shortness of breath in the past 12 months.

Discussion

While asthma prevalence was higher in Poland compared to Belarus and Ukraine, spastic bronchitis diagnosis, an alternative to asthma diagnosis in some countries, was higher in Belarus and Ukraine compared to Poland. While chest wheeze in the past 12 months was lower in Poland than in the other two countries and report of diagnosed rhinitis and rhinitis symptoms

Table 3 Adjusted [a] associations between respiratory health risk factors and outcomes of report of diagnosed asthma, wheeze in the past 12 months, and diagnosed spastic bronchitis

	Diagnosed asthma OR (95 % CI)	Wheeze in the past 12 months OR (95 % CI)	Diagnosed spastic bronchitis OR (95 % CI)
Country			
Belarus	1.00	1.00	1.00
Ukraine	1.32 (0.86–2.01)	1.20 (1.02–1.43)	0.99 (0.81–1.24)
Poland	2.40 (1.67–3.44)	0.42 (0.34–0.51)	0.36 (0.28–0.47)
Sex			
Male	1.00	1.00	1.00
Female	0.70 (0.53–0.92)	0.81 (0.70–0.94)	0.76 (0.64–0.91)
Mother with > high school			
No	1.00	1.00	1.00
Yes	1.15 (0.81–1.65)	0.91 (0.77–1.09)	1.09 (0.88–1.36)
Father with > high school			
No	1.00	1.00	1.00
Yes	0.93 (0.62–1.38)	1.06 (0.88–1.27)	1.11 (0.88–1.39)
Any parental history of allergic disease			
No	1.00	1.00	1.00
Yes	3.01 (2.25–4.04)	1.62 (1.34–1.96)	2.72 (2.20–3.36)
Either parent currently smoking			
No	1.00	1.00	1.00
Yes	1.18 (0.89–1.57)	1.03 (0.89–1.19)	0.95 (0.79–1.15)
Maternal smoking during pregnancy			
No	1.00	1.00	1.00
Yes	2.42 (1.42–4.11)	0.98 (0.61–1.56)	1.50 (0.90–2.53)
Using coal or wood for cooking or heating			
No	1.00	1.00	1.00
Yes	1.01 (0.67–1.51)	1.02 (0.80–1.29)	1.01 (0.75–1.31)
Any mold or dampness in the home			
No	1.00	1.00	1.00
Yes	1.33 (1.01–1.77)	1.35 (1.16–1.56)	1.28 (1.07–1.55)
With a cat			
No	1.00	1.00	1.00
Yes	0.84 (0.62–1.15)	0.93 (0.79–1.09)	1.04 (0.85–1.27)
With a dog			
No	1.00	1.00	1.00
Yes	0.78 (0.57–1.06)	0.94 (0.80–1.11)	0.77 (0.62–0.96)
Residence			
Rural	1.00	1.00	1.00
Urban	0.95 (0.71–1.27)	0.97 (0.83–1.13)	0.98 (0.80–1.19)
Age	1.11 (1.03–1.20)	0.93 (0.90–0.97)	0.95 (0.90–0.99)

[a]Adjusted for each variable in the table

were higher in Poland, there were inconsistent patterns in symptom prevalence. With the exception of the country of residence and its association with the outcomes considered, the associations between suspected asthma risk factors and asthma were generally consistent between locations where there was an increased risk of asthma associated with parental history of allergy and presence of home mold or dampness along

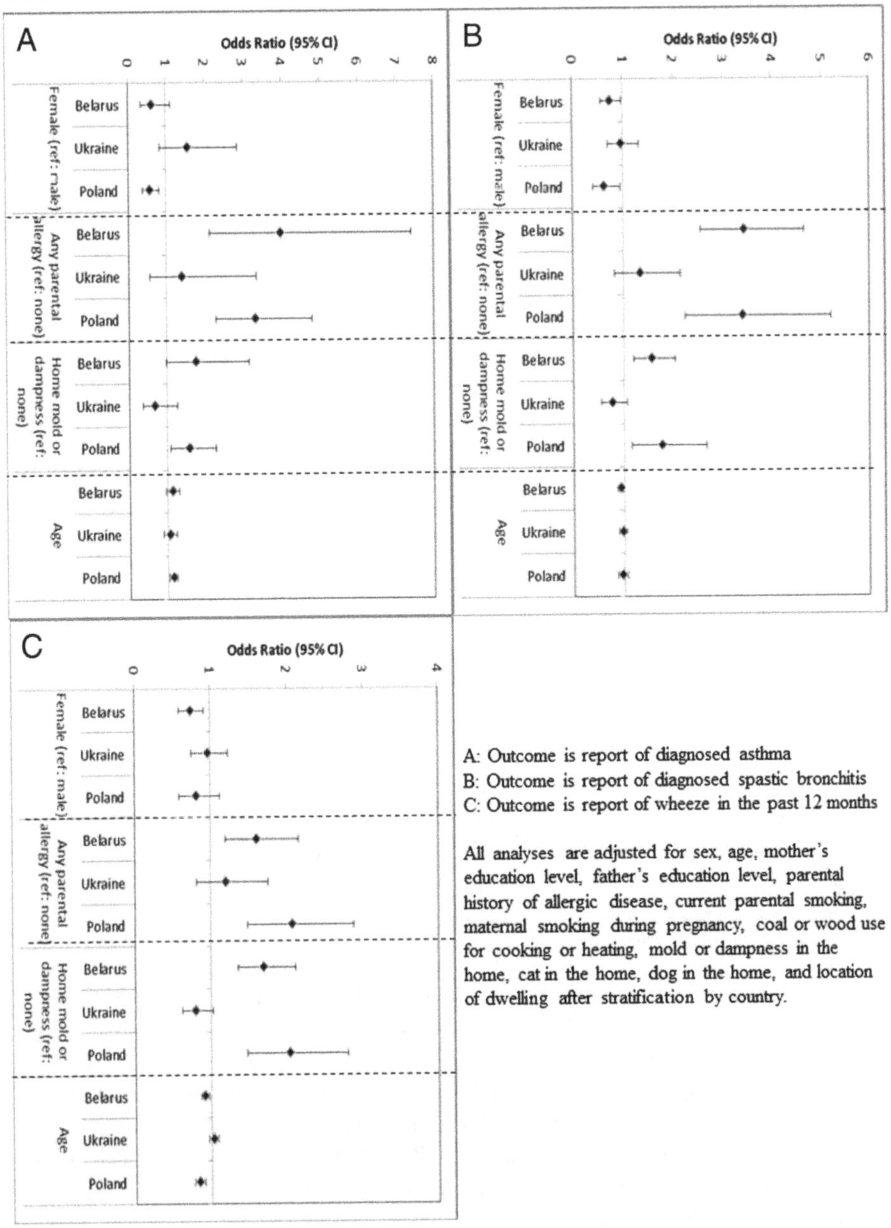

Fig. 1 Adjusted associations between personal and environmental characteristics with report of diagnosed asthma, diagnosed spastic bronchitis, and wheeze in the past 12 months. **a** Outcome is report of diagnosed asthma. **b** Outcome is report of diagnosed spastic bronchitis. **c** Outcome is report of wheeze in the past 12 months. All analyses are adjusted for sex, age, mother's education level, father's education level, parental history of allergic disease, current parental smoking, maternal smoking during pregnancy, coal or wood use for cooking or heating, mold or dampness in the home, cat in the home, dog in the home, and location of dwelling after stratification by country

with an inverse association with sex. Our results suggest that differences in diagnostic labeling may be occurring. Symptom characteristics of children who had a report of a diagnosis of asthma between countries were not consistent. In light of this, it is important to further examine regional variation in diagnostic labeling and management practices among children with asthma as well as those without asthma but with conditions labels which may be used in place of asthma.

Our findings confirm those of global and regional investigations of childhood asthma prevalence where geographic variation has been observed [1–3, 11]. Generally, Westernized nations have experienced a higher prevalence of asthma than non-Westernized nations. While global differences have been relatively clear based on the ISAAC studies, more regionally, within Europe, differences have also been shown to exist. One previous study following ISAAC protocols found that there was higher

Table 4 Distribution of symptoms, allergic conditions, health care utilization, and morbidity by country and location of residence among those with a previous diagnosis of asthma

	Urban			Rural		
	Belarus ($n = 30$)	Ukraine ($n = 54$)	Poland ($n = 84$)	Belarus ($n = 29$)	Ukraine ($n = 27$)	Poland ($n = 70$)
Asthma attacks in the past 12 months	50.0	42.3	42.7*	51.7	37.0	26.9
Woken by asthma attacks in the past 3 months	33.3	16.3	35.5*	24.1	17.4	16.9
Ever diagnosed with spastic bronchitis	76.7*	58.3	38.1**	48.3	53.8	37.9
Chest wheeze in the past 12 months	73.3	70.4*	45.5	62.1	44.4	40.9
SOB with exercise in the past 12 months	46.7	53.7	36.6	37.9	44.4	24.6
Nocturnal SOB in the past 12 months	30.0	23.1	37.3*	24.1	29.6	22.4
Cough in the past 12 months	83.3	90.7*	92.7	86.2	74.1	88.1
Productive cough in the past 12 months	80.0	70.0	67.1	58.6	63.0	62.5
Ever diagnosed with rhinitis	43.3*	31.9	76.0*, **	13.8	25.0	55.9***
Ever diagnosed with eczema	56.7*	30.6	37.1	10.3	37.5	24.6
Ever diagnosed with any allergy	80.0*	46.0	66.2**	41.4	68.0	49.3
Ever had symptoms of allergic rhinitis or hayfever	50.0*	49.1	61.4	13.8	60.0	48.5‡
Ever had sneezing with congestion or intense runny nose apart from a cold	76.7	66.7	65.1	62.1	77.8	55.2
Ever had skin allergy or itching	50.0	23.1	28.6**	37.9	44.4	21.7
Ever used medication for asthma	86.7	42.0	65.8**	93.1	55.6	60.3***
Hospitalization due to breathing troubles in the past 12 months	20.0	28.8	6.0**	20.7	20.0	4.8***
Visited a doctor for breathing troubles in the past 12 months	60.0	45.3	50.6	51.7	55.6	41.2
Spirometry testing in the past 12 months	43.3	16.7	26.2**	24.1	18.5	37.1
Skin prick testing in the past 12 months	30.0	20.4	22.6	20.7	18.5	31.4

*$p < 0.05$ comparing urban to rural within country
**$p < 0.05$ comparing across countries among urban children
***$p < 0.05$ comparing across countries among rural children

wheeze prevalence in Scandinavian centres compared to Eastern European centers [11]. In addition to this, there was a gradient where the highest prevalence was observed in Scandinavia (Sweden and Finland; 11–19 %) followed by Estonia, Latvia, and Poland (7.5–8.5 %), countries with increasingly Westernized culture, and lowest in Albania, Romania, Russia, Georgia, and Uzbekistan (2.6–5.9 %), countries with the least amount of Western influence [11]. In a separate study of Eastern and Central Europe, similar patterns of asthma prevalence were observed with a high between-country variation but lower within-country variation in asthma prevalence [3]. However, from this study, it was suggested that diagnostic differences may explain some of the differences in asthma prevalence with bronchitis being used as a label more frequently in these centres compared to Western centres [3]. In our study, we advance this concept by showing that even within relatively close geographic proximity, these labeling differences occur where we see increased risk of asthma in Poland but a significant inverse association with spastic bronchitis in Poland.

Regardless of the outcome considered (asthma, wheeze in the past 12 months, or spastic bronchitis), consistent associations were observed personal and genetic factors. A parental history of allergic disease suggests a strong genetic component, which is well known to occur in asthma and allergic disease [12, 13]. Given that wheeze and spastic bronchitis are not thought to be as linked to allergic disease and family history as asthma, this provides some evidence that there may be some labelling issues, especially among those with spastic bronchitis given the similarity in odds ratio with asthma (2.72 vs. 3.01, respectively).

Associations between the environment and asthma have been less consistent. With regard to home mold or dampness, each association was statistically significant with a similar strength of association (odds ratios = 1.28–1.35). Mold and dampness has been associated with asthma and wheeze fairly consistently in recent years [14, 15]. While having a dog showed a consistent inverse association with each of the three outcomes considered, it was only statistically significant with spastic bronchitis and a trend towards statistical significance with asthma. However, the strength of each of these associations was almost identical (odds ratios = 0.78 vs 0.77). With the similarity in associations, it again adds some evidence that some children with spastic bronchitis may truly be children with asthma. Several other studies have reported a protective effect. However, these associations are not consistent and can be complex, often depending on other factors, and timing of exposure.

There was also an inverse association between age with wheeze in the past 12 months and age with ever diagnosed with spastic bronchitis. This association is easily explainable for wheeze in the past 12 months since a high proportion of children have wheeze while they are young but will grow out of this transient wheeze later in life. It is a little more difficult to explain the inverse association with spastic bronchitis. Given that the prevalence of this outcome is a cumulative indicator (ever diagnosed), we would expect that the risk of having this diagnosis would increase with age. Speculatively, it could be that the true prevalence of asthma is increasing but there is mislabelling where those with asthma are being labelled with spastic bronchitis. In younger children, there will be more labeling than had occurred with older children, leading to an inverse association.

The consistency between countries in the relationship between the various exposures and outcomes was encouraging and adds strength to our study. However, we did find that some of the associations were dependent on country. In general, while the associations were relatively consistent, results from the Ukraine were weaker and not statistically significant. A notable and consistent exception was that of home mold or dampness which showed significant effect modification with country regardless of outcome. In each case, associations in Belarus and Poland showed statistically significant increased risk while in Ukraine, non-significant inverse associations were observed. In a previous Canadian study, similar differences in effect were observed between two south Saskatchewan regions when considering mold and dampness [16]. While interesting, some caution must be taken since the results in Ukraine were weak and not statistically significant for this variable. However, differences in the housing or environment may be leading to different types of mould exposure, either in quantity or diversity, which may then be leading to differential associations with the outcomes. Those dwelling in Ukraine were much more likely to report home mold or dampness in the home compared to those in Belarus or Poland. A more rigorous investigation with objective measures would help explain these observations.

One of our research foci was to examine the association between rural living and asthma. We did not find statistically significant associations between rural residence and any of the considered outcomes. While not entirely consistent, previous research has suggested less asthma prevalence in rural areas compared to urban areas [17, 18] In our multivariate analyses we did not observe this association with asthma, wheeze in the past 12 months, or spastic bronchitis. In previous studies, farm dwelling has generally showed a stronger, more consistent, association with asthma than the more general rural dwelling. It may be that in our analyses, we did not capture the environmental effect associated with asthma through our definition of rural. Despite this, we found many differences in environmental exposures between urban and rural dwellers within each country and that based on crude analyses, the prevalence of diagnosed allergic disease and symptoms (e.g., eczema, rhinitis, general allergy) were almost always significantly higher in urban compared to rural dwellers, regardless of country. This is consistent with the existing literature which has shown more consistent associations with allergic disease than with asthma.

When we considered symptom characteristics among those with asthma by country, few consistent patterns emerged. One difficulty was that our statistical power in this phase of the analysis was greatly reduced. Despite this, among children with asthma, those living in Poland consistently had a lower likelihood of being diagnosed with spastic bronchitis or being hospitalized due to breathing problems but an increased risk of having ever been diagnosed with rhinitis. These differences may be related to better identification and labelling of asthma, avoiding terms such as spastic bronchitis, which may lead to better outpatient management. It is important to consider that in these comparisons, we are considering children who had a previous diagnosis of asthma and who were then possibly better managed, which makes interpretation of this part of the analysis difficult, explaining some of the inconsistency. In addition to this, the health care systems themselves may have a role in the diagnostic policies and management following a diagnosis, adding an extra layer of complexity to the interpretation of results comparing children with a previous diagnosis of asthma.

The current study has several strengths and limitations. First, this was a cross-sectional study, which limits our ability to investigate associations between risk factors and asthma. However, cross-sectional studies are ideally suited for the assessment of the prevalence of disease, which was a major focus of our study. The response rate was excellent in each region making reported prevalence representative of these populations, although not of the entire countries involved. A high response rate is necessary to complete studies of asthma prevalence. The sample size in each region was also high reducing the likelihood of low statistical power and Type II error. While we could not assess the temporality of the associations investigated, we used identical questionnaires and protocols in each of the regions while completing the study at the same point in time. In addition to this, our study allows us to consider the associations in a consistent manner between locations so that in the event of bias, it will be consistent across study locations.

Asthma diagnosis lacks on objective gold standard and questionnaire report of a doctor's diagnosis of asthma is used very frequently in epidemiological studies. This method has reasonable levels of agreement with other methods of assessment and has been suggested as the method of choice for large epidemiologic studies [19] given its validity and practical application. Third, this study was based on self-report and used a proxy reporter. This may result in some misclassification. However, previously, the sensitivity and specificity of this method to assess asthma has been high compared to blinded physician assessment [20]. Also, respiratory symptoms have been found to be accurately reported by the adolescent and strongly agree with parental reports in terms of asthma diagnoses [21]. Another possibility is that the participant experienced respiratory symptoms and did not seek medical attention. However, we examined differences in prevalence of symptoms in addition to diagnosed conditions, which should minimize biases due to labeling. Within Poland, an area included in the current study, we previously found high agreement between survey reported asthma and clinical evaluation of asthma among those children where asthma was already reported suggesting that asthma diagnosis is relatively accurate when applied but that among those without a label of asthma but with respiratory symptoms in the past year, there may be substantial underdiagnosis of asthma [22]. Additionally, language barriers may bias the study results. Efforts were made to ensure accurate translation by European members of the study team who each speak multiple languages, including those included in the study regions. Part of our analysis considered rural vs. urban comparisons. It is possible that the design we used did not truly capture the individual's exposure based on rural settings. For example, if an urban dweller frequently visited a farm or had farm type exposures in town. There are many methods of defining rural [23] and we chose to use one that would capture exposures based on agricultural activity. Finally, potential confounding factors that were not addressed in the current analysis are the management practices and health care systems in each of the countries considered. The type and frequency of medication use may be dependent on differences in the healthcare system and asthma medication reimbursement procedures. According to our knowledge, in Ukraine, Belarus and Poland, children's health care is free with open access to physicians. Also a high proportion of asthma medication is reimbursed. These problems are beyond the current publication and deserve a more detailed and separate analysis.

Future work in this area will include further investigation of diagnostic labeling and presenting patterns in the region. As part of this, work must be completed to assess and implement practice guidelines for the diagnosis and management of childhood asthma. This would include education and awareness programs aimed physicians and health care professionals as well as the general population. Results from Poland showing increases in asthma prevalence over a 21 year span [6] may serve as an example of changes that can occur after implementation of guidelines. While we were unable to directly link individual results with implementation of asthma consensus guidelines within countries, the timing allows us some interpretation linking the increases in asthma prevalence and improved asthma management Over this time, the proportion of those with asthma who were treated also improved [6] suggesting that these improvements could occur.

Conclusion

In conclusion, we found that there was significant variation in asthma prevalence between the three BUPAS countries and that some of this variation is likely due to diagnostic differences between centres. By understanding patterns of geographic variation in asthma prevalence, we will be in a better position to study the etiology and better plan for asthma management.

Abbreviations

ANOVA: Analysis of variance; BMI: Body mass index; BUPAS: Belarus, Ukraine, Poland Asthma Study; CI: Confidence Interval; cm: Centimeter; ISAAC: International study of asthma and allergies in childhood; Kg: Kilogram; OR: Odds ratio; p-value: Probability value; SOB: Shortness of breath; SPSS: Statistical package for the social sciences.

Competing interests

The authors declare that they have no competing interests.

Authors' contributions

GB was part of the research team who helped conceive and design the study. In addition to this, GB co-led the international coordination as well as data collection in Poland. GB was also involved in the data analysis and interpretation, initial drafting of the manuscript, and critical review of the manuscript. JL worked on the statistical analysis, interpretation of results, initial drafting, and critical review of the manuscript. AS was part of the research team who helped conceive and design the study, led the data collection in Belarus, and critically reviewed the manuscript. OF was part of the research team who helped conceive and design the study, led the data collection in Ukraine, and critically reviewed the manuscript. LH was part of the research team who helped conceive and design the study, helped coordinate data collection in Ukraine, and critically reviewed the manuscript. DR aided in the interpretation of results and critical review of the manuscript. JZ was part of the research team who helped conceive and design the study. JZ was also involved in a leadership role with all aspects of the study including leading the international collaboration, facilitated communication and study team development, advised on data collection, provided interpretation of results and critical review of the manuscript. All authors have read and approved the final manuscript.

Acknowledgements

We wish to acknowledge the technical help provided by: Volianska Liubov, Voroncova Tamara, Kubey Inga, Levenets Sofia, Luchyshyn Natalia, Moroz Irina, Stetsenko Vira, Yarema Natalia, Andrei Stryzhak, Tatsiana Neviartovich, Aliaksey Abialesky, Volha Pavluc, Aksana Volkova and Sylwia Sowa.

Author details

[1]Department of Epidemiology, School of Medicine in Katowice, Medical University of Silesia, Katowice, Poland. [2]Department of Medicine and Canadian Center for Health and Safety in Agriculture, University of Saskatchewan, Saskatoon, Canada. [3]Department of Sport Medicine and Rehabilitation, Yanka Kupala State University of Grodno, Grodno, Belarus.

[4]Department of Paediatrics with Children Surgery №1, Horbachevsky State Medical University, Ternopil, Ukraine. [5]Department of Tuberculosis, Horbachevsky State Medical University, Ternopil, Ukraine. [6]College of Nursing and Canadian Center for Health and Safety in Agriculture, University of Saskatchewan, Saskatoon, Canada.

References

1. Asher MI, Monteforte S, Bjorksten B, Lai CKW, Strachan DP, Weiland SK, et al. Worldwide time trends in the prevalence of symptoms of asthma, allergic rhinoconjunctivitis, and eczema in childhood: ISAAC Phases One and Three repeat multicountry cross-sectional surveys. Lancet. 2006;368:733–43.
2. The International Study of Asthma and Allergies in Childhood (ISAAC) Steering Committee. Worldwide Variations in the Prevalence of Asthma Symptoms: The International Study of Asthma and Allergies in Childhood (ISAAC). Eur Respir J. 1998;12:315–35.
3. Leonardi GS, Houthuijs D, Nikiforov B, Volf J, Rudnai P, Zejda JE, et al. Respiratory symptoms, bronchitis, and asthma in children of central and eastern Europe. Eur Resp J. 2002;20:890–8.
4. Fedortsiv O, Brozek GM, Luchyshyn N, Kubey I, Lawson JA, Rennie DC, et al. Prevalence of childhood asthma, rhinitis, and ecema in the Ternopil region of Ukraine - results of BUPAS study. Advances in Medical Sciences. 2012;57:282–9.
5. Shpakou A, Brozek G, Stryzhak A, Neviartovich T, Zejda J. Allergic disease and respiratory symptoms in urban and rural children in Grodno Region (Belarus). Pediatr Allergy Immunol. 2012;23:339–46.
6. Brozek G, Lawson J, Szumilas D, Zejda J. Increasing prevalence of asthma, respiratory symptoms, and allergic diseases: Four repeated surveys from 1993–2014. Respir Med. 2015;109:982–90.
7. Asher MI, Anderson HR, Beasley R, Crane J, Martinez FD, Mitchell EA, et al. International study of asthma and allergies in childhood (ISAAC): rationale and methods. Eur Resp J. 1995;8:483–91.
8. Ellwood P, Williams H, Ait-Khaled N, Bjorksten B, Robertson C, ISAAC Phase III Study Group. Translation of questions: the International Study of Asthma and Allergies in Childhood (ISAAC) experience. Int J Tuberc Lung Dis. 2009;13:1174–82.
9. Centers for Disease Control. Percentiles for Body Mass Index 2000. Available from: http://www.cdc.gov/growthcharts. Accessed 12 Jan 2016.
10. Cole TJ, Bellizzi MC, Flegal KM, Dietz WH. Establishing a standard definition for child overweight and obesity worldwide: an international survey. BMJ. 2000;320:1240–3.
11. Bjorksten B, Dumitrascu D, Foucard T, Khetsurian N, Khaitov R, Leja M, et al. Prevalence of childhood asthma, rhinitis, and eczema in Scandanavia and Eastern Europe. Eur Resp J. 1998;12:432–7.
12. Ober C. Do Genetics Play a Role in Asthma? J Allergy Clin Immunol. 1998;101(2):S417–20.
13. Sandford A, Weir T, Pare P. The Genetics of Asthma. Am J Respir Crit Care Med. 1996;153:1749–65.
14. Dick S, Friend A, Dynes K, Alkandari F, Doust E, Cowie H, et al. A systematic review of associations between environmental exposures and development of asthma in children aged up to 9 years. BMJ Open. 2014;4:e006554 (14 pages).
15. Reponen T, Vesper SJ, Levin L, Johansson E, Ryan P, Burkle J, et al. High environmental relative moldiness index during infancy as a predictor of asthma at 7 years of age. Ann Allergy Asthma Immunol. 2011;107:120–6.
16. Lawson JA, Rennie DC, Senthilselvan A, Cockcroft DW, McDuffie HH. Regional variations in risk factors for asthma in school children. Can Resp J. 2005;12:321–6.
17. Lawson JA, Janssen I, Bruner MW, Madani K, Pickett W. Urban–rural differences in asthma prevalence among young people in Canada: the roles of health behaviours and obesity. Ann Allergy Asthma Immunol. 2011;10:220–8.
18. Riedler J, Eder W, Oberfeld G, Schreuer M. Austrian children living on a farm have less hay fever, asthma and allergic sensitization. Clin Exp Allergy. 2000;30:194–200.
19. Kemp T, Pearce N, Crane J, Beasley R. Problems of measuring asthma prevalence. Respirology. 1996;3:183–8.
20. Jenkins MA, Clarke JR, Carlin JB, Robertson CF, Hopper JL, Dalton MF, et al. Validation of questionnaire and bronchial hyperresponsiveness against respiratory physician assessment in the diagnosis of asthma. Int J Epidemiol. 1996;25:609–16.
21. Hedman L, Lindgren B, Perzanowski M, Ronmark E. Agreement between parental and self-completed questionnaires about asthma in teenagers. Pediatr Allergy Immunol. 2005;16:176–81.
22. Brozek G, Farnik M, Lawson J, Zejda J. Underdiagnosis of childhood asthma: A comparison of survey estimates to clinical evaluation. Int J Occup Med Environ Health. 2013;26:900–9.
23. Du Plessis V, Beshiri R, Bollman R, Clemenson H. Definitions of rural. Ottawa, Ontario, Canada: 2002 Contract No.: Catalogue no. 21-601-MIE — No. 061 - Working paper No 61.

Impact of occupational exposures on exacerbation of asthma: a population-based asthma cohort study

Jeong-Lim Kim[1*], Paul K. Henneberger[2], Susanna Lohman[1], Anna-Carin Olin[1], Anna Dahlman-Höglund[1], Eva Andersson[1], Kjell Torén[1] and Mathias Holm[1]

Abstract

Background: Asthma is a prevalent chronic disease and occupation contributes to approximately 15 % of cases among adults. However, there are still few studies on risk factors for work-exacerbated asthma. The current study investigated the association between asthma exacerbations and occupational exposures.

Methods: The study comprised all currently working adults ($n = 1356$) who reported ever asthma in prior population-based cohorts. All subjects completed a questionnaire about exposures, occupations and exacerbations of asthma. Exposure to high and low molecular weight agents, irritating agents and asthmagens were classified using the asthma-specific job exposure matrix for northern Europe (N-JEM). Severe exacerbation of asthma was defined as sought emergency care at a hospital, admitted to a hospital overnight, or made an urgent visit to a primary care physician or district medical office due to breathing problems during the last 12 months. Moderate exacerbation was defined as both being not severe exacerbation and an additional visit to a primary care physician or district medical office, or had extra treatments with corticosteroid tablets. Mild exacerbation was defined as being neither severe nor moderate exacerbation, and increasing usage of inhaled corticosteroids.

Multiple logistic regression was applied to investigate the association between exacerbation of asthma and occupational exposures while adjusting for potential confounders.

Results: Approximately 26 % of the working asthmatics reported exacerbation, and more than two-thirds of them had moderate or severe exacerbation. From 23 to 49 % of the asthmatics reported occupational exposure to a variety of different types of agents. Exposure to any gas, smoke or dust (OR 1.7[95 % CI 1.2–2.6]) was associated with severe exacerbation of asthma, as were organic dust (OR 1.7[1.2–2.5]), dampness and mold (OR 1.8[1.2–2.7]), cold conditions (OR 1.7[1.1–2.7]), and a physically strenuous job (OR 1.6[1.03–2.3]). Asthmagens and low molecular weight agents classified by the N-JEM were associated with mild exacerbation, with OR 1.6[1.1–2.5] and OR 2.2[1.1–4.4], respectively.

Conclusions: Self-reported exposure to any gas, smoke or dust, organic dust, dampness and mold, cold conditions and physically strenuous work, and jobs handling low molecular weight agents were associated with exacerbation of asthma. Reduction of these occupational exposures may help to reduce exacerbation of asthma.

Keywords: Asthma, Exacerbation, Job exposure matrix, Occupational exposure, Work exacerbated asthma, Workplace

* Correspondence: jeong-lim.kim@amm.gu.se
[1]Section of Occupational and Environmental Medicine, Sahlgrenska Academy at University of Gothenburg, Box 414S-405 30 Gothenburg, Sweden
Full list of author information is available at the end of the article

Background

Asthma is a prevalent chronic disease and occupational contribution to asthma has been reported as approximately 15 % among adult population [1]. Asthma due to occupational exposures is mainly separated into occupational asthma (asthma caused by work) and work-exacerbated asthma (WEA). Recent reviews have estimated that occupational exposures are causing 18 % of all adult-onset asthma [2] and that work-exacerbated asthma occurs in 22 % of adults with asthma [3, 4]. Exposures to irritant gases, fumes, dusts, chemicals, abnormal temperatures, poor indoor air quality and physically strenuous work have all been associated with WEA [5–8]. In contrast to occupational asthma, however, there are still few studies on risk factors for work-exacerbated asthma. In most of these studies, the subjects were asked if their aggravated asthma symptoms were associated with their work. This kind of question can cause bias by giving some information on the aim of the study.

Those with WEA seem to have a more severe asthma than workers with occupational asthma [9]. One recent study regarding work-exacerbated asthma showed that approximately 30 % of participants reported severe exacerbation [10]. They found a 2.5 fold-significantly increased risk for being exposed to inorganic dust among men and a 2-fold increased risk for low molecular weight reactive agents among women.

In the current study, we aimed to investigate WEA in a large study population by separating questions about specific occupational exposures from those used to define asthma exacerbation in a large study population. Also, we aimed to investigate WEA in relation to both several items on self-reported occupational exposures and the Nordic asthma-specific job exposure matrix (JEM) called the N-JEM [11, 12].

Methods

Study design and study population

The present study is based on an asthma cohort called Asthma-X that was derived from four different Swedish population-based studies: ADONIX [13], ALL000 [14, 15], MAP [16] and the Gothenburg part from the RHINE study [17], and one case-control study called M10 [18].

In brief, the ADONIX study includes a general population of men and women aged 25 to 75 years that were investigated between year 2001 and 2003. In total, 2,200 subjects completed a questionnaire and were clinically examined. The ALL000 study was carried out in all schoolchildren aged 15 and living in a county of West Sweden in year 2000. A questionnaire including items regarding respiratory symptoms was completed by 10,837 subjects. The MAP study included a random sample of the general population ($n = 15{,}813$), aged 20 to 50 years in 1993. The subjects completed a questionnaire regarding respiratory symptoms and smoking, of which 5.3 % reported asthma. The RHINE study was a follow-up of the random population samples in the European Respiratory Health Survey in Sweden, Norway, Denmark, Iceland and Estonia. For the RHINE study, a questionnaire including a self-reported asthma question was completed in a population aged 30–54 years ($n = 14{,}731$) during the follow-up period 1999–2001. The M10 study was carried out with a case-control design in 1996 and which consists of 321 adult asthmatics and 1,459 controls who completed a comprehensive questionnaire that included items regarding respiratory symptoms and details on occupation.

From these five previous studies, 2887 subjects who had reported that they have or ever had asthma were identified. In 2009, all of them were invited to participate in the current questionnaire-based survey and 1753 of them who agreed to participate completed the questionnaire and sent it back (response rate 61 %). Subjects with missing data on age or sex, or with a name that did not fully match were excluded ($n = 7$). We further restricted the study sample with complete data on subjects who had worked during the last year, smoking and exacerbation of asthma. This gave a final study population of 1356 subjects. Details of the study population are presented in Fig. 1.

Questionnaire

The questionnaire comprised items about work and occupational exposure, acute breathing problems, respiratory problems, atopy and allergy, asthma medications, tobacco use and second-hand smoking (SHS), spare time and home environment.

Information on occupations and work tasks with at least 1 month of duration was requested, including the month and year of start and end for each occupation. We also asked about occupational exposures during the past 12 months, i.e., gas, smoke or dust; smell of frying; car exhaust fumes/engine fumes; mineral dust; organic dust (flour dust, wood dust, paper dust or textile dust); inorganic dust (grinding, milling, turning, mineral wool, glass wool or rock wool); welding or metal smoke; chemicals (strong acids, ammonia, formalin, cleaning chemicals, quick dry glue, cyanoacrylates, painting, lacquering or solvents); animals; dampness and mold (visible water damage, visible mold or smell of mold); cold (in cold store or outside during the winter); and physically strenuous job or frequent heavy lifting.

Second-hand smoke (SHS) was assessed by asking about regular exposure to other peoples' tobacco smoke in the past 12-month period. *Atopy and allergy in childhood* were defined as an affirmative answer to the question, "Did you as a child have any form of allergy, for instance atopic dermatitis, asthma or hay fever?"

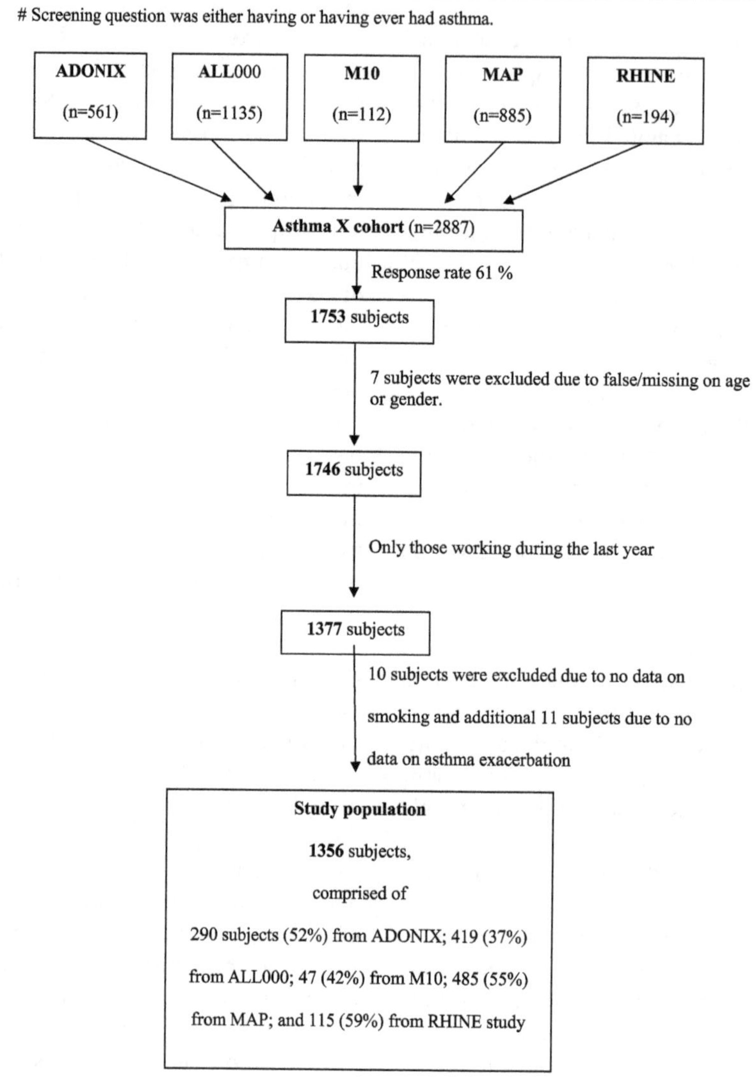

Fig. 1 Flow diagram illustrating the study population

Main outcome variables

The exacerbation variables were based on responses to questionnaire items that inquired about asthma-related care in the last 12 months. *Severe exacerbation of asthma* was defined as having sought emergency care at a hospital, admission to a hospital overnight, or having made an urgent visit to a primary care physician or district medical office due to breathing problems.

Moderate exacerbation of asthma was defined as both being *not severe exacerbation of asthma* and having made an additional visit to a primary care physician or district medical office, or taken any extra treatments with corticosteroids tablets due to breathing problems.

Mild exacerbation of asthma was defined as being not *severe* or *moderate exacerbation asthma*, and an affirmative answer to increasing usage of inhaled corticosteroids.

Any participant who fulfilled the criteria for one of the above-defined levels of exacerbation was considered as positive for "Overall exacerbation" and compared to those without exacerbation.

Job Exposure Matrix (JEM)

The reported occupations were coded by an experienced occupational hygienist (ADH) according to the International Standard Classification of Occupations (ISCO-88) [19]. These codes were then linked to the newly developed N-JEM [11] (JEM for new onset of asthma in the countries in northern Europe) which included six main groups: high molecular weight agents (HMW); low molecular weight agents (LMW); irritating agents; accidental peak exposure to irritants; uncertain or low exposed group; and unexposed reference group. Moreover, we combined those who belonged to any of the following categories: HMW, LMW, irritating agents or accidental peak exposure into "Asthmagens" to investigate an overall exposure effect on respiratory health. In all the analyses, we used occupations held during the last 12 months. Subjects were allowed to belong to more than one JEM group if they had more than one occupation in the last year or more than one type of exposure in their job.

Statistical methods

The continuous variables are presented as arithmetic mean with standard deviation (SD) and/or median with interquartile range (IQR), and categorical variables as frequency with percentages. Age was treated as a continuous variable in all regression models. Dummy variables were created for smoking status (never smoker versus ex-smoker and never smoker versus current smoker).

Chi-square test or Fisher's exact test was performed to test differences in those with self-reported occupational exposures and in JEM groups with regard to exacerbation of asthma. To study associations between asthma exacerbation and potential predictors, multiple logistic regression models were performed with mutual adjustments for potential confounding factors. The reference group in each regression model was restricted to subjects who were not exposed to the specific occupational exposure, which means they might have had other types of work exposures. Multicollinearity was tested to detect the effect of inter-correlation among explanatory variables by using the variance inflation factor (VIF) and the results presented here were obtained by models with VIF values below 2. Hosmer–Lemeshow goodness-of-fit statistics were used to assess the calibration of the models, and all models which met the criteria ($p > 0.05$) are presented in either text or tables. The results of regression analyses are presented as odds ratios with 95 % confidence intervals (CI). All statistical analyses were performed using version 9.3 of SAS for Windows (SAS Institute, Inc., Cary, NC, USA), applying two-tailed tests and a 5 % level of significance.

Results

Demographic characteristics of the study population are presented in Table 1. Approximately 47 % were men and the mean age was 43 years (SD 14.2) and the median was 44 (range 25–77 and IQR 25–55). Eleven per cent of the subjects were current smokers and a similar proportion had regularly been exposed to SHS. However, the rate of regular SHS at work was low (1.9 %). Onset of asthma after the age of 15 was reported by 21 % and current asthma, which is defined as either asthma symptoms or medication during the last 12 months, was reported by 52 %.

Mild exacerbation of asthma during the past 12 months was reported by 8.1 %, moderate exacerbation by 8.7 % and severe by 9.8 %. (Table 1). Severe exacerbation of asthma was more common among females ($p < 0.01$), current smokers ($p < 0.05$) and those exposed to SHS ($p < 0.01$) (data not shown). There was no such pattern regarding mild or moderate exacerbation of asthma.

Table 1 Demographic characteristics of the study population and exacerbation of asthma

	Study population ($n = 1356$) N (%)
Sex	
Women	723 (53.3)
Men	633 (46.7)
Age	
Mean (standard deviation)	42.5 (14.2)
Median (interquartile range)	44.0 (25–55)
Smoking status	
Never smoker	794 (58.6)
Ex- smoker	411 (30.3)
Current smoker	151 (11.1)
Regular second hand smoke exposure in the past 12 months	150 (11.1)
Atopy and allergy in childhood	981 (72.9)
Onset of asthma after the age of 15	284 (20.9)
Exacerbation of asthma	
Mild	107 (8.1)
moderate	118 (8.7)
Severe	133 (9.8)

Based on crude comparisons, both self-reported and N-JEM classified occupational exposures did not differ between those with overall exacerbation and without exacerbation (Table 2). By dividing into different definition categories of exacerbation, however, moderate exacerbation of asthma was more common in those with self-reported exposure to animals (only 5 % exposed, $p < 0.05$) and severe exacerbation was more common in those with self-reported exposures to any gas, smoke or dust ($p < 0.05$), organic dust ($p < 0.01$), dampness and mold ($p < 0.01$) and working in cold conditions ($p < 0.05$). These exposures were reported by a large proportion of the study population, ranging from 23 to 50 %.

According to N-JEM, our study population was allocated into approximately 17 % exposed to HMW, 7 % LMW and 21 % irritating agents. (Table 2). From comparisons of the crude data, the prevalence of asthma exacerbation did not significantly differ by the different N-JEM categories. For further analyses in the current investigation, the category of accidental peak exposure to irritants was excluded due to too few subjects.

Table 2 Self-reported work exposure during the past 12 months and Job Exposure matrix (JEM)

	Study population (*n* = 1356)	Asthma exacerbation							
		Mild (*n* = 107)		Moderate (*n* = 118)		Severe (*n* = 133)		Overall (*n* = 358)	
	N (%)	N (%)	*p*-value*	N (%)	*p*-value*	N (%)	*p*-value*	N (%)	*p*-value*
Self-reported work exposure in the past 12 months									
Gas, smoke or dust	593 (44.6)	52 (50.0)	0.22	48 (40.7)	0.49	69 (53.5)	0.03	169 (48.2)	0.15
Smell of frying	179 (13.7)	16 (15.8)	0.44	18 (15.4)	0.50	20 (15.6)	0.50	54 (15.6)	0.25
Car exhaust fumes/engine fumes	311 (23.7)	23 (23.0)	0.86	26 (22.2)	0.71	31 (24.2)	0.88	80 (23.2)	0.82
Mineral dust	154 (11.7)	12 (12.1)	0.99	14 (12.0)	0.98	13 (10.2)	0.57	39 (11.3)	0.71
Organic dust[a]	461 (34.9)	34 (34.0)	0.88	41 (35.3)	0.68	60 (46.5)	<0.01	135 (39.1)	0.05
Inorganic dust[b]	211 (16.0)	17 (16.7)	0.93	18 (15.4)	0.81	19 (15.0)	0.74	54 (15.6)	0.75
Welding or metal smoke	166 (12.6)	12 (11.9)	0.79	16 (13.6)	0.78	14 (11.1)	0.61	42 (12.2)	0.76
Chemicals[c]	512 (38.9)	46 (45.5)	0.17	46 (39.3)	0.88	52 (40.6)	0.67	144 (41.6)	0.28
Animals	157 (11.9)	16 (15.5)	0.28	6 (5.2)	0.02	19 (15.2)	0.24	41 (12.0)	0.97
Dampness and mold[d]	299 (22.6)	23 (22.3)	0.96	22 (18.8)	0.46	42 (32.3)	<0.01	87 (24.9)	0.30
Cold (in cold store/outside during the winter)	314 (23.7)	26 (25.2)	0.57	29 (25.0)	0.58	40 (30.8)	0.05	95 (27.2)	0.10
Physically strenuous job[e]	649 (48.8)	54 (52.4)	0.41	50 (42.4)	0.21	73 (56.6)	0.06	177 (50.6)	0.45
Job Exposure Matrix (JEM) by the job in the last 12 months									
Unexposed any of exposure below	704 (51.9)	50 (46.7)	0.21	59 (50.0)	0.63	66 (49.6)	0.58	175 (49.0)	0.17
Asthmagens[f]	530 (39.1)	50 (46.7)	0.07	48 (40.7)	0.69	54 (40.6)	0.71	152 (42.5)	0.13
High molecular weight agents (HMW)	235 (17.3)	25 (23.4)	0.09	20 (17.0)	0.91	23 (17.3)	0.99	68 (19.0)	0.34
Low molecular weight agents (LMW)	100 (7.4)	12 (11.2)	0.14	8 (6.8)	0.74	8 (6.0)	0.53	28 (7.8)	0.71
Irritating agents	286 (21.1)	22 (20.6)	0.99	29 (24.6)	0.32	30 (22.6)	0.66	81 (22.6)	0.41
Accidental peak exposure to irritants	15 (1.1)	3 (2.8)	N.A	1 (0.9)	N.A	2 (1.5)	N.A.	6 (1.7)	0.27
Uncertain/low exposed	132 (9.7)	7 (6.5)	0.26	11 (9.3)	0.89	14 (10.5)	0.75	32 (8.9)	0.58

*P-value was obtained by Chi-square test or Fisher's exact test comparing differences in those with yes vs. no in different categories of exacerbation
[a]Flour/wood/paper/ textile dust
[b]Grinding/milling/turning/mineral wool/glass wool/rock wool
[c]Cleaning chemicals/ strong acids/ammonia/formalin/quick dry glue or cyanoacrylates/painting or lacquering/solvents
[d]Visible water damage, visible mold or smell of mold
[e]Physically strenusous job/frequent heavy lifting
[f]Any of exposure to HMW, LMW, Irritating agents or peak exposure to irritants

When performing multiple logistic regression, overall asthma exacerbation was associated with self-reported exposures to any gas, smoke or dust (OR 1.4, 95 % CI 1.1–1.8), organic dust (OR 1.4, 95 % CI 1.0–1.8) and working in cold conditions (OR 1.6, 95 % CI 1.2–2.2) (Table 3). When restricting analyses to severe exacerbation of asthma, these associations were even stronger with ORs of approximately 1.7. Moreover, severe exacerbation of asthma was more pronounced among those who reported a workplace with dampness and mold (OR 1.8, 95 % CI 1.2–2.7), and a physically strenuous job (OR 1.6, 95 % CI 1.0–2.3). None of these associations was found among those with mild or moderate exacerbation.

When all the self-reported occupational exposures associated with severe exacerbation in prior analyses were included in one regression model, severe exacerbation of asthma was still associated with exposure to organic dust (OR 1.5, 95 % CI 1.0–2.4) and to dampness and mold (OR 1.7, 95 % CI 1.1–2.6) but far from significant association to exposure to any gas, smoke or dust, working in cold conditions or physically strenuous job ($p > 0.1$) (data not shown). However, overall exacerbation of asthma was no longer significantly associated with any self-reported occupational exposures in analysis with all exposures in one model. When the model was stratified by sex, the main findings remained similar but the association between severe exacerbation of asthma and self-reported physically strenuous job was significant only in males (OR 1.9, 95 % CI 1.0–3.8) but not in females (OR 1.4, 95 % CI 0.8–2.3) (data not shown).

From multiple regression models with covariate for exposure categories, asthmagens (OR 1.6, 95 % CI 1.01–2.5) and LMW (OR 2.2, 95 % CI 1.1–4.4) classified by the N-JEM were associated with mild exacerbation of asthma, and asthmagens (OR 1.3, 95 % CI .1.01–1.7) was associated with overall exacerbation (Table 4). However,

Table 3 Multiple logistic regression models for exacerbation of asthma in relation to self-reported work exposure in the last 12 months ($n = 1356$)

Predictor categories	Mild OR (95 % CI)	Moderate OR (95 % CI)	Severe OR (95 % CI)	Overall OR (95 % CI)
Exposure in the past 12 months[a]				
Gas, smoke or dust	1.48 (0.96–2.28)	0.94 (0.62–1.42)	**1.74 (1.17–2.58)**	**1.39 (1.07–1.81)**
Smell of frying	1.33 (0.74–2.38)	1.38 (0.78–2.42)	0.92 (0.53–1.60)	1.20 (0.83–1.74)
Car exhaust fumes/engine fumes	1.03 (0.61–1.76)	1.09 (0.67–1.77)	1.12 (0.70–1.77)	1.10 (0.80–1.51)
Mineral dust	1.23 (0.63–2.42)	1.10 (0.58–2.10)	1.10 (0.58–2.08)	1.15 (0.76–1.74)
Organic dust	1.10 (0.71–1.71)	1.17 (0.77–1.77)	**1.72 (1.18–2.51)**	**1.36 (1.04–1.76)**
Inorganic dust	1.30 (0.71–2.39)	0.92 (0.51–1.68)	1.25 (0.70–2.21)	1.15 (0.79–1.67)
Welding or metal smoke	1.14 (0.58–2.25)	1.07 (0.57–2.00)	1.12 (0.59–2.12)	1.12 (0.74–1.68)
Chemicals	1.52 (0.99–2.34)	1.12 (0.74–1.70)	1.10 (0.74–1.63)	1.25 (0.96–1.62)
Animals	1.53 (0.84–2.78)	0.48 (0.20–1.13)	1.07 (0.61–1.90)	1.00 (0.67–1.50)
Dampness and mold	1.08 (0.66–1.78)	0.96 (0.59–1.57)	**1.79 (1.19–2.67)**	1.25 (0.93–1.68)
Cold (in cold store/outside during the winter)	1.48 (0.95–2.31)	1.44 (0.89–2.34)	**1.74 (1.12–2.69)**	**1.59 (1.17–2.15)**
Physically strenuous job	1.48 (0.95–2.31)	0.86 (0.56–1.31)	**1.55 (1.03–2.32)**	1.29 (0.99–1.69)

[a]Each model was separately performed for each type of self-reported work exposure adjusting for gender (reference = female), age (continuous variable), current smoker, Second-hand smoke (SHS) and history of self-reported allergy. The reference group in each model was the unexposed subjects for the specific occupational exposure category which means they might have had other types of work exposures. *P*-values <0.05 are marked bold

neither moderate nor severe exacerbation of asthma was associated with an exposure category by the N-JEM.

Discussion

In the current cohort of working asthmatics, the prevalence of exacerbation of asthma during the last 12 months was approximately 26 % and more than two-thirds of them had moderate or severe exacerbation. The 9.8 % of current participants with severe exacerbation was only somewhat greater than the 7.7 % of working adults with asthma who fulfilled similar criteria for severe exacerbation in the European Community Respiratory Health Survey II [6]. A substantial proportion of the study population reported occupational exposures to chemicals, gas, smoke, dust, fumes, dampness and mold, and work in the cold conditions. Females and current smokers reported more exacerbations of asthma, which is in good agreement with previous findings [6, 20]. Those exposed to SHS were also more prone to report asthma exacerbations.

Self-reported exposure to any gas, smoke or dust, and organic dust, and working in cold conditions, were associated with overall exacerbation of asthma. Moreover, self-reported exposure to dampness and mold, and physically strenuous job were associated with severe exacerbation of asthma. Exposure to "asthmagens" and "low molecular weight agents" in the N-JEM were significantly associated with mild exacerbation of asthma but no significant association with the other categories in the N-JEM was found.

The strength of the current study of asthma exacerbation is the detailed questioning on work exposures regardless of any respiratory symptoms and recent job history in a large cohort of asthmatics. Moreover, the reported occupations were coded and linked to a newly

Table 4 Multiple logistic regression models for exacerbation of asthma in relation to JEM in the last 12 months[a]

Predictor categories	Mild OR (95 % CI)	Moderate OR (95 % CI)	Severe OR (95 % CI)	Overall OR (95 % CI)
Unexposed (reference, $n = 704$)	1	1	1	1
Asthmagens ($n = 530$)[b]	**1.62 (1.06–2.49)**	1.17 (0.77–1.78)	1.07 (0.72–1.59)	**1.32 (1.01–1.72)**
High molecular weight agents (HMW, $n = 235$)	1.68 (0.98–2.88)	1.02 (0.58–1.82)	0.96 (0.57–1.62)	1.22 (0.86–1.74)
Low molecular weight agents (LMW, $n = 100$)	**2.16 (1.05–4.44)**	0.97 (0.42–2.26)	0.91 (0.39–2.12)	1.35 (0.82–2.25)
Irritating agents ($n = 286$)	1.29 (0.73–2.30)	1.36 (0.81–2.30)	1.25 (0.75–2.09)	1.36 (0.96–1.92)
Uncertain/low exposed ($n = 132$)	0.77 (0.33–1.76)	1.08 (0.54–2.14)	1.40 (0.75–2.63)	1.10 (0.70–1.71)

[a]Each model was separately performed for each type of work exposure adjusting for sex (reference = female), age (continuous variable), current smoker, second hand smoke (SHS) and atopy and allergy in childhood. *P*-values <0.05 are marked bold
[b]Any of exposure to HMW, LMW or Irritating agents

developed asthma-specific JEM that was intended for use in northern Europe [11, 12]. Thus, both self-reported and JEM-assessed occupational exposures were analyzed in relation to exacerbations of asthma.

Our study also has some potential methodological limitations. The cross-sectional design of the study implies a risk of recall bias. In order to reduce this type of bias, we separated the exposure questions from those used to define asthma exacerbation. In order to establish an unbiased assessment of occupational exposure we also used the N-JEM. Another potential limitation is that exacerbation of asthma was defined by using a self-administered questionnaire although this approach is commonly used in epidemiological studies. However, the questions we used to define asthma exacerbation are distinct, and especially the questions used to define a severe exacerbation (achieving the highest risk-estimates), i.e., to seek acute help from a health care provider seem easy to remember and we think the answers to the questions match the real circumstances well.

Another possible limitation is that subjects in the current asthma cohort study were derived from five different studies and one of them was carried out among relatively young adults (15 years old in the year 2000) [14, 15]. The total response rate was approximately 61 % but in the young adult population study it was as low as 44 %, which may cause some under-representation of young asthmatics in the present study. Also, the low participation percentage among young adults might imply that selection bias may be more likely than among older participant groups. Nonetheless, there might be sufficient accumulation of young participants with asthma since a large proportion of the current asthma cohort was derived from the young population study ALL000. Since age distribution varies among the five studies, consequently, we controlled for potential confounding by this factor in all the models. Furthermore, we have studied subjects that reported "ever asthma" in previous surveys, of which a large proportion reported onset of asthma before the age of 16. Consequently, it follows that individuals with asthma in remission were included, and some participants may only have had transient asthma during childhood. This probably resulted in a lower prevalence of asthma exacerbation than if only subjects with an ongoing asthma had been studied.

The definition of *severe asthma exacerbation* has not been constant in the literature. However, in a recent American Thoracic Society (ATS)/European Respiratory Society (ERS) statement severe asthma exacerbations were defined as events that require use, or an increase from a stable dose, of systemic corticosteroids and/or hospitalization or emergency room visit [21] which is close to our definition. Less severe exacerbations seem more difficult to define and it is hard to draw a distinct line between moderate exacerbations and normal fluctuations in the asthma disease, especially in questionnaire-based studies. In the ATS/ERS consensus statement [21], a moderate asthma exacerbation was defined as an event that result in a temporary change in treatment that is intended to prevent the exacerbation from becoming severe. For the current study, we have a large number of events which allowed us to use the modified ATS/ERS consensus statement to three severity grades: Severe, Moderate and Mild; and overall asthma exacerbation regardless of severity grades. We also found the strongest associations for the severe exacerbations, where the definition is most precise.

So far, relatively few studies have attempted to demonstrate work-related risk factors for severe exacerbation of asthma or aggravated asthma symptoms [6, 8, 10]. An increased risk of severe exacerbation of asthma among those exposed to gas/fume, mineral dust or any dust at work has been shown [5–7]. A recent study showed that high exposure to gas, dust or fumes was significantly associated with severe exacerbation of asthma (relative risk 2.5 with 95 % CI 1.2–5.5) [6]. In the current study, we found similar results with a significant association between severe exacerbation of asthma and self-reported exposure to any gas, smoke or dust. Moreover, self-reported exposure to organic dust was associated with severe exacerbation of asthma. We also found that self-reported problems with dampness/mold at work were significantly associated with severe exacerbation of asthma, which is in good agreement with previous literature. Numerous studies have shown that exposure to dampness and biological contaminants in indoor environment can be adversely associated with asthma and respiratory symptoms [22, 23]. Self-reported work in cold conditions and physically strenuous job were both associated with asthma exacerbations, which is in line with results from a study by Saarinen et al. 2003 [8], where such exposures were associated with work-aggravated asthma symptoms. We found slightly different pictures of association between occupational exposure and exacerbation of asthma, when comparing self-reported and N-JEM categories. That is, the self-reported "any exposure to gas, smoke or dust" and "exposure to organic dust" are exposures that fit under the "irritating agents" and "asthmagens" N-JEM category. A possible explanation for the finding may be information bias. Previously, it was shown that the prevalence of self-reported occupational exposure depended on asthmatic health status [24]. In other words, subjects with severe asthma might be more likely to report their occupational exposure than others. The association of N-JEM "asthmagens" with mild exacerbation alone might indicate that the exposure was sufficient to result in this mild response but not moderate or severe exacerbation. It is also possible that some imprecision in the exposure metric compromised the ability to detect an association with the moderate or severe outcome. One has to bear in mind that the N-JEM is an asthma-specific JEM that was developed with special focus on detection of new-onset asthma rather than exacerbation of asthma. The vast majority of participants in the current study probably did not have occupational asthma, but rather asthma caused by factors outside their work. Apart from the fact that agents that are causing asthma do not necessarily trigger exacerbations of the disease, it can be that those who are already suffering from asthma are likely to develop exacerbations at lower levels of exposures than those levels needed to initiate new-onset asthma. In fact, Lemiere and co-authors concluded in a recent study [9] that subjects with work-exacerbated asthma appeared to have greater asthma severity than those with occupational asthma. In short, there is a possibility that both exposures and exposure levels of interest for WEA are not fully covered by the JEM we used, consistent with the fact that it is challenging to accurately assess occupational exposures in a questionnaire-based setting.

Conclusion

Adults with asthma who reported occupational exposure to any gas, smoke or dust; organic dust; dampness and mold; cold conditions; or physically strenuous work, and who had jobs working with low molecular weight agents had increased risk of exacerbation of asthma. To diminish exacerbation of asthma, it may help to reduce such exposures in workplaces.

Abbreviations

ATS: American thoracic society; CI: Confidence interval; ERS: European respiratory society; HMW: High molecular weight agents; IQR: Interquartile range; JEM: Job exposure matrix; LMW: Low molecular weight agents; N-JEM: The Nordic asthma-specific job exposure matrix; SD: Standard deviation; SHS: Second-hand smoking; VIF: Variance inflation factor; WEA: Work-exacerbated asthma

Acknowledgements

Not applicable.

Funding

The study was supported by the Swedish Research Council for Health, Working Life and Welfare (FORTE).

Authors' contributions

JLK, SL, ACO, ADH, EA, KT and MH made substantial contributions to study design and data collection and interpretation. JLK performed all statistical analyses, interpreted the results with PKH, KT and MH, and a major contributor in writing the manuscript. All the other authors were involved in drafting the manuscript and/or revising it critically for important intellectual content. All authors have given final approval of the version to be published.

Competing interests

The authors declare that they have no competing interests.

Consent of publication

Not applicable.

Disclaimer

The findings and conclusions in this report are those of the authors and do not necessarily represent the views of the National Institute for Occupational Safety and Health (NIOSH). Mention of any company or product does not constitute endorsement by NIOSH.

Author details

[1]Section of Occupational and Environmental Medicine, Sahlgrenska Academy at University of Gothenburg, Box 414S-405 30 Gothenburg, Sweden.
[2]National Institute for Occupational Safety and Health, Centers for Disease Control and Prevention, Morgantown, WV, USA.

References

1. Balmes J, Becklake M, Blanc P, Henneberger P, Kreiss K, Mapp C, Milton D, Schwartz D, Toren K, Viegi G. American thoracic society statement: occupational contribution to the burden of airway disease. Am J Respir Crit Care Med. 2003;167:787–97.
2. Toren K, Blanc PD. Asthma caused by occupational exposures is common - a systematic analysis of estimates of the population-attributable fraction. BMC Pulm Med. 2009;9:7.
3. Henneberger PK, Redlich CA, Callahan DB, Harber P, Lemiere C, Martin J, Tarlo SM, Vandenplas O, Toren K. An official american thoracic society statement: work-exacerbated asthma. Am J Respir Crit Care Med. 2011;184:368–78.
4. Fishwick D. Work aggravated asthma; a review of the recent evidence. Br Med Bull. 2014;110:77–88.
5. Berger Z, Rom WN, Reibman J, Kim M, Zhang S, Luo L, Friedman-Jimenez G. Prevalence of workplace exacerbation of asthma symptoms in an urban working population of asthmatics. J Occup Environ Med. 2006;48:833–9.
6. Henneberger PK, Mirabelli MC, Kogevinas M, Anto JM, Plana E, Dahlman-Hoglund A, Jarvis DL, Kromhout H, Lillienberg L, Norback D, et al. The occupational contribution to severe exacerbation of asthma. Eur Respir J. 2010;36:743–50.
7. Goe SK, Henneberger PK, Reilly MJ, Rosenman KD, Schill DP, Valiante D, Flattery J, Harrison R, Reinisch F, Tumpowsky C, et al. A descriptive study of work aggravated asthma. Occup Environ Med. 2004;61:512–7.
8. Saarinen K, Karjalainen A, Martikainen R, Uitti J, Tammilehto L, Klaukka T, Kurppa K. Prevalence of work-aggravated symptoms in clinically established asthma. Eur Respir J. 2003;22:305–9.
9. Lemiere C, Boulet LP, Chaboillez S, Forget A, Chiry S, Villeneuve H, Prince P, Maghni K, Kennedy WA, Blais L. Work-exacerbated asthma and occupational asthma: do they really differ? J Allergy Clin Immunol. 2013;131:704–10.
10. Henneberger PK, Liang X, Lillienberg L, Dahlman-Hoglund A, Toren K, Andersson E. Occupational exposures associated with severe exacerbation of asthma. Int J Tuberc Lung Dis. 2015;19:244–50.
11. Lillienberg L, Andersson E, Janson C, Dahlman-Hoglund A, Forsberg B, Holm M, Glslason T, Jogi R, Omenaas E, Schlunssen V, et al. Occupational exposure and new-onset asthma in a population-based study in Northern Europe (RHINE). Ann Occup Hyg. 2013;57:482–92.
12. Lillienberg L, Dahlman-Hoglund A, Schioler L, Toren K, Andersson E. Exposures and asthma outcomes using two different job exposure matrices in a general population study in northern Europe. Ann Occup Hyg. 2014;58:469–81.
13. Olin AC, Rosengren A, Thelle DS, Lissner L, Toren K. Increased fraction of exhaled nitric oxide predicts new-onset wheeze in a general population. Am J Respir Crit Care Med. 2010;181:324–7.
14. Kim JL, Winkvist A, Aberg MA, Aberg N, Sundberg R, Toren K, Brisman J. Fish consumption and school grades in Swedish adolescents: a study of the large general population. Acta Paediatr. 2010;99:72–7.
15. Kim JL, Brisman J, Aberg MA, Forslund HB, Winkvist A, Toren K. Trends in the prevalence of asthma, rhinitis, and eczema in 15 year old adolescents over an 8 year period. Respir Med. 2014;108:701–8.

16. Toren K, Hermansson BA. Incidence rate of adult-onset asthma in relation to age, sex, atopy and smoking: a Swedish population-based study of 15813 adults. Int J Tuberc Lung Dis. 1999;3:192–7.
17. Toren K, Gislason T, Omenaas E, Jogi R, Forsberg B, Nystrom L, Olin AC, Svanes C, Janson C. A prospective study of asthma incidence and its predictors: the RHINE study. Eur Respir J. 2004;24:942–6.
18. Toren K, Balder B, Brisman J, Lindholm N, Lowhagen O, Palmqvist M, Tunsater A. The risk of asthma in relation to occupational exposures: a case-control study from a Swedish city. Eur Respir J. 1999;13:496–501.
19. ILO. International Standard Classification of Occupations: ISCO-88. Geneva: International Labor Office; 1991.
20. Weber EJ, Silverman RA, Callaham ML, Pollack CV, Woodruff PG, Clark S, Camargo Jr CA. A prospective multicenter study of factors associated with hospital admission among adults with acute asthma. Am J Med. 2002;113:371–8.
21. Reddel HK, Taylor DR, Bateman ED, Boulet LP, Boushey HA, Busse WW, Casale TB, Chanez P, Enright PL, Gibson PG, et al. An official American Thoracic Society/European Respiratory Society statement: asthma control and exacerbations: standardizing endpoints for clinical asthma trials and clinical practice. Am J Respir Crit Care Med. 2009;180:59–99.
22. Park JH, Cox-Ganser JM. Mold exposure and respiratory health in damp indoor environments. Front Biosci (Elite Ed). 2011;3:757–71.
23. Mendell MJ, Mirer AG, Cheung K, Tong M, Douwes J. Respiratory and allergic health effects of dampness, mold, and dampness-related agents: a review of the epidemiologic evidence. Environ Health Perspect. 2011;119:748–56.
24. de Vocht F, Zock JP, Kromhout H, Sunyer J, Anto JM, Burney P, Kogevinas M. Comparison of self-reported occupational exposure with a job exposure matrix in an international community-based study on asthma. Am J Ind Med. 2005;47:434–42.

19

A case–control study of innate immunity pathway gene polymorphisms in Puerto Ricans reveals association of toll-like receptor 2 +596 variant with asthma

Mario G. Ortiz-Martínez[1,2,3], Orquídea Frías-Belén[4], Sylvette Nazario-Jiménez[5], María López-Quintero[6], Rosa I. Rodríguez-Cotto[1,3] and Braulio D. Jiménez-Vélez[1,3*]

Abstract

Background: For many years, African Dust Storms (ADE) has been thought to be associated with high prevalence of asthma in Puerto Rico (PR). Endotoxins (ENX) have been associated with ADE particulate matter (PM) and are known to promote pro-inflammatory responses in lung cells of susceptible individuals through the Toll-like receptor (TLR2/4) signaling pathways. Genetic variants are plausible contributors to such susceptibility. Therefore, we have evaluated a series of nine single nucleotide polymorphisms (SNPs) in TLR genes, which have been correlated positive and negatively to asthma prevalence and/or risk, in the Puerto Rican asthmatic population.

Methods: The following SNPs were evaluated in 62 asthmatics and 61 controls through Taqman® Real Time PCR Assay: TLR4 (+896A/G, +1196C/T, −6687A/G); TLR2 (+596C/T, −16934 T/A, +399A/G, +1349C/T) and CD14 (−159C/T, +1188C/G). Genotypes were assessed for asthma association employing an odds ratio (OR) analysis.

Results: Minor allele frequencies ($n = 123$) were determined for those variants as 0.07, 0.06, 0.35, 0.35, 0.37, 0.29, 0.04, 0.35 and 0.11, respectively. Two (+596C/T, +399A/G) TLR2 SNPs showed to be more represented in the asthmatic group by 89 % and 65 %, respectively. TLR4 SNP +896A/G analysis revealed only 1 G/G genotype (2 %) on the asthmatic group. The CD14 SNPs were similarly represented in the Puerto Rican population. Only the TLR2 +596 SNP was found to be significantly associated to asthma (*OR = 3.24 for CT, 2.71 for TT*) and particularly to females.

Conclusions: The identification of TLR SNPs will reveal potential candidates for gene-environment interactions in Puerto Ricans. As far as we know this is the first study to evaluate this type of TLR gene polymorphisms in Puerto Rican asthmatics, contributing to the current knowledge in the Hispanic population.

Keywords: Asthma, Puerto Ricans, Toll-like receptors, Single nucleotide polymorphisms, Odds ratio, Genotyping, Toll-like receptor 2 +596 variant

* Correspondence: braulio.jimenez@upr.edu
[1]Department of Biochemistry, University of Puerto Rico-Medical Sciences Campus Main Bldg Lab B-210, San Juan 00935, Puerto Rico, USA
[3]Center for Environmental and Toxicological Research, University of Puerto Rico-Medical Sciences Campus, San Juan, Puerto Rico, USA
Full list of author information is available at the end of the article

Background

Asthma is an influential chronic illness in children and youth in the United States (US) and worldwide. Over the last decades it has been estimated that 300 million individuals are affected with asthma all over the world [1]. Asthma poses a heavy burden, which has steeply increased in minorities, particularly in Puerto Rican children [2]. Puerto Ricans exhibit the highest asthma prevalence (current: 16.6 % vs. 11.1 %/Non-Hispanic blacks, 8.2 %/ Non-Hispanic whites and 6.3 %/total Hispanics for 2009 in US) than any other racial or ethnic group [3–6]. Recent statistics from the *National Health Interview Survey (NHIS)*, 2013 indicate that Puerto Ricans (18.8 %) had the higher asthma prevalence in the US; particularly in adult females (15.6 %). Not only in the island but also in the US, Puerto Ricans have high asthma prevalence [3] which suggests a genetic association. Ledogar et al. [7] found that Puerto Ricans living in New York City had asthma prevalence very similar to those living in the island (~16-18 %), especially pediatric patients from 0–12 yrs of age.

The striking racial and ethnic disparities in asthma prevalence cannot be solely attributed to one specific factor but to the interaction among many factors including genetic background, environmental exposures, nutrition, as well as socioeconomic status and access to health care [8, 9]. Indeed, genetic variation along with early-life environmental and lifestyle exposures correlated to admixture influences (African ancestry) can affect lung development and growth in Puerto Rican children [10]. A literature review for 2000–2009 revealed a list of 127 genes and respective proteins linked to asthma in which TLR pathway intermediaries are influential members [11]. Puerto Ricans are heavily exposed to PM airborne constituents such as ENX in constant African Dust Storms (ADE) [12–14]. Endotoxins are known ligands to Toll-like receptors (TLR2/4) and its co-receptor, the Cluster of Differentiation 14 (CD14) [15, 16]. The possible modification of ENX-receptor interaction and its link to specific single nucleotide polymorphisms (SNPs) could play significant role with asthma susceptibility [17]. Epidemiological studies have evaluated numerous polymorphisms in TLR2, TLR4 and CD14 in relation to asthma and similar phenotypes and some were significantly associated with high asthma prevalence, risk or severity. Two SNPs in the CD14 gene (–260C/T and -159C/T) have been shown to be associated with asthma susceptibility in French, Dutch and English populations [18–20]. The CD14 -159C/T variant was found to be as frequent as 0.67 in Puerto Ricans [21]. The TLR2 +596C/T variant was related to lower asthma risk in a French population [18]. Another group reports -16934 T/A to link significantly to a less tendency to have asthma diagnosis, symptoms and atopy between others [22]. Other TLR2 SNPs have been associated with allergic asthma [23] and TLR4 SNPs (Asp299Gly and T399I) with asthma pathogenesis in a German population [24]. Interestingly, the Asp299Gly SNP was found to be associated with 4-fold higher asthma prevalence and 7-fold higher prevalence of atopic asthma in a Swedish children population [25]. However, these findings have not been consistent in all studies [26]. Raby et al. [27] found no association of six different TLR4 SNPs and asthma susceptibility in three different ethnic groups from US and Canada. Furthermore, Nishimura et al. [28] observed no association between CD14 -159C/T SNP and asthma in a Japanese population. The variability in the association of the aforementioned SNPs to asthma outcomes may be attributed to inherent factors that are different among the populations studied and it has been suggested that gene-environment interactions may also explain the variable association [26, 29]. Choudry et al. [21] found association of the CD14 + 1437C/G SNP and asthma severity in Mexican and Puerto Rican asthmatics exposed to Environmental Tobacco Smoke, ETS and suggested a gene-environment interaction between ETS and that gene variant together with the -159C/T SNP. Exposure of Puerto Rican individuals with those variants showed a significant reduction in pulmonary function and immunoglobulin E (IgE) levels [21].

There has been no study performed on the Puerto Rican asthmatic population living in the island with particular interest in the frequency of polymorphisms in the TLR2/4 genes. This study evaluates specific SNPs in TLR2 (4 variants), TLR4 (3 variants) and CD14 (2 variants) genes in a Puerto Rican asthmatic population. The SNP selection was based on literature findings and their functionality in terms of significant associations to the condition of asthma.

Methods

Case–control study

Sixty-two Puerto Rican asthmatics 14 years old or more born from Puerto Rican parents and residents of Puerto Rico were recruited for the study. These subjects were diagnosed with asthma by a physician. The control group was represented by sixty-one Puerto Rican subjects without asthma, rhinosinusitis or any other chronic allergic and/or pro-inflammatory condition, including Chronic Obstructive Pulmonary Disease (COPD). A questionnaire containing personal, lifestyle, health, asthma family history, African Dust awareness and knowledge (perception) was completed by all subjects for descriptive and analytical purposes. Information about atopic status of subjects was not considered. Experimental and control subjects were recruited from the University of Puerto Rico, School of Medicine Clinics. Eligibility of all subjects was evaluated applying the inclusion/exclusion criteria established. Selected candidates were asked to sign an informed consent document, interviewed and asked to provide a saliva sample. The experimental design protocol (#A8570111) used in this study was reviewed and approved by the University of Puerto Rico – Medical Sciences Campus Institutional Review Board (UPR MSC IRB).

DNA extraction and genotyping

Saliva samples were obtained from subjects using Saliva Collection Kits (SalivaGene® from B-Bridge International, Inc.). Genomic DNA extractions from these samples were performed following the manufacturer instructions. Extracted DNA was then diluted to 7 ng/μl and used for SNP genotyping assays through Real-Time Polymerase Chain Reaction (PCR) and Taqman® probes (Applied Biosystems) following the corresponding recommendations from the manufacturer. A total of 9 SNPs from three genes were analyzed. These were the TLR4 gene: +896A/G (rs4986790), +1196C/T (rs4986791) and -6687G/A (rs2737190); the TLR2 gene: +596C/T (rs3804099), −16934 T/A (rs4696480), +399A/G (rs13150331) and +1349 T/C (rs3804100); and in the CD14 gene: −159G/A (rs2569190), +1188C/G (rs4914).

Statistical analyses

Three major parameters were used for sample size calculation: asthma prevalence (12.5-13 %, Continuous Health Survey for the Municipalities of Puerto Rico, 2003), the study site scenario of 696 patients (derived from 13–16 patients per week, where half or a third are asthmatics) and a confidence interval of 95 %. The *Epi-Info 6.04d software* was used as an instrument for that estimation, providing an approximate population size of 60 cases and 60 controls. Descriptive statistics (means, frequencies and standard deviations) were used to describe the studied population. Differences in the distribution of socio-demographic characteristics between asthmatics and controls were also evaluated. Multivariate analysis was performed to compare the following variables: 1) having asthma or not and 2) the presence or absence of one of the polymorphisms previously stated. Differences in proportions between groups were assessed by Pearson chi-square distribution, *t* test or Fisher's exact test as appropriate. The magnitude of these associations was determined estimating prevalence odds ratio (OR) along with 95 % confidence intervals (CI) and p values for significance using a simple logistic regression model. Significant associations were adjusted by the potential confounding interaction variable of gender. Interaction terms formed by all combination pairs of the predictor variables within the multivariate model were tested with the likelihood ratio test. Data analysis was performed using the Data Analysis and Statistical Software STATA® 11.

Minor allele frequency (MAF) was calculated for each SNP in the experimental and control groups using the following equation: (N minor allele)/(total N × 2). Hardy-Weinberg equilibrium was tested through the X^2 goodness-of-fit test to compare the observed SNP genotype frequencies with the expected ones. The Online Encyclopedia for Genetic Epidemiology Studies (OEGE) 2006-2011© Hardy Weinberg calculator tool (www.oege.org/software/hardy-weinberg.html) was used to perform this test [30].

Results

Descriptive profiles

Sixty-two Puerto Rican asthmatics and sixty-one non-asthmatic control subjects were recruited for this case–control study. Table 1 illustrates the characteristic profiles for both study groups. The mean age for the asthmatic group was 41.2 ± 13.5 years and 46 ± 16.4 for the control. This particular characteristic was the only one that exhibited a statistically significant difference between the proportions of asthmatics and controls (p 0.035). Eighteen percent of the asthmatics were males while 82 % were females. In the controls, 34 % were males while 66 % were females. Most of the population studied lived in the metropolitan area, 64 % of asthmatics and 56 % controls. In terms of smoking habits, 31 % of the asthmatics and 23 % of the controls have smoke; and 83 % of the experimental group and 62 % of the control group were current smokers. A 54 % (asthmatics) vs. 51 % (controls) reported to have pets in their homes. Eighty-six percent of the asthmatics stated to have family history of asthma (first line relatives: parents and brothers/sisters) as compared to 81 % of the controls. A 48 % of the asthmatics reported to have experienced asthma exacerbations and the majority of them suffered the effects frequently. Eighty-nine percent of the asthmatics reported the use of asthma prescribed medications.

As part of exposure to environmental events, the subjects were asked some questions about African Dust knowledge and perception. Almost all the subjects knew what the African Dust was: 95 % of the asthmatics and 98 % of the controls. Only, 47 % of the asthmatics experienced an adverse effect caused by the dust.

SNP genotyping

Three TLR4, 4 TLR2 and 2 CD14 gene polymorphisms were evaluated in this study. The distribution of each SNP among asthmatics and controls is presented in Tables 2, 3 and 4. All gene variants were in Hardy Weinberg equilibrium as indicated by chi-square values at *p*-values >0.05 shown on Tables 2, 3 and 4.

TLR4 +896 AA and AG genotypes were similar between the groups and only 1 homozygote GG was observed in the asthmatics. Minor allele frequencies were practically the same (Table 2). In the case of TLR4 +1196, the distribution of genotypes and MAF was similar in both groups. The TLR4 -6687 presented

Table 1 Characteristic profiles of asthmatic and control subjects

Characteristic [N (%) or otherwise stated]	Puerto Rican[a] Asthmatic Group N = 62	Puerto Rican Control Group N = 61
Age in years [Mean (SD)][d]	41.2 (13.5)	46 (16.4)
Age by Category		
14–24	5 (8.1)	3 (4.9)
25–35	20 (32.3)	20 (32.8)
36–45	13 (20.9)	5 (8.2)
46+	24 (38.7)	33 (54.1)
Gender [*N* (%) Males/*N* (%) Females]	11 (17.7)/51 (82.3)	21 (34.4)/40 (65.6)
Residence in Metropolitan (Urban) Area	40 (64.5)	34 (55.7)
Smoking[c]	19 (30.6)	14 (22.9)
Indoor Pets	33 (54.1)	31 (50.8)
Family Asthma History[b]	49 (86)	34 (80.9)
Asthma Exacerbations	30 (48.4)	
Asthma Medication Usage	55 (88.7)	
African Dust Knowledge	59 (95.2)	60 (98.4)
Asthma symptoms caused by African Dust	29 (46.8)	

Legend: [a]Puerto Rican ancestry (European, West African and Native American); [b]first line relatives: parents, sons (daughters) and/or brothers (sisters) have or had asthma; SD means standard deviation and [c]the smoking characteristic is based on the answer to the question, have you ever smoked in your life? [d]The only characteristic that showed a statistically significant difference between the proportions of asthmatics and controls was age with a *p* value of 0.035

more AG genotypes in asthmatics, but more AA in controls. Minor allele frequency (G) was somewhat higher in asthmatics (37 % vs. 33 %).

TLR2 gene variant +596 showed more heterozygotes CT (58 %), more homozygotes TT (31 %) and less homozygotes CC (11 %) in asthmatics compared to controls (Table 3). Minor allele (C) was equally distributed in asthmatics and controls. Other 2 TLR2 variants, −16934 and +1349 revealed more heterozygotes in the asthmatic group, although more CC and AA homozygotes, respectively in the control group. The +1349 SNP showed only 1 CC homozygote in controls. Lastly, the +399 SNP presented more AG and less AA in asthmatics than among controls and the same GG in both groups. Minor allele frequency (G) was higher among asthmatics (32 % vs. 26 %).

The CD14 polymorphism, −159 was characterized by more AG genotypes in the control group and more AA genotypes in the asthmatic group (Table 4). The minor

Table 2 TLR4 SNP Genotypes and Minor Allele Frequencies (MAF) along with Hardy Weinberg Equilibrium Values in Asthmatic and Control Groups

SNP Genotypes	Asthmatics N (%)	Controls N (%)	Total N (%)	Hardy Weinberg Equilibrium (X^2, $p > 0.05$)
TLR4 +896				0.11
AA	54 (87.1)	51 (83.6)	105 (85.4)	
AG	7 (11.3)	10 (16.4)	17 (13.8)	
GG	1 (1.6)	0	1 (0.8)	
MAF (G)	0.06 (6)	0.08 (8)		
TLR4 +1196				0.52
CC	55 (88.7)	53 (86.9)	108 (87.8)	
CT	7 (11.3)	8 (13.1)	15 (12.2)	
MAF (T)	0.06 (6)	0.07 (7)		
TLR4 -6687				0.69
GG	10 (16.1)	11 (18.0)	21 (17.1)	
AG	36 (58.1)	29 (47.5)	65 (52.2)	
AA	16 (25.8)	21 (34.4)	37 (30.1)	
MAF (G)	0.37 (37)	0.33 (33)		

Hardy Weinberg equilibrium chi-square values were acquired under a *p*-value >0.05

Table 3 TLR2 SNP Genotypes and Minor Allele Frequencies (MAF) along with Hardy Weinberg Equilibrium Values in Asthmatic and Control Groups

SNP Genotypes	Asthmatics N (%)	Controls N (%)	Total N (%)	Hardy Weinberg Equilibrium (X^2, $p > 0.05$)
TLR2 +596				0.14
CC	7 (11.3)	17 (27.9)	24 (19.5)	
CT	36 (58.1)	27 (44.3)	63 (51.2)	
TT	19 (30.6)	17 (27.8)	36 (29.3)	
MAF (C)	0.35 (35)	0.36 (36)		
TLR2 -16934				0.65
TT	17 (27.4)	14 (23.0)	31 (25.2)	
AT	32 (51.6)	26 (42.6)	58 (47.2)	
AA	13 (21.0)	21 (34 .4)	34 (27.6)	
MAF (A)	0.35 (35)	0.38 (38)		
TLR2 +399				0.88
AA	23 (37.1)	29 (47.5)	52 (42.3)	
AG	33 (53.2)	26 (42.6)	59 (48.0)	
GG	6 (9.7)	6 (9.8)	12 (9.7)	
MAF (G)	0.32 (32)	0.26 (26)		
TLR2 +1349				2.53
TT	56 (90.3)	57 (93.4)	113 (91.9)	
CT	6 (9.7)	3 (4.9)	9 (7.3)	
CC	0	1 (1.6)	1 (0.8)	
MAF (C)	0.05 (5)	0.03 (3)		

Hardy Weinberg equilibrium chi-square values were acquired under a *p*-value >0.05

allele frequency (A) was the same in asthmatics and non-asthmatic controls. CD14 +1188 SNP was represented with more CG genotypes and higher MAF (G) in controls and more CC genotypes among asthmatics.

Logistic regression and interaction analyses

A logistic regression analysis was performed to assess the association of each socio-demographic trait and having the condition of asthma (Table 5). Gender, age, education, marital status, residence, lifestyle (smoking and having pets) and asthma history were considered in the analysis. An OR of 2.43 resulted for the significant association of gender, specifically in females with asthma (p 0.038). Furthermore, asthma was associated to the age category of 36–45 years with an OR of 3.57 (p 0.031).

The analysis revealed a significant association between the TLR2 +596 CT genotype and asthma in the Puerto Rican population with an OR of 3.24, p 0.023 (Table 6). Moreover, the TT genotype was marginally associated to

Table 4 CD14 SNP Genotypes and Minor Allele Frequencies (MAF) along with Hardy Weinberg Equilibrium Values in Asthmatic and Control Groups

SNP Genotypes	Asthmatics N (%)	Controls N (%)	Total N (%)	Hardy Weinberg Equilibrium (X^2, $p > 0.05$)
CD14 -159				0.05
GG	20 (32.2)	19 (31.2)	39 (31.7)	
AG	29 (46.8)	31 (50.8)	60 (48.8)	
AA	13 (21.0)	11 (18.0)	24 (19.5)	
MAF (A)	0.35 (35)	0.35 (35)		
CD14 +1188				1.72
CC	51 (82.3)	46 (75.4)	97 (78.9)	
CG	11 (17.7)	15 (24.6)	26 (21.4)	
MAF (G)	0.26 (26)	0.12 (12)		

Hardy Weinberg equilibrium chi-square values were acquired under a *p*-value >0.05

Table 5 Logistic Regression Analysis for the association of each socio-demographic trait and asthma. "Yes/No" categories were based on the answer of having or not the respective trait. Abbreviations: CI = confidence interval

Characteristics	OR	95 % CI	P-value
Gender			
Male	1.00		
Female	2.43	1.05-5.63	0.038
Age			
14-24	2.29	0.50-10.53	0.286
25-35	1.37	0.61-3.10	0.443
36-45	3.57	1.12-11.38	0.031
46+	1.00		
Education			
High School or less	2.00	0.67-5.99	0.216
Post-secondary Studies	1.22	0.45-3.28	0.694
Graduate Studies	1.00		
Marital Status			
Single	1.00		
Married/Living with someone	0.65	0.30-1.41	0.274
Widow	0.50	0.08-3.26	0.469
Divorced	0.64	0.09-2.20	0.481
Metropolitan Area Residence			
No	1.00		
Yes	1.44	0.70-2.98	0.321
Smoking Anytime in Life			
No	1.00		
Yes	1.48	0.66-3.32	0.337
Currently Smoking			
No	1.00		
Yes	3.13	0.59-16.58	0.181
Passive Smoking			
No	1.00		
Yes	1.50	0.50-4.52	0.471
First Line Asthmatic Relative			
No	1.00		
Yes	1.44	0.49-4.22	0.504
Indoor Pets			
No	1.00		
Yes	1.14	0.56-2.32	0.717

Legend: *OR* odds ratio, *CI* confidence interval

Table 6 Logistic Regression Analysis for the association of each TLR4, TLR2 and CD14 SNPs and asthma

SNP Genotypes	OR	95 % CI	P-value
TLR4 +896			
AA	1.00		
AG	0.66	0.23-1.87	0.435
TLR4 +1196			
CC	1.00		
CT	0.84	0.29-2.49	0.757
TLR4 -6687			
GG	1.00		
AG	1.37	0.51-3.66	0.536
AA	0.84	0.29-2.46	0.748
TLR2 +596			
CC	1.00		
CT	3.24	1.18-8.91	0.023
TT	2.71	0.91-8.13	0.074
TLR2 -16934			
TT	1.00		
AT	1.01	0.42-2.43	0.976
AA	0.51	0.19-1.37	0.182
TLR2 +399			
AA	1.00		
AG	1.60	0.76-3.39	0.220
GG	1.26	0.36-4.43	0.718
TLR2 +1349			
TT	1.00		
CT	2.04	0.49-8.54	0.331
CD14 -159			
GG	1.00		
AG	0.89	0.49-2.00	0.774
AA	0.12	0.41-3.11	0.824
CD14 +1188			
CC	1.00		
CG	0.66	0.28-1.59	0.354
GG			

Legend: *OR* odds ratio, *CI* confidence interval

asthma with an OR of 2.71 (p 0.074). There was no association of any other TLR pathway SNPs with asthma.

Analysis of the genotypes adjusted by gender also resulted in significant associations of TLR2 +596 genotypes and asthma in the Puerto Rican population (Table 7). Females with the CT genotype were strongly associated to asthma with an OR of 6.53 (p 0.004). The TT genotype, which was initially marginal in significance when using the crude OR analysis was statistically significant after the gender adjustment, where females exhibited an OR of 6.04 (p 0.008). Males with the CT genotype presented an OR of 0.67 but it was not significant (p 0.665). Another TLR2 SNP, −16934 turned to be significant in males with the AA genotype (OR 0.13/ p 0.039).

The likelihood ratio test revealed interaction between 2 of the 9 SNPs and asthma, TLR2 +596 (X^2 = 10.21,

Table 7 Logistic Regression Analysis adjusted by gender of the association between TLR4, TLR2 and CD14 SNPs and asthma

	Males			Females		
	Adjusted OR	95 % CI	*P*-value	Adjusted OR	95 % CI	*P*-value
TLR4 +896						
AG	2.25	0.37-13.67	0.378	0.41	0.11-1.51	0.181
TLR4 +1196						
CT	3.56	0.50-25.56	0.206	0.48	0.13-1.84	0.286
TLR4 -6687						
AG	3.00	0.26-34.57	0.378	1.20	0.39-3.66	0.748
AA	0.33	0.02-7.14	0.482	1.11	0.33-3.75	0.865
TLR2 +596						
CT	0.67	0.11-4.17	0.665	6.53	1.82-23.40	0.004
TT				6.04	1.59-23.01	0.008
TLR2 -16934						
AT				2.40	0.85-6.73	0.096
AA	0.13	0.02-0.90	0.039	0.90	0.27-3.00	0.864
TLR2 +399						
AG	0.60	0.12-2.89	0.525	2.30	0.93-5.67	0.070
GG				0.74	0.18-3.05	0.678
TLR2 +1349						
CT				2.47	0.47-12.95	0.286
CD14 -159						
AG	1.94	0.29-13.19	0.496	0.73	0.29-1.85	0.503
AA	2.79	0.36-21.73	0.325	1.00	0.28-3.54	1
CD14 +1188						
CG				0.72	0.28-1.90	0.513

Legend: *OR* odds ratio, *CI* confidence interval

p 0.0061) and TLR2 + 399 ($X^2 = 7.84$, p 0.0199). Others did not present a significant interaction [TLR4 + 896 ($X^2 = 2.24$, p 0.1348); TLR4 + 1196 ($X^2 = 2.77$, p 0.0961); TLR4 -6687 ($X^2 = 3.66$, p 0.1607) and CD14 -159 ($X^2 = 1.02$, p 0.5999)].

Discussion

The TLR2 +596 SNP (genotypes: CT and TT) was associated to asthma within the Puerto Rican population as demonstrated among French atopic subjects carrying the allele C, while non-atopic subjects revealed a positive but not significant association [18]. More importantly, the authors discovered a gene-environment interaction, where non-atopic subjects with the C allele were protected from asthma by means of living in a country environment. This variant was also studied in Korean patients of allergic rhinitis where no significant difference was found compared to controls and no correlation to total serum IgE levels, but it was associated to peripheral blood eosinophil counts [31]. Interestingly, MAFs (C) found in that study (cases: 0.32; controls: 0.31) correlate well with our findings in Puerto Rican asthmatics in spite of notable differences in sample size (cases: 0.35; controls: 0.36) [31, 32]. This polymorphism was associated to protection to non-atopic asthma in children from the International Study of Asthma and Allergy in Childhood (ISAAC) phase II [33]. A haplotype involving TLR +596 C and TLR2 +1349 C was also not related to allergic asthma in Norwegian asthmatic children [23].

The TLR2 +596 SNP was particularly associated to females after gender adjustments. The fact that this SNP was significantly predominant in Puerto Rican asthmatic females is consistent with a higher prevalence asthma reported for females vs. males: 20.4 vs. 12.7 by Akinbami et al. [6]. This marked difference can also be attributed to female steroid sex hormones. Bonds and Midoro-Horiuti [34] described estrogens involvement in allergic sensitization as well as lung function and mechanics, where for example they can relax airway smooth muscle and increase ciliary beat frequency. Sex hormones have been implicated in the interaction and modulation of TLR expression and function, where lipopolysaccharide-induced airway inflammation is reduced in female rats and increased after stimulation with testosterone [35, 36].

Other study has shown inhibition of TLR agonist-induced interleukin (IL-8) release by estradiol in cystic fibrosis bronchial epithelial cells [37].

The TLR2 +596 SNP is characterized as a synonymous or silent mutation (sSNP) whose functional mechanism is unknown. The concept of this type of SNPs of being "silent" is questionable since in some cases these mutations are responsible of more profound effects than non-synonymous SNPs and their importance relies on the comparable occurrence 1.1 % vs. 1.5 % for non-synonymous in coding regions [38]. Based on studies of other sSNPs it could create a translational pause or affect protein folding, mRNA splicing, mRNA structure and stability, protein abundance, microRNAs binding sites, co-translational protein folding and post-translational modifications via mRNA-RNA and mRNA protein interactions [38–42]. Speculations exist about how the +596 SNP could lower TLR2 expression in innate immune cell membranes [18, 43]. It has been hypothesized that this sSNP can alter function of the integrin β3 (ITGB3)-TLR2 complex, increasing mold sensitization; decrease cytokine production (TNF-α) in monocytes (CC genotype); increase (decrease in haplotype with other variants) TNF-α, IL-10 and IL-8 in peripheral blood leukocytes (T allele) stimulated with bacterial lipoprotein [43–45]. Finally, it has been suggested that TLR2 SNPs in its heterodimeric network is a major factor mediating inter-individual variation in in vitro cytokine responses to lipopeptide, Pam_3CSK_4 [33, 46].

The TLR2 SNP, +399A/G and TLR2 -16934 SNP (in males) also presented an interaction with asthma, but it was not considered important since the previous analysis did not reveal any significant associations. In support of this result, this SNP has not been associated with childhood asthma [47].

Our results for the TLR2, TLR4 and CD14 SNPs frequencies are similar to those that have been reported for Hispanic and Caucasian populations found in the National Center for Biotechnology Information (*NCBI)* SNP database (details about the comparison of the allele frequencies in the present Puerto Rican population with other racial groups included in Additional file 1: Table S1). Compared to Hispanics as a group, the +596 SNP presented more heterozygotes and TT homozygotes; but compared to Caucasians the frequency of TT was the same. Surprisingly, the TLR4 +1196 SNP frequencies obtained for the studied population are exactly the same as that found in Mexicans even though these two Hispanic groups present asthma disparities in terms of asthma prevalence, Puerto Ricans presenting the highest and Mexicans the lowest compared to non-Hispanic whites and blacks [4, 6]. The AA genotype of the TLR2 -16934 SNP was more representative in Puerto Ricans as compared to Caucasians and Hispanics. Frequencies for the TLR4 +896 and TLR2 +1349 SNP genotypes in Puerto Ricans are very similar to African Americans. Genotype frequencies for TLR4 +896, TLR2 +1349 and CD14 +1188 variants were somewhat similar to those reported for the African population. Frequencies for the CD14 SNP in asthmatics (AA = 0.32, AG = 0.47, GG = 0.21) relate well with that previously reported by Choudry, et al. [21] (0.29, 0.50 and 0.21, respectively). A significant association to asthma was not encountered possibly due to age differences between the two designs (childhood against adulthood). O'Donnell et al. [48] described an increased OR for atopy and airway hyper-responsiveness in children carriers of the CD14 -159CC genotype, while the association was not identified among adults, suggesting an age-dependent modulation of the atopic phenotype.

The analysis of genetic association to complex diseases (e.g. asthma) often exhibits result inconsistency. In fact, we found the TLR2 +596 SNP to be associated to asthma in Puerto Ricans, but others did not obtain any association with asthma in farmers/non-farmers European children [22]. Noguchi et al. [49] did not detect association to the development of asthma and total IgE serum levels in the presence of the +596 variant but stated that low frequency of some haplotypes including it as well as +1349 SNP impeded the relation to asthma development. These variable findings may be related to a number of factors which may represent limitations. Discrepancies in status of the risk/association of TLR variants in asthma can be explained by differences in ethnicity or admixture, environmental exposures such as dust allergens and endotoxins and even gene-gene and gene-environment interactions [50–57]. Low gene penetrance, low allele frequency and linkage disequilibrium are other factors that may avoid interactions of SNPs with disease [32, 33, 41, 50, 52, 58]. These properties probably explain why some of the other SNPs with relatively low MAF evaluated in our study did not result significant (TLR4 +896 and +1196 SNPs). Although a sample size calculation was performed, insufficient power [54, 59] could possibly prevent any link between the other SNPs and asthma. Replication of the presented genetic analysis is advised in an effort to account for those limitations and consider other unmeasured confounding factors.

Genetic variation in genes responsible for ENX recognition (TLRs) could modify their respective signaling pathway. Asthma susceptibility caused by this variation could be developed as an increase or reduction in NF-kB signaling that ultimately leads to an increase or reduction in the production of the pro-inflammatory mediators such as cytokines: interleukins IL-6 and IL-8. The expression of genetic variants can be modified by environmental effects of pollution, allergen exposure, social stressors and other conditions [60]. Interests in this aspect are seen in studies from Kerkhof et al. [61] where TLR2 -16934 (rs4696480) was shown to modify the effect of

$PM_{2.5}$ exposure (traffic-related) on doctor-diagnosed asthma prevalence in the age range of birth to 8 years in a population from Netherlands. The TLR2 +596 SNP was also evaluated too but did not interact with particle pollution. Nonetheless, increasing the sample size of the present study which is characterized by a different ethnic population could reveal a different biological scenario. Further studies are needed to confirm the functionality of this particular SNP in vitro.

Conclusions

Our study demonstrates an association between the TLR2 +596 SNP and asthma in Puerto Ricans. This variant is a potential gene-environment interaction candidate that may be able to modify the biological effects generated by exposure to environmental endotoxins in particle pollution, which are known to exacerbate asthmatic symptoms, and in that way modulate negative or positively the pro-inflammatory response in asthmatic individuals. Overall, the study represents a step forward not only in searching causes to explain the characteristic high prevalence of asthma in the Puerto Rican population, but also in identifying SNPs that could be considered as targets for the advancement of the pharmacogenomics field. In the future, it will help in the improvement of current asthma therapy and will provide the basis for the effectiveness of personalized medicine in Puerto Rican asthmatics.

Additional file

Additional file 1: Table S1. Comparison of TLR2, TLR4 and CD14 SNP frequencies among the analyzed Puerto Rican population with other racial groups - This table presents a comparison of the SNP genotype frequencies found in the studied Puerto Rican population (asthmatics and controls as one group) with other population heritages (Hispanic = HISP1; Caucasian = CAUC1; African American = AFR1; Mexican = HapMap MEX; Chinese = HapMap CHD; Japanese = HapMap JPT; Italian = HapMap TSI; African = HapMap YRI). The NCBI database was used as a source for those frequencies and ancestral alleles are highlighted.

Abbreviations

ADE, african dust storms or events; CI, confidence interval; COPD, chronic obstructive pulmonary disease; ENX, endotoxins; ETS, environmental tobacco smoke; ISAAC, international study of asthma and allergy in childhood; MAF, minor allele frequency; NCBI, national center for biotechnology information; NHIS, national health interview survey; OEGE, online encyclopedia for genetic epidemiology studies; OR, odds ratio; PCR, polymerase chain reaction; PM, particulate matter; PR, Puerto Rico; SNPs, single nucleotide polymorphisms; sSNP, silent single nucleotide polymorphism; TLR, toll-like receptor; US, United States

Acknowledgements

We would like to give thanks to Mariely Nieves from the Clinical Research Center (CRC) from the University of Puerto Rico-Medical Sciences Campus for her help in the IRB protocol preparation. Also to Evelyn Patiño and the Administration of the School of Medicine Clinics from the University of Puerto Rico-Medical Sciences Campus for allowing the study to be performed on site. We appreciate the help in the recruitment procedure of Drs. Mark Vergara, Ángel Laureano and the Pneumologists Group from the same Clinics.

Funding

This study was supported by the National Institute of General Medical Sciences of the National Institutes of Health (NIH) under award R25GM061838. Infrastructure support was offered in part by grant from the National Institute on Minority Health and Health Disparities (8G12MD007600). The University of Puerto Rico-Medical Sciences Campus, Deanship of Biomedical Sciences also provided support.

Authors' contributions

MO wrote the manuscript and actively participated in the subject recruitment, did all the subject interviews and analysis of answers. He also carried out all DNA sample handling (extractions and genotyping experiments) and analyzed the results. OF helped in the design and development of the statistical analysis. SN and ML helped in the development of the recruitment protocol and manuscript draft revisions. RR was involved in analysis and interpretation of results. BJ designed the research study and was actively involved in the analysis and interpretation of results, manuscript draft revisions and research supervision. All authors read and approved the final manuscript.

Competing interests

All authors declare that they have no competing interests.

Consent for publication

Even though we presented the characteristic profiles of subjects as a group and not independently, consent for publication was taken as part of the consent for participation in the study.

Author details

[1]Department of Biochemistry, University of Puerto Rico-Medical Sciences Campus Main Bldg Lab B-210, San Juan 00935, Puerto Rico, USA. [2]Department of Biology, University of Puerto Rico at Humacao, Humacao, Puerto Rico, USA. [3]Center for Environmental and Toxicological Research, University of Puerto Rico-Medical Sciences Campus, San Juan, Puerto Rico, USA. [4]School of Public Health, University of Puerto Rico, Medical Sciences Campus, San Juan, Puerto Rico, USA. [5]Department of Allergy and Immunology and School of Medicine Clinics, University of Puerto Rico-Medical Sciences Campus, San Juan, Puerto Rico, USA. [6]Department of Internal Medicine and School of Medicine Clinics, University of Puerto Rico-Medical Sciences Campus, San Juan 00935, Puerto Rico, USA.

References

1. Tesse R, Pandey RC, Kabesch M. Genetic variations in toll-like receptor pathway genes influence asthma and atopy. Allergy. 2011;66:307–16. http://dx.doi.org/10.1111/j.1398-9995.2010.02489.x.
2. Canino G, McQuaid EL, Rand CS. Addressing asthma health disparities: a multilevel challenge. J Allergy Clin Immunol. 2009;123(6):1209–17. http://dx.doi.org/10.1016/j.jaci.2009.02.043.
3. Hunninghake GM, Weiss ST, Celedón JC. Asthma in Hispanics. Am J Respir Crit Care Med. 2006;173:143–63. http://dx.doi.org/10.1164/rccm.200508-1232SO.
4. Lara M, Akinbami L, Flore G, Morgenstern H. Heterogeneity of childhood asthma among Hispanic children: Puerto Rican children bear a disproportionate burden. Pediatrics. 2006;117(1):43–53. http://dx.doi.org/10.1542/peds.2004-1714.
5. Choudry S, Ung N, Avila PC, Ziv E, Nazario S, Casal J, Torres A, Gorman JD, Salari K, Rodriguez-Santana JR, Tosacano M, Sylvia JS, Alioto M, Castro RA, Salazar M, Gomez I, Fagan JK, Salas J, Clark S, Lilly C, Matallana H, Selman M, Chapela R, Sheppard D, Weiss ST, Ford JG, Boushey HA, Drazen JM, Rodriguez-Cintron W, Silverman EK and González Burchard E on behalf of the Genetics of Asthma in Latino Americans, (GALA) Study. Pharmacogenetic differences in response to albuterol between Puerto Ricans and Mexicans with asthma. Am J Respir Crit Care Med. 2005a;171: 563–570. http://dx.doi.org/10.1164/rccm.200409-1286OC
6. Akinbami LJ, Moorman JE, Liu X. Asthma prevalence, health care use, and mortality: United States, 2005–2009. Natl Health Stat Rep. 2011;32:1–16.

7. Ledogar R, Penchaszadeh A, Iglesias-Garden C, Garden-Acosta L. Asthma and Latino cultures: different prevalence reported among groups sharing the same environment. Am J Public Health. 2000;90(6):929–35. http://dx.doi.org/10.2105/AJPH.90.6.929.
8. Canino G, Koinis-Mitchell D, Ortega AN, McQuaid EL, Fritz GK, Alegría M. Asthma disparities in the prevalence, morbidity, and treatment of Latino children. Soc Sci Med. 2006;63(11):2926–37. http://dx.doi.org/10.1016/j.socscimed.2006.07.017.
9. Current asthma prevalence percents by age; United States: National Health Interview Survey (NHIS). National Center for Chronic Disease Prevention and Health Promotion (CDC). 2013. Retrieved from http://www.cdc.gov
10. Brehm JM, Acosta-Pérez E, Klei L, Roeder K, Barmada MM, Boutaoui N, Forno E, Cloutier MM, Datta S, Kelly R, Paul K, Sylvia J, Calvert D, Thornton-Thompson S, Wakefield D, Litonjua AA, Alvarez M, Colón-Semidey A, Canino G, Celedón JC. African ancestry and lung function in Puerto Rican children. J Allergy Clin Immunol. 2012;129(6):1484–90. http://dx.doi.org/10.1016/j.jaci.2012.03.035.
11. Renkonen J, Joenväärä S, Parviainen V, Mattila P, Renkonen R. Network analysis of single nucleotide polymorphisms in asthma. J Asthma Allergy. 2010;3:177–86. http://dx.doi.org/10.2147/JAA.S14459.
12. Rodríguez Cotto RI, Ortiz Martínez MG, Rivera Ramírez E, Méndez LB, Dávila JC, Jiménez Vélez BD. African dust storms reaching Puerto Rican coast stimulate the secretion of IL-6 and IL-8 and cause cytotoxicity to human bronchial epithelial cells (BEAS-2B). Health. 2013;5(10A2):14–28. doi:10.4236/health.2013.510A2003.
13. Rodríguez-Cotto RI, Ortiz-Martínez MG, Jiménez-Vélez BD. Organic extracts from African dust storms stimulate oxidative stress and induce inflammatory responses in human lung cells through Nrf2 but not NF-kB. Environ Toxicol Phar. 2014;39(2):845–56. http://dx.doi.org/10.1016/j.etap.2015.02.015.
14. Ortiz-Martínez, MG, Rodríguez-Cotto, RI, Ortiz-Rivera, MA, Pluguez-Turull, CW, & Jiménez-Vélez, BD. Linking Endotoxins, African Dust PM10 and Asthma in an Urban and Rural Environment of Puerto Rico. Mediators Inflamm. 2015. http://dx.doi.org/10.1155/2015/784212.
15. Ferwerda B, McCall MBB, Verheijen K, Kullberg B, van der Ven AJAM, Van der Meer JWM, Netea MG. Functional consequences of toll-like receptor 4 polymorphisms. Mol Med. 2008;14(5–6):346–52. doi:10.2119/2007-00135. Ferwerda.
16. Kawasaki T. and Kawai T. Toll-like receptor signaling pathways. Front Immunol. 2014;5(461). http://dx.doi.org/10.3389/fimmu.2014.00461
17. Lazarus R, Vercelli D, Palmer LJ, Klimecki WJ, Silverman EK, Richter B, Riva A, Ramoni M, Martinez FD, Weiss ST, Kwiatkowsk DJ. Single nucleotide polymorphisms in innate immunity genes: abundant variation and potential role in complex human disease. Immunol Rev. 2002;190:9–25. http://dx.doi.org/10.1034/j.1600-065X.2002.19002.x.
18. Smit LAM, Siroux V, Bouzigon E, Oryszczyn M, Lathrop M, Demenais F, Kauffman F, on behalf of the Epidemiological Study on Genetics and Environment of Asthma, Bronchial Hyperresponsiveness, and Atopy (EGEA). CD14 and Toll-like receptor gene polymorphisms, country living and asthma in adults. Am J Respir Crit Care Med. 2009;179:363–8. http://dx.doi.org/10.1164/rccm.200810-1533OC.
19. Koppelman G, Reijmerink N, Stine OC, Howard TD, Whittaker PA, Meyers DA, Postma DS, Bleecker ER. Association of a promoter polymorphism of the CD14 gene and atopy. Am J Respir Crit Care Med. 2001;163:965–9. http://dx.doi.org/10.1164/ajrccm.163.4.2004164.
20. Simpson A, John S, Jury F, Niven R, Woodcock A, Ollier WER, Custovic A. Endotoxin exposure, CD14, and allergic disease. Am J Respir Crit Care Med. 2006;174:386–92. http://dx.doi.org/10.1164/rccm.200509-1380OC.
21. Choudry S, Avila PC, Nazario S, Ung N, Kho J, Rodríguez-Santana JR, Casal J, Tsai H, Torres A, Ziv E, Toscano M, Sylvia JS, Alioto M, Salazar M, Gomez I, Fagan JK, Salas J, Lilly C, Matallana H, Castro RA, Selman M, Weiss ST, Ford JG, Drazan JM, Rodriguez-Cintron W, Chapela R, Silverman EK and González Burchard E on behalf of the Genetics of Asthma in Latino Americans (GALA) Study. CD14 tobacco gene-environment interaction modifies asthma severity and immunoglobulin E levels in Latinos with asthma. Am J Respir Crit Care Med. 2005b;172:173–182. http://dx.doi.org/10.1164/rccm.200409-1232OC
22. Eder W, Klimecki W, Yu L, von Mutius E, Riedler J, Braun-Fahrländer C, Nowak D, Martinez FD. and the ALEX study team. Toll-like receptor 2 as a major gene for asthma in children of European farmers. J Allergy Clin Immunol. 2004;113(3):482–8. http://dx.doi.org/10.1016/j.jaci.2003.12.374.
23. Bjørnvold M, Munthe-Kaas MC, Egeland T, Joner G, Dahl-Jørgensen K, Njølstad PR, Akselsen HE, Gervin K, Carlsen KCL, Carlsen KH, Undlien DE. A TLR2 polymorphism is associated with type 1 diabetes and allergic asthma. Genes Immun. 2009;10:181–7. http://dx.doi.org/10.1038/gene.2008.100.
24. Werner M, Topp R, Wimmer K, Richter K, Bischof W, Wjst M, Heinrich J. TLR4 gene variants modify endotoxin effects on asthma. J Allergy Clin Immunol. 2003;112(2):323–30. http://dx.doi.org/10.1067/mai.2003.1648.
25. Fagerås-Böttcher M, Hmani-Aifa M, Lindström A, Jenmalm MC, Mai X, Nilsson L, Zdolsek HA, Björkstén B, Söderkvist P, Vaarala O. A TLR4 polymorphism is associated with asthma and reduced lipopolysaccharide-induced interleukin-12(p70) responses in Swedish children. J Allergy Clin Immunol. 2004;114(3):561–7. http://dx.doi.org/10.1016/j.jaci.2004.04.050.
26. Martínez FD. CD14, endotoxin and asthma risk. Proc Am Thorac Soc. 2007;4: 26–31. http://dx.doi.org/10.1513/pats.200702-035AW.
27. Raby BA, Klimecki WT, Laprise C, Renaud Y, Faith J, Lemire M, Greenwood C, Weiland KM, Lange C, Palmer LJ, Lazarus R, Vercelli D, Kwiatkowski DJ, Silverman EK, Martinez FD, Hudson TJ, Weiss ST. Polymorphisms in Toll-like receptor 4 are not associated with asthma or atopy-related phenotypes. Am J Respir Crit Care Med. 2002;166(11):1449–56. http://dx.doi.org/10.1164/rccm.200207-634OC.
28. Nishimura F, Shibasaki M, Ichikawa K, Arinami T, Noguchi E. Failure to find an association between CD14–159 C/T polymorphism and asthma: a family-based association test and meta-analysis. Allergol Int. 2006;55(1):55–8. http://dx.doi.org/10.2332/allergolint.55.55.
29. Kleeberger SR, Peden D. Gene-environment interactions in asthma and other respiratory diseases. Annu Rev Med. 2005;56:383–400. http://dx.doi.org/10.1146/annurev.med.56.062904.144908.
30. Rodríguez S, Gaunt T, Day I. Hardy Weinberg Equilibrium Testing of Biological Ascertainment for Mendelian Randomization Studies. Am J Epidemiol. 2009;169:505–14. http://dx.doi.org/10.1093/aje/kwn359.
31. Kang I, Oh Y, Lee SH, Jung HM, Chae S, Lee JH. Identification of polymorphisms in the Toll-like receptor gene and the association with allergic rhinitis. Eur Arch Otorhinolaryngol. 2010;267:385–9. http://dx.doi.org/10.1007/s00405-009-1103-8.
32. Gao Z, Rennie DC, Senthilselvan A. Allergic rhinitis and genetic components: focus on Toll-like receptors (TLRs) gene polymorphism. Appl Clin Genet. 2010;3:109–20. https://dx.doi.org/10.2147/TACG.S8380.
33. Kormann MSD, Depner M, Hartl D, Klopp N, Illig T, Adamski J, Vogelberg C, Weiland SK, von Mutius E, Kabesch M. Toll-like receptor heterodimer variants protect from childhood asthma. J Allergy Clin Immunol. 2008; 122(1):86–92. http://dx.doi.org/10.1016/j.jaci.2008.04.039.
34. Bonds RS, Midoro-Horiuti T. Estrogen effects in allergy and asthma. Curr Opin Allergy Clin Immunol. 2013;13:92–9. http://dx.doi.org/10.1097/ACI.0b013e32835a6dd6.
35. Card JW, Carey MA, Bradbury JA, DeGraff LM, Morgan DL, Moorman MP, Flake GP, Zeldin DC. Gender differences in murine airway responsiveness and lipopolysaccharide-induced inflammation. J Immunol. 2006;177:621–30. doi:10.4049/jimmunol.177.1.621.
36. Li J, Ao L, Zhai Y, Cleveland JCJ, Fullerton DA, Meng X. Gender disparity in the role of TLR2 in post-ischemic myocardial inflammation and injury. Int J Clin Exp Med. 2015;8(7):10537–47. PMC4565226.
37. Chotirmall SH, Greene CM, Oglesby IK, Thomas W, O'Neill SJ, Harvey BJ, McElvaney NG. 17Beta-estradiol inhibits IL-8 in cystic fibrosis by up-regulating secretory leucoprotease inhibitor. Am J Respir Crit Care Med. 2010;182:62–72. http://dx.doi.org/10.1164/rccm.201001-0053OC.
38. Hunt R, Sauna ZE, Ambudkar SV, Gottesman MM and Kimchi-Sarfaty C. Silent (synonymous) SNPs: should we care about them? Single Nucleotide Polymorphisms, Methods in Molecular Biology 578. Humana Press. 2009. p. 23–39. http://dx.doi.org/10.1007/978-1-60327-411-1_2
39. Fung K, Gottesman M. A synonymous polymorphism in a common MDR1 (ABCB1) haplotype shapes protein function. Biochim Biophys Acta. 2009; 1794:860–71. http://dx.doi.org/10.1016/j.bbapap.2009.02.014.
40. Parmley J, Hurst L. How do synonymous mutations affect fitness? Bioessays. 2007;29:515–9. http://dx.doi.org/10.1002/bies.20592.
41. Shabalina SA, Spiridonov NA, Kashina A. Sounds of silence: synonymous nucleotides as a key to biological regulation and complexity. Nucleic Acids Res. 2013;41(4):2073–94. http://dx.doi.org/10.1093/nar/gks1205.
42. Sauna ZE, Kimchi-Sarfaty C. Understanding the contribution of synonymous mutations to human disease. Nat Rev Genet. 2011;12:683–91. http://dx.doi.org/10.1038/nrg3051.
43. Smit LAM, Bouzignon E, Bousquet J, Le Moual N, Nadif R, Pin I, Lathrop M, Demenais F, Kauffman F, Siroux V. on behalf of the Epidemiological Study

on the Genetics and Environment of Asthma. Mold allergen sensitization in adult asthma according to integrin β3 polymorphisms and Toll-like receptor 2/+596 genotype. J Allergy Clin Immunol. 2011;128(1):185–91. http://dx.doi.org/10.1016/j.jaci.2011.04.007.

44. Pimentel-Nunes P, Teixeira AL, Pereira C, Gomes M, Brandão C, Rodrigues C, Gonçalves N, Boal-Carvalho I, Roncon-Albuquerque Jr R, Moreira-Dias L, Leite-Moreira AF, Medeiros R, Dinis-Ribeiro M. Functional polymorphisms of Toll-like receptors 2 and 4 alter the risk for colorectal carcinoma in Europeans. Dig Liver Dis. 2013;45:63–9. http://dx.doi.org/10.1016/j.dld.2012.08.006.

45. Chen K, Gu W, Ling Z, Jiang D, Zhang L, Zhou J, Du D, Hu P, Liu Q, Huang S, Jiang J. Identification of haplotype tag SNPs within the entire TLR2 gene and their clinical relevance in patients with major trauma. Shock. 2010;35(1):35–41. http://dx.doi.org/10.1097/SHK.0b013e3181eb45b3.

46. Mikacenic C, Reiner AP, Holden TD, Nickerson DA, Wurfel MM. Variation in the TLR10/TLR1/TLR6 locus is the major genetic determinant of interindividual difference in TLR1/2-mediated responses. Genes Immun. 2013;14:52–7. http://dx.doi.org/10.1038/gene.2012.53.

47. Klaassen EMM, Thönissen BEJT, van Eys G, Dompeling E, Jöbsis Q. A systematic review of CD14 and toll-like receptors in relation to asthma in Caucasian children. Allergy Asthma Clin Immunol. 2013;9:1–10. doi:10.1186/1710-1492-9-10.

48. O'Donnell AR, Toelle BG, Marks GB, Hayden CM, Laing IA, Peat JK, Goldblatt J, Le Souëf PN. Age-specific relationship between CD14 and atopy in a cohort assessed from age 8 to 25 years. Am J Respir Crit Care Med. 2004;169:615–22. http://dx.doi.org/10.1164/rccm.200302-278OC.

49. Noguchi E, Nishimura F, Fukai H, Kim J, Ichikawaw K, Shibasakiz M, Arinami T. An association study of asthma and total serum immunoglobin E levels for Toll-like receptor polymorphisms in a Japanese population. Clin Exp Allergy. 2004;34:177–83. http://dx.doi.org/10.1111/j.1365-2222.2004.01839.x.

50. Bottema RWB, Kerkhof M, Reijmerink NE, Thijs C, Smit HA, van Schayck CP, Brunekreef B, van Oosterhout AJ, Postma DS, Koppelman GH. Gene-gene interaction in regulatory T-cell function in atopy and asthma development in childhood. J Allergy Clin Immunol. 2010;126(2):338–46. http://dx.doi.org/10.1016/j.jaci.2010.04.024.

51. Kumar R, Nguyen EA, Roth LA, Oh SS, Gignoux CR, Huntsman S, Eng C, Moreno-Estrada A, Sandoval K, Pe-alosa-Espinosa RI, López-López M, Avila PC, Farber HJ, Tcheurekdjian H, Rodriguez-Cintron W, Rodriguez-Santana JR, Serebrisky D, Thyne SM, Williams LK, Winkler C, Bustamante CD, Pérez-Stable EJ, Borrell LN, Burchard EG. Factors associated with degree of atopy in Latino children in a nationwide pediatric sample: The Genes-environments and Admixture in Latino Asthmatics (GALA II) study. J Allergy Clin Immunol. 2013;132(4):896–905. http://dx.doi.org/10.1016/j.jaci.2013.02.046.

52. Hussein YM, Awad HA, Shalaby SM, Ali AA, Alzahrani SS. Toll-like receptor 2 and Toll-like receptor 4 polymorphisms and susceptibility to asthma and allergic rhinitis: a case–control analysis. Cell Immunol. 2012;274:34–8. http://dx.doi.org/10.1016/j.cellimm.2012.02.006.

53. Choudry S, Seibold MA, Borrell LN, Tang H, Serebrisky D, Chapela R, Rodriguez-Santana JR, Avila PC, Ziv E, Rodriguez-Cintron W, Risch NJ, González BE. Dissecting complex diseases in complex populations Asthma in Latino Americans. Proc Am Thorac Soc. 2007;4:226–33. doi:10.1513/pats.200701-029AW.

54. Zhang G, Candelaria P, Mäkelä JM, Khoo S, Hayden MC, von Hertzen L, Laatikainen T, Vartiainen E, Goldblatt J, Haahtela T, LeSouëf NP. Disparity of innate immunity–related gene effects on asthma and allergy on Karelia. Pediatr Allergy Immunol. 2011;22:621–30. http://dx.doi.org/10.1111/j.1399-3038.2011.01186.x.

55. Leung T, Tang NLS, Wong GWK, Fok T. CD14 and Toll-like receptors: potential contribution of genetic factors and mechanisms to inflammation and allergy. Curr Drug Targets Inflamm Allergy. 2005;4(2):169–75. http://dx.doi.org/10.2174/1568010053586336.

56. March ME, Sleiman PMA, Hakonarson H. Genetic polymorphisms and associated susceptibility to asthma. Int J Gen Med. 2013;6:253–65. doi:10.2147/IJGM.S28156.

57. Ege MJ, Strachan DP, Cookson WOCM, Moffatt MF, Gut I, Lathrop M, Kabesch M, Genuneit J, Büchele G, Sozanska B, Boznanski A, Cullinan P, Horak E, Bieli C, Braun-Fahrländer C, Heederik D, von Mutius E. and the GABRIELA study group. Gene-environment interaction of childhood asthma and exposure to farming in Central Europe. J Allergy Clin Immunol. 2010;127(1):138–44. http://dx.doi.org/10.1016/j.jaci.2010.09.041.

58. Reijmerink NE, Bottema RWB, Kerkhof M, Gerritsen J, Stelma FF, Thijs C, van Schayck CP, Smit HA, Brunekreef B, Koppelman GH, Postma DS. TLR-related pathway analysis: novel gene-gene interactions in the development of asthma and atopy. Allergy. 2010;65:199–207. http://dx.doi.org/10.1111/j.1398-9995.2009.02111.x.

59. Qian FH, Zhang Q, Zhou LF, Jin GF, Bai JL, Yin KS. Polymorphisms in the Toll-like receptor 2 subfamily and risk of asthma: a case–control analysis in a Chinese population. J Investig Allergol Clin Immunol. 2010;20(4):340–6.

60. Reibman J, Liu M. Genetics and asthma disease susceptibility in the US Latino population. Mt Sinai J Med. 2010;77:140–8. http://dx.doi.org/10.1002/msj.20171.

61. Kerkhof M, Postma DS, Brunekreef B, Reijmerink NE, Wijga AH, de Jongste JC, Gehring U, Koppelman GH. Toll-like receptor 2 and 4 genes influence susceptibility to adverse effects of traffic-related air pollution on childhood asthma. Thorax. 2010;65:690–7. http://dx.doi.org/10.1136/thx.2009.119636.

Automated chart review utilizing natural language processing algorithm for asthma predictive index

Harsheen Kaur[1,2,3†], Sunghwan Sohn[4†], Chung-Il Wi[1,2], Euijung Ryu[2,4], Miguel A. Park[5], Kay Bachman[5], Hirohito Kita[5], Ivana Croghan[6], Jose A. Castro-Rodriguez[7], Gretchen A. Voge[1,2,8], Hongfang Liu[4*] and Young J. Juhn[1,2*]

Abstract

Background: Thus far, no algorithms have been developed to automatically extract patients who meet Asthma Predictive Index (API) criteria from the Electronic health records (EHR) yet. Our objective is to develop and validate a natural language processing (NLP) algorithm to identify patients that meet API criteria.

Methods: This is a cross-sectional study nested in a birth cohort study in Olmsted County, MN. Asthma status ascertained by manual chart review based on API criteria served as gold standard. NLP-API was developed on a training cohort ($n = 87$) and validated on a test cohort ($n = 427$). Criterion validity was measured by sensitivity, specificity, positive predictive value and negative predictive value of the NLP algorithm against manual chart review for asthma status. Construct validity was determined by associations of asthma status defined by NLP-API with known risk factors for asthma.

Results: Among the eligible 427 subjects of the test cohort, 48% were males and 74% were White. Median age was 5.3 years (interquartile range 3.6–6.8). 35 (8%) had a history of asthma by NLP-API vs. 36 (8%) by abstractor with 31 by both approaches. NLP-API predicted asthma status with sensitivity 86%, specificity 98%, positive predictive value 88%, negative predictive value 98%. Asthma status by both NLP and manual chart review were significantly associated with the known asthma risk factors, such as history of allergic rhinitis, eczema, family history of asthma, and maternal history of smoking during pregnancy (p value < 0.05). Maternal smoking [odds ratio: 4.4, 95% confidence interval 1.8–10.7] was associated with asthma status determined by NLP-API and abstractor, and the effect sizes were similar between the reviews with 4.4 vs 4.2 respectively.

Conclusion: NLP-API was able to ascertain asthma status in children mining from EHR and has a potential to enhance asthma care and research through population management and large-scale studies when identifying children who meet API criteria.

Keywords: Asthma, API, Epidemiology, Informatics, NLP

* Correspondence: liu.hongfang@mayo.edu; juhn.young@mayo.edu
[†]Equal contributors
[4]Division of Biomedical Statistics and Informatics, Mayo Clinic, 200 1st Street SW, Rochester, MN 55905, USA
[1]Department of Pediatric and Adolescent Medicine, Mayo Clinic, 200 1st Street SW, Rochester, MN 55905, USA
Full list of author information is available at the end of the article

Background

According to a report from the Agency for Healthcare Research and Quality, asthma is one of the five most burdensome diseases in the United States [1]. Asthma is the most common chronic illness in childhood, affecting 4–17% of children in the United States [2] and 2.8–37% of children worldwide depending on countries [3] with significant healthcare, social, and academic burden. [4, 5] Despite the availability of evidence-based guidelines for asthma management and effective asthma therapies, there has been virtually no change between 1990 and 2010 in years lived with asthma-related morbidity in the United States [2].

One of the major challenges in the current asthma research is inconsistency in study results reported in genome-wide association studies [6], clinical trials [7, 8], and studies addressing heterogeneity of asthma [9, 10], making it difficult to apply these results to clinical practice and advancement of the field. Apart from the true biological heterogeneity of asthma, other important sources of variability in the above studies include inconsistent asthma criteria (physician diagnosis vs. subjective determination based on diverse asthma criteria) and ascertainment processes (chart review vs. surveys), which may obscure a better understanding of biological heterogeneity of asthma. As an example, literature showed asthma status according to parental report was associated with significant misclassification bias [11], and studies including younger children (e.g., < 3 years old) for whom asthma diagnosis rarely occur may not use physician diagnosis nor International Classification of Diseases (ICD) codes for asthma. The latter is very important for many reasons. First, the burden of disease is greatest in preschoolers with a significantly higher proportion of emergency department visits, more hospitalizations, more sleep disturbances, and more limitation of family activities/play than older children [12, 13]. Second, the irreversible impairment in lung function may occur during the preschool period, suggesting a window of opportunity to perhaps prevent irreversible damage [14]. It is possible that the repeated and cumulative lung injury caused by various respiratory infections that are frequent at this age may be causal or important intercurrent factors affecting lung growth and asthma persistence. Despite these limitations, these approaches are still frequently used for large-scale asthma studies. While implementing laboratory tests can be considered, it can be impractical for studies based on large cohorts.

Until today, manual chart review is the most accurate method to identify asthma cases regardless of physician diagnosis of asthma, but this becomes a challenge for large-scale studies. There is an emerging need for developing a medical informatics approach like natural language processing (NLP) that processes free-text and classifies asthma status at a patient level in the era of electronic health records (EHR).

In the medical community, Asthma Predictive Index (API) [15] is a validated criterion and can be a potential option for asthma studies and help to reduce the variability described above in the future research work for asthma in children. We recently demonstrated feasibility of using NLP algorithms for an existing other asthma criteria, Predetermined Asthma Criteria [16–18], which was originally developed by Yunginger et al. [19] and has been used extensively in research for asthma epidemiology [20, 21]. At present, given the potential suitability of API to a retrospective study [22, 23], the recommended use of API by National Asthma Education and Prevention Program guidelines [24], and unavailability of NLP algorithm for API, developing and validating an NLP-based API algorithm would be worthwhile.

To date, there is no NLP algorithm enabling automated chart review for EHR to ascertain asthma status in children based on API. Therefore, the main aim of this study was to develop and validate an NLP algorithm to identify patients that meet API positive criteria by assessing criterion and construct validity in a retrospective study.

Methods

The study was approved by the institutional review boards at the Mayo Clinic and Olmsted Medical Center, located in Olmsted County, Minnesota.

Study setting

Demographic characteristics of the population of Rochester and Olmsted County were similar to those of the U.S. Caucasian population, with the exception of a higher proportion of the working population of this community being employed in the health care industry [19]. Olmsted County has a few important epidemiological advantages for conducting retrospective studies such as this because medical care is virtually self-contained within the community. In addition, research authorization for using medical records for research purposes is obtained from the patients the first time they ever register with a provider in the community. The rate of granting this authorization is about 95% in Olmsted County [25]. Once this permission is granted, each patient is assigned a unique identifier under the auspices of the Rochester Epidemiology Project, which has been continuously funded by the National Institute of Health (NIH) since 1966 [26]. Using this unique identifier, all clinical diagnoses and events, and detailed information from every interaction among the patients and providers are retrieved from detailed patient-based medical records [26]. As this resource has been electronically available since 1997 (i.e., the inception of the EHR at Mayo Clinic), it enables us to retrieve all asthma-related events and associated free-text information (e.g., symptoms, visits, and medications) electronically to ascertain asthma status based on API [15].

Study design

This is a cross-sectional study nested in a birth cohort study, which was designed to develop and validate an NLP algorithm for ascertaining asthma status by API (NLP-API) using convenience samples. The NLP algorithm was developed on the training cohort and evaluated on an independent test cohort for which asthma status by manual chart review (CW) was already available based on API. Criterion validity was assessed by determining concordance of asthma status by API between NLP-API and manual chart review. Construct validity of NLP-API was assessed by determining the association between asthma status ascertained by NLP algorithms and the known risk factors for asthma.

Study subjects

There were two cohorts enrolled in this study. The first cohort was used to develop the NLP algorithm (i.e., training cohort, $n = 87$) and the second one was used for validating the results (i.e., test cohort, $n = 427$). The training cohort was made up of subjects who were all born after the implementation of the EHR at the Mayo Clinic (i.e.1998–2002) [16]. Briefly, the training cohort were children who were enrolled in the Mayo Clinic sick child care program and their parents agreed to participate in a previous study assessing factors associated with parents' care-seeking behavior for mild acute illness of young children. Of the original 115 children, subjects were excluded due to the following reasons: 1) change of research authorization status ($n = 3$), 2) adopted children ($n = 4$; one of the major criteria of API is parental history of asthma), and 3) primary care at a non-Mayo site ($n = 21$; NLP was only available for Mayo EHR during the study period).

The validation part of the study utilized a random sample of the 2002–2006 population-based birth cohort who had been enrolled in a previous asthma study and had medical records mainly at Mayo Clinic, Rochester, Minnesota [27]. Briefly, the original study enrolled 579 subjects comprised of 282 late-preterm infants (34 0/7 to 36 6/7 weeks of gestation) and 297 gender- and birth year-matched term infants (37 0/7 to 40 6/7 weeks of gestation) randomly selected from the 2002–2006 birth cohort born in Olmsted County, Minnesota. In this study, a total of 152 subjects were excluded due to the following reasons: 1) change in research authorization status ($n = 17$), 2) adopted children ($n = 3$), and 3) primary care outside Mayo Clinic ($n = 132$), leaving 427 study subjects for this present study.

Asthma predictive index (API)

The presence of asthma was defined if frequent wheezing episodes (i.e., two or more wheezing episodes within one year) AND either one of the major criteria or two of the minor criteria are satisfied (Table 1) [15, 22, 23]; otherwise, study subjects were considered non-asthmatics. An index date of asthma was defined as the earliest date when the API criteria were met. The operational procedures for API for retrospective studies were described in a previous study [23].

Development of NLP algorithm for API

The overall process for the NLP-API algorithm to ascertain asthma status is depicted in Fig. 1. Our NLP algorithm used three different sources of data—i.e., clinical notes, laboratory data, and patient-provided information. Parents' asthma information (one of major criteria) was identified from both clinical notes (family history section of the patient's chart) and patient-provided information, and an eosinophil value was extracted from the lab data if tested for any reason. The other items of API criteria (i.e., eczema, allergic rhinitis, and wheezing ± colds) were extracted from clinical notes using pattern-based rules, assertion status (e.g., non-negated, associated with patient), and section constraints (e.g., diagnosis section). Then, we developed expert rules implementing API criteria (Table 1). Our algorithm was built in the open-source NLP pipeline MedTagger (https://sourceforge.net/projects/ohnlp/files/MedTagger/) developed by Mayo Clinic [16]. In this pipeline, there are two basic conceptual blocks to identify API-positive asthmatics. 1) A text processing component which finds evidence text in EHRs to match specific API criteria, and 2) A patient classification component which decides the patient's API status based on available evidence.

Asthma risk factor variables

These variables were collected during the previous study [27] and utilized for this study to assess construct validity (i.e., association between NLP-API (vs. manual chart review) and asthma risk factors for comparison purpose). These included birth weight, small for gestational age,

Table 1 Asthma Predictive Index (API) for asthma[a] ascertainment

Major Criteria	Minor criteria
1. Physician diagnosis of asthma for parents	1. Physician diagnosis of allergic rhinitis for patient
2. Physician diagnosis of eczema for patient	2. Wheezing apart from colds
	3. Eosinophilia (≥ 4%)

[a]Asthma is determined by frequent wheezing episodes (two or more wheezing episodes within one year) plus at least one of major criteria or two of minor criteria

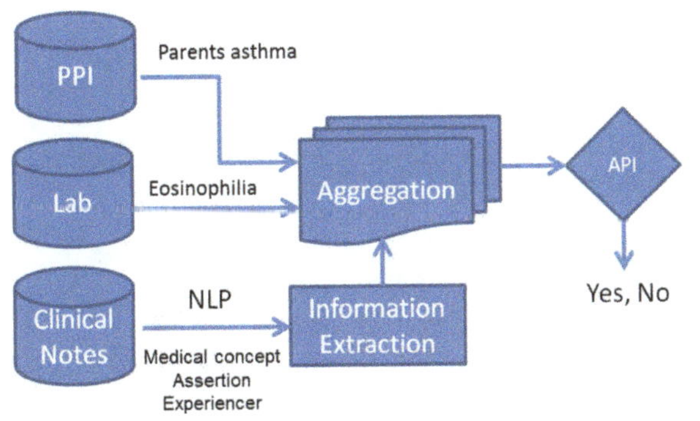

Fig. 1 Overview of NLP-API algorithm (Abbreviation: PPI – Patient Provided Information)

Table 2 Demographics of the test cohort

	Test cohort ($n = 427$)
Age at the last follow-up date, years, median (interquartile range)	5.3 (3.6, 6.7)
Male, n (%)	209 (48%)
White, n (%)	315 (74%)
Asthma (ascertained by abstractors), n (%)	36 (8%)
Allergic rhinitis, n (%)	39 (9%)
Eczema, n (%)	102 (24%)
Family history of asthma, n (%)	101 (23%)
Maternal smoking during pregnancy, n (%)	33 (7%)
History of breastfeeding, n (%)	354 (84%)

mode of delivery (Cesarean section vs. vaginal delivery), gestational age, a family history of asthma and other atopic conditions such as allergic rhinitis or atopic dermatitis, a history of patient's allergic rhinitis or eczema, maternal smoking during pregnancy, passive smoking exposure after birth (up to the first 6 years of life), and breast-feeding history. As all asthmatics did not fulfill the same criteria, we also assessed individual items included in API as risk factors for determining construct validity.

Statistical analysis

Performance of NLP-API was assessed for both criterion and construct validity. For criterion validity, we calculated agreement rate, Kappa index, and validation index (sensitivity, specificity, positive predictive value, and negative predictive value) for concordance in asthma status between NLP-API and manual chart review as gold standard. Using logistic regression models, construct validity was assessed by determining the association of asthma status ascertained by NLP-API with the known risk factors for asthma as NLP-API is expected to be correlated with the known risk factors if NLP algorithm reflects true asthma. The associations were summarized by odds ratios and their corresponding 95% confidence intervals. All analyses were performed using JMP statistical software package (Ver 10; SAS Institute, Inc., Cary, NC).

Results

Study subjects

Characteristics of the test cohort are summarized in Table 2. 209 (48%) were male, and 315 (74%) were female. The median age (interquartile range) at the last follow-up date was 5.3 years (3.6, 6.7). 36 (8%) met the API by manual chart review, and 39 (9%) and 102 (24) had history of allergic rhinitis and eczema by physician diagnosis during the study period.

Concordance in asthma status between NLP-API and manual chart review (criterion validity)

For the test cohort, Kappa index and agreement for asthma status between NLP algorithm and manual chart review were 0.86 and 97%, respectively. Sensitivity, specificity, positive predictive value, and negative predictive value for NLP algorithm in predicting asthma status were 86%, 98%, 88%, and 98%, respectively. Overall, these results were similar with regard to gender, ethnicity and gestational age (Table 3).

Association of asthma status of NLP-API with the known risk factors (construct validity)

The results for construct validity are summarized in Table 4. A correlation analysis of each of the risk factors with asthma status by NLP and manual chart review was run on the test cohort independently. Asthma status by both NLP and manual chart review were significantly associated with the known asthma risk factors. For example, children with asthma compared to those without asthma had higher odds for having a history of allergic rhinitis, eczema, family history of asthma, and maternal history of smoking during pregnancy (p value < 0.05). For the factors of family history of other atopic conditions, passive smoking exposure, gestational age, birth weight, childcare attendance, and breastfeeding history, the direction and effect sizes were comparable between manual chart review and NLP-API, although the associations were not statistically significant.

Discussion

Our study results suggest that developing an NLP algorithm for API mining from EHR was feasible, as demonstrated by both criterion and construct validity. Our NLP-API algorithm has a potential to overcome the current challenges for asthma ascertainment in asthma care and research, enabling large-scale asthma studies by identifying children who meet API, current asthma guideline-recommended criteria [24].

Table 3 Agreement of asthma ascertainment between NLP and manual chart review (criterion validity)

Test cohort ($n = 427$)	Kappa-index	Overall agreement rate	Sensitivity	Specificity	PPV[a]	NPV[b]
Overall	0.86	97%	86%	98%	88%	98%
Sex						
Male ($n = 209$)	0.89	98%	90%	98%	90%	98%
Female ($n = 218$)	0.82	97%	80%	99%	85%	98%
Race						
Caucasian ($n = 315$)	0.83	97%	81%	98%	88%	98%
Non-Caucasian ($n = 106$)	0.94	99%	100%	98%	90%	100%
Gestational age						
Late Preterm ($n = 197$)	0.82	96%	84%	98%	84%	98%
Term ($n = 230$)	0.90	98%	88%	99%	93%	99%

[a]PPV: Positive Predictive Value
[b]NPV: Negative Predictive Value

Table 4 Associations of asthma status determined by NLP and manual chart review with known risk factors for asthma (construct validity)

	By NLP				By manual chart review			
	No asthma ($n = 392$)	Asthma ($n = 35$)	OR[d] (95% CI)	*p*-value	No asthma ($n = 391$)	Asthma ($n = 36$)	OR[d] (95% CI)	*p*-value
Age,[a] years, median (IQR)	5.2 (3.4, 6.7)	6.2 (4.6, 6.8)	1.2 (1.0, 1.4)	.01	5.1 (3.5, 6.7)	6.3 (4.4, 6.8)	1.2 (1.0, 1.4)	.02
Male, *n* (%)	188 (47%)	21 (60%)	1.6 (0.8, 3.2)	.17	188 (48%)	21 (58%)	1.5 (0.7, 3.0)	.23
White, *n* (%)	290 (75%)	25 (71%)	0.8 (0.3, 1.7)	.62	288 (75%)	27 (75%)	1.0 (0.4, 2.2)	.97
Birth weight, median (IQR)	3.14 (2.5,3.5)	2.8 (2.3,3.4)	0.9 (0.9, 1.0)	.08	3.1 (2.5–3.5)	2.8 (2.4–3.4)	0.9 (0.9, 1.0)	.14
Cesarean section, *n*(%)	115 (29%)	11 (31%)	1.1 (0.5,2.3)	.79	116 (30%)	10 (28%)	0.9 (0.4–1.9)	.81
Gestational age, median (IQR)	37 (36,39)	36 (36,37)	0.8 (0.6, 1.0)	.07	37 (36,39)	36 (36,38)	0.8 (0.7, 1.0)	.15
Allergic rhinitis, *n* (%)	31 (8%)	8 (23%)	3.4 (1.4, 8.2)	< .01	31 (8%)	8 (22%)	3.3 (1.3, 7.8)	< .01
Eczema, *n* (%)	87 (22%)	15 (44%)	2.7 (1.3, 5.6)	< .01	86 (22%)	16 (44%)	2.8 (1.3, 5.6)	< .01
Family history of asthma, *n* (%)	80 (20%)	21 (60%)	5.8 (2.8, 12.0)	< .01	80 (20%)	21 (58%)	5.4 (2.6,11.0)	< .01
Family history of atopic diseases, *n*(%)	150 (38%)	14 (40%)	1.0 (0.5–2.1)	.83	148 (37%)	16 (44%)	1.3 (0.6–2.6)	.43
Passive smoke exposure, *n* (%)	51 (14%)	8 (24%)	1.9 (0.8–4.5)	.11	51 (14%)	8 (24%)	1.8 (0.8–4.3)	.13
Maternal smoking,[b] *n* (%)	25 (6%)	8 (23%)	4.4 (1.8, 10.7)	< .01	25 (7%)	8 (23%)	4.2 (1.7,10.3)	< .01
Childcare attendance,[c] *n* (%)	165 (42%)	18 (51%)	1.4 (0.7, 2.9)	.28	164 (42%)	19 (53%)	1.5 (0.7, 3.0)	.21
Breastfeeding, *n* (%)	327 (85%)	27 (82%)	0.8 (0.3, 2.0)	.66	325 (84%)	29 (85%)	1.0 (0.3, 2.8)	.89

[a]Age at the last follow-up date
[b]maternal smoking status during pregnancy
[c]Childcare attendance before 3 years
[d]Unadjusted Odds ratio

Our study results show that the NLP-API asthma status was highly correlated with manual chart review, and this concordance was not affected by gender, ethnicity, or gestational age, suggesting criterion validity (Table 3). The study findings suggest 88% positive predictive value and 99% negative predictive value for ascertaining asthma. Discrepancies between NLP-API and manual chart review were in part because 1) the abstractors reviewed *parental* records for parental history of asthma, but NLP used only child's medical records (e.g., the note section of Family history), and 2) NLP often misinterpreted "cold" in "wheezing without cold" although both NLP and human abstractor used the pre-defined definition of "cold" [22, 23]. Also, the associations of known risk factors for asthma (e.g., maternal smoking during pregnancy) with the NLP-API determined asthma status were similar to those determined by manual chart review, suggesting construct validity. In contrast, the widely used method of ascertaining asthma status such as ICD-9 codes showed poor sensitivity as noted in our previous study—sensitivity of ICD codes was 31% whereas the NLP had 97% sensitivity although different asthma criteria was used [16, 28]. Studies based on self-reporting of asthma status such as questionnaire and survey data are subject to significant misclassification bias. For example, almost a quarter of parents whose children were admitted to the hospital for asthma did not report a history of asthma in their children [11]. There have been studies based on ascertaining asthma status with the help of lab tests (e.g., eosinophils) or biomarkers for asthma ascertainment [29], but these tests are impractical when a large number of patients or large study cohorts are involved. Importantly, our study results suggest that the NLP algorithm for API not only ascertains asthma status but also identifies associated individual risk factors such as a family history of asthma, allergic rhinitis, and atopic dermatitis which are part of API [30].

EHRs have been around since the 1960s when they were introduced as a technique to guide and teach medical professionals about how to handle medical knowledge [31]. In the early twenty-first century, a need for standardizing national data, as transmitting health information across organizational and regional boundaries was brought forth [32]. The Health Information Technology for Economic and Clinical Health (HITECH) Act of 2009 directed the Office of the National Coordinator for Health Information Technology (ONC) to promote the adoption and meaningful use of electronic health records. By 2014, 3 out of 4 (76%) hospitals had adopted at least a basic EHR system [33], and there are growing trends of applying EHR to clinical and translational research. For example, clinical studies are facilitating investigators in identifying the characteristics of patients and discovering phenotypes from EHR such as Electronic Medical Records and Genomics (eMERGE) [34]. NLP algorithms have been used for automated encoding of text data into structured data [35], extraction of molecular pathways from articles [36], translation of information from chest radiographs [37] as well as identification of medical complications in postoperative patients from EHR [38]. Thus, given the growing worldwide deployment of EHR systems and the usefulness of free-text embedded in medical records in capturing text-based events, an NLP algorithm will be an important tool to overcome the current challenges of processing large-scale data in disease ascertainment or phenotypic characterization.

Indeed, in our previous studies [16–18], we were able to establish the application of NLP algorithms for asthma ascertainment using an existing other asthma criteria, and to our knowledge, this was the first exploration to apply NLP algorithms to asthma ascertainment as other algorithms using NLP for asthma were for identifying physician diagnosis of asthma or asthma guideline, but not for applying existing asthma criteria [39–41]. This current study is an extension of our previous work by adding an NLP algorithm for API. Given the lack of gold standard to ascertain asthma status, National Asthma Education and Prevention Program guidelines suggest using API for asthma management. API has been used for prospective as well as retrospective studies [22, 42]. As EHRs are likely to continue to be used in clinical research described above, an NLP algorithm for API can be beneficial in the future.

Our study results have several implications in clinical practice, research, and public health. In clinical practice, it enables clinicians and health care systems to apply NLP-API for population management strategies. Using NLP-API, health care systems may identify children who meet API during early childhood (e.g., < 3 years old) on a regular basis for their better access to preventive and therapeutic interventions for asthma, and temporal and geographic trends of outcomes to these interventions may be assessed and monitored at a population level. The impact of a delay in diagnosis of asthma on asthma outcomes can also be examined. Allocation of resources could then be guided by this surveillance system. In research, while NLP-API addresses the limitations of the current methods of asthma ascertainment, it is an innovative approach enabling large-scale clinical studies minimizing methodological heterogeneity of asthma ascertainment due to human biases and mistakes when they review medical records, especially for a large volume of patients. There is a noteworthy finding in our error analysis to examine discrepancies of patient's API status between NLP-API and manual chart review. Independent third reviewer (an allergist) assessed the discrepancies, and we found that the NLP-API was able to capture API-positive patients that were missed by manual chart review as humans could miss or overlook asthma-related events during the review of large volumes of medical records. Thus, the NLP approach might potentially open up a venue to improve or correct human errors in processing a large volume of data or text review, and this needs to be further studied. Use of a computer based algorithm for ascertaining asthma becomes helpful in public health surveillance as it allows health care systems to monitor the trends of asthma prevalence and incidence in real-time and assess the impact of asthma on serious health outcomes (e.g., susceptibility to serious and common infections including vaccine preventable diseases) [21].

The main strength of our study is the epidemiological advantages of conducting retrospective studies in a study setting that is virtually a self-contained health care environment. In addition, under the auspices of the Rochester Epidemiology Project, we were able to capture all inpatient and outpatient asthma-related events for this present study from birth to the last follow-up date [26]. Our NLP algorithm has a unique capability to determine asthma index (inception) date, which helps researchers discern temporality [22]. An additional strength of this study is the unique aspect of NLP algorithm incorporating free-text data (e.g., asthma symptoms), lab data (e.g., eosinophil count), and structured data (e.g., self-reported response collected at clinic visit).

Limitations of our study includes a retrospective study design with a relatively small sample size, and thus, we were not able to fully address the associations between asthma status and certain risk factors such as second-hand smoking exposure and breastfeeding history. Although it was not statistically significant, NLP-API still showed strong associations with the expected direction for these factors. Another potential limitation is the portability of applying NLP-API to different EHR and health care systems. Appropriate adjustments to NLP algorithms may be necessary to address the intrinsic heterogeneity of EHR in order to produce a desirable performance of NLP algorithms at a different study setting. While our previous study demonstrated the portability of NLP asthma ascertainment tool based on a different asthma criteria using EHR [18, 43], the study result of NLP-API needs to be validated in different clinical settings to ensure the portability. In addition, there were the difficulties of semantic understanding of complex assertion status in clinical narratives (e.g., identifying asthma-related concepts that are negated, hypothetical, or associated with other family members), resulting in false negatives and false positives. Intrinsic limitation of EHR reliability collected from the sources may not represent complete history of patient's conditions (eg, parents' asthma collected from family history section and patient provided information) and thus affect the final asthma ascertainment. Our earlier work based on a prospective cohort study showed a close correlation between medical events (mild acute illnesses) in EMR and those captured by prospective follow up [44, 45]. Lastly, our cohorts used for the training (Mayo Clinic sick child care cohort) and test (preterm-weighted cohort) from a single center may not represent general population in children.

Conclusion

In conclusion, our NLP-API algorithm may prove to be valuable not only in the research realm where it can aid with large-scale clinical studies, but it also has the ability to help the clinician as a population management tool as well becoming a method of surveillance for the public health sector.

Abbreviations
API: Asthma Predictive Index; EHR: Electronic Health Record;
ICD: International Classification of Diseases; NIH: National Institute of Health;
NLP: Natural Language Processing

Acknowledgements
We thank Ms. Kelly Okeson for her administrative assistance.

Funding
This was supported by National Institute of Health (NIH)-funded R01 grant (R01 HL126667). This study also utilized the resources of the Rochester Epidemiology Project, which is supported by the National Institute on Aging of the National Institutes of Health under Award Number R01 AG034676.

Authors' contributions
YJ had full access to all of the data in the study and take responsibility for the integrity of the data and the accuracy of the data analysis. HK: contributed to the acquisition, analysis, and interpretation of the data; drafting the manuscript and revising it for important intellectual content; and approving the final manuscript. SS: contributed to the study concept and design; acquisition, analysis, and interpretation of the data; drafting the manuscript and revising it for important intellectual content; and approving the final manuscript. CW: contributed to the study concept and design; acquisition, analysis, and interpretation of the data, revising the manuscript for important intellectual content, and approving the final version. ER: contributed to the study concept and design; acquisition, analysis, and interpretation of the data, revising the manuscript for important intellectual content, and approving the final version. MP: contributed to the study concept and design; revising the manuscript for important intellectual content, and approving the final version. KB: contributed to the study concept and design; revising the manuscript for important intellectual content, and approving the final version. HK: contributed to the study concept and design; revising the manuscript for important intellectual content, and approving the final version. IC: contributed to the study concept and design; revising the manuscript for important intellectual content, and approving the final version. JC: contributed to the study concept and design; revising the manuscript for important intellectual content, and approving the final version. GV: contributed to the acquisition of data, revising the manuscript for important intellectual content, and approving the final version. HL: contributed to the study concept and design; analysis and interpretation of the data; revising the manuscript for important intellectual content, and approving the final version. All authors read and approved the final manuscript.

Ethics approval and consent to participate
This study was approved by the institutional review boards at the Mayo Clinic (14-009934) and Olmsted Medical Center (008-OMC-15). General

authorization to review medical records for research in accordance with Minnesota Statute was checked, and no medical records were reviewed of any child for whom the general research authorization has been refused. As some of the subjects have left the community, it is practically impossible to locate all subjects who are eligible to the study and obtain consent for this proposed study. Therefore, the need for consent was waived by the institutional review boards at two institutions mentioned above.

Consent for publication
Not applicable

Competing interests
Dr. Young Juhn is the Principal Investigator (PI) of the Innovative Asthma Research Methods Award from Genentech and the PI of Real World Evidence Pediatric Asthma Study supported by Roche/Genentech. Otherwise, the authors have nothing to disclose that pose a conflict of interest.

Author details
[1]Department of Pediatric and Adolescent Medicine, Mayo Clinic, 200 1st Street SW, Rochester, MN 55905, USA. [2]Asthma Epidemiology Research Unit, Mayo Clinic, Rochester, MN, USA. [3]Departement of Pediatrics, University of New Mexico, Albuquerque, NM, USA. [4]Division of Biomedical Statistics and Informatics, Mayo Clinic, 200 1st Street SW, Rochester, MN 55905, USA. [5]Division of Allergic Disease, Mayo Clinic, Rochester, MN, USA. [6]Department of Medicine Research, Mayo Clinic, Rochester, MN, USA. [7]Division of Pediatrics, School of Medicine, Pontificia Universidad Catolica de Chile, Santiago, Chile. [8]Division of Neonatology, Children's Hospitals and Clinics of Minnesota, Minneapolis, MN, USA.

References

1. Stanton MW. The High Concentration of U.S. Health Care Expenditures. Agency for Healthcare Research and Quality 2006. https://meps.ahrq.gov/data_files/publications/ra19/ra19.pdf. Accessed 23 Jan 2018. Research in Action.
2. Centers for Disease Control and Prevention. Vital signs: asthma prevalence, disease characteristics, and self-management education: United States, 2001–2009. MMWR Morb Mortal Wkly Rep. 2011;60(17):547–52.
3. Asher MI, et al. Worldwide time trends in the prevalence of symptoms of asthma, allergic rhinoconjunctivitis, and eczema in childhood: ISAAC phases one and three repeat multicountry cross-sectional surveys. Lancet. 2006; 368(9537):733–43.
4. Nurmagambetov T, et al. State-level medical and absenteeism cost of asthma in the United States. J Asthma. 2017;54(4):357–70.
5. Mukherjee M, et al. The epidemiology, healthcare and societal burden and costs of asthma in the UK and its member nations: analyses of standalone and linked national databases. BMC Med. 2016;14(1):113.
6. Deborah AM. Genetics of asthma and allergy: what have we learned? J Allergy Clin Immunol. 2010;126(3):439–46.
7. Ducharme FM, et al. Preemptive use of high-dose Fluticasone for virus-induced wheezing in young children. N Engl J Med. 2009;360(4):339–53.
8. Panickar J, et al. Oral Prednisolone for preschool children with acute virus-induced wheezing. N Engl J Med. 2009;360(4):329–38.
9. Fitzpatrick AM, et al. Heterogeneity of severe asthma in childhood: confirmation by cluster analysis of children in the National Institutes of Health/National Heart, Lung, and Blood Institute severe asthma research program. J Allergy Clin Immunol. 2011;127(2):382–9. e13
10. Moore WC, et al. Identification of asthma phenotypes using cluster analysis in the severe asthma research program. Am J Respir Crit Care Med. 2010; 181(4):315–23.
11. Miller JE, Gaboda D, Davis D. Early childhood chronic illness: comparability of maternal reports and medical records. Vital Health Stat 2. 2001;131:1–10.
12. Radhakrishnan DK, et al. Trends in the age of diagnosis of childhood asthma. J Allergy Clin Immunol. 2014;134(5):1057–62. e5
13. Kuehni CE, Frey U. Age-related differences in perceived asthma control in childhood: guidelines and reality. Eur Respir J. 2002;20(4):880–9.
14. Morgan WJ, et al. Outcome of asthma and wheezing in the first 6 years of life: follow-up through adolescence. Am J Respir Crit Care Med. 2005;172(10):1253–8.
15. Castro-Rodriguez JA, et al. A clinical index to define risk of asthma in young children with recurrent wheezing. Am J Respir Crit Care Med. 2000;162(4 Pt 1):1403–6.
16. Wu ST, et al. Automated chart review for asthma cohort identification using natural language processing: an exploratory study. Ann Allergy Asthma Immunol. 2013;111(5):364–9.
17. WI CI, et al. Application of a natural language processing algorithm to asthma ascertainment. An automated chart review. Am J Respir Crit Care Med. 2017;196(4):430–7.
18. Wi, C.I., et al., Natural Language Processing for Asthma Ascertainment in Different Practice Settings. J Allergy Clin Immunol Pract, 2017. In Press; doi https://doi.org/10.1016/j.jaip.2017.04.041.
19. Yunginger JW, et al. A community-based study of the epidemiology of asthma. Incidence rates, 1964-1983. Am Rev Respir Dis. 1992;146(4):888–94.
20. Yawn BP, et al. Allergic rhinitis in Rochester, Minnesota residents with asthma: frequency and impact on health care charges. J Allergy Clin Immunol. 1999; 103(1 Pt 1):54–9.
21. Juhn YJ. Risks for infection in patients with asthma (or other atopic conditions): is asthma more than a chronic airway disease? J Allergy Clin Immunol. 2014;134(2):247.
22. Wi CI, et al. Risk of herpes zoster in children with asthma. Allergy Asthma Proc. 2015;36(5):372–8.
23. Wi CI, Park MA, Juhn YJ. Development and initial testing of asthma predictive index for a retrospective study: an exploratory study. Journal Asthma. 2015;52(2):183–90.
24. National Asthma Education and Prevention Program. Expert Panel Report 3 (EPR-3): Guidelines for the Diagnosis and Management of Asthma-Summary Report 2007. J Allergy Clin Immunol. 2007;120(5 Suppl):S94–138.
25. Yawn BP, et al. The impact of requiring patient authorization for use of data in medical records research. J Fam Pract. 1998;47(5):361–5.
26. Rocca WA, et al. History of the Rochester epidemiology project: half a century of medical records linkage in a US population. Mayo Clinic Proc. 2012;87(12):1202–13.
27. Voge GA, et al. What accounts for the association between late preterm births and risk of asthma? Allergy Asthma Proc. 2017;38(2):152–6.
28. Wi CI, et al. Application of a natural language processing algorithm to asthma ascertainment: an automated chart review. Am J Respir Crit Care Med. 2017;196(4):430–7.
29. Klaassen EM, et al. Exhaled biomarkers and gene expression at preschool age improve asthma prediction at 6 years of age. Am J Respir Crit Care Med. 2015;191(2):201–7.
30. Castro-Rodriguez, J.A., et al., Risk and Protective Factors for Childhood Asthma: What Is the Evidence? J Allergy Clin Immunol Pract. 2016. 4(6): p. 1111-1122.
31. Weed LL. Medical records that guide and teach. N Engl J Med. 1968;278(11): 593–600.
32. Jha AK. Meaningful use of electronic health records: the road ahead. JAMA. 2010;304(15):1709–10.
33. Dustin Charles, M.M.G., PhD; Talisha Searcy, MPA, MA Adoption of Electronic Health Record Systems among U.S. Non Federal Acute Care Hospitals: 2008–2014, in ONC Data Brief. 2015, Office of the National Coordinator for Health Information Technology (ONC).
34. Kirby JC, et al. PheKB: a catalog and workflow for creating electronic phenotype algorithms for transportability. Journal of the American Medical Informatics Association: JAMIA. 2016;23(6):1046–52.
35. Heinze, D.T. and M.L. Morsch, Automatically assigning medical codes using natural language processing. 2005, Google Patents.
36. Friedman C, et al. GENIES: a natural-language processing system for the extraction of molecular pathways from journal articles. Bioinformatics. 2001; 17(suppl 1):S74–82.
37. Hripcsak G, et al. Use of natural language processing to translate clinical information from a database of 889,921 chest radiographic reports 1. Radiology. 2002;224(1):157–63.
38. Murff HJ, et al. Automated identification of postoperative complications within an electronic medical record using natural language processing. JAMA. 2011;306(8):848–55.
39. Zeng QT, et al. Extracting principal diagnosis, co-morbidity and smoking status for asthma research: evaluation of a natural language processing system. BMC Med Inform Decis Mak. 2006;6:30.

40. Pacheco JA, et al. A highly specific algorithm for identifying asthma cases and controls for genome-wide association studies. AMIA Annu Symp Proc. 2009;2009:497–501. AMIA Symposium
41. Ertle, A.R., E.M. Campbell, and W.R. Hersh, Automated application of clinical practice guidelines for asthma management. Proceedings : a conference of the American Medical Informatics Association / ... AMIA Annual Fall Symposium. AMIA Fall Symposium, 1996: p. 552–6.
42. Huffaker MF, Phipatanakul W. Utility of the asthma predictive index in predicting childhood asthma and identifying disease-modifying interventions. Ann Allergy Asthma Immunol. 2014;112(3):188–90.
43. Sohn, S., et al., Clinical documentation variations and NLP system portability: a case study in asthma birth cohorts across institutions. J Am Med Inform Assoc 2017 (Epub ahead of print).
44. Juhn YJ, et al. The potential biases in studying the relationship between asthma and microbial infection. J Asthma. 2007;44(10):827–32.
45. Voigt RG, et al. Why parents seek medical evaluations for their children with mild acute illnesses. Clin Pediatr (Phila). 2008;47(3):244–51.

Permissions

All chapters in this book were first published in PM, by BioMed Central; hereby published with permission under the Creative Commons Attribution License or equivalent. Every chapter published in this book has been scrutinized by our experts. Their significance has been extensively debated. The topics covered herein carry significant findings which will fuel the growth of the discipline. They may even be implemented as practical applications or may be referred to as a beginning point for another development.

The contributors of this book come from diverse backgrounds, making this book a truly international effort. This book will bring forth new frontiers with its revolutionizing research information and detailed analysis of the nascent developments around the world.

We would like to thank all the contributing authors for lending their expertise to make the book truly unique. They have played a crucial role in the development of this book. Without their invaluable contributions this book wouldn't have been possible. They have made vital efforts to compile up to date information on the varied aspects of this subject to make this book a valuable addition to the collection of many professionals and students.

This book was conceptualized with the vision of imparting up-to-date information and advanced data in this field. To ensure the same, a matchless editorial board was set up. Every individual on the board went through rigorous rounds of assessment to prove their worth. After which they invested a large part of their time researching and compiling the most relevant data for our readers.

The editorial board has been involved in producing this book since its inception. They have spent rigorous hours researching and exploring the diverse topics which have resulted in the successful publishing of this book. They have passed on their knowledge of decades through this book. To expedite this challenging task, the publisher supported the team at every step. A small team of assistant editors was also appointed to further simplify the editing procedure and attain best results for the readers.

Apart from the editorial board, the designing team has also invested a significant amount of their time in understanding the subject and creating the most relevant covers. They scrutinized every image to scout for the most suitable representation of the subject and create an appropriate cover for the book.

The publishing team has been an ardent support to the editorial, designing and production team. Their endless efforts to recruit the best for this project, has resulted in the accomplishment of this book. They are a veteran in the field of academics and their pool of knowledge is as vast as their experience in printing. Their expertise and guidance has proved useful at every step. Their uncompromising quality standards have made this book an exceptional effort. Their encouragement from time to time has been an inspiration for everyone.

The publisher and the editorial board hope that this book will prove to be a valuable piece of knowledge for researchers, students, practitioners and scholars across the globe.

List of Contributors

Deimante Hoppenot, Simona Lavinskiene and Raimundas Sakalauskas
Department of Pulmonology and Immunology, Medical Academy, Lithuanian University of Health Sciences, Kaunas, Lithuania

Kestutis Malakauskas
Laboratory of Pulmonology, Department of Pulmonology and Immunology, Medical Academem, Lithuanian University of Health Sciences, Kaunas, Lithuania

Céline El Baou
GSK, Middlesex, Stockley Park, Uxbridge, UK

David Stempel
GSK, Research Triangle Park, NC, USA

Rafael Alfonso-Cristancho
GSK, Upper Providence, PA, USA
University of Washington, School of Medicine, Seattle, WA, USA

Elizabeth A Suarez
New England Research Institutes, Watertown, MA, USA
University of North Carolina at Chapel Hill, Chapel Hill, NC, USA

Mark L Everard
The University of Western Australia, Crawley, WA 6009, Australia

Neil Barnes
GSK, Brentford, UK
William Harvey Research Institute, Barts and The London School of Medicine and Dentistry, London, UK

Rachael L. Di Santostefano
Janssen Pharmaceuticals, Titusville, NJ, USA
GSK, Research Triangle Park, NC, USA

Christine R. Jenkins
Department of Thoracic Medicine, Concord Hospital and The George Institute for Global Health, Sydney, NSW 2050, Australia

Göran Eriksson
Department of Respiratory Medicine and Allergology, University Hospital, Lund, Sweden

Eric D. Bateman
Division of Pulmonology, Department of Medicine, University of Cape Town, Cape Town, South Africa

Helen K. Reddel
Clinical Management Group, Woolcock Institute of Medical Research, University of Sydney, Sydney, Australia

Paul M. O'Byrne and Malcolm R. Sears
Michael G DeGroote School of Medicine, Faculty of Health Sciences, McMaster University, Hamilton, Canada

Magnus Lindberg
Biometrics and Information Sciences (B&I), AstraZeneca R&D, Mölndal, Sweden

Jean Bousquet
Fondation MACVIA-LR, Contre les Maladies Chroniques pour un Vieillissement Actif en Languedoc-Roussillon, European Innovation Partnership on Active and Healthy Ageing Reference Site, University of Montpellier, Montpellier, France
INSERM, VIMA: Ageing and Chronic Diseases, Epidemiological and Public Health Approaches, U1168, Paris, France
UVSQ, UMR-S 1168, Université Versailles St-Quentin-en-Yvelines, Paris, France

Michael Gibbs
Global Respiratory Franchise, GSK House, Brentford, Middlesex, UK

Xin Zhou
Shanghai First People's Hospital, Shanghai, China

Susan A Tomkins and Nadeem Gul
Quantitative Science, Clinical Statistics, GSK, Stockley Park, Middlesex, UK

Young-Joo Cho
Ewha Womans University, School of Medicine, Seoul, South Korea

Hae-Sim Park
Ajou University Medical Center, Suwon, South Korea

William Busse
University of Wisconsin, School of Medicine and Public Health, Madison, WI, USA

Nanshan Zhong
State Key Laboratory of Respiratory Disease, Guangzhou Institute of Respiratory Disease, First Affiliated Hospital of Guangzhou Medical University, Guangzhou, China

Roy H. E. Cloots, Selvakumari Sankaranarayanan, Els Terwindt, Paul van Dijk and S. Eleonore Köhler
Department of Anatomy & Embryology and NUTRIM School of Nutrition and Translational Research in Metabolism, Maastricht University, 6200, MD, Maastricht, The Netherlands

Wouter H. Lamers
Tytgat Institute for Liver and Intestinal Research, Academic Medical Center, Amsterdam, The Netherlands

Matthew E. Poynter
Division of Pulmonary Disease and Critical Care, Department of Medicine, College of Medicine, University of Vermont, Burlington, VT, USA

Collin R. Brooks, Christine J. Van Dalen, Elizabeth Harding and Jeroen Douwes
Centre for Public Health Research, Massey University Wellington Campus, Private, Wellington 6140, New Zealand

Ian F. Hermans
Malaghan Institute of Medical Research, Wellington, New Zealand

Yanting Zhu, Xin Yan, Cui Zhai, Lan Yang and Manxiang Li
Department of Respiratory Medicine, The First Affiliated Hospital of Xi'an Jiaotong University, No.277, West Yanta Road, Xi'an 710061, Shaanxi, People's Republic of China

Ma'en Obeidat, Bryna A. Arsenault, Yunlong Nie, Stephanie Warner, Dorota Stefanowicz, Samuel J. Wadsworth, S. Jasemine Yang and Delbert R. Dorscheid
UBC Institute for Heart Lung Health, St. Paul's Hospital, 1081 Burrard St, Vancouver, BC, Canada

Peter D. Paré
UBC Department of Medicine, Division of Respirology, University of British Columbia, Vancouver, BC, Canada
University of British Columbia Centre for Heart Lung Innovation, St. Paul's Hospital, 1081 Burrard St, Vancouver, BC, Canada

Chris Carlsten
UBC Chan-Yeung Centre for Occupational and Environmental Respiratory Disease, Gordon & Leslie Diamond Health Care Centre, Vancouver General Hospital, 2775 Laurel Street, 7th floor, Vancouver, BC, Canada
UBC School of Population and Public Health, University of British Columbia, Vancouver, BC, Canada

Tillie L. Hackett
UBC Department of Anesthesiology, Pharmacology and Therapeutics, University of British Columbia, Vancouver, BC, Canada

Chun Y. Seow
UBC Department of Pathology and Laboratory Medicine, University of British Columbia, Vancouver, BC, Canada

Jeremy A. Hirota
Division of Respirology, Department of Medicine, McMaster University, Hamilton, ON, Canada

Christopher D. Pascoe
Children's Hospital Research Institute of Manitoba, 513-715 McDermot Avenue, Winnipeg, MB R3E 3P4, Canada

Euijung Ryu
Asthma Epidemiology Research Unit, Mayo Clinic, Rochester, MN, USA

Hongfang Liu, Sunghwan Sohn and Euijung Ryu
Division of Biomedical Statistics and Informatics, Mayo Clinic, 200 1st Street SW, Rochester, MN 55905, USA

Miguel A. Park, Kay Bachman and Hirohito Kita
Division of Allergic Disease, Mayo Clinic, Rochester, MN, USA

Ivana Croghan
Department of Medicine Research, Mayo Clinic, Rochester, MN, USA

Jose A. Castro-Rodriguez
Division of Pediatrics, School of Medicine, Pontificia Universidad Catolica de Chile, Santiago, Chile

Mark D. DeBoer and W. Gerald Teague
University of Virginia School of Medicine, Charlottesville, VA 22908, USA

Brenda R. Phillips and David T. Mauger
Pennsylvania State University School of Medicine, Hershey, USA

Joe Zein and Serpil C. Erzurum
Lerner Research Institute, Cleveland Clinic Foundation, Cleveland, USA

Anne M. Fitzpatrick and Min Jie Lee
Emory University School of Medicine, Atlanta, USA

David Langton, Kim Bennetts and Virginia Plummer
Department of Thoracic Medicine, Frankston Hospital, Peninsula Health, 2 Hastings Road, Frankston, VIC 3199, Australia

Wei Wang
Faculty of Medicine, Nursing and Health Sciences, Monash University, Clayton, Vic, Australia

Claude Farah
Faculty of Medicine and Health Sciences, Macquarie University, Sydney, NSW, Australia
Sydney Medical School, University of Sydney, Sydney, NSW, Australia

Matthew Peters and Alvin Ing
Department of Thoracic Medicine, Concord Hospital, Concord, NSW, Australia

Francis Thien
Department of Respiratory Medicine, Eastern Health, Vic, Boxhill, Australia

Sophie Demarche, Florence Schleich, Monique Henket, Virginie Paulus and Renaud Louis
Department of Respiratory Medicine, CHU Liege, Sart-Tilman B35, 4000 Liege, Belgium
GIGA I3 Research Group, University of Liege, Liege, Belgium

Signe Timm
Department of Public Health, Danish Ramazzini Center, Aarhus University, Aarhus, Denmark

Benjamin M. Gaston, Ross Myers, Kristie R. Ross and James Chmiel
Rainbow Babies and Children's Hospital, Cleveland, USA

John V. Fahy, Michael Peters and Ngoc P. Ly
San Francisco School of Medicine, University of California, San Francisco, USA

Sally E. Wenzel, Merritt L. Fajt and Fernando Holguin
University of Pittsburgh School of Medicine, Pittsburgh, USA

Deborah Meyers, Eugene R. Bleecker, Wendy C. Moore and Stephen P. Peters
Wake Forest University School of Medicine, Winston-Salem, USA

Mario Castro, Leonard B. Bacharier and Andrea M. Coverstone
Washington University School of Medicine, St. Louis, USA

Nizar N. Jarjour, Ronald L. Sorkness and Sima Ramratnam
University of Wisconsin School of Medicine, Madison, USA

Anne-Marie Irani
Virginia Commonwealth University School of Medicine, Richmond, USA

Wanda Phipatanakul, Jonathan M. Gaffin, Elliot Israel and Bruce Levy
Harvard University School of Medicine, Boston, USA

Hesham Tarraf
The Medical School, Cairo University, Cairo, Egypt

Omur Aydin and Dilsad Mungan
Department of Chest Diseases, Division of Allergy and Immunology, Ankara University, School of Medicine, Ankara, Turkey

Mohammad Albader
Chest Medicine Department, Zain Hospital, Kuwait City, Kuwait

Bassam Mahboub
College of Medicine, University of Sharjah, Sharjah, United Arab Emirates

Bassam Mahboub
Department of Pulmonary Medicine, Rashid Hospital, Dubai, United Arab Emirates

Adam Doble
Foxymed, Paris, France

Aaicha Lahlou
MS Health, Rabat, Morocco

Fayaz Aziz, Luqman Tariq and Abdelkader El Hasnaoui
GlaxoSmithKline, Dubai, United Arab Emirates

Vicky Thomas, Priyanka Raju, Daryl Freeman, Carole Nicholls, Iain R. Small, Erika Sims and Henry Chrystyn
Observational and Pragmatic Research Institute Pte Ltd, Singapore, Singapore

David B. Price
University of Aberdeen, Aberdeen, UK

P. N. Richard Dekhuijzen
Radboud University Nijmegen Medical Center, Nijmegen, The Netherlands

Sinthia Bosnic-Anticevich
Woolcock Institute, University of Sydney and Sydney Local Health District, Sydney, NSW, Australia

Nicolas Roche
University Paris Descartes, Paris, France

Federico Lavorini
University of Florence, Florence, Italy

Erika Sims
Norwich Medical School, University of East Anglia, Norwich, UK

Guilherme Safioti and Janice Canvin
Teva Pharmaceuticals Europe BV, Amsterdam, The Netherlands

Henry Chrystyn
Inhalation Consultancy Ltd, Leeds, Yeadon, UK

Song-Ying Shen, Wan-Qing Xiao, Jin-Hua Lu, Ming-Yang Yuan, Jian-Rong He and Xiu Qiu
Division of Birth Cohort Study, Guangzhou Women and Children's Medical Center, Guangzhou Medical University, 9 Junsui Road, Zhujiang Newtown, Tianhe District, Guangzhou 510623, China

Hui-Min Xia
Department of Pediatric Surgery, Guangzhou Women and Children's Medical Center, Guangzhou Medical University, Guangzhou, China

Kar Keung Cheng
Institute of Applied Health Research, University of Birmingham, Birmingham, UK

Kin Bong Hubert Lam
Clinical Trial Service Unit and Epidemiological Studies Unit, Nuffield Department of Population Health, University of Oxford, Oxford, UK

Ralf Schubert, Stefan Zielen and Martin Rosewich
Department for Children and Adolescents, Division for Allergology, Pneumology and Cystic Fibrosis, University Hospital Goethe University, Theodor-Stern-Kai 7, 60590 Frankfurt am Main, Germany

Sinem Koc-Günel
Department of Internal Medicine, Division of Pneumology, University Hospital Goethe University, Theodor-Stern-Kai 7, Frankfurt am Main 60590, Germany

Ingrid N. Kuiper and Randi J. Bertelsen
Department of Occupational Medicine, Haukeland University Hospital, N-5021 Bergen, Norway

Cecilie Svanes and Ane Johannessen
Centre for International Health, Department of Global Public Health and Primary Care, University of Bergen, Bergen, Norway

Bryndis Benediktsdottir
Faculty of medicine, University of Iceland, Reykjavik, Iceland

Lennart Bråbäck
Occupational and Environmental Medicine, Umeå University, Umeå, Sweden

Randi J. Bertelsen
Department of Clinical Science, University of Bergen, Bergen, Norway

Francisco Gómez Real
Department of Gynecology and Obstetrics, Haukeland University Hospital, Bergen, Norway

Miguel A. Park, Kay Bachman and Hirohito Kita
Division of Allergic Disease, Mayo Clinic, Rochester, MN, USA

José Luis Sánchez-Ramos
Facultad de Enfermeria, University of Huelva, Huelva, Spain

Vivi Schlünssen
National Research Center for the Working Environment, Copenhagen, Denmark

Thierry Van Hees
Department of Clinical and Hospital Pharmacy, University of Liege, Liege, Belgium

Grzegorz Brozek and Jan Zejda
Department of Epidemiology, School of Medicine in Katowice, Medical University of Silesia, Katowice, Poland

Joshua Lawson
Department of Medicine and Canadian Center for Health and Safety in Agriculture, University of Saskatchewan, Saskatoon, Canada

Andrei Shpakou
Department of Sport Medicine and Rehabilitation, Yanka Kupala State University of Grodno, Grodno, Belarus

Olga Fedortsiv
Department of Paediatrics with Children Surgery №1, Horbachevsky State Medical University, Ternopil, Ukraine

Leonid Hryshchuk
Department of Tuberculosis, Horbachevsky State Medical University, Ternopil, Ukraine

Donna Rennie
College of Nursing and Canadian Center for Health and Safety in Agriculture, University of Saskatchewan, Saskatoon, Canada

Jeong-Lim Kim, Susanna Lohman, Anna-Carin Olin, Anna Dahlman-Höglund, Eva Andersson, Kjell Torén and Mathias Holm
Section of Occupational and Environmental Medicine, Sahlgrenska Academy at University of Gothenburg, 30 Gothenburg, Sweden

Paul K. Henneberger
National Institute for Occupational Safety and Health, Centers for Disease Control and Prevention, Morgantown, WV, USA

Rosa I. Rodríguez-Cotto and Braulio D. Jiménez-Vélez
Department of Biochemistry, University of Puerto Rico-Medical Sciences Campus Main Bldg Lab B-210, San Juan 00935, Puerto Rico, USA
Center for Environmental and Toxicological Research, University of Puerto Rico-Medical Sciences Campus, San Juan, Puerto Rico, USA

Mario G. Ortiz-Martínez
Department of Biology, University of Puerto Rico at Humacao, Humacao, Puerto Rico, USA

Orquídea Frías-Belén
School of Public Health, University of Puerto Rico, Medical Sciences Campus, San Juan, Puerto Rico, USA

Sylvette Nazario-Jiménez
Department of Allergy and Immunology and School of Medicine Clinics, University of Puerto Rico-Medical Sciences Campus, San Juan, Puerto Rico, USA

María López-Quintero
Department of Internal Medicine and School of Medicine Clinics, University of Puerto Rico-Medical Sciences Campus, San Juan 00935, Puerto Rico, USA

Harsheen Kaur
Department of Pediatric and Adolescent Medicine, Mayo Clinic, 200 1st Street SW, Rochester, MN 55905, USA
Asthma Epidemiology Research Unit, Mayo Clinic, Rochester, MN, USA
Departement of Pediatrics, University of New Mexico, Albuquerque, NM, USA

Chung-Il Wi and Young J. Juhn
Department of Pediatric and Adolescent Medicine, Mayo Clinic, 200 1st Street SW, Rochester, MN 55905, USA
Asthma Epidemiology Research Unit, Mayo Clinic, Rochester, MN, USA

Euijung Ryu
Asthma Epidemiology Research Unit, Mayo Clinic, Rochester, MN, USA
Division of Biomedical Statistics and Informatics, Mayo Clinic, 200 1st Street SW, Rochester, MN 55905, USA

Sunghwan Sohn and Hongfang Liu
Division of Biomedical Statistics and Informatics, Mayo Clinic, 200 1st Street SW, Rochester, MN 55905, USA

Ivana Croghan
Department of Medicine Research, Mayo Clinic, Rochester, MN, USA

Jose A. Castro-Rodriguez
Division of Pediatrics, School of Medicine, Pontificia Universidad Catolica de Chile, Santiago, Chile

Gretchen A. Voge
Department of Pediatric and Adolescent Medicine, Mayo Clinic, 200 1st Street SW, Rochester, MN 55905, USA
Asthma Epidemiology Research Unit, Mayo Clinic, Rochester, MN, USA
Division of Neonatology, Children's Hospitals and Clinics of Minnesota, Minneapolis, MN, USA

Index

www.ingramcontent.com/pod-product-compliance
Lightning Source LLC
LaVergne TN
LVHW080913210926
848485LV00004B/643
* 9 7 8 1 6 3 9 2 7 4 5 5 0 *